# THE BIPOLAR BRAIN

# THE BIPOLAR BRAIN

## Integrating Neuroimaging and Genetics

**EDITED BY**

## Stephen M. Strakowski, MD

SENIOR ASSOCIATE DEAN FOR RESEARCH

VICE-PRESIDENT OF RESEARCH, UC HEALTH

UNIVERSITY OF CINCINNATI COLLEGE OF MEDICINE

CINCINNATI, OH

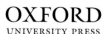

OXFORD

UNIVERSITY PRESS

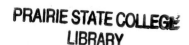

# OXFORD
#### UNIVERSITY PRESS

Oxford University Press, Inc., publishes works that further
Oxford University's objective of excellence
in research, scholarship, and education.

Oxford   New York
Auckland   Cape Town   Dar es Salaam   Hong Kong   Karachi
Kuala Lumpur   Madrid   Melbourne   Mexico City   Nairobi
New Delhi   Shanghai   Taipei   Toronto

With offices in
Argentina   Austria   Brazil   Chile   Czech Republic   France   Greece
Guatemala   Hungary   Italy   Japan   Poland   Portugal   Singapore
South Korea   Switzerland   Thailand   Turkey   Ukraine   Vietnam

Copyright © 2012 Oxford University Press

Published by Oxford University Press, Inc.
198 Madison Avenue, New York, New York 10016
www.oup.com

Oxford is a registered trademark of Oxford University Press

Library of Congress Cataloging-in-Publication Data

The bipolar brain: integrating neuroimaging and genetics/edited by Stephen M. Strakowski.
    p.; cm.
Includes bibliographical references and index.
ISBN 978-0-19-979760-8 (hardback)
I. Strakowski, Stephen M.
[DNLM: 1. Bipolar Disorder—diagnosis. 2. Bipolar Disorder—genetics. 3. Brain—physiology.
4. Brain Mapping—methods. 5. Magnetic Resonance Imaging—methods. WM 207]
LC classification not assigned
616.89'5—dc23                                          2011038676

9 8 7 6 5 4 3 2 1

Printed in China on acid-free paper

# CONTENTS

# FOREWORD

Edited books about bipolar disorder abound. To my knowledge, however, this one stands out as unique. Steve Strakowski and his colleagues have assembled a hugely ambitious scholarly project that brings together two fields on the leading edge of neurobiological research on bipolar disorders—neuroimaging and genetics.

Herein, the reader will find a treasure trove of new data from these two rapidly growing fields. Equally valuable is that the individual chapter authors were clearly encouraged to push the envelope conceptually by articulating models for framing an understanding, however tentative, of the exploding data in these fields.

A common critique of edited books is that there is too much overlapping, redundant, or even contradictory material. But here some overlap, even redundancy, is helpful because most readers will find, as I did, that so many of the studies being reviewed are so new and fresh that repetition of the same data from different perspectives actually enhances the learning experience.

If anyone still needs to be convinced that our field is moving rapidly beyond the classical and iconic rheostatic monoamine hypotheses of depression and mania (still prominent in advertisements for psychoactive drugs), this book will convince them.

Of the many new emerging fields covered here, one of the most fascinating is represented by the data nicely pulled together in Chapter 4 by Kim and colleagues, Chapter 11 by Clay and colleagues, and in Steve Strakowski's Integration Chapter 13: these data point to the likely involvement of mitochondrial dysfunction in the pathophysiology of bipolar disorder. As summarized by Strakowski: "[we hypothesize that] bipolar disorder arises from genetic variations in the control of monoaminergic or glutamatergic regulation, mitochondrial function, brain development, or circadian rhythm regulation that disrupt the neurochemistry, structure, and function of prefrontal–amygdala brain networks that are responsible for maintaining emotional homeostasis."

Thus, the evidence from imaging studies marshaled to support this broad hypothesis (in addition to the genetic evidence) comes not only from structural and functional imaging but also from the relatively new field of *neurochemical* imaging principally through magnetic resonance spectroscopy (MRS) that can directly assess *in vivo* key chemical components of mitochondria such as *N*-acetyl-aspartate (NAA), as outlined by Kim et al. in Chapter 4.

Drawing on structural imaging studies reviewed by Matsuo et al. in Chapter 2, and functional imaging studies reviewed by Altshuler and Townsend in Chapter 3, Strakowski goes on to hypothesize, "that mania results from the loss of ventral prefrontal modulation of amygdala and other limbic brain areas due to developmental errors in brain structure (e.g., striatal overgrowth, disrupted prefrontal/amygdala connectivity), coupled with excessive (or incorrectly modulated) dopaminergic neurotransmission to striatum and prefrontal cortex. These abnormalities in neurotransmission might arise directly from genetic lesions or indirectly through ineffective metabolic processes," by which he means abnormalities in cellular energetics involving mitochondrial dysfunction, abnormalities that have been demonstrated directly in bipolar patients using MRS; direct evidence of mitochondrial dysfunction in bipolar patients is made all the more compelling by the preliminary findings (reviewed by Clay and colleagues in Chapter 11) suggesting altered mitochondria-related gene expression in bipolar disorder.

Commenting on what is often the worsening course of bipolar illness through the first several episodes, Strakowski draws on data outlined in several of the individually authored chapters to suggest that neurons with abnormal mitochondrial metabolism are compromised in their "ability to manage reactive oxygen species that arise in the course of metabolism . . . [and therefore they] may be particularly susceptible to injury or death during periods of hypermetabolism or excessive glutamate neurotransmission (e.g., mood episodes)."

As with all research in bipolar disorder, so-called "well state" studies are the most intriguing because they have the potential to reflect underlying, genetically influenced vulnerability factors. For example, in their chapter on functional brain imaging, Altshuler and Townsend suggest that response inhibition mediated through the inferior frontal cortex appears to represent a trait marker perhaps correlating with the pre-morbid trait of impulsivity in bipolar subjects. Altshuler and Townsend note some other functional imaging abnormalities that persist beyond the episode and suggest that they are correlated with the well known persistence of neuropsychological impairment among bipolar patients after recovery from an acute episode.

Of course most well state or trait data are obtained from patients after recovery from an episode, making it difficult to distinguish true pre-morbid trait markers from the persistence of an impact of an affective episode. In this regard, it is interesting that a few imaging studies have been able to find abnormalities in subjects at high risk but without evidence of the illness.

Given the complexity of the imaging data, it is quite useful that many of the authors make efforts to link imaging findings to clinical observations. It is also helpful that the authors generally take care to point out the limitations of the studies they review, including the paucity of 1) longitudinal studies employing imaging strategies, and 2) imaging studies in relation to treatment response.

Here it might also be appropriate to observe that the history of neurobiological research on bipolar disorder teaches us that the clinical phenomenology is all too often the weak link. Imprecise diagnostic criteria, achieving reliability at the cost of validity, can cloud the meaning of even the most sophisticated neurobiological techniques, confounding efforts at replication.

One area particularly relevant here is the examination of differential neurobiological findings in bipolar compared to unipolar patients. While the value of attempting this is obvious, the field is hampered by an overly broad definition of unipolar, which essentially means little more than "not bipolar". In the current diagnostic system the unipolar group includes patients with one lifetime depressive episode along with those with a history of highly recurrent cyclic depressions (with an episode frequency comparable to the average bipolar patient). *DSM-IV* attempts to address this heterogeneity by creating a category of recurrent unipolar depression but since this designation requires only two lifetime episodes to qualify, it does very little to reduce the heterogeneity of the unipolar group. Given a diagnostic system which relegates cyclicity to a secondary position behind polarity, it is little wonder that replications among studies of unipolar–bipolar differences are hard to come by.

Another area of differential diagnosis is the age-old question: Are schizophrenia and bipolar disorder fundamentally different expressions of the same underlying illness or are they separate, albeit overlapping, disorders? Two chapters are devoted to this question. In Chapter 7, Whalley and colleagues review neuroimaging differences in bipolar disorder and schizophrenia. My reading of this chapter is that the data, albeit incomplete and in places not internally consistent, tend to support the two illness model, with substantial areas of symptomatic and functional overlap. On the other hand, the genetics findings, reviewed by Talkowski and colleagues in Chapter 10, are not yet sufficiently definitive for either group to allow even a tentative answer to the one illness–two illness question.

Finally, as a companion to Strakowski's integration chapter, Perlis and Blumberg address how imaging and genetics might inform more personalized treatment decisions. In today's environment where "personalized medicine" has taken on the status of the Holy Grail about to rescue a troubled healthcare system, Perlis and Blumberg are to be commended for their careful blend of vision and caution as they lay out a roadmap for the future development of imaging and genetic biomarkers.

Frederick K. Goodwin, MD

# PREFACE

Bipolar disorder is a common psychiatric illness that affects up to 3% of the global population. It is the sixth leading cause of disability worldwide and causes substantial morbidity and mortality among its sufferers. The estimated costs of bipolar disorder are enormous, approaching $50 billion annually in the United States alone. The societal and personal suffering caused by this condition is immeasurable. Nonetheless, despite its public health significance, bipolar disorder remains difficult to diagnosis and complicated to manage.

A major factor contributing to these difficulties is a lack of an established neurophysiological model for bipolar disorder. Such a model would provide objective measures for diagnosing the condition, as well as physiological parameters to monitor and predict treatment response. During the previous decade, neuroimaging and genetic techniques have rapidly advanced and proliferated, so that these technologies are providing important new leads toward models of the neurophysiological basis of bipolar illness. Modern neuroimaging techniques, particularly magnetic resonance imaging, have rapidly emerged as the most important tool for the study of the living human brain in general, and in bipolar disorder specifically, leading to accumulating evidence to guide the creation of brain-based models of bipolar disorder. In the absence of meaningful animal models of this uniquely human condition, neuroimaging has truly revolutionized the study of the neurophysiology of bipolar disorder. Moreover, because bipolar disorder is clearly familial, genetic studies are revealing the inherited molecular basis of the condition, complementing advances in neuroimaging. Consequently, we have now arrived at a point where integration of neuroimaging and genetic findings is possible and may position us to identify the very neurophysiological models needed to support the next generation of studies that translates research observations into clinical realities. The goal of this book is to provide a contemporary, focused review of neuroimaging and genetic research in bipolar disorder in order to develop an integrated neurophysiological model of this illness. This model can then serve to advance future studies toward improving the clinical management of this condition. The book is organized so that each chapter builds upon historical and recent advances toward an integrative model. Additionally, the authors selected to write each chapter represent international experts in the respective topics, so that the top minds in the world in these areas have contributed to this text.

Part I of this book is focused on neuroimaging findings in bipolar disorder. Chapter 1, by Caleb Adler and Michael Cerullo, provides a description of the principal brain imaging techniques used to study bipolar disorder, namely structural and functional magnetic resonance imaging (sMRI and fMRI respectively) and positron emission tomography (PET). This moderately technical overview of approaches to imaging the bipolar brain provides context for subsequent chapters in this section.

The next three chapters build from this introduction. In Chapter 2, Koji Matsuo, Marsal Sanches, Paulo Brambilla, and Jair Soares develop a neuroanatomy of bipolar disorder based on structural magnetic resonance imaging findings. In Chapter 3, Lori Altshuler and Jennifer Townsend extend this neuroanatomic substrate by examining how functional neuroimaging studies, using a variety of cognitive probes, identify where in the brain bipolar disorder may reside. Chapter 4, by Jieun Kim, In Kyoon Lyoo, and Perry Renshaw, builds from these previous chapters to incorporate neurochemical brain measures obtained through magnetic resonance spectroscopy into an evolving model of bipolar neurophysiology. In particular, problems with mitochondrial function and brain metabolism are identified and described.

Bipolar disorder typically begins in adolescence. In Chapter 5, Manpreet Singh, Melissa DelBello, and Kiki Chang explore brain imaging findings in children and adolescents with bipolar disorder or who are at risk for bipolar disorder due to having bipolar parents. This chapter identifies features of brain developmental abnormalities that may be part of the early progression of bipolar illness.

Chapter 6, by Amelia Versace, Jorge Almeida, and Mary Phillips, identifies brain imaging abnormalities that may be unique for bipolar depression by examining studies that compared bipolar and unipolar depressed subjects. The goal of this comparison is to add specificity to the evolving bipolar illness model. This specificity is further expanded in Chapter 7 by Heather Whalley, Jessika Sussmann, and Andrew McIntosh through examining neuroimaging differences between people with bipolar disorder and schizophrenia.

Part II of the book shifts to genetics. As with the neuroimaging discussion, this section begins with a review of genetic techniques that have been applied in studies of bipolar disorder, by way of providing context for the rest of the chapters in this section. Aaron Vederman and Melvin McInnis provide a moderately technical overview of these techniques in Chapter 8, to allow readers to understand the measurements provided and their limitations. Following this introduction, in Chapter 9 John Nurnberger provides an overview of the current literature of genetic findings in bipolar disorder, with particular focus on findings that have been replicated several times. These findings can then be integrated into potential molecular models of the illness. Indeed, one such model is proposed in Chapter 11 by Hayley Clay, Satoshi Fuke, Tadafumi Kato, and Christine Konradi, who discuss the potential of a mitochondrial basis for bipolar disorder based upon genetic findings, a discussion of mitochondrial function, and a reference back to findings discussed in Chapter 4. In Chapter 10, Michael Talkowski, Kodavali Chowdari, Hader Mansour, K. M. Prasad, Joel Wood, and Vishwajit Nimgaonkar compare and contrast the different genetic findings in bipolar disorder and schizophrenia in order to identify any specific genetic lesions that are unique to bipolar disorder, in order to refine genetic models of this illness.

Part III of the book is composed of two chapters that integrate the separate genetic and neuroimaging literature to better understand bipolar illness. In Chapter 12, Roy Perlis and Hilary Blumberg discuss how these advances in neuroimaging and genetics might be integrated in future studies to develop specific measures that can guide diagnostic and treatment decisions in clinical samples. Although we are not at this point yet, this chapter provides examples on how these techniques are used within the context of treatment studies to achieve this ultimate goal. Finally, in Chapter 13, I integrate and consolidate the previous chapters in order to describe a neurophysiological model of bipolar disorder, based upon both genetic and neuroimaging findings. The goal of the final chapter is to provide an over-arching neurophysiological model of bipolar disorder to guide future studies for many years.

We hope that readers of this text will find each of the chapters to be valuable overviews and intellectually stimulating, in order to encourage additional investigation into the neural basis of this common, fascinating, and too often tragic human condition. It is our further hope that one or more readers will build from our work and advance a bipolar neurophysiology that leads to novel treatment interventions that truly revolutionize the lives of our patients. Indeed, in the end, we hope that it is our patients who will ultimately benefit from this publication.

Stephen M. Strakowski, MD

# CONTRIBUTORS

**Caleb M. Adler, MD**
Department of Psychiatry and Behavioral Neuroscience
University of Cincinnati College of Medicine
Cincinnati, OH

**Jorge R. C. Almeida, MD**
Department of Psychiatry
Western Psychiatric Institute and Clinic
University of Pittsburgh School of Medicine
Pittsburgh, PA

**Lori L. Altshuler, MD**
Department of Psychiatry and Biobehavioral Sciences
David Geffen School of Medicine at UCLA; and
Department of Psychiatry
VA Greater Los Angeles Healthcare System
West Los Angeles Health Care Center
Los Angeles, CA

**Hilary P. Blumberg, MD**
Department of Psychiatry
Yale School of Medicine
New Haven, CT

**Paolo Brambilla, MD**
Department of Experimental Clinical Medicine
Inter-University Center for Behavioral Neurosciences
University of Udine
IRCCS Scientific Institute "E. Medea"
Udine, Italy

**Michael A. Cerullo, MD**
Department of Psychiatry and Behavioral Neuroscience
University of Cincinnati College of Medicine
Cincinnati, OH

**Kiki D. Chang, MD**
Department of Psychiatry and Behavioral Sciences
Stanford University School of Medicine
Stanford, CA

**Kodavali V. Chowdari, PhD**
Western Psychiatric Institute and Clinic
University of Pittsburgh School of Medicine
Western Psychiatric Institute and Clinic
Pittsburgh, PA

**Hayley B. Clay**
Neuroscience Graduate Program
Vanderbilt University
Nashville, TN

**Melissa P. DelBello, MD**
Department of Psychiatry and
    Behavioral Neuroscience
University of Cincinnati College of Medicine
Cincinnati, OH

**Satoshi Fuke, PhD**
Laboratory for Molecular Dynamics of
    Mental Disorders
RIKEN Brain Science Institute
Saitama, Japan

**Frederick K. Goodwin, MD**
Professor of Psychiatry
George Washington University Medical Center
Chevy Chase, MD

**Tadafumi Kato, MD, PhD**
Laboratory for Molecular Dynamics of
    Mental Disorders
RIKEN Brain Science Institute
Saitama, Japan

**Jieun E. Kim, MD, PhD**
Department of Brain and
    Cognitive Sciences
Ewha Womans University
Seoul, South Korea

**Christine Konradi, PhD**
Departments of Pharmacology and Psychiatry
Center for Molecular Neuroscience
Kennedy Center for Research on Human Development
Vanderbilt University
Nashville, TN

**In Kyoon Lyoo, MD, PhD**
Departments of Psychiatry and Neuroscience
Seoul National University
Seoul, South Korea; and
The Brain Institute
The University of Utah
Salt Lake City, UT

**Hader Mansour, MD, PhD**
Western Psychiatric Institute and Clinic
University of Pittsburgh School of Medicine
Pittsburgh, PA

**Koji Matsuo, MD, PhD**
Division of Neuropsychiatry
Department of Neuroscience
Yamaguchi University Graduate School of Medicine
Yamaguchi, Japan

**Melvin G. McInnis, MD**
Department of Psychiatry
University of Michigan Health System
Ann Arbor, MI

**Andrew M. McIntosh, MD, MRCPsych**
Division of Psychiatry
University of Edinburgh
Royal Edinburgh Hospital, Morningside Park
Edinburgh, UK

**Vishwajit L. Nimgaonkar, MBBS, PhD**
Western Psychiatric Institute and Clinic
University of Pittsburgh School of Medicine
Department of Human Genetics
Graduate School of Public Health
University of Pittsburgh
Pittsburgh, PA

**John I. Nurnberger, Jr., MD, PhD**
Joyce and Iver Small Professor of Psychiatry
Professor of Medical Neuroscience and
    Medical and Molecular Genetics
Director, Institute of Psychiatric Research
Indiana University School of Medicine
Indianapolis, IN

**Roy H. Perlis**
Department of Psychiatry
Bipolar Clinic and Research Program
Massachusetts General Hospital
Boston, MA

**Mary L. Phillips, MD**
Western Psychiatric Institute and Clinic
University of Pittsburgh School of Medicine
Pittsburgh, PA

**Konasale M. Prasad, MD, MRCPsych**
Western Psychiatric Institute and Clinic
University of Pittsburgh School of Medicine
Pittsburgh, PA

**Perry F. Renshaw, MD, PhD**
The Brain Institute
The University of Utah
Salt Lake City, UT

**Marsal Sanches, MD, PhD**
Department of Psychiatry and Behavioral Sciences
University of Texas Houston Medical School
Houston, TX

**Manpreet K. Singh, MD**
Department of Psychiatry and Behavioral Sciences
Stanford University School of Medicine
Stanford, CA

**Jair C. Soares, MD**
Department of Psychiatry and Behavioral Sciences
University of Texas Houston Medical School
Houston, TX

**Stephen M. Strakowski, MD**
Senior Associate Dean for Research
Vice-President of Research, UC Health
University of Cincinnati College of Medicine
Cincinnati, OH

**Jessika E. Sussmann, MBChB, MRCPsych**
Division of Psychiatry
University of Edinburgh
Royal Edinburgh Hospital, Morningside Park
Edinburgh, UK

**Michael E. Talkowski, PhD**
Center for Human Genetic Research
Massachusetts General Hospital
Department of Neurology
Harvard Medical School
Boston, MA; and
Program in Medical and Population Genetics
Broad Institute of Harvard and M.I.T
Cambridge, MA

**Jennifer D. Townsend**
Department of Psychiatry and Biobehavioral Sciences
David Geffen School of Medicine at UCLA
Los Angeles, CA

**Aaron C. Vederman, PhD**
Department of Psychiatry
University of Michigan Health System
Ann Arbor, MI

**Amelia Versace, MD**
Western Psychiatric Institute and Clinic
University of Pittsburgh School of Medicine
Pittsburgh, PA

**Heather C. Whalley, PhD**
Division of Psychiatry
University of Edinburgh
Royal Edinburgh Hospital, Morningside Park
Edinburgh, UK

**Joel Wood**
Western Psychiatric Institute and Clinic
University of Pittsburgh School of Medicine
Pittsburgh, PA

# PART I

## HOW NEUROIMAGING INFORMS MODELS OF BIPOLAR DISORDER

# 1.

# BRAIN IMAGING TECHNIQUES AND THEIR APPLICATION TO BIPOLAR DISORDER

## Caleb M. Adler and Michael A. Cerullo

## NEUROSTRUCTURAL IMAGING

Although efforts to examine the structure and function of the human brain stretch back centuries (Paluzzi et al., 2007), only recently have techniques been developed to allow these studies to be safely conducted in living human subjects. Early investigators confined themselves to studying external features, with eighteenth-century methodologies such as phrenology purporting to link extracranial proxies for brain size and structure to specific personality traits (Livianos-Aldana et al., 2007). These techniques were not useful for either clinical or research purposes. Two-dimensional x-ray imaging, while constituting an important medical advance, also did not provide sufficient soft tissue contrast to be useful for studying functional psychiatric disorders such as bipolar disorder; techniques to enhance contrast, such as ventriculography and pneumoencephalography were similarly limited (Figure 1.1). Widespread *in vivo* studies of brain morphometry had to await the development of computed tomography imaging (CT) in the early 1970s. By the early 1980s, CT was already being applied to the study of bipolar disorder (Pearlson et al., 1981).

Conventional x-ray involves collapsing a three-dimensional picture into a two-dimensional view. In CT imaging, two-dimensional x-ray images are acquired from multiple angles and used to reconstruct a three-dimensional image, which allows a detailed examination of brain structures. Early CT studies of patients with bipolar disorder typically examined overall brain volume; ventricular fissure, or sulcal size; or specific structures that could be reliably identified and measured. Many of these early measurements were made by hand on hard copies of the CT scans (Nasrallah et al., 1982a; Nasrallah et al., 1982b; Pearlson et al., 1981; Tanaka et al., 1982). Nonetheless, the relatively poor resolution and contrast of CT scans limited their usefulness; many structures could be identified only with difficulty, and small structures of particular relevance to bipolar disorder, such as the amygdala, could not be consistently delineated.

## STRUCTURAL MAGNETIC RESONANCE IMAGING

It was the advent of structural magnetic resonance imaging (MRI) in the late 1970s that ultimately led to the current profusion of structural brain imaging studies across a wide range of psychiatric conditions including bipolar disorder (Damadian et al., 1977). MRI constitutes a major technical break from previous imaging techniques. Rather than direct visualization or ionizing radiation, MRI takes advantage of the quantum mechanical properties of the spin angular momentum of the single proton of the hydrogen atom (Bushong, 2003; Huettal et al., 2003). A standard MRI scan generates an image by emitting and receiving radio signals that interact with the spinning protons of hydrogen atoms within water molecules. Most clinical MRI scanners currently in use generate a permanent magnetic field of 1 to 3 Teslas (the earth's magnetic field is $\sim 5 \times 10^{-5}$ Tesla), but scanners up to 7 Tesla may be used for research purposes. Although early MRI scans sometimes used a permanent magnet, the higher fields employed today are generated by an electromagnetic using a superconductor wound around the bore of the MRI machine (Figure 1.2) (Bushong, 2003; Huettal et al., 2003). During the MRI scan, protons align with the high magnetic field in the scanner; these protons are targeted by radio waves emitted at a specific frequency determined by multiplying the strength of the magnetic field by the gyro-magnetic ratio (called the Larmor frequency) (Bushong, 2003; Huettal et al., 2004). Proton spin is altered by the absorbed energy; when the protons return to their original state, the energy released is detected by the MRI scanner. Anatomic localization is accomplished using two magnetic gradients parallel to the permanent magnetic field.

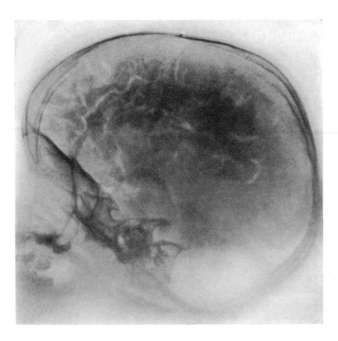

*Figure 1.1* EXAMPLE OF PNEUMOENCEPHALOGRAPHY (Source: Available online at http://en.wikipedia.org/wiki/Pneumoencephalography; listed as public domain.)

The first structural MRI scans were analyzed much like earlier structural CT scans, focusing on ventricle size and discrete anatomic structures (Besson et al., 1987; Nasrallah et al., 1989). Volumetric studies of this kind are still widely performed and are arguably the gold standard for examining changes in specific brain structures. Today, the majority of these studies involve computer tracing of anatomic features across multiple slices of the MRI scan (Hallahan et al., 2011). These structural studies may yield fairly precise measurements of brain structures, but are not without significant disadvantages. The labor involved limits the number of scans tested and some structures have more clearly delineated boundaries than others-limiting examination of some potentially important brain regions,

including portions of the prefrontal cortex (Strakowski et al., 1999). In addition, relatively small morphological differences in larger structures may be missed.

More recently, many structural studies in bipolar disorder have been analyzed using voxel-by-voxel analysis techniques such as voxel-based morphometry (VBM). A "voxel" or volume element is a three-dimensional analog of a pixel or picture element, familiar to most people as the limit of resolution of their television or digital camera. A voxel similarly constitutes the limit of resolution for an MRI scan. By normalizing MRI scans to a standard brain template, groups may be analyzed and compared across individual voxels, rather than larger brain structures. To minimize the anatomic distortion inevitably introduced by this process, the standard brain template must be as representative as possible. Although many studies still use the brain from the Talairach atlas published in 1988, recent templates based on a larger cross section of brains, such as that distributed by the Montreal Neurologic Institute, are coming into more widespread use (Hammers et al., 2003). VBM techniques may be used to compare tissue density, and using methodologies developed by Good and others, to measure local volumetric differences as well (Bora et al., 2010; Good et al., 2001).

VBM has several distinct advantages over traditional structural analyses. Because VBM is largely automated, large numbers of images may be more easily examined. In addition, potential problems with determining regional boundaries are avoided; areas of significant density or volume difference are localized to a region after the comparison is made (Figure 1.3). Voxel-based techniques have their own potential limitations, however. The thousands of voxels tested introduce significant risk of type I statistical error; that is, they may identify a significant difference when one does not really exist. A simple Bonferroni correction is not feasible given the number of comparisons typically made; study analyses instead employ combinations of statistical threshold and cluster size in which groups of contiguous voxels below a specific number are excluded from consideration. Several different techniques may be employed to set appropriate significance criteria, the discussion of which is beyond the scope of this chapter (Ashburner, 2009). Although the majority of studies applying voxel-based analyses to patients with bipolar disorder have explored differences over the entire brain, voxel-by-voxel tests can be limited to specific brain regions-potentially limiting the necessary corrections for multiple comparisons and thereby increasing power.

Increasingly novel VBM-base techniques are being employed to study brain structure in patients with bipolar

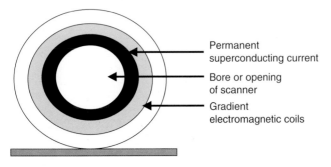

Permanent superconducting current

Bore or opening of scanner

Gradient electromagnetic coils

*Figure 1.2* SCHEMATIC OF MRI SCANNER. The superconducting current creates the permanent magnetic field while the gradient coils generate temporary magnetic field gradients in two directions perpendicular to the permanent magnetic field.

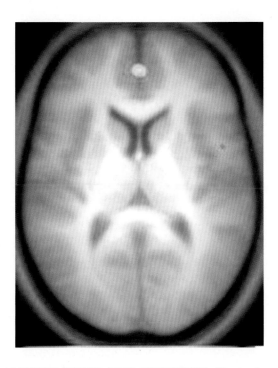

Figure 1.3 EXAMPLE OF VOXEL-BASED MORPHOMETRY. Structural differences are centered in the anterior cingulate cortex.

disorder. In deformation-based morphometry, the degree of deformation required to register a brain to the normalized template is studied to determine morphological changes (Soares et al., 2005). Another automated technique involves measuring cortical thickness across the brain (Foland-Ross et al., 2011) (Figure 1.4). Together, these automated structural imaging techniques are allowing more detailed analyses of regional differences in the brains of bipolar patients from comparison groups and better analyses of how demographic, clinical and longitudinal influences may affect the neuroanatomy of bipolar patients (Bora et al., 2010).

## MAGNETIZATION TRANSFER IMAGING

MRI technology has proven to be extremely versatile. Newer magnetic resonance-based techniques outside of traditional structural MRI are being increasingly employed to study the neuroanatomy of bipolar patients. Magnetization transfer imaging (MTI) takes advantage of energy differences between bound and free protons. Because of the immobility of hydrogen bonds, the former are preferentially

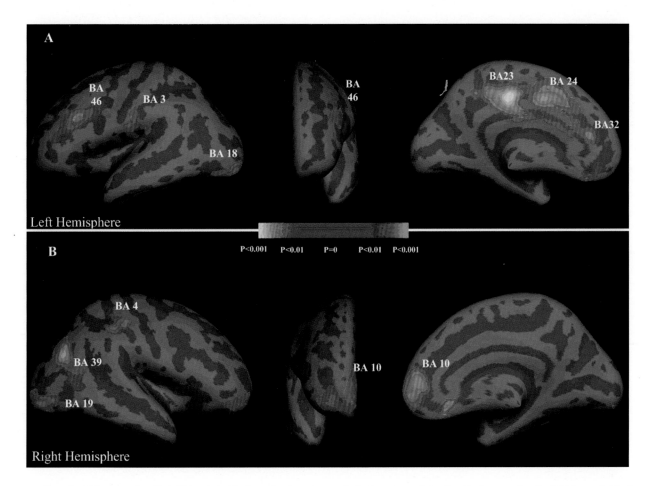

Figure 1.4 Example of decreased cortical thickness in bipolar patients; red areas indicate regions of significantly decreased cortical thickness in bipolar versus healthy subjects. (Source: Lyoo et al., 2006.)

saturated by off-frequency radio frequency pulses; energy is transferred to the free protons in neighboring water molecules. The resulting signal loss corresponds with macromolecular density. The magnetization transfer ratio (MTR) represents the degree of signal loss; MTR may provide sharp contrasts between tissue types, and alterations in MTR may represent underlying changes in the neural substrate. In patients with bipolar disorder, MTI has for the most part been used to study white matter (Bruno et al., 2004).

### DIFFUSION TENSOR IMAGING

Diffusion tensor imaging (DTI) is another magnetic-resonance based technique that is primarily employed to study white matter changes in patients with bipolar disorder. As noted previously, magnetic resonance imaging involves measuring signal decay after exciting protons using short-duration radio-frequency pulses. Because signal decay increases with the movement of water molecules, applying an additional magnetic gradient allows measurement of water diffusion in the gradient direction. With multiple gradients a more complete picture of diffusion can be obtained; a minimum of six gradients is necessary for DTI, but increased numbers of diffusion vectors allow improved resolution (Beaulieu, 2002).

In the absence of any constraints, water molecules diffuse outward in a spherical pattern, or "isotropically". Diffusion in cerebrospinal fluid (CSF) for example, is essentially isotropic. Where water diffusion is restricted however, the overall diffusion may decrease, and if the restriction is asymmetric the pattern of diffusion may be altered. Both of these phenomena are observed in white matter tracts. The former phenomenon is often reported as "mean diffusivity" or "trace apparent diffusion coefficient." Decreases in these measures suggest a loss of structural integrity within the axons comprising white matter pathways. It is the latter phenomenon, however, that may be particularly prominent in white matter tracts. Water diffusion within and around the closely packed axons is more restricted perpendicular to the neuronal fibers than parallel, largely because of intracellular structures, the cellular membrane, and myelin sheath. As a result, water molecules diffuse in an ellipsoid or "anisotropic" pattern (Figure 1.5). White matter changes (for example, a loss of organizational structure), may allow water molecules to move more freely and result in a partial loss of this anisotropic pattern. Measures such as fractional and relative anisotropy are calculated from the main axes of the diffusion ellipsoid and may be used as proxies of white matter integrity (Beaulieu, 2002).

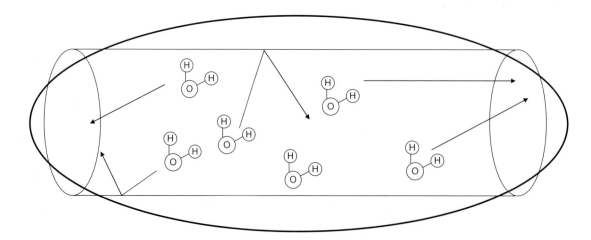

*Figure 1.5.* Water molecules in and around the axons comprising white matter tracts diffuse more freely parallel to cell membranes, forming an ellipsoid, or "anisotropic" pattern. A partial loss of this anisotropic diffusion suggests evidence of white matter pathology, such as loss of structural integrity.

DTI can be used for intergroup comparisons of white matter integrity in several ways. Some of the earliest uses of DTI to study patients with bipolar disorder measured averaged anisotropy or mean diffusivity across a specified region of white matter (Adler et al., 2004; 2006). In placing individual regions-of-interest (ROIs) it is important that investigators ensure that there is no mixing of voxels containing gray matter or cerebrospinal fluid (CSF) within the region; because of the nature of neuronal organization, water diffusion is substantially more rapid and less anisotropic in the former and is approximately isotropic in the latter. As a result, a lack of care in ROI placement can wildly skew DTI findings. Other studies of bipolar patients have employed a voxel-wise approach like that used in studies of brain morphometry. The anatomic distortions inevitably introduced by normalizing individual brains to a standard template limit this approach somewhat because introduction of DTI data from neighboring gray matter or CSF may adversely effect the validity of findings, for reasons previously mentioned (Bruno et al., 2008).

DTI also allows tracing of individual white matter tracts. Tractography studies of this kind have impacted our understanding of healthy neuroanatomy and are now allowing identification of anatomically abnormal white matter networks in patients with bipolar disorder (McCrea, 2008; Mori et al., 1999). In these studies, an initial seed volume is chosen, and the white matter tracts leading from this region are assumed to follow the path of greatest diffusion (Basser et al., 2000) (Figure 1.6). Potential problems arise however, at voxels in which the average diffusion might distort the underlying values, for instance at voxels in which two white matter tracts cross (Assaf and Pasternak, 2008).

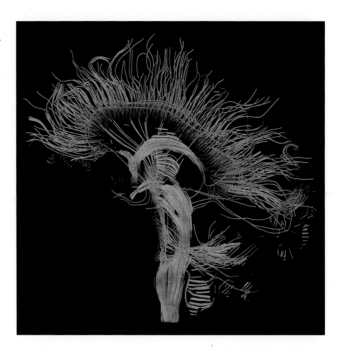

Figure 1.6 EXAMPLE OF WHITE MATTER TRACTS OBTAINED USING DIFFUSION TENSOR IMAGING. (Source: Available from http://commons.wikimedia.org/wiki/File:DTI-sagittal-fibers.jpg with the following notation: Permission is granted to copy, distribute and/or modify this document under the terms of the GNU Free Documentation License, Version 1.2 or any later version published by the Free Software Foundation; with no Invariant Sections, no Front-Cover Texts, and no Back-Cover Texts. A copy of the license is included in the section entitled GNU Free Documentation License. www.gnu.org/copyleft/fdl.htmlGFDLGNU Free Documentation Licensetruetrue. This file is licensed under the Creative Commons Attribution-Share Alike 3.0 Unported license.)

> **Diffusion Tensor Imaging (DTI)**
>
> · Is a magnetization resonance-based technique
>
> · Measures changes in patterns of water diffusion
>
> · Is primarily employed to study white matter changes
>
> · May be analyzed by regions on a voxel-wise basis
>
> · Allows tracing of white matter tracts, called tractography

## MAGNETIC RESONANCE SPECTROSCOPY

With magnetic resonance spectroscopy (MRS), magnetic resonance technology can be used to study localized brain chemistry in subjects with bipolar disorder. Nuclear magnetic resonance (NMR), the precursor to MRI, was originally employed to examine the chemical constitution of experimental samples. This technology was later modified as described earlier, to allow structural MRI and the many other magnetic resonance techniques now in use. MRS arguably represents a partial return to the original application of NMR with the chemical characterization of brain samples, albeit without first extracting the neuronal tissue.

MRS allows detection of certain specific atomic nuclei that contain unpaired nucleons. These nuclei demonstrate magnetic properties that result in their spins aligning with the strong magnetic field of the MRI scanner. A radiofrequency pulse is applied during MRS imaging, disturbing the equilibrium of the nuclei. The local chemical environment influences the resonance frequency, with molecule-specific variations in chemical shift. The resultant chemical shift data are represented by a spectrum in which specific peaks correspond to each measured neurochemical; the area under the curve (AUC) is proportional to the local concentration (Figure 1.7). Imaging parameters can be optimized to maximize the signal for specific molecules of

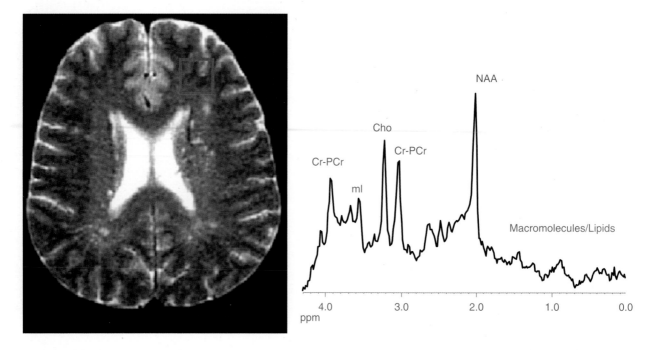

*Figure 1.7* Magnetic resonance spectroscopy data are represented by a spectrum in which specific peaks correspond to measured neurochemicals. Data are often obtained from single voxels (illustrated by the blue square in the image on the left), often localized to areas hypothesized to be relevant to bipolar disorder, such as the prefrontal cortex. *Abbreviations*: Cr-PCr = creatine/phosphocreatine; mI = myo-inositol; Cho = choline; NAA = n-acetyl-aspartate.

interest. A variety of external factors however, may influence spectra obtained; to compare these values across scans, concentrations need to be normalized to an external or internal standard such as chemical ratios or a water signal. Multiple software packages are commonly used to quantify MRS output, with LCmodel and Magnetic Resonance User Interface (MRUI) being arguably the most popular (Dager et al., 2008; Naressi et al., 2001; Provencher, 1993).

While several atomic nuclei can be imaged using MRS, including $^{31}$Ph, $^{13}$C, $^{19}$F, and $^{7}$Li, [$^{1}$H] MRS is the most wide-spread application of this technique and is most commonly used to study a fairly limited number of neurochemicals that include N-acetylaspartate (NAA), choline (Cho), creatine (cr), myo-inositol (mI), and glutamate/glutamine/γ-aminobutyric acid (Glx). The precise interpretation of MRS findings is not without controversy, but some suggestions have been widely accepted. NAA for instance, is present only in the nervous system and has long been employed as a proxy for neuronal integrity (DelBello & Strakowski, 2004); NAA concentrations might be a more sensitive indicator of tissue loss than structural MRI (Deicken et al., 2003). More recently, NAA has been hypothesized to be a marker of neuronal metabolism as well, or a combination of neuronal integrity and metabolism (DelBello & Strakowski, 2004; Tallan et al., 1956).

Myo-inositol may hold particular importance for studies of bipolar disorder because of longstanding suggestions

that the mechanism of action for lithium involves inhibition of inositol monophosphastase (IMPase) and effects on the phosphoinositide cycle. As a result, myo-inositol concentrations may be reduced with a concomitant reduction in neuronal signaling during lithium treatment (Berridge, 1989). Myo-inositol has also been identified as a marker of glial proliferation and a potential marker of inflammation (Rosen & Lenkinski, 2007). The choline (Cho) signal is comprised of four membrane constituents, phosphorylethanolamine, phosphorylcholine, glycerophosphorylethanolamine, and glycerophosphorylcholine (Dager et al., 2008); it appears to arise from membrane turnover and may therefore represent a marker of membrane integrity (Soares & Law, 2009). Creatine is comprised of signal from both creatine (Cr) and phosphocreatine (PCr). Because only the ratio of Cr/PCr is thought to change with changing cellular energy demands while the combined concentration remains stable, the Cr peak has been used as an internal control for chemical ratios.

The Glx peak is comprised of several chemicals with closely overlapping peaks, including glutamate, glutamine, and γ-aminobutyric acid (GABA). At lower field strengths, individual components can be difficult to disentangle, but glutamate is thought to make the largest contribution to the signal (Kreis et al., 1993). As a result, changes in Glx are often interpreted to reflect underlying changes in glutamate concentrations (Moore et al., 2007). At higher field strengths however, distinct glutamate and GABA signals can be obtained (Schubert et al., 2004; Shen et al., 2002). Glutamate is both an important structural amino acid and the most common excitatory neurotransmitter in the brain, as well as a potential neurotoxin (Bergles et al., 1999; Rodríguez et al., 2000).

As noted, other atomic nuclei are amenable to imaging with MRS by virtue of unpaired nucleons. Of these, $^{31}$phosphorus is the most commonly studied (Gujar et al., 2005). [$^{31}$Ph] MRS allows the measurement of several molecules involved in neuronal energetics and has been applied to studies of bipolar patients for several years (Kato et al., 1998; Stork & Renshaw, 2005). Although lithium is not naturally found in the body, [$^{7}$Li] MRS has been employed to study brain lithium concentrations in patients receiving clinical treatment with lithium carbonate (Soares et al., 2000). Limited data suggest that direct brain measures of lithium may better correlate with clinical efficacy than proxy measurements of serum lithium concentrations (Kato et al., 1994). [$^{13}$C] (carbon) and [$^{19}$F] (fluorine) MRS are also not naturally present in the brain, but may be administered and then used to mark glucose, amino acids or medications in order to measure *in vivo* concentrations of these compounds (Kato et al., 1998). Neither of these has been widely used to study patients with bipolar disorder.

Like other neuroimaging techniques, MRS may be analyzed in multiple ways, each with its own advantages and disadvantages. Most commonly, data are obtained from single voxels located in brain regions hypothesized to play a role in affective symptoms, such as portions of the prefrontal cortex and anterior cingulate. Some potentially important regions, including the subgenual anterior cingulate, are difficult to image with single voxel MRS because their location makes establishing a homogenous magnetic field technically difficult (Yildiz-Yesiloglu & Ankerst, 2006). The size of these individual voxels may vary considerably depending on scan time and scanner specifications, but often encompass fairly large regions of interest in the brain, potentially complicating the interpretation of findings. A minority of MRS studies has obtained data from two- or even three-dimensional slabs of brain that cut across multiple regions, though few data from studies using this approach in patients with bipolar disorder have been published (Shahana et al., 2011).

## NEUROFUNCTIONAL IMAGING

Although indirect measurements of brain activity date back centuries, including those of reaction time from both manual and behavioral tasks, modern efforts to examine human brain function lagged structural imaging by decades. As early as 1890, however, William James described experiments in which intellectual activity was correlated with increased blood flow to the brain (James, 1890). Electroencephalography (EEG), first demonstrated in humans in 1924, was arguably the next significant advance in functional imaging. Essentially representing measurements of the electrical activity associated with brain activity, EEG can be considered a functional imaging modality, but is outside the focus of this chapter.

As previously discussed, a standard CT or structural MRI scan delivers a static picture of the anatomic structure of the brain. Functional imaging by contrast generates a series of three-dimensional images projected across time. An analogy (in two dimensions) is that a structural image represents a single photograph while a functional image is a video recording. There are currently three major techniques for generating functional images: functional magnetic resonance imaging (fMRI), single photon emission computed tomography (SPECT), and positron emission tomography (PET) (Pardo et al., 2008). The advances in functional imaging represented by these techniques have revolutionized cognitive neuroscience by opening up non-invasive methodologies for studying the working human brain and have found widespread use in psychiatric research (Carter, 2001; Malhi & Lagopoulos 2008 Pardo et al., 2008). While there are currently few clinical applications for functional imaging in psychiatry, many active research programs are hoping to develop these tools for use in diagnosis and treatment assignment. Over the next few decades functional neuroimaging has the potential to become a useful diagnostic tool and facilitate selection of appropriate treatment

---

**Magnetic Resonance Spectroscopy (MRS)**

- Is similar to *in vivo* NMR

- Allows detection of certain specific atomic nuclei including $^{1}$H, $^{31}$Ph, $^{13}$C, $^{19}$F, and $^{7}$Li

- Based on [$^{1}$H] is the most widespread application of this technique

- Based on [$^{31}$Ph] allows measurement of molecules involved in neuronal energetics

- Based on [$^{7}$Li] has been employed to study brain lithium concentrations

- Data are usually obtained from single brain voxels

modalities (Cannon, 2007; Malhi & Lagopoulos 2007; Philips, 2007).

## SINGLE-PHOTON EMISSION COMPUTED TOMOGRAPHY

Single-photon emission computed tomography (SPECT) is the first functional imaging technique to produce what was generally regarded as a picture of brain function. The earliest use of SPECT scanning to study bipolar disorder dates to approximately 1989, and although SPECT is less commonly used to study bipolar disorder than positron emission tomography (PET), the typically lower cost and wider availability of SPECT have lead to continued application of this technology (Reischies et al., 1990).

SPECT generates an image by introducing radioactive isotopes into molecules of known biological relevance and then injecting these molecules into the bloodstream. These radionuclides generate a single gamma ray upon decay. The gamma rays are detected by a gamma camera that rotates around the patient's head and generates multiple two-dimensional (2-D) images. These 2-D images are then used to create three-dimensional images using reconstruction algorithms similar to those employed in CT scanning. Newer systems may have multi-headed gamma detectors that allow for much greater spatial resolution.

It has been understood for decades that active neurons demonstrate increased oxygen demand; blood vessels around these neurons dilate in response to increased brain activity, to increase blood flow to that region. The early experiments described by James (1890) relied on measuring changes in an individual's center of mass with increased blood flow to the brain. Some of the earliest modern studies of the effects of cognition on intracranial blood flow used inhaled $^{133}$Xenon to crudely localize areas of increased perfusion. SPECT scanning allows for an estimation of brain activity using technetium 99m-hexamethylpropylene amine oxime ($^{99m}$Tc-HMPAO), the most commonly used radionuclide in SPECT brain scans (Malison & Innis 2000; Camarago, 2001). $^{99m}$Tc-HMPAO is taken up by brain tissue in proportion to blood flow, which is correlated with brain activity. Analysis can be done either regionally or on a voxel-wise basis as described for structural imaging. In the former, regions-of-interest may be identified on specific scans or a group of scans normalized to a standard space as previously discussed. In the latter, normalization of the scans to a standard template is required.

In addition to blood flow, SPECT allows scanning of a variety of labeled radiotracers. Most commonly, these tracers consist of receptor ligands, molecules that bind to specific neuroreceptors (Zipursky et al. 2007). While SPECT has historically been most commonly used to study perfusion, Anand et al. (2000) and others have used $^{123}$I-Iodobenzamide (IBZM), an iodine-labeled dopamine receptor ligand, to study amphetamine-induced changes in $D_2$ binding in bipolar disorder (Anand et al., 2000). More recently, investigators used tracers such as $^{123}$I-labeled 2-((2-((dimethylamino)methyl)phenyl)thio)-5-iodophenylamine ($^{123}$I-ADAM) and [99mTc] TRODAT-1 to demonstrate differences in serotonin and dopamine transporter binding (Chang et al., 2010; Chou et al., 2010).

---

**Single-Photon Emission Computed Tomography (SPECT)**

- Use in bipolar disorder research dates back to 1989

- Uses radio-labeled molecules that generate a single gamma ray

- Multiple 2-dimensional images are used to construct a 3-dimensional picture

- May be used to measure perfusion, which may correlate with brain activity

- Using radio-labeled ligands, SPECT may be used to study neuroreceptors

- Analysis may be voxel-wise or by region-of-interest

---

## POSITRON EMISSION TOMOGRAPHY (PET)

Like SPECT, PET depends on emission of radioactive isotopes introduced into the body to generate an image. Isotopes are chosen that emit positrons (the positively charged antiparticle of the electron). When the generated positrons encounter an electron, very rapidly after isotope delay, their mutual annihilation produces two gamma rays that travel 180 degrees in opposite directions. Although the distance travelled by the positron prior to annihilation is less than three millimeters, it inevitability limits the minimum spatial resolution of a PET scan. Photomultipliers line the cylinder of the PET scanner so that the two gamma rays may be detected on opposite sides of the scanner as coincident events. The geometry of this detection allows determination of the collision location. The other two spatial dimensions needed to create the three dimensional image are obtained by a mathematical transformation of the angle of release and distance traveled by each photon. The final representation is created using the information from the totality of photon pairs. The number of photon pairs detected in each voxel directly correlates with the concentration of the labeled compound. In PET scan images, these data are usually represented by an arbitrary color scale (Phelps & Mazziotta 1985; Wahl, 2002; Saha, 2005).

The four most commonly used isotopes in PET are $^{11}$C, $^{13}$N, $^{15}$O and $^{18}$F (Saha 2005. These isotopes may be used to label water or glucose and hence to measure brain activity as described subsequently, or incorporated into ligands that bind to specific molecular receptors. In this chapter we will only review a few of the most common molecules used in psychiatric research (Pardo et al. 2008; Smith & Jakobsen, 2009).

One common method in PET is to determine brain activity by measuring perfusion or even direct uptake of glucose using $^{15}$O labeled water or $^{18}$F labeled fluorodeoxyglucose (FDG), respectively. $^{15}$O labeled water has a very short half-life (~2 minutes), but it quickly diffuses through the body, serving as a good indicator of blood flow (Dunn et al., 2005; Saha, 2005). $^{18}$F-Fluorodeoxyglucose (FDG) has a much longer half-life (over an hour) and is actively taken up by cells in place of glucose. Deoxyglucose, however, is incompletely metabolized, allowing it to be used as a direct marker of neuronal metabolism. These differences dictate the nature of the study designs for $^{15}$O labeled water and FDG. The short half-life of the former allows for a blocked approach, in which subjects perform separate tasks while PET images are obtained. In contrast, FDG is often used to measure neuronal metabolism at rest or during a task administered while the agent is taken up by the brain; this task can even be performed outside the scanner, given FDG's long half-life. Like SPECT, analysis of these data can be performed based on specific regions-of-interest or voxel-by-voxel.

Also like SPECT, PET may be used to measure receptor binding using radio-labeled ligands. For instance, PET scanning has been used to study both dopamine and serotonin receptors in patients with bipolar disorder using a

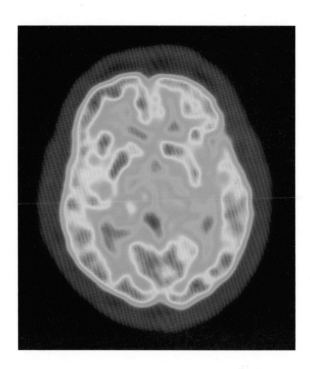

*Figure 1.8* BRAIN METABOLISM MEASURED WITH $^{18}$F LABELED FLUORODEOXYGLUCOSE (FDG); BRIGHT AREAS INDICATE INCREASED GLUCOSE UTILIZATION. (Source: Available from http://en.wikipedia.org/wiki/File:PET-image.jpg with the following notation: This work has been released into the public domain by its author, I, Jens Langner. This applies worldwide.)

variety of radio-ligands (Sargent et al., 2009; Yatham et al., 2002) (Figure 1.8). While PET scans have clear limitations to their resolution, the lower limits of these radiotracer studies is significantly better than that achieved by SPECT, as are perfusion data acquired with PET. Because of the short half-lives of some of the isotopes involved however, many of these radio-ligands, as well as $^{15}$O labeled water require a nearby cyclotron. Not surprisingly, the cost may also be somewhat higher than most SPECT scans. A final limitation of both SPECT and PET is that the number of repeat scans is limited by the necessary exposure to ionizing radiation (Malhi & Lagopoulos 2007).

### BLOOD OXYGEN LEVEL-DEPENDENT FUNCTIONAL MAGNETIC RESONANCE IMAGING (fMRI)

Functional magnetic resonance imaging (fMRI) represents another use of magnetic resonance imaging techniques. In contrast to structural MRI, fMRI is a functional methodology that builds on the standard techniques described earlier. FMRI requires the rapid acquisition of MRI images, typically using an echo-planner imaging (EPI) sequence that allows multiple images to be acquired over a short period of time (Huettel et al., 2004). This rapid acquisition

**Positron Emission Tomography (PET)**

- Relies on radioactive isotopes introduced into the body to generate an image

- Gamma rays are produced when emitted positrons strike electrons with mutual annihilation

- Detection of the gamma rays allows localization of labeled compounds

- PET may be used to measure cerebral perfusion and neuronal metabolism

- Radiolabled compounds also allow measurement of neuronal transporters and receptors

is traded against resolution, which is much lower than a standard structural MRI image that may take significantly longer to collect.

Most fMRI depends on the blood oxygen level-dependent (BOLD) response which allows the correlation of these rapid EPI images with ongoing brain activation (Huettel et al., 2003 Pardo et al., 2008). As noted earlier, it has long been understood that blood vessels around active neurons dilate in response to brain activity to increase blood flow to that region. BOLD fMRI takes advantage of this phenomenon to measure brain activity. The magnetic properties of hemoglobin in the MRI scanner vary; deoxygenated hemoglobin is paramagnetic, while oxygenated hemoglobin is diamagnetic. Increased blood flow with increased neuronal activity changes the ratio of oxy- to deoxyhemoglobin and thus the local magnetic signal. To the degree that increased blood flow reflects increased neuronal metabolism, changes in the local magnetic environment serve as an indirect measurement of brain activity (Huettel et al., 2003 Pardo et al., 2008).

Unlike some PET scanning, BOLD fMRI does not measure the absolute amount of blood flow or energy metabolism in the brain. FMRI depends on "subtraction" to determine relative brain activity across regions (Huettel et al., 2004). Subtraction involves comparing the signal strength of two different fMRI images. In a classic block design, tasks are presented alternately, typically over a period of several minutes. The active portion might consist of a motor or cognitive task, which is matched to a control task that ideally incorporates unwanted aspects of the active task. The signal from the active and control tasks are compared; because the magnetic environment varies with blood flow, signal differences between tasks presumably represent areas that are active during the former, but not latter portions of the fMRI scan. Study design may be somewhat more complicated however. In event-related designs, active trials are intermixed with control regions. Event-related studies often allow more sophisticated analyses at the expense of a loss of power. Functional magnetic resonance imaging analysis is not entirely straightforward and a full discussion is well beyond the scope of this chapter. Good reviews can be found in Huettal et al. (2004), Sarty (2007), Lazar (2008), and Lindquist (2008).

The nature of fMRI scanning, including as it does the acquisition of many images over a short period of time, introduces some potentially significant problems. A typical fMRI image may consist of 20 or more image slices across the brain that are collected in 2 to 3 seconds. For technical reasons, these images are often collected in an interleaved pattern that may create slight distortions that must be corrected (Huettal et al., 2004; Sarty, 2007; Lazar, 2008). In addition, inadvertent head motion can introduce significant noise, requiring correction (Huettal et al., 2004; Sarty, 2007; Lazar, 2008; Lindquist, 2008). Once the raw imaging data have been reconstructed, they may be analyzed in multiple ways. Most commonly, a voxel-wise analysis is performed, as discussed earlier. Individual scans are usually aligned with a contemporaneously acquired structural scan. As in structural VBM, this structural scan is mapped onto a common brain template; the mapping parameters may then be applied to the aligned functional scans (Huettal et al., 2004; Lazar, 2008). This approach has similar advantages and disadvantages to those discussed earlier with regard to VBM. A large number of scans may be compared, and the process is structurally agnostic, no *a priori* brain regions need be defined. Some distortion is inevitable however, and this technique requires controlling for the large number of comparisons (Figure 1.9).

Another approach to analysis involves choosing specific regions-of-interest (ROIs) and comparing the average signal

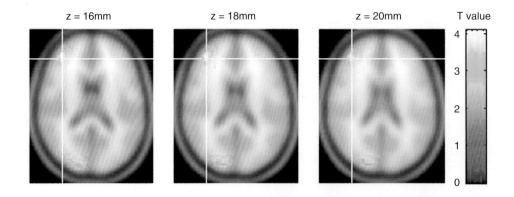

*Figure 1.9* FUNCTIONAL MAGNETIC RESONANCE IMAGING (fMRI) VOXEL-BASED ANALYSIS IMPLEMENTED IN SPM8. PERFORMANCE OF A VISUAL CONTINUOUS PERFORMANCE ATTENTION TASK (CPT) WAS ASSOCIATED WITH ACTIVITY IN THE RIGHT PREFRONTAL CORTEX. (Image courtesy of the Division of Bipolar Disorders Research, of the University of Cincinnati College of Medicine.)

THE BIPOLAR BRAIN

strength across each region. This method potentially allows for more specific testing of *a priori* hypotheses and may have greater power to detect differences by limiting the number of comparisons (Lazar, 2008). ROI analyses may be made on non-normalized scans, but more commonly use automated methods applied to scans that have been normalized to a specific brain template.

Recently there has also been increased interest in newer analysis techniques such as functional connectivity and structural equation modeling (Sarty, 2007; Lazar, 2008). Functional connectivity examines correlations in activity between brain regions. An initial seed region is chosen and

brain activation in this region is compared to the rest of the brain, with a correlation value computed for each voxel outside the seed region. Cluster thresholding is used to avoid multiple comparison errors, as previously described. These data can identify regions showing increased or decreased correlation with the original seed region, suggesting that brain regions with high correlations are functionally linked. Connectivity may be determined during a putative resting state or as steady state data obtained during performance of a specific task, or type of task (Figure 1.10). The interpretation of functional connectivity however, remains somewhat controversial as the field becomes accustomed

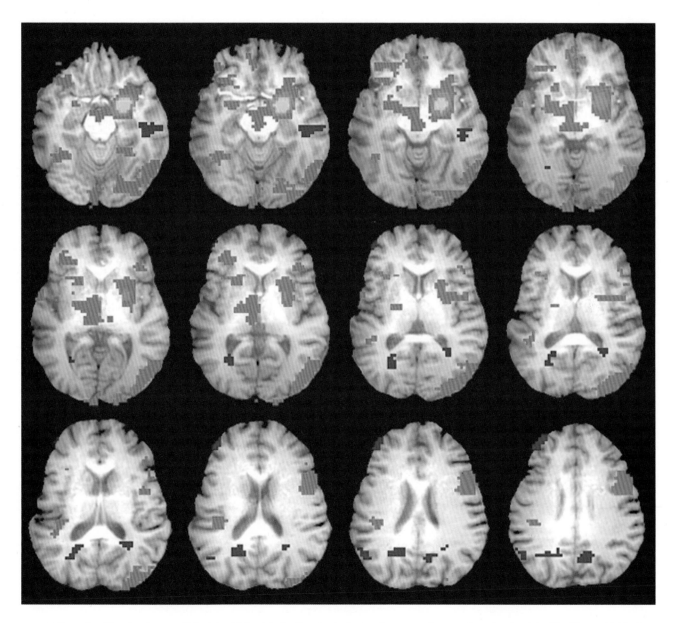

*Figure 1.10* Example of functional connectivity data obtained during the steady-state performance of an emotion-related task in 15 subjects with bipolar disorder during mania. The left amygdala was used as the seed region. Orange regions represent clusters of brain activation that were significantly positively correlated with left amygdala activation. (Image courtesy of the Division of Bipolar Disorders Research and Center for Imaging Research, of the University of Cincinnati College of Medicine.)

to this new technique. Moreover, there continues to be potential issues with determining causal relationships, although newer analytic techniques, such as structural equation modeling, may at least partially remedy some of these problems. These analyses are also subject to potentially significant technical confounds. It is essential to remove physiologic variables such as pulse and respiration which may drive spurious correlations. Techniques using physiologic measures recorded while scanning and others involving post-processing have been advanced to control for these effects.

Although fMRI has arguably become the most widespread functional imaging technique, there are several potential issues that must be considered. The increase in blood flow coupled to increased regional brain activity takes several seconds to peak and fade, which limits the temporal resolution of this technique to several seconds. Similarly, because BOLD fMRI measures changes in blood flow rather than directly measuring neuronal activity, spatial resolution is limited to a few millimeters. Furthermore, because it is an indirect measure, BOLD fMRI may be subject to other confounds, including effects of medications and vascular pathology on blood flow. Most importantly however, the link between brain activity and blood flow remains poorly understood.

---

**Functional Magnetic Resonance Imaging (fMRI)**

- Allows analysis of brain activity without ionizing radiation

- Takes advantage of differences between the magnetic qualities of oxy- and deoxyhemoglobin

- Requires contrast between active and control tasks

- Studies may be done voxel-wise or by region

- May be affected by neurovascular pathology or other changes in neural blood flow

---

## PERFUSION-BASED FUNCTIONAL MAGNETIC RESONANCE IMAGING

As observed earlier, both SPECT and PET can be used to measure brain perfusion using radiolabeled tracers. Although not commonly used in bipolar disorder research, magnetic resonance imaging may also measure brain perfusion using an exogenous tracer. Arterial spin labeling (ASL) allows measurement of perfusion without addition of exogenous compounds. Although there are several forms of ASL, in each of them water molecules are labeled using a radio-frequency pulse that saturates their spin. Comparing MRI scans taken as the labeled blood enters the area of interest with control scans allows determination of cerebral blood flow (CBF) (Huettel et al., 2004; Petcharunpaisan et al., 2010).

ASL can be used for fMRI under the same principles as BOLD. Rather than relying on differences in the paramagnetic qualities of hemoglobin however, perfusion-based fMRI compares more direct measures of CBF. This more direct measure may account for suggestions of decreased variability in perfusion-based fMRI findings. This technique however, may be less sensitive and is associated with less temporal resolution than BOLD fMRI (Petcharunpaisan et al., 2010).

## CONCLUSIONS

The significant technological advances of the last century have left their mark on psychiatric imaging, as they have on medicine in general. Structural imaging has progressed from examining gross specimens in an anatomy laboratory to high-resolution imaging and techniques allowing analysis of white matter tracts and neurochemistry. Over this same time period, functional imaging has gone from purely behavioral testing to sophisticated techniques for measuring brain activity and receptor density. As a result, we appear to be at the beginning of a revolution in our understanding of the neural basis of bipolar symptoms that has already impacted our understanding of the disorder in profound ways, as discussed in detail in chapters 2–7 of this book. Neuroimaging will almost certainly lead the way toward both a better understanding of bipolar neurophysiology as well as the development of novel, more effective treatments.

## REFERENCES

Adler, C. M., Adams, J., DelBello, M. P., Holland, S. K., Schmithorst, V., Levine, A., . . . Strakowski, S. M. 2006. Evidence of white matter pathology in first-episode manic adolescents with bipolar disorder: a diffusion tensor imaging study. *American Journal of Psychiatry*, 163: 322–324.

Adler, C. M., Holland, S. K., Schmithorst, V., Wilke, M., Weiss, K. L., Pan, H., & Strakowski, S. M. 2004. Abnormal frontal white matter tracts in bipolar disorder: a diffusion tensor imaging study. *Bipolar Disorders*, 6: 197–203.

Aguirre, G., & D'Esposito, M. 2000. Experimental design for brain fMRI. In C. Moonen & T. W. Bandettini, (eds.), *Functional MRI* (pp. 369–380). Heidelberg, Berlin: Springer-Verlag.

Anand, A., Verhoeff, P., Seneca, N., Zoghbi, S. S., Seibyl, J. P., Charney, D. S., & Innis, R. B. 2000. Brain SPECT imaging of amphetamine-induced dopamine release in euthymic bipolar disorder patients. *American Journal of Psychiatry*, 157(7): 1108–1114.

Ashburner, J. 2009. Computational anatomy with the SPM software. *Magnetic Resonance Imaging*, 27(8): 1163–1174.

Assaf, Y., & Pasternak, O. 2008. 3Diffusion tensor imaging (DTI)-based white matter mapping in brain research: a review. *Journal of Molecular Neuroscience*, 34(1): 51–61.

Basser, P.J., Pajevic, S., Pierpaoli, C., Duda, J., & Aldroubi, A. 2000. In vivo fiber tractography using DT-MRI data. *Magnetic Resonance in Medicine*, 44(4):625–632.

Beaulieu, C. 2002. The basis of anisotropic diffusion in the nervous system—a technical review. *NMR in Biomedicine*, 15: 435–455.

Bergles, D. E., Diamond, J. S., & Jahr, C. E. 1999. Clearance of glutamate inside the synapse and beyond. *Current Opinion in Neurobiology*, 9(3): 293–298.

Berridge, M. J. 1989. The Albert Lasker Medical Awards. Inositol tris-phosphate, calcium, lithium, and cell signaling. *JAMA*, 262(13): 1834–1841.

Besson, J. A., Henderson, J. G., Foreman, E. I., & Smith, F. W. 1987. An NMR study of lithium responding manic depressive patients. *Magnetic Resonance Imaging*, 5(4): 273–277.

Bora, E., Fornito, A., Yücel, M., & Pantelis, C. 2010. Voxelwise meta-analysis of gray matter abnormalities in bipolar disorder. *Biological Psychiatry*, 67(11): 1097–1105.

Bruno, S., Cercignani, M., & Ron, M. A. 2008. White matter abnormalities in bipolar disorder: a voxel-based diffusion tensor imaging study. *Bipolar Disorders*, 10(4): 460–468.

Bruno, S. D., Barker, G. J., Cercignani, M., Symms, M., & Ron, M. A. 2004. A study of bipolar disorder using magnetization transfer imaging and voxel-based morphometry. *Brain* 127(11): 2433–2440.

Bushong, S. 2003. *Magnetic Resonance Imaging: Physical and Biological Principles*. St. Louis, MO: Mosby.

Camargo, E. E. 2001. Brain SPECT in Neurology and Psychiatry. *Journal of Nuclear Medicine*, 42(4): 611–623.

Cannon, D. 2007. Neuroimaging in psychiatry. *International Journal of Psychiatry in Medicine*, 24(3): 86–88.

Carter, C. S. 2001. Cognitive neuroscience: The new neuroscience of the mind and its implication for psychiatry. In Morisha, J. M (ed.) *Advances In Brain Imaging* (pp. 25–52). Washington, DC: American Psychiatric Publishing.

Chang, T. T., Yeh, T. L., Chiu, N. T., Chen, P. S., Huang, H. Y., Yang, Y. K., . . . Lu, R. B. 2010. Higher striatal dopamine transporters in euthymic patients with bipolar disorder: a SPECT study with [Tc] TRODAT-1. *Bipolar Disorersd*. Feb. 12(1): 102–106.

Chou, Y. H., Wang, S. J., Lin, C. L., Mao, W. C., Lee, S. M., & Liao, M. H. 2010. Decreased brain serotonin transporter binding in the euthymic state of bipolar I but not bipolar II disorder: a SPECT study. *Bipolar Disorders*, 12(3): 312–318.

Cox, R. W., & Jesmanowicz, A. 1999. Real-time 3D image registration for functional MRI. *Magnetic Resonancein Medicine*, 42(6): 1014–1018.

D'Esposito, M., Zarahn, E., & Aguirre, G. 1999. *Event-related functional MRI: implications for cognitive psychology*. *Psychological Bulletin*, 125(1): 155–164.

Dager, S. R., Corrigan, N. M., Richards, T. L., & Posse S. 2008. Research applications of magnetic resonance spectroscopy to investigate psychiatric disorders. *Topics in Magnetic Resonance Imaging*, 19(2): 81–96.

Damadian, R., Goldsmith, M., & Minkoff, L. 1977. NMR in cancer: XVI. FONAR image of the live human body. *Physiological Chemistry and Physics*, 9(1): 97–100,108.

Deicken, R. F., Pegues, M. P., Anzalone, S., Feiwell, R., & Soher, B. 2003. Lower concentration of hippocampal N-acetylaspartate in familial bipolar I disorder. *American Journal of Psychiatry*. 160(5): 873–882.

DelBello, M. P., & Strakowski, S. M. 2004. Neurochemical predictors of response to pharmacologic treatments for bipolar disorder. *Current Psychiatry Reports*, 6(6): 466–472.

Dunn, R., Willis, M., Benson, B., Repella, J., Kimbrell, T., Ketter, T., . . . Post, R. 2005. Preliminary findings of uncoupling of flow and metabolism in unipolar compared with bipolar affective illness and normal controls. *Psychiatry Research*, 140: 181–198.

Reischies, FM, Hedde, J. P., & Drochner, R. 1989. Clinical correlates of cerebral blood flow in depression. *Psychiatry Research*, 29(3): 323–326.

Foland-Ross, L. C., Thompson, P. M., Sugar, C. A., Madsen, S. K., Shen, J. K., Penfold, C., . . . Altshuler, L. L. 2011. Investigation of cortical thickness abnormalities in lithium-free adults with bipolar I disorder using cortical pattern matching. *American Journal of Psychiatry*, 168(5): 530–539.

Good, C. D., Johnsrude, I. S., Ashburner, J., Henson, R. N., Friston, K. J., & Frackowiak, R. S. 2001. A voxel-based morphometric study of ageing in 465 normal adult human brains. *Neuroimage*, 14: 21–36.

Gujar, S. K., Maheshwari, S., Björkman-Burtscher, I., Sundgren, P. C. 2005. Magnetic resonance spectroscopy. *Journal of Neuroophthalmology*, 25(3): 217–226.

Haas, L. F. 2003. Hans Berger (1873–1941), Richard Caton (1842–1926), and electroencephalography. *Journal of Neurology, Neurosurgery & Psychiatry*, 74(1): 9.

Hallahan, B., Newell, J., Soares, J. C., Brambilla, P., Strakowski, S. M., Fleck, D. E., . . . McDonald, C. 2011. Structural magnetic resonance imaging in bipolar disorder: an international collaborative mega-analysis of individual adult patient data. *Biological Psychiatry*, 69(4): 326–335.

Hammers, A., Allom, R., Koepp, M. J., Free, S. L., Myers, R., Lemieux, L., . . . Duncan, J. S. 2003. Three-dimensional maximum probability atlas of the human brain, with particular reference to the temporal lobe. *Human Brain Mapping*, 19(4): 224–247.

Huettal, S., Song, A., & McCarthy, G. 2003. *Functional Magnetic Resonance Imaging*. Sunderland, MA: Sinauer Associates.

James, W. 1890. *The Principles of Psychology*. Cambridge, MA: Harvard University Press.

Kato, T., Inubushi, T., & Kato N. 1998. Magnetic resonance spectroscopy in affective disorders. The *Journal of Neuropsychiatry and Clinical Neurosciences*, 10(2): 133–147.

Kato, T., Inubushi, T., & Takahashi, S. 1994. Relationship of lithium concentrations in the brain measured by lithium-7 magnetic resonance spectroscopy to treatment response in mania. *Journal of Clinical Psychopharmacology* 14(5): 330–335.

Kreis, R., Ernst, T., & Ross, B. D. 1993. Development of the human brain: in vivo quantification of metabolite and water content with proton magnetic resonance spectroscopy. *Magnetic Resonance in Medicine*, 30(4): 424–437.

Lazar, N. 2008. *The Statistical Analysis of Functional MRI Data*. Athens, GA: Springer.

Lindquist, M. A. 2008. The statistical analysis of fMRI data. *Statistical Science*, 23(4): 439–464.

Livianos-Aldana, L., Rojo-Moreno, L., & Sierra-SanMiguel, P. 2007. F. J. Gall and the phrenological movement. *American Journal of Psychiatry*, 164(3): 414.

Lyoo, I. K., Sung, Y. H., Dager, S. R., Friedman, S. D., Lee, J. Y., Kim, S. J., . . . Renshaw, P. F. 2006. Regional cerebral cortical thinning in bipolar disorder. *Bipolar Disorders*., 8(1): 65–74.

Malhi, G. S., & Lagopoulos, J. 2008. Making sense of neuroimaging in psychiatry. *Acta Psychiatrica Scandinavica*, 117(2): 100–117.

Malison, R. T., & Innis, R. B. 2000. Principles of Neuroimaging: Radiotracer Techniques. 154–162. In Sadock, B. J., & Sadock, V. A (eds.) Kaplan and Sadock's *Comprehensive Textbook of Psychiatry*. Philadelphia: Lippincott Williams and Wilkins.

McCrea, S. M. 2008. Bipolar disorder and neurophysiologic mechanisms. *Journal of Neuropsychiatric Disease and Treatment*, 4(6): 1129–1153.

Moore, C. M., Biederman, J., Wozniak, J., Mick, E., Aleardi, M., Wardrop, M., . . . Renshaw, P. F. 2007. Mania, glutamate/glutamine and risperidone in pediatric bipolar disorder: a proton magnetic resonance spectroscopy study of the anterior cingulate cortex. *Journal of Affective Disorders*, 99(1–3): 19–25.

Mori, S., Crain, B. J., Chacko, V. P., & van Zijl, P. C. 1999. Three-dimensional tracking of axonal projections in the brain by magnetic resonance imaging. *Annals of Neurology*, 45(2): 265–269.

Naressi, A., Couturier, C., Devos, J. M., Janssen, M., Mangeat, C., de Beer, R., & Graveron-Demilly, D. 2001. Java-based graphical user interface for the MRUI quantitation package. *Magnetic Resonance Materials in Physics, Biology and Medicine*, 12: 141–152.

Nasrallah, H. A., Coffman, J. A., & Olson, S. C. 1989. Structural brain-imaging findings in affective disorders: an overview. *Journal of Neuropsychiatry and Clinical and Neurosciences*, 1(1): 21–26.

Nasrallah, H. A., McCalley-Whitters, M., & Jacoby, C. G. 1982. Cortical atrophy in schizophrenia and mania: a comparative CT study. *Journal of Clinical Psychiatry*, 43(11): 439–441.

Nasrallah, H. A., McCalley-Whitters, M., & Jacoby, C. G. 1982. Cerebral ventricular enlargement in young manic males. A controlled CT study. *Journal of Affecivet Disorders*, 4(1): 15–19.

Obrist, W. D., Thompson, H. K. Jr., Wang, H. S., & Wilkinson, W. E. 1975. Regional cerebral blood flow estimated by 133-xenon inhalation. *Stroke*, 6(3): 245–256.

Paluzzi, A., Belli, A., Bain, P., & Viva, L. 2007. Brain "imaging" in the Renaissance. *Journal of the Royal Society of Medicine,* 100(12): 540–543.

Pardo, P. J., Olman, C. A., & Pardo, J. V. 2008. Neuroimaging in psychiatry. 695–723. In Fatemi, S.H. & Clayton, P. J (eds.) *The Medical Basis of Psychiatry*. Totowa, NJ: Human Press.

Pearlson, G. D., Veroff, A. E., & McHugh, P. R. 1981. The use of computed tomography in psychiatry: recent applications to schizophrenia, manic-depressive illness and dementia syndromes. *Johns Hopkins Medical Journal*, 149(5): 194–202.

Petcharunpaisan, S., Ramalho, J., & Castillo, M. 2010. Arterial spin labeling in neuroimaging. *World Journal of Radiology*, 2(10): 384–398.

Phelps, M., & Mazziotta, J. 1985. Positron emission tomography: human brain function and biochemistry. *Science*, 228(4701): 799–809.

Phillips, M. 2007. The emerging role of neuroimaging in psychiatry: characterizing treatment-relevant endophenotypes. *American Journal of Psychiatry*, 164(5): 697–699.

Provencher, S. W. 1993. Estimation of metabolite concentrations from localized in vivo proton NMR spectra. *Magnetic Resonance in Medicine,* 30: 672.

Rodríguez, M. J., Bernal, F., Andrés, N., Malpesa, Y., & Mahy, N. 2000. Excitatory amino acids and neurodegeneration: a hypothetical role of calcium precipitation. *International Journal of Developmental Neuroscience*, 18(2–3): 299–307.

Rosen, Y., & Lenkinski, R. E. 2007. Recent advances in magnetic resonance neurospectroscopy. *Neurotherapeutics*, 4(3): 330–345.

Saha, G. 2005. *Basics of PET Imaging: Physics, Chemistry, and Regulations.* New York: Springer.

Sargent, P., Rabiner, E., Bhagwager, Z., Clark, L., Cowen, P., Goodwin, G., & Grasby, P. 2009. 5-HT$_{1A}$ receptor binding in euthymic bipolar patients using positron emission tomography with [*carbonyl*-$^{11}$C] WAY-100635. *Journal of Affective Disorders*, 123: 77–80.

Sarty, G. 2007. *Computing brain activity maps.* Cambridge: Cambridge University Press.

Schubert, F., Gallinat, J., Seifert, F., & Rinneberg, H. 2004. Glutamate concentrations in human brain using single voxel proton magnetic resonance spectroscopy at 3 Tesla. *Neuroimage*, 21(4): 1762–1771.

Shahana, N., DelBello, M., Chu, W-J., Jarvis, K., Fleck, D., Welge, J., Strakowski, S.,. . . Adler, C. 2011. Neurochemical alteration in the caudate: implications for the pathophysiology of bipolar disorder. *Psychiatry Research*, 193(2): 107–112.

Shen, J., Rothman, D. L., & Brown, P. 2002. In vivo GABA editing using a novel doubly selective multiple quantum filter. *Magnetic Resonance in Medicine*, 47(3): 447–454.

Smith, D., & Jakobsen, S. 2009. Molecular tools for assessing human depression by positron emission tomography. *European Neuropsychopharmacology*, 19(9): 611–628.

Soares, D. P., & Law, M. 2009. Magnetic resonance spectroscopy of the brain: review of metabolites and clinical applications. *Clinical Radiology*, 64(1): 12–21.

Soares, J. C., Boada, F., & Keshavan, M. S. 2000. Brain lithium measurements with (7)Li magnetic resonance spectroscopy (MRS): a literature review. *European Neuropsychopharmacology*, 10(3): 151–158.

Soares, J. C., Kochunov, P., Monkul, E. S., Nicoletti, M. A., Brambilla, P., Sassi, R. B., . . . Fox, P. 2005. Structural brain changes in bipolar disorder using deformation field morphometry. *NeuroReport*, 16(6): 541–544.

Stork, C., & Renshaw, P. F. 2005. Mitochondrial dysfunction in bipolar disorder: evidence from magnetic resonance spectroscopy research. *Molecular Psychiatry*, 10(10): 900–919.

Strakowski, S. M., DelBello, M. P., Sax, K. W., Zimmerman, M. E., Shear, P. K., Hawkins, J. M., & Larson, E. R. 1999. Brain magnetic resonance imaging of structural abnormalities in bipolar disorder. *Archives of General Psychiatry*, 56(3): 254–260.

Tallan, H. H., Moore, S., & Stein, W. H. 1956. N-Acetyl-L-aspartic acid in brain. *The Journal of Biological Chemistry*, 219(1): 257–264.

Tanaka, Y., Hazama, H., Fukuhara, T., & Tsutsui, T. 1982. Computerized tomography of the brain in manic-depressive patients—a controlled study. *Folia Psychiatrica et Neurologica Japonica*, 36(2): 137–143.

Wahl, R. L., Buchanan, J. W. (eds.) 2002. *Principles and Practice of Positron Emission Tomography*. Philadelphia: Lippincott Williams & Wilkins.

Yatham, L., Liddle, P., Lam, R., Shiah, I., Lane, C., Stoessl, A., Sossi, V., & Ruth, 2002. T. PET study of the effects of valproate on dopamine D$_2$ receptors in neuroleptic- and mood-stabilizer-naïve patients with nonpsychotic mania. *American Journal of Psychiatry*. 159(10): 1718–1723.

Yildiz-Yesiloglu, A., & Ankerst, D. P. 2006. Neurochemical alterations of the brain in bipolar disorder and their implications for pathophysiology: a systematic review of the in vivo proton magnetic resonance spectroscopy findings. *Progress in Neuropsychopharmacology & Biological Psychiatry*, 30(6): 969–995.

Zipursky, R. B., Meyer, J. H., & Verhoeff, N. P. 2007. PET and SPECT imaging in psychiatric disorders. *Canadian Journal of Psychiatry*, 52(3): 146–157.

# 2.

# STRUCTURAL BRAIN ABNORMALITIES IN BIPOLAR DISORDER

## Koji Matsuo, Marsal Sanches, Paolo Brambilla, and Jair C. Soares

## INTRODUCTION

Considerable evidence points to disruptions in neural circuits that underpin emotional and cognitive processes as a potential cause of the symptoms of bipolar disorder (Price & Drevets, 2010; Savitz & Drevets, 2009; Drevets, 2001; Adler et al., 2006; Strakowski et al., 2005; Soares & Mann, 1997; Phillips et al., 2008; Keener & Phillips, 2007). Additionally, since bipolar disorder is highly heritable (Goodwin & Jamison, 2007), a pressing question is whether some of the brain abnormalities associated with bipolar disorder, and observed with neuroimaging, may serve as endophenotypes—that is, intermediate phenotypes that fill the gap in the causal chain between gene dysfunction and disease manifestation (Gottesman & Shields, 1973). Over the last few decades, structural neuroimaging assessments have been widely used to investigate the hypothesis that these disruptions in emotional and cognitive circuitry underlie bipolar disorder.

The earliest neuroimaging studies of bipolar disorder emerged in the 1980s, and used computerized tomography (CT). These studies focused on whole brain and ventricular volumes (Nasrallah et al., 1981; Yates et al., 1987; Rothschild et al., 1989). In the 1990s, however, magnetic resonance imaging (MRI) became the main method used to investigate structural brain findings in living human subjects, given its better resolution and accuracy, particularly in the distinction between gray and white matter, as well as in the assessment of infratentorial structures.

In addition, progress was made in measurement techniques. In the past decade, manual tracing methods for gray-matter quantification were frequently used for regional volumetric brain measurements. Those approaches are being gradually replaced by semi-automated methods that are less labor intensive and that, in conjunction with computerized statistical programs such as statistical parametric mapping (SPM), have allowed investigators to analyze larger samples in order to provide statistically robust evidence of structural abnormalities.

More recently, higher-resolution MRI technology has allowed identification of more subtle abnormalities in smaller regions of the brain. A newer technique, diffusion tensor imaging (DTI), is now available to measure the integrity of white matter tracts and water diffusion in brain tissue to elucidate white-matter abnormalities.

This chapter contains a critical review of the controlled structural MRI studies from adult patients with bipolar disorder, with emphasis on associations between structural findings and clinical variables, as well as integration with genetic studies. Further, we discuss a putative model of the neuroanatomic basis for bipolar disorder in light of available evidence.

## MORPHOMETRIC ABNORMALITIES IN BIPOLAR DISORDER

Given the large number of structural MRI studies in patients with bipolar disorder and the heterogeneity of their results, meta-analyses are a useful and highly desirable way to summarize the main findings of the studies (Table 2.1). For example, an early meta-analysis (Hoge et al., 1999) analyzed whole brain volumes of patients with bipolar disorder compared to healthy subjects using six MRI and one CT study and found no significant differences between the groups. Another meta-analysis focused on a brain region thought to be specifically relevant to mood and cognitive regulation, namely the amygdala (Hajek et al., 2008; 2009). This analysis included nine amygdala structural MRI studies consisting of 215 patients with bipolar disorder and 275 healthy subjects. Enlarged amygdala has been considered a replicable finding among adults with bipolar disorder. However, no significant differences between bipolar and healthy subjects was found for left or right amygdala volumes in the

## TABLE 2.1 META-ANALYSES OF VOLUMETRY AND HYPERINTENSITIES STUDIES IN BIPOLAR DISORDER

| No | Study | Publication year | Sample studies | Years of database | Subjects | Mean age |
|----|-------|------------------|----------------|-------------------|----------|----------|
| | **BRAIN VOLUME** | | | | | |
| 1 | Hallahan et al. | 2010 | Regional structure studies in 11 research groups | 1980–2009 | 321 BDI vs. 442 HC | BDI 34.07 ±12.18 HC 34.21±13.01 |
| 2 | Ellison-Wright et al. | 2010 | 14 VBM studies of BD  42 VBM studies of SCZ | 1995–2009 | 366 BD vs. 497 HC  2058 SCZ vs. 2131 HC | BD 32.5 vs. HC 32.2  SCZ 33.4 vs. HC 32.6 |
| 3 | Bora et al. | 2010 | 21 VBM studies | 1995–2009 | 660 BD vs. 770 HC | BD 35.2 HC 33.9 |
| 4 | Hajek et al. | 2009 | 9 structural MRI studies | 1992–2008 | 215 BD vs. 275 HC | |
| 5 | Vita et al. | 2009 | 22 structural and VBM studies | 1993–2008 | 221 first-episode BD vs. 321 HC | |
| 6 | Arnone et al. | 2009 | 65 structural MRI studies | 1990–2008 | 661 BD vs. 723 HC | 29.4±11.8 |

| Female % | Patients characteristics | Medicated | MRI | ROIs | Findings of BD |
|---|---|---|---|---|---|
| BDI 52.6 HC 51.1 | Mean onset of illness, 21y Mean duration of illness, 12y Median number of hospitalization, 3 (range 0–20) | Li 50.4% VPA 30.6% CBZ 8.9% MS 77.5% AP 44.3% AD 24.3% | 1T or greater | Total brain Temporal Amygdala Hippocampus Anterior cingulate Caudate Putamen Thalamus Lateral ventricles Third ventricle | BD > HC Total temporal lobe Left temporal lobe Right putamen Right lateral ventricles |
| BD 53% vs. HC 53%  SCZ 31% vs. HC 40% | Duration of illness BD 12.3y vs. SCZ 8.0y | BD No medication 25% Li 29% AE 28% AP 37% SCZ No medication 14% AP 85% | 1.5T 64.3% >1.5T 35.7% | N/A | BD < HC Bilateral insula Perigenual anterior cingulate Subgenual anterior cingulate |
| BD 55.9% HC 54.2% | | Medicated 376/344 Li 124/282 AP 188/425 AE 70/215 AD 86/320 | 1.5T 76.2% >1.5T 23.8% | N/A | BD < HC Right anterior insula (including inferofrontal cortex) Left rostral anterior [perigenual] cingulate Left inferior frontal cortex/ anterior insula  BDI < HC Right anterior insula (including inferofrontal cortex) Left rostral anterior [perigenual] cingulate Left inferior frontal cortex/ anterior insula |
| | | | 1.5T 87.5% >1.5 12.5% | Amygdala | N.S. |
| | | Medication naïve | 1.5T 100% | Intracranial Whole brain GM WM | BD < HC Intracranial and total WM |
| BD 49% | | | | Whole brain Frontal cortex Subgenual PFC Temporal Amygdala Hippocampus Amygdala-hippocampus complex Superior temporal gyri Anterior cingulate Posterior cingulate Pituitary grand Caudate Putamen Thalamus Cerebellar vermis region 1–3 Lateral ventricles Third ventricle Intracranial Globus pallidus | BD < HC Whole brain  BD > HC Bilateral lateral ventricles Globus pallidus |

(Continued)

| No | Study | Publication year | Sample studies | Years of database | Subjects | Mean age |
|---|---|---|---|---|---|---|
| 7 | Hajek et al. | 2008 | 8 structural MRI studies | 1997–2007 | 99 BD vs. 160 HC | |
| 8 | Kempton et al. | 2008 | 8 CT and 90 MRI studies in the database (Database of 125 MRI and 16 CT studies) | 1981–2007 | In database 3509 BD vs. 4687 HC (1961 BDI and 215 BDII) | BD 32.6±8.0 HC 31.7±7.6 |
| 9 | Bora et al. | 2008 | 5 structural MRI studies | 1989–2007 | 91 BD vs. 114 HC | BD 30.2 HC 29.5 |
| 10 | McDonald et al. | 2004 | 26 structural MRI studies | 1990–2003 | 440 BD vs. 696 HC | |
| 11 | Hoge et al. | 1999 | 6 structural MRI and 1 CT studies | 1989–1997 | 160 BD vs. 212 HC | |

| Female % | Patients characteristics | Medicated | MRI | ROIs | Findings of BD |
|---|---|---|---|---|---|
| | | | 1.5T 92%<br>>1.5T 7% | Subgenual anterior cingulate | N.S. |
| BD 46.0<br>HC 42.0 | | No medication 25.0%<br>MS 68.9%<br>Li 53.1%<br>VPA 21.7%<br>CBZ 5.8%<br>AP 22.7%<br>AD 14.5%<br>BZP 3.1%<br>ECT 11.6% | 1.5T 78%<br><1.5T 18%<br>>1.5T 3% | Brain<br>Cerebrum<br>Temporal<br>Amygdala<br>Hippocampus<br>Amygdala-hippocampus complex<br>Anterior cingulate<br>Posterior cingulate<br>Caudate<br>Putamen<br>Thalamus<br>Subgenual PFC<br>Cerebellar vermis region 1–3<br>Lateral ventricles<br>Third ventricle<br>Intracranial<br>GM<br>WM<br>Globus pallidus<br>Corpus callosum (length and cross sectional area) | BD < HC<br>Corpus callosum (cross sectional area)<br>BD > HC<br>Total lateral ventricles<br>Right lateral ventricle<br>Third ventricle<br><br>BD < SCZ<br>Left lateral ventricle<br>Third ventricle<br>BD > SCZ<br>Right and left hippocampus |
| BD 49.0%<br>HC 44.7% | | | <1.5T 20.0%<br>1.5T 80.0% | Corpus callosum | BD > HC |
| | | | <1.5T 15.4%<br>1.5T 80.8%<br><1.5T 3.8% | Whole brain<br>GM<br>WM<br>Prefrontal cortex<br>Subgenual PFC<br>Temporal<br>Amygdala<br>Hippocampus<br>Amygdala-hippocampus complex<br>Superior temporal gyri<br>Caudate<br>Putamen<br>Thalamus<br>Globus pallidus<br>Lateral ventricles<br>Third ventricle | BD > HC<br>Right lateral ventricular |
| | | | | Total brain volume and area | N.S. |

(Continued)

| No | Study | Publication year | Sample studies | Years of database | Subjects | Mean age |
|---|---|---|---|---|---|---|
| WHITE MATTER HYPERINTENSITIES | | | | | | |
| 1 | Beyer et al. | 2010 | 21 structural MRI studies | 1990–2005 | 573 BD vs. 850 HC | BD 35.0 HC 33.2 |
| 2 | Kempton et al. | 2008 | 141 structural MRI and CT studies (125 MRI and 16 CT) 23 structural studies for BD vs. SCZ | 1981–2007 | 3509 BD vs. 4687 HC (1961 BDI and 215 BDII) | BD 32.6±8.0 HC 31.7±7.6 |
| 3 | Altshuler et al. | 1995 | 8 structural MRI studies | 1990–1995 | 198 BDI vs. 307 HC | BD 40.8 HC 39.6 |

Abbreviations: BD = bipolar disorder; BDI = bipolar disorder type I; BDII = bipolar disorder type II; SCZ = schizophrenia; HC = healthy comparision subjects; CT = computed tomography; MRI = magnetic resonance imaging; VBM = voxel-based morphometry; GM = gray matter; WM = white matter; Li = lithium; VPA = valproate; CBZ = carbamazepine; MS = mood stabilizers; AP = antipsychotics; AD = antidepressants; AE = antiepileptics; BZP = benzodiazepines; ECT = electroconvulsive therapy.

whole sample, although children and adolescents with bipolar disorder showed smaller left amygdala volumes compared with healthy subjects. Additionally, adults with bipolar disorder showed a trend toward smaller amygdala volumes compared with healthy adults. There were no significant differences in amygdala volumes between medicated and unmedicated patients with bipolar disorder (Hajek et al., 2009).

Furthermore, even though the classical studies by Drevets and colleagues demonstrated the potential role of the anterior subgenual cingulate in the pathophysiology of mood disorders (Drevets et al., 1997; Drevets et al, 2008), a meta-analysis of eight structural studies measuring subgenual cingulate volume in patients with mood disorders showed no significant differences between bipolar and healthy subjects. Nevertheless, the subgenual cingulate volumes were significantly smaller among patients with unipolar depression than in healthy subjects (Hajek et al., 2008).

The studies included in this meta-analysis used the "region of interest" approach, in which volumes of specific areas of the brain are obtained through a manual or semi-automatic tracing method. An alternative technique is voxel-based morphometry (VBM) that allows fully automatic comparisons of subject groups in regard to generalized and regional brain volumes. Two meta-analyses of VBM studies have been performed (Ellison-Wright & Bullmore, 2010; Bora et al., 2010). In the first (Ellison-Wright & Bullmore, 2010), lower gray matter volumes in the right and left insula, perigenual anterior cingulate and subgenual anterior cingulate were found in bipolar patients, with no evidence of higher gray-matter volumes in any region compared with healthy subjects. In the second meta-analysis, bipolar patients were found to have decreased gray-matter volumes of right insula-inferior frontal cortex, left rostral anterior (pregenual) cingulate cortex, and left anterior insular-inferior frontal cortex; gray-matter volume again was not greater than healthy subjects in any region. An example of a VBM study is provided in Figure 2.1.

On the other hand, Kempton and colleagues (Kempton et al., 2008) created a database for neuroimaging studies of bipolar disorder (BiND, available at http://www.bipolar-database.org). They performed a mega-analysis (i.e., directly merging raw datasets) comparing the volumes of 47 regions of interest using 3,509 patients with bipolar disorder and 4,687 healthy subjects, and found that bipolar patients had significantly larger lateral ventricles and smaller corpus callosum. Surprisingly, no significant differences were found in subgenual and perigenual anterior cingulate cortex,

| Female % | Patients characteristics | Medicated | MRI | ROIs | Findings of BD |
|---|---|---|---|---|---|
| | | | <1.5T 95.2%<br>>1.5 4.8% | | BD > HC<br>Deep white matter<br>Subcortical<br>Periventricular |
| BD 46.0<br>HC 42.0 | | No medication 25.0%<br>MS 68.9%<br>Li 53.1%<br>VPA 21.7%<br>CBZ 5.8%<br>AP 22.7%<br>AD 14.5%<br>BZP 3.1%<br>ECT 11.6% | 1.5T 78%<br><1.5T 18%<br>>1.5T 3% | Any<br>Deep white matter<br>Periventricular<br>Subcortical gray matter<br>Left hemisphere<br>Right hemisphere<br>Frontal lobe<br>Parietal lobe | BD > HC<br>Any<br>Deep white matter<br>Subcortical gray matter<br>Left hemisphere<br>Right hemisphere<br>Frontal lobe<br>Parietal lobe |
| | | | | T2 hyperintensities | BD > HC |

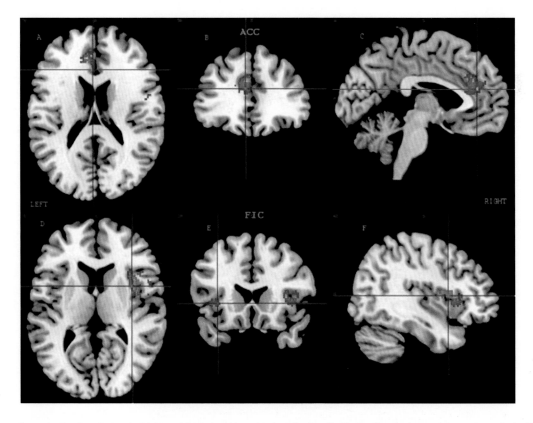

*Figure 2.1* Gray matter reduction in anterior cingulate and fronto-insular cortex in patients with bipolar disorder by voxelwise meta-analysis. (Reprinted from *Biological Psychiatry* 67(11), Bora E, Fornito A, Yucel M, Pantelis C, 'Voxelwise Meta-Analysis of Gray Matter Abnormalities in Bipolar Disorder,' pages 1097-1105, copyright 2010, with permission from Elsevier.)

amygdala, and hippocampus. It was hypothesized that these negative findings were in part due to the heterogeneity of the subjects included in the analysis, some of which were receiving lithium, a medication with reported effects on brain structural volumes. In order to overcome some of these methodological issues, Hallahan and colleagues (2011) conducted another mega-analysis including data from 11 research groups. They found larger total and left temporal lobe, right putamen and right lateral ventricles in bipolar patients compared to healthy subjects.

Finally, very recent structural MRI studies of bipolar disorder, which were not included in recent meta-analyses, support prior findings of enlarged third ventricle (Cousins et al., 2010), and decreased volumes of temporal lobes (Javadapour et al., 2010; Takahashi et al., 2010; Savitz et al., 2010), prefrontal lobe (Penttila et al., 2009), orbitofrontal lobe (Nery et al., 2009), anterior cingulate (Fornito et al., 2009), pituitary (Cousins et al., 2010; Takahashi et al., 2010). and cerebellar vermis (Womer et al., 2009).

Overall, current evidence points to larger lateral ventricles, smaller corpus callosum, decreased subgenual anterior cingulate cortex. and larger amygdala volumes among adult patients with bipolar disorder when compared to healthy control subjects. In young bipolar patients, however, smaller amygdala volumes seem to be present, which may indicate that disruptions in the maturation of the central nervous are involved in the pathophysiology of pediatric bipolar disorder (Sanches et al., 2008).

## CLINICAL VARIABLES AND STRUCTURAL ABNORMALITIES

### COURSE OF ILLNESS

Neuroimaging findings among first-episode patients are of high interest given their potential to identify endophenotypes, since these findings are less likely to have been caused by medication effects and neurodegenerative factors. Vita and colleagues (2009) performed a meta-analysis of VBM studies from first-episode bipolar subjects. The meta-analysis included 22 studies comprising 221 first-episode bipolar disorder and 321 healthy subjects. Patients with bipolar disorder had significantly smaller intracranial and total white-matter volumes, but no significant differences in gray-matter volumes. In contrast, another analysis revealed that first-episode bipolar disorder patients had smaller gray-matter content in the anterior cingulate

> **Structural (Morphometric) Studies in Bipolar Disorder vs. Healthy Subjects**
>
> - Include enlarged lateral ventricles and putamen in bipolar disorder
>
> - Include decreased volumes in prefrontal cortex (particularly ventral PFC), insula, cerebellar vermis, and corpus callosum in bipolar disorder
>
> - Suggest inconsistent differences in amygdala, with possible enlargement in bipolar adults, but decreased volumes in bipolar youth

cortex (Bora et al., 2010), total brain, and left and right amygdala. They also seem to have smaller mean cerebral volumes compared with healthy subjects (Hallahan et al., 2011). Other findings among first-episode patients with bipolar disorder include reduced amygdala volume (Rosso et al., 2007) and increased thickness in the right subcallosal limbic anterior cingulate cortex (Fornito et al., 2009).

With respect to duration of illness, some cross sectional studies found it to be directly related to the gray-matter volume of left putamen, globus pallidus, bilateral caudate, left amygdala, and thalamus (Bora et al., 2010; Arnone et al., 2009). However, duration of illness is also inversely associated with gray-matter volume of left fronto-insular cortex (Bora et al., 2010), temporal lobe (Arnone et al., 2009), hippocampus, fusiform gyrus, cerebellum (Moorhead et al., 2007), and mean cerebral volume (Hallahan et al., 2011). Furthermore, longitudinal neuroimaging studies exhibited progressive reduction of anterior cingulate volume in bipolar patients (Farrow et al., 2005; Koo et al., 2008; Kalmar et al., 2009). Together, these findings suggest that neuroanatomic abnormalities change during the course of bipolar illness.

These findings seem to be consonant with studies that addressed the number of episodes among bipolar patients. Those with fewer episodes seem to have larger left hippocampal volumes than healthy subjects (Javadapour et al., 2010). In addition, a higher lifetime number of manic episodes in patients with bipolar disorder was found to be associated with smaller gray-matter volumes of inferior frontal gyrus. Curiously, this association was not found in regard to the number of depressive episodes or illness duration (Ekman et al., 2010). In contrast, Hallahan et al., (2011) did not find an association between number of hospitalizations and regional brain volume.

Finally, early onset of bipolar disorder was associated with smaller mean cerebral volumes and left thalamus, but larger total and left-side amygdala (Hallahan et al., 2011). Older age at illness onset, on the other hand, was linked to larger differences in hippocampal volumes between bipolar and healthy subjects (Arnone et al., 2009). Moreover, age of onset was positively associated with gray-matter volume in the left putamen (Bora et al., 2010), and intermediate-onset (25–45 yrs) bipolar patients had reduced local sulcal index in the right dorsolateral prefrontal cortex (as well as lower global sulcal indices) compared to early-onset (<25 yrs) bipolar patients and healthy subjects (Penttila et al., 2009).

Overall, whereas first-episode studies suggest that some brain abnormalities seem to be present early in the course of the disease (supporting the involvement of neurodevelopmental factors in the pathogenesis of bipolar disorder), the available literature points to inverse relationships between length of illness and the volume of several brain structures among bipolar disorder patients, suggesting that degenerative processes might also be involved in the course of this illness.

## MEDICATION EFFECTS

Several medications commonly used in the treatment of bipolar disorder have been shown to affect the volumes of brain structures. For example, neurobiological studies in animals suggest that lithium affects multiple cellular signaling pathways in the brain (Phiel & Klein, 2001) and has neurotrophic and neuroprotective effects (Manji et al., 2000; Chuang & Manji, 2007). Longitudinal human studies also demonstrated a relationship between lithium administration and increased gray-matter volume in whole brain (Moore et al., 2000; Sassi et al., 2002; Monkul et al., 2007) and total gray matter volume (Kempton et al., 2008). Furthermore, lithium-treated bipolar patients were found to have larger gray-matter volumes in the right subgenual anterior cingulate gyrus, postcentral gyrus, hippocampus/amygdala complex, and left insula when compared to bipolar patients treated with anticonvulsants and antipsychotics (Germana et al., 2010; Bearden et al., 2007; Foland et al., 2008; Yucel et al., 2008). In another study, the daily dose of lithium treatment was positively correlated with the volume of right planum polare and rostral superior temporal gyrus in patients with bipolar I disorder (Takahashi et al., 2010).

Using a different study design, Lyoo et al. (2010) recruited drug-naïve bipolar disorder patients and healthy subjects in order to assess putative differences in regard to changes in the brain volume after lithium or valproate treatment (Lyoo et al., 2010). Patients treated with lithium displayed significant increases in their gray matter volumes, which peaked at weeks 10 to 12 and persisted through 16 weeks of treatment. Furthermore, this increase in volume was associated with clinical improvement. On the other hand, valproate-treated patients and healthy subjects did not show gray matter volume changes over time. In another longitudinal study of depressed bipolar subjects (Moore et al., 2009), total brain gray matter, prefrontal gray matter, and left subgenual prefrontal gray matter volumes were compared at baseline (prior to medication exposure) and after four weeks of lithium administration. Significant increases in total brain gray matter volumes were observed after 4 weeks of lithium administration compared to the baseline. Of note, lithium-responders showed a significant increase in the prefrontal cortex gray-matter volume compared with non-responders.

In addition, two meta-analyses examined neuroimaging findings related to lithium treatment of bipolar disorder. According to the first (Hallahan et al., 2011), lithium-treated bipolar patients exhibited larger hippocampal and amygdala volumes, as well as larger total brain volumes, than non-lithium-treated bipolar patients and healthy subjects. The second meta-analysis (Bora et al., 2010) revealed that lithium use among patients with bipolar disorder was associated with larger gray matter volumes in rostral anterior cingulate cortex, while no differences were associated with treatment with antipsychotics, antidepressants, and anticonvulsants.

Finally, medication-naïve patients with bipolar disorder had smaller left anterior and posterior cingulate volumes compared to patients medicated with valproate and quetiapine and healthy subjects (Atmaca et al., 2007). Another group described larger temporal lobe white matter volumes among bipolar patients treated with antipsychotics (Jones et al., 2009), whereas the use of antipsychotics and antidepressants seems to be associated with decreases in the right amygdala and temporal lobe volume, according to a meta-analysis (Arnone et al., 2009). The same authors concluded that the widely described differences between patients with bipolar disorder and healthy subjects in regard to amygdala volumes tend to be magnified with the use of mood stabilizers, which were also associated with larger right globus pallidus and temporal lobe.

Together, these findings suggest that medications may influence the volume of brain structures among bipolar patients. The evidence is particularly robust in regard to the use of lithium, and there seems to be a correlation between these putative brain changes and the therapeutic effects of that medication.

Structural neuroimaging findings have been associated with other clinical variables such as mood state and subtype of bipolar disorder. Total gray matter volumes of the orbitofrontal cortex were significantly smaller in depressed than euthymic patients with bipolar disorder, and were inversely correlated with the intensity of the depressive symptoms (Nery et al., 2009). In another study, bipolar I (but not bipolar II) patients had widespread gray-matter reductions in the frontal, temporal, parietal and parahippocampal regions when compared to healthy subjects (Ha et al., 2009). In contrast, no significant differences in brain volumes occur between bipolar patients with and without psychosis (Hallahan et al., 2011).

---

**Structural (Morphometric) Abnormalities in Bipolar Disorder**

- Are present, but relatively modest at the time of the first episode

- Appear to progress with illness duration and affective episode recurrence

- Differ between early- and late-onset bipolar disorder

- Change with the course of illness, supporting a model of neuroanatomic progression as part of the neuropathogenesis of bipolar disorder

- Appear to be linked with treatment and treatment response, particularly for lithium; lithium is associated with increases in gray matter volumes

---

## WHITE MATTER HYPERINTENSITIES IN BIPOLAR DISORDER

White-matter hyperintensities are commonly found among people over 60 years of age (Wen & Sachdev, 2004; Sachdev et al., 2005). Although considered a nonspecific finding, they seem to be particularly prominent among bipolar patients. Several studies comparing bipolar and healthy subjects described more hyperintensities among the bipolar group in frontal/parietal areas, the subependymal region, subcortical nuclei, and deep white matter (Gulseren et al., 2006; Aylward et al., 1994; Dupont et al., 1995; Pillai et al., 2002; Lyoo et al., 2002; Figiel et al., 1991; McDonald et al., 1999). In addition, two meta-analyses (Kempton et al., 2008; Beyer et al., 2009) addressed differences between bipolar and healthy subjects in regard

to white matter hyperintensities. Bipolar patients have significantly more hyperintensities than healthy subjects in deep white matter and subcortical and periventricular regions, as well as in the frontal and temporal lobes.

## HYPERINTENSITIES, CLINICAL FEATURES, AND MEDICATION EFFECTS

Bipolar patients over 60 years of age were found to have significantly higher rates of hyperintensities in frontal deep white matter and subcortical gray regions compared with age-matched healthy subjects (de Asis et al., 2006). In addition, higher rates of right frontal hyperintensities were associated with later age of onset of manic episodes. These findings agree with previous reports suggesting that patients with late-onset (age 50 years or older) bipolar disorder seem to have a higher number of large subcortical hyperintensities, particularly in the middle third of the brain parenchyma, when compared with healthy subjects (McDonald et al., 1991). In contrast, in one meta-analysis (Beyer et al., 2009), the odds ratio for hyperintensities (any region) among bipolar patients was higher for children and adolescents (5.7) than for adults (2.2), whereas in the other (Kempton et al., 2008) no signifcant associations were found between the rates of white matter hyperintensities and age or age at onset of bipolar disorder.

With respect to course of illness, there seems to be a direct relationship between the rate of white matter hyperintensities and the number of manic (but not depressive) episodes (Gulseren et al., 2006). Similarly, a higher incidence of periventricular white matter hyperintensities was directly related to the number of previous hospitalizations (Altshuler et al., 1995). Furthermore, bipolar patients with poor outcomes had more deep subcortical hyperintensities, but not periventricular or white-matter hyperintensities compared with bipolar patients with favorable outcomes and healthy subjects (Moore et al., 2001).

Studies have also explored possible relationships between psychotropic medications and hyperintensities. There was no significant association between lithium use and frequency of deep white matter hyperintensities in patients with bipolar disorder (Kempton et al., 2008). Similarly, antidepressant use in patients with bipolar disorder was not associated with the presence of hyperintensities (Persaud et al., 1997). These findings are in contrast with another study in which cardiovascular disease, old age, history of re-hospitalizations, and lithium use were considered strong predictors of the presence of hyperintensities in patients with psychiatric diseases, although not specifically in bipolar disorder (Breeze et al., 2003),

Overall, white-matter hyperintensities seem to occur at higher rates among bipolar patients than healthy subjects. Even though their pathophysiological meaning has not yet been elucidated, it has been hypothesized that these nonspecific findings reflect disruptions in white matter connections among key brain regions and circuits involved in emotional processing, therefore contributing to mood dysregulation in bipolar disorder (Soares & Mann, 1997).

## MICROSCOPIC STRUCTURE OF WHITE MATTER IN BIPOLAR DISORDER

Diffusion tensor imaging (DTI) is a technique used to measure the rate and directionality of water diffusion, which can be used to evaluate the microscopic structure of white matter and specific interconnectivity of white-matter tracts. Diffusion is measured using parameters such as fractional anisotropy (FA), mean diffusivity, and the apparent diffusion coefficient, as reviewed in chapter 1 (see section titled *Diffusion Tensor Imaging*). Although the specific causes and pathophysiology underlying high and low values are not fully understood, they are likely to reflect changes in the density, diameter, alignment, and myelination of white matter tracts (Bruno et al., 2008). High FA values are observed in richly myelinated tracts, whereas low FA values indicate axonal loss or destruction of myelin sheaths, found in several degenerative white-matter disorders such as multiple sclerosis, dementias, and infections (Benedetti et al., 2011).

A small number of DTI studies have been performed among patients with bipolar disorder (Table 2.2). Among other positive findings, bipolar patients seem to have significantly lower FA values in brain areas above the anterior commissure (Adler et al., 2004), in the anterior cingulum, (Wang et al., 2008; Wang et al., 2008), and in the middle corpus callosum (Wang et al., 2008) when compared to healthy subjects, as well as higher apparent diffusion coefficient in the left and right orbital frontal white matter (Beyer et al., 2005). On the other hand, a recent meta-analysis reviewed 10 whole-brain DTI studies comparing bipolar and healthy subjects (Vederine et al., 2011). According to that review, decreased FA seems to be consistently found in two main brain regions, both in the right white matter. The first is located close to the parahippocampal gyrus, whereas the second is located close to the right anterior cingulate cortex and subgenual prefrontal cortex. Further, DTI tractography allows the virtual reconstruction of whole white-matter bundles and their microstructural properties (Houenou et al., 2007) (see Figure 2.2). In this sense, a recent study described significant differences between bipolar and healthy subjects in the white matter tracts connecting the frontal cortex with the temporal and parietal cortices, as well as in subcortical circuits (Lin et al., 2011).

In summary, although findings from DTI studies of bipolar disorder are diverse, they suggest that the white matter structure is disrupted in bipolar patients, particularly in prefrontal regions and tracts connecting sub-regions of frontal lobe with subcortical and temporal structures (Brambilla et al., 2009). These findings suggest that impaired connectivity among key brain regions involved in the regulation of mood (frontolimbic circuitry) may be involved in the pathogenesis of bipolar disorder.

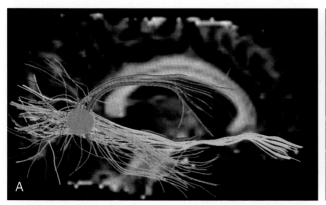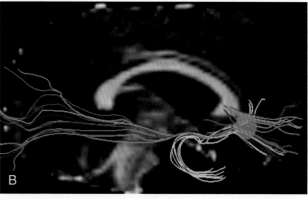

*Figure 2.2* WHITE MATTER TRACTS CROSSING THE CLUSTER (IN GREEN) OF DECREASED FA IN PATIENTS WITH BIPOLAR DISORDER BY META-ANALYSIS. (A) The cluster was colored in green: inferior longitudinal fasciculus (ILF) in orange, superior longitudinal fasciculus (SLF) in purple, inferior fronto-occipital fasciculus (IFOF) in yellow, posterior thalamic radiations in blue. (B) The cluster was colored in green: inferior fronto-occipital fasciculus (IFOF) in blue, uncinate in yellow and forceps minor in purple (white matter tracts extracted with DTI query from the data for a single normal individual, projected on a right parasagittal view of a FA map). (Reprinted from *Progress in Neuro-Psychopharmacology and Biological Psychiatry*, Vol 35, François-Eric Vederine, Michèle Wessa, Marion Leboyer, Josselin Houenou, 'A meta-analysis of whole-brain diffusion tensor imaging studies in bipolar disorder,' 1820-1826, 2011, with permission from Elsevier.)

## CLINICAL VARIABLES, MEDICATION STATUS, AND DTI FINDINGS

One study found significant negative correlations between age and FA values in different regions among bipolar patients, but not in healthy subjects (Versace et al., 2008). Longer duration of illness and earlier age at onset were associated with lower FA and higher mean diffusivity in diverse brain locations (Versace et al., 2008; Zanetti et al., 2009). Similarly, lower FA values have been described in depressed bipolar patients when compared to remitted ones (Zanetti et al., 2009). These results suggest that white matter disruption may integrate putative degenerative processes involved in the pathophysiology of bipolar disorder, and that these disruptions can, to a certain extension, be maximized during acute mood episodes, in contrast to the periods of remission.

With respect to medication status and DTI findings, scant evidence is currently available. There seems to be some association between use of psychotropics (mood stabilizers, antidepressants, and benzodiazepines) and differences in the FA and high mean diffusivity values in different regions (Versace et al., 2008; Benedetti et al., 2011). These findings may represent direct effects of medications on the integrity of the white matter tracts or, alternatively, may be the downstream result of the main pharmacological effects of these agents. Additional studies are necessary to clarify these relationships.

Overall, although the findings above are suggestive, the literature in regard to relationships between medication effects, clinical features, and DTI findings are far from conclusive at this point. The large variability of results in the topography of the findings makes the available evidence difficult to interpret. Further exploration of these possible associations represents a promising area for research.

**Brain White Matter Abnormalities in Bipolar Disorder**

- Include MRI T2-weighted hyperintensities that are the most consistent neuroimaging finding in bipolar disorder; however, these abnormalities are nonspecific

- Include abnormalities in white matter structure within ventral prefrontal networks that modulate mood, as measured with diffusion tensor imaging (DTI) methods

- May worsen during the course of illness, as measured by decreases in fractional anisotropy, i.e., integrity of white matter tracts

## GENETIC IMAGING STUDIES IN BIPOLAR DISORDER

Studies conducted among relatives of patients with bipolar disorder have documented a 6%–15% genetic risk for bipolar disorder (Goodwin & Jamison, 2007). Reports from controlled family studies show an average ten-fold increased risk of bipolar disorder among adult relatives of probands with bipolar disorder, compared to relatives of healthy probands. Therefore, structural imaging of family members of bipolar patients might elucidate genetic influences on potential structural brain markers in bipolar disorder. Here we review several structural studies of twins and relatives of patients with bipolar disorder. As a second step, we summarize the findings of the few genetic-imaging studies that analyzed associations between gene variants and structural abnormalities in bipolar disorder.

### TWIN STUDIES

Neuroimaging studies of twins represent a method to investigate heritability of structural brain abnormalities. Those studies, nonetheless, are difficult to conduct, given the numerous obstacles for recruiting an adequate number of twins with and without bipolar disorder, as well as matched healthy twins. To date, a few bipolar disorder studies using twin-pairs have been reported (Kieseppa et al., 2003; Noga et al., 2001; van der Schot et al., 2010; van der Schot et al., 2009) (Table 2.3). The results of these studies suggest that some of the structural findings among bipolar subjects seem to be directly related to the genetic load for bipolar disorder and are found not only among bipolar patients, but also in their healthy co-twins. As examples, decreases in left hemispheric white matter volumes were observed by Kieseppa et al. (2003), enlarged caudate by Noga et al. (2001), and decreased white matter volume and decreased grey matter density in the right medial frontal gyrus, precentral gyrus and insula by van der Schot et al. (2010). On the other hand, some findings seem to be present only in bipolar subjects and not in their affected co-twins. These findings include decreased hippocampal volumes and asymmetry (Kieseppa et al., 2003), as well as decreased total cortical volume (van der Schot et al., 2009).

### STUDIES WITH FIRST-DEGREE RELATIVES OF BIPOLAR PATIENTS

Unaffected relatives of bipolar probands seem to share neurocognitive deficits with bipolar patients, including impairments in response inhibition, executive function, verbal memory, and sustained attention (Bora et al., 2008; Bora et al., 2009). In this section we discuss some of the structural neuroimaging studies of first-degree relatives of patients with bipolar disorder (Table 2.3; Figure 2.3).

Compared with healthy subjects, first-degree relatives of bipolar patients were found to have reduced gray-matter volume of left insula (Matsuo et al., 2011), left anterior thalamus, and body of caudate (McIntosh et al., 2004). However, other studies point to larger left insula among these subjects, in addition to larger caudate, amygdala, and hippocampal volumes (Boccardi et al., 2010; Kempton et al., 2009; Hajek et al., 2009). Other findings include decreased gray-matter volume of pituitary (Takahashi et al., 2010) and left substantia nigra (Kempton et al., 2009), as well as increased mean callosal area (Walterfang et al., 2009).

Moreover, in an early and noteworthy study, McDonald et al. (2004) examined associations between brain volumetric findings and a genetic liability scale using patients with bipolar I disorder, their first-degree relatives without psychosis, patients with schizophrenia and their first-degree relatives without psychosis. The authors found that the genetic risk of bipolar disorder was associated with gray and white-matter deficits in several brain areas, including prefrontal cortex. In a DTI study (Chaddock et al., 2009), unaffected relatives of bipolar patients and healthy subjects were found to have FA values in a whole brain analysis. Finally, in regard to white matter hyperintensities, while one study described a higher frequency of hyperintensities among patients with bipolar disorder and unaffected family members (Ahearn et al., 1998), another study found no differences between bipolar disorder patients, unaffected relatives, and healthy subjects (Gunde et al., 2011).

In summary, there is evidence of some structural brain abnormalities among twins and unaffected relatives of bipolar patients, although the results are inconsistent in regard to the brain regions most likely to be involved. Nevertheless, these studies suggest that some volumetric findings in bipolar disorder may represent endophenotypes separate from the clinical course itself and therefore, may be present in individuals at high genetic risk for bipolar disorder prior to the onset of the mood symptoms. A better characterization of these findings is highly desirable, not only to better understand the pathophysiology of bipolar illness, but also because of the potential clinical applications of these measures for identifying individuals vulnerable to develop bipolar disorder. Such measures might, in the future, lead to the implementation of preventive measures in identified at-risk individuals.

## GENOTYPE AND NEUROIMAGING STUDIES IN BIPOLAR DISORDER

Recently, possible relationships between volumetric brain findings and gene polymorphisms in bipolar disorder have been examined. These studies usually focus on candidate genes for bipolar disorder, such as the genes encoding

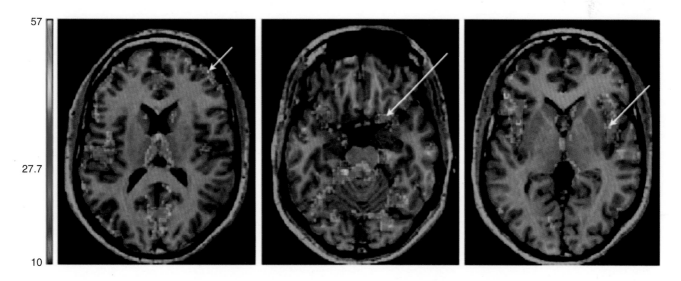

*Figure 2.3* NEGATIVE PHENOTYPIC ASSOCIATIONS BETWEEN LIABILITY TO BIPOLAR DISORDER AND GREY MATTER DENSITY (RPH). Phenotypic correlations between liability to bipolar disorder and grey matter density. Areas with a significant genetic contribution are indicated by an arrow. For visualization purposes, _2 values in this picture range from 15 to 57 (significant _2427.7). Left: right medial/dorsolateral prefrontal gyrus. Brodmann areas 9, 46. Peak value _2 = 44, rph = _0.33, rg = _0.18, re = _0.81. Middle: right medial orbital gyrus. Brodmann area 11. Peak value _2 = 32, rph = _0.17, rg = 0.22, re = _0.95. Right: right insula, Brodmann area 13. Peak value _2 = 44, rph = _0.33, rg = _0.17, re = _0.83. (Reprinted from Astrid C. van der Schot et al., 'Genetic and environmental influences on focal brain density in bipolar disorder,' *Brain*, 2010, vol. 133, issue 10, 3080-3092, by permission of Oxford University Press.)

TABLE 2.2 DIFFUSION TENSOR IMAGING STUDIES OF BIPOLAR DISORDER

| No | Study | Publication year | Subjects | Mean age | Female % |
|----|-------|------------------|----------|----------|----------|
| 1 | Benedetti et al. | 2011 | 40 BD (Depressed) 21 HC | BD; Li medicated 47.8±13.3 Unmedicated 45.1±9.8 HC 39.9±11.1 | BD; Li medicated 64.3% Unmedicated 80.8% HC 47.6% |
| 2 | Lin et al. | 2011 | 18 BD 16 HC | BD 28.5±11.1 HC 29.9±9.2 | BD 66.7% HC 75.0% |
| 3 | Chan et al. | 2010 | 16 BD 16 HC | BD 36.9±10.3 HC 37.3±10.3 | BD 25.0% HC 25.0% |
| 4 | Chaddock et al. | 2009 | 19 BDI 21 unaffected 1st-degree relatives 18 HC | BD 43.3±10.2 UAR 42.5±13.6 HC 41.7±12.2 | BD 52.6% UAR 42.9% HC 44.4% |
| 5 | Mahon et al. | 2009 | 30 BD 38 HC | BD 33.4±8.7 HC 31.9±8.6 | BD 50.0% HC 42.1% |

| Patients characteristics | Medicated | MRI | Analysis | Findings |
|---|---|---|---|---|
| | 14 Li 26 Unmedicated | 3.0T | TBSS | BD vs. HC<br>Low FA; genu of corpus callosum, right dorsal cingulum<br>High RD; right posterior corona radiata<br>High MD; splenium of corpus callosum/ posterior corona radiata<br><br>Unmedicated BD vs. HC<br>High RD; right dorsal cingulum, right superior longitudinal fasciculus<br>High MD; splenium of corpus callosum, body of corpus callosum<br><br>BD with Li vs. HC<br>Low FA; right anterior corona radiata, right superior longitudinal fasciculus, genu of corpus callosum, left posterior corona radiata<br>High RD; right superior longitudinal fasciculus<br>High MD; right posterior corona radiata, right posterior thalamic radiation |
| | 11 Li 11 AD 2 VPA | 1.5T | Tractography ROIs WM tract connecting the frontal cortex; anterior thalamic radiation, uncinate fasciculus, superior longitudinal fasciculus, cingulum, inferior fronto-occipital fasciculus | Low FA; left anterior thalamic radiation, left uncinate fasciculus, left superior longitudinal fascicules, left cingulum |
| | 6 Li 7 Other MS 12 AP | 3.0T | TBSS | Low FA; right posterior thalamic radiation, left and right temporal WM, left cingulum, left and right sagittal striatum, left anterior WM, left genu corpus callosum<br>High RD; left and right sagittal striatum, right posterior thalamic radiation, right genu corpus callosum, left anterior frontal WM, left cingulum |
| | 4 Unmedicated 9 Li 8 VPA 5 AD 3 AP | 1.5T | Voxel-based | BD vs. HC<br>Low FA; bilateral deep frontal WM, the genu of the corpus callosum and a left lateralized portion of the internal capsule, right temporal WM superiorly towards the parietal lobe, superior frontal cluster<br><br>UAR vs. HC<br>N.S. |
| | All medicated | 1.5T | Voxel-based tractography | High FA; right and left frontal WM corresponding to fibers of the corticopontine tract/corticospinal tract and the superior longitudinal fasciculus as well as superior thalamic radiation fibers<br>Low FA; left cerebellum corresponding to the pontine crossing tract |

(Continued)

| No | Study | Publication year | Subjects | Mean age | Female % |
|----|-------|------------------|----------|----------|----------|
| 6 | Sussmann et al. | 2009 | 42 BD<br>28 SCZ<br>38 HC | BD 39.6±10.1<br>SCZ 38.0±9.9<br>HC 37.2±11.9 | BD 47.6%<br>SCZ 46.4%<br>HC 50.0% |
| 7 | Zanetti et al. | 2009 | 37 BD<br>26 HC | BD 34.1±9.0<br>HC 28.8±9.5 | BD 64.9%<br>HC 53.8% |
| 8 | Bruno et al. | 2008 | 25 BDI<br>11 BDII<br>28 HC | BDI 37.4<br>BDII 42.8 | BDI 60.0%<br>BDII 72.7% |
| 9 | McIntosh et al. | 2008 | 40 BD<br>25 SCZ<br>49 HC | BD 39.9±10.1<br>SCZ 37.2±9.2<br>HC 35.3±11.0 | BD 47.5%<br>SCZ 44.0%<br>HC 42.9% |
| 10 | Versace et al. | 2008 | 31 BD<br>25 HC | BD 35.9±8.9<br>HC 29.5±9.4 | BD 64.5%<br>HC 56.0% |
| 11 | Wang et al. | 2008 | 33 BD<br>40 HC | BD 32.6±10.1<br>HC 29.2±9.2 | BD 69%<br>HC 64% |
| 12 | Wang et al. | 2008 | 33 BD<br>40 HC | BD 32±10.1<br>HC 29.2±9.2 | BD 73%<br>HC 68% |
| 13 | Houenou et al. | 2007 | 16 BD (Remitted)<br>16 HC | BD 41.9±12.8<br>HC 40.5±12.8 | BD 50.0%<br>HC 43.8% |

| Patients characteristics | Medicated | MRI | Analysis | Findings |
|---|---|---|---|---|
| | BD<br>24 Li<br>19 AP<br>21 AD<br><br>SCZ<br>28 AP<br>8 AD | 1.5T | Voxel-based<br>ROIs<br>Prefrontal lobe and anterior limb of the internal capsule<br>The frontal portion of the uncinate fasciculus. | BD vs. HC<br>Low FA; superior thalamic radiation, left uncinate fasciculus, anterior thalamic radiation, left anterior limb of the internal capsule |
| | 12 Li<br>8 VPA<br>5 LTG<br>19 AP<br>16 AD<br>3 CBZ | 3T | TBSS | Low FA; left and right external capsule, right superior and inferior longitudinal fasciculi<br>High MD; right superior and inferior longitudinal fasciculi |
| | 2 Unmedicated<br>23 Li<br>3 VPA<br>4 CBZ<br>3 LTG<br>11 AD<br>9 AP<br>5 ECT | 1.5T | Voxel-based | High MD; prefrontal WM in part of anterior fronto-occipital fasciculus, right posterior frontal WM in part of posterior fronto-occipital fasciculus and the corpus callosum<br>Low FA; inferior longitudinal fasciculus |
| | BD<br>22 Li<br>18 AP<br>21 AD<br><br>SCZ<br>25 AP<br>8 AD | 1.5T | Tractography<br>ROI<br>Uncinate fasciculi<br>Anterior thalamic radiations | Low FA; uncinate fasciculi, anterior thalamic radiations |
| | 11 Li<br>22 MS<br>17 AP<br>15 AD | 3.0T | TBSS | Low FA; left uncinate fasciculus corresponding to orbito-medial frontal cortex or insula, left optic radiation corresponding to cuneus and temporal cortex, right anterothalamic radiation corresponding to thalamus |
| | 7 unmedicated<br>11 Li<br>20 AE<br>19 AP<br>17 AD | 3T | ROIs<br>Anterior and posterior cingulum | Low FA; anterior cingulum |
| | 6 unmedicated<br>8 Li<br>17 AE<br>16 AP | 3T | ROI, voxel-based<br>Corpus callosum | Low FA; anterior and middle corpus callosum, genu, rostral body, and anterior midbody of corpus callosum |
| | 2 unmedicated<br>5 Li<br>9 combined therapy (Li, AP, SSRI) | 1.5T | Tractography<br>Reconstructed fibers of connecting pairs: right subgenual cingulate and right amygdalo-hippocamus, left subgenual cingulate and left amygdalo-hippocampus,<br>pons and right cerebellum, pons and left cerebellum,<br>pons and right subgenual cingulate,<br>pons and left subgenual cingulate | Increase of the virtual reconstructed fibres between left subgenual cingulate and left amygdalo-hippocampus |

(Continued)

| No | Study | Publication year | Subjects | Mean age | Female % |
|----|-------|------------------|----------|----------|----------|
| 14 | Yurgelun-Todd et al. | 2007 | 11 BD (Remitted)<br>10 HC | BD 32.9±10.5<br>HC 32.4±9.1 | BD 45.5%<br>HC 60.0% |
| 15 | Beyer et al. | 2005 | 14 BD<br>21 HC | BD 44.0±17.6<br>HC 44.6±13.5 | BD 71.4%<br>HC 81.0% |
| 16 | Haznedar et al. | 2005 | 17 BDI<br>7 BDII<br>16 Cyclothymia<br>36 HC | BDI 39.8±13.4<br>BDII 43.8±6.7<br>Cyclothymia 43.9±9.2<br>HC 40.7±11.6 | |
| 17 | Adler et al. | 2004 | 9 BD<br>9 HC | BD 32±8<br>HC 31±7 | BD 55.6%<br>HC 33.3% |

Abbreviations: BD = bipolar disorder; BDI = bipolar disorder type I; BDII = bipolar disorder type II; SCZ = schizophrenia; HC = healthy comparison subjects; UAR = unaffected relatives; ROI = region of interest; TBSS = tract based spatial statistics; Li = lithium; VPA = valproate or divalproate; CBZ = carbamazepine or oxcarbazepine; LTG = lamotrigine; MS = mood stabilizers AP = antipsychotics; AD = antidepressants; AE = antiepileptics; ECT = electroconvulsive therapy; FA = fractional anisotropy; RD = radial diffusivity; MD = mean diffusivity; ADC = apparent diffusion coefficient; OFC = orbitofrontal cortex.

| Patients characteristics | Medicated | MRI | Analysis | Findings |
|---|---|---|---|---|
| | 2 unmedicated<br>3 Li<br>6 AE<br>4 AP | 1.5T | ROIs<br>Genu and the midline of the splenium of the corpus callosum | High FA; genu of corpus callosum |
| | | 1.5T | ROIs<br>OFC<br>middle and superior<br>frontal gyri | High ADC; orbitofrontal WM |
| | BDI<br>3 drug-naïve<br>3 MS<br>1 AP<br>13 MS + AP<br>BDII and<br>cyclothymia<br>All unmedicated | 1.5T | ROIs<br>Anterior and posterior<br>limb of the internal capsule<br>Anterior frontal WM<br>Fasciculus longitudinalis superior<br>Anterior fronto-occipital fasciculus<br>Posterior fronto-occipital fasciculus | Bipolar spectrum vs. HC<br>Decrease of asymmetry bilaterally in the anterior genu<br>Low FA; right and left internal capsule, posterior internal capsule, anterior fronto-occipital fasciculus,<br>High FA; anterior frontal WM |
| | Medicated | 3T | ROIs<br>Anterior commissure | Low FA; anterior comissure |

TABLE 2.3 FAMILY STUDIES OF BIPOLAR DISORDER

TWIN STUDY

| No | Study | Publication year | Subjects | Mean age | Female % |
|---|---|---|---|---|---|
| 1 | van der Schot et al. | 2010 | 23 BD MZ<br>26 BD DZ<br>39 HC MZ twin pairs<br>28 HC DZ twin pairs | BD MZ 36.9±10.5<br>BD DZ 43.8±8.5<br>HC MZ 39.0±9.9<br>HC DZ 39.0±7.5 | BD MZ 73.9%<br>BD DZ 67.3%<br>HC MZ 59.0%<br>HC DZ 55.4% |
| 2 | van der Schot et al. | 2009 | 9 BD MZ concordant<br>15 BD MZ discordant<br>4 BD DZ concordant<br>22 BD DZ discordant<br>39 HC MZ twin pairs<br>28 HC DZ twin pairs | BD MZ 37.4±10.6<br>BD DZ 43.8±8.5<br>HC MZ 39.0±9.9<br>HC DZ 39.0±7.5 | BD MZ 72.9%<br>BD DZ 67.3%<br>HC MZ 59.0%<br>HC DZ 55.4% |
| 3 | Keiseppa et al. | 2003 | 2 BD MZ concordant<br>1 BD MZ discordant<br>2 BD DZ concordant<br>11 BD DZ discordant<br>7 HC MZ twin pairs<br>20 HC DZ twin pairs | BD twins 44.4<br>Healthy<br>co-twins 44.5<br>Control twins 46.7 | BD twins 45.8%<br>Healthy co-twins 60.0%<br>Control twins 48.1% |
| 4 | Noga et al. | 2001 | 6 pairs of MZ twins discordant for BD<br>6 HC pairs of MZ twins | BD MZ 34.5±10.5<br>HC MZ 34.7±11.0 | BD MZ 83.3%<br>HC MZ 16.7% |

| Patients characteristics | Medicated | MRI | Measurement | Matter | Findings of BD |
|---|---|---|---|---|---|
| | Li BD of MZ 61.9% BD of DZ 66.6% | 1.5T | VBM | GM and WM | BD was associated with decreased GM density in the inferior/medial-dorsolateral/superior frontal gyri, anterior cingulate, precentral, inferior temporal gyrus and lingual gyri, bilateral insula and thalamus. <br><br> BD was associated with decreased WM density in superior longitudinal fasciculus, the left inferior frontal and postcentral gyrus and the right optic radiation, and with increased white matter density in the right inferior frontal gyrus. <br><br> Genetic contribution <br> Decreased GM density of right medial frontal gyrus and right insula <br> Increased GM density of right orbitofrontal gyrus <br> Decreased WM density of superior frontal/precentral gyrus. |
| | Li BD of MZ 78.8% BD of DZ 66.6% | 1.5T | ROIs Intracranium Cerebrum GM WM Lateral ventricle Third ventricle Cortical Prefrontal lobe Temporal lobe Parietal lobe Occipital | GM and WM | Decrease of WM was related to the genetic risk of developing BD. <br> BD was associated with decrease of total cortical volume. Adjusted for the effect of Li, BD was positively associated with ventricular and intracranial volumes and was negatively associated with all other volumes. |
| | 67% AP | 1.0T | ROIs; GM WM Left hemisphere Right hemisphere Frontal Temporal Left and right ventricular Frontal CSF Temporal CSF | GM and WM | BDI and their co-twins < healthy twins <br> Left hemispheric WM <br><br> BDI < healthy twins <br> Right hemispheric and bilateral frontal WM <br> Frontal CSF |
| | | 1.5T | ROIs Caudate Putamen Globus pallidus Amygdala-hippocampus complex | GM | Affected BD twins > Unaffected twins BD and HC twins <br> Right caudate <br> BD MZ > HC MZ <br> Left caudate <br> Affected BD twins > Unaffected BD twins <br> Right hippocampus |

(Continued)

TABLE 2.3 FAMILY STUDIES OF BIPOLAR DISORDER (CONTINUED)

**RELATIVE STUDY**

| No | Study | Publication year | Subjects | Mean age | Female % |
|----|-------|------------------|----------|----------|----------|
| 1 | Matsuo et al. | 2011 | 35 BDI<br>20 unaffected first-degree relatives of BD<br>40 HC | BD 40.8±9.2<br>UAR 46.2±10.7<br>HC 41.6±9.1 | BD 77.1%<br>UAR 75.0%<br>HC 60.0% |
| 2 | Baccardi et al. | 2010 | 1 BD and 4 MDD in a family<br>10 their unaffected relatives<br>15 HC | BD and MDD 58.7±17.0<br>UAR 45.1±14.0<br>HC for BD and MDD 58.9±17.3<br>HC for UAR 45.0±13.2 | BD and MDD 100%<br>UAR 60%<br>HC for BD and MDD 100%<br>HC for UAR 60% |
| 3 | Takahashi et al. | 2010 | 29 BD<br>49 first-degree relatives of BD<br>(15 relatives with MDD)<br>52 HC | BD 39.6±9.9<br>Relatives 33.9±12.7<br>HC 35.8±13.6 | BD 48.3%<br>Relatives 53.1%<br>HC 46.2% |
| 4 | Chaddock et al. | 2009 | 19 BDI<br>21 their unaffected first-degree relatives<br>18 HC | BDI 43.3±10.2<br>Their unaffected first-degree relatives 42.5±13.6<br>HC 41.7±12.2 | BDI 52.6%<br>Their unaffected first-degree relatives 42.9%<br>HC 44.4% |
| 5 | Kempton et al. | 2009 | 30 BD<br>50 siblings and offspring of BD<br>(14 relatives with MDD)<br>52 HC | BD 39.4±9.8<br>Relatives 33.8±12.7<br>HC 35.2±13.0 | BD 50%<br>Relatives 52%<br>HC 48.1% |

| Patients characteristics | Medicated | MRI | Measurement | Matter | Findings of BD |
|---|---|---|---|---|---|
| | 22 unmedicated 13 medicated | | VBM in SPM8 | GM and WM | GM<br>Main effect of diagnosis; left insula, right inferior frontal gyrus<br><br>BD and UAR < HC<br>Left insula<br><br>BD < HC<br>Right inferior gyrus<br><br>WM<br>Main effect of diagnosis; right medical frontal gyrus<br><br>UAR < HC<br>Right medical frontal gyrus |
| | | 1.0T | Hippocampus Amygdala | GM | BD and MDD < HC<br>Right hippocampus, eft amygdala<br><br>UAR > HC<br>Right hippocampus, left and right amygdala, hippocampal asymmetry |
| | 27 medicated BD (8 AP, 26 MS, 14 AD) | 1.5T | Pituitary | GM | BD > Relative and HC |
| | 15 BD medicated 4 BD unmedicated | 1.5T | Voxel-based analysis in fractional anisotropy in SPM2 | WM | BD < HC<br>Bilateral deep frontal WM and genu of the corpus callosum<br>Superior frontal WM<br>Parietotemporal junction<br><br>UAR vs. HC<br>N.S.<br><br>Regions with low FA associated with genetic risk of BD<br>The cerebellum and brainstem, bilateral inferior and superior longitudinal fasciculi and uncinate, bilateral anterior regions of the fronto-occipital fasciculus, superior longitudinal fasciculus, superior fronto-occipital fasciculus, bilateral portions of the inferior fronto-occipital and inferior longitudinal fasciculi, splenium of the corpus callosum and corona radiata |
| | 29 medicated BD (12 AP, 19 MS, 13 AD, 2 hypnotics) | | VBM in SPM5 | GM | Main effect of diagnosis<br>Left insula, left cerebellum, left substantial nigra<br><br>BD and relatives > HC<br>Left insula<br><br>BD > relatives and HC<br>Left substantial nigra |

(Continued)

TABLE 2.3 FAMILY STUDIES OF BIPOLAR DISORDER (CONTINUED)

| No | Study | Publication year | Subjects | Mean age | Female % |
|---|---|---|---|---|---|
| 6 | Walterfang et al. | 2009 | 70 BDI<br>45 their unaffected siblings and offspring of BDI<br>75 HC | BD 43.6±11.8<br>UAR 34.8±12.5<br>HC 36.1±13.5 | BD 52.9%<br>UAR 51.1%<br>HC 48% |
| 7 | Hajek et al. | 2009 | 26 unaffected offspring with second degree relatives with BDI or first- or second-degree relatives with BDII<br>20 affected offspring with second degree relatives with BDI or first- or second-degree relatives with BDII<br>11 MDD, 3 BDI,<br>1 BDNOS, 3 BDII,<br>1 dysthymia,<br>1 psychosis NOS<br>31 HC | Unaffected offspring 19.6±3.1<br>Affected offspring 21.0±3.7<br>HC 20.6±3.3 | Unaffected offspring 65.4%<br>Affected offspring 75.0%<br>HC 64.5% |
| 8 | Hajek et al. | 2009 | 26 unaffected offspring with second degree relatives with BDI or first- or second-degree relatives with BDII<br>20 affected offspring with second degree relatives with BDI or first- or second-degree relatives with BDII<br>11 MDD, 3 BDI,<br>1 BDNOS, 3 BDII,<br>1 dysthymia,<br>1 psychosis NOS<br>31 HC | Unaffected offspring 19.6±3.1<br>Affected offspring 21.0±3.7<br>HC 20.6±3.3 | Unaffected offspring 65.4%<br>Affected offspring 75.0%<br>HC 64.5% |
| 9 | Hajek et al. | 2008 | 26 unaffected offspring with second degree relatives with BDI or first- or second-degree relatives with BDII<br>19 affected offspring with second degree relatives with BDI or first- or second-degree relatives with BDII<br>10 MDD, 3 BDI,<br>1 BDNOS, 3 BDII,<br>1 dysthymia,<br>1 psychosis NOS<br>31 HC | Unaffected offspring 19.8±3.2<br>Affected offspring 21.3±3.5<br>HC 20.6±3.3 | Unaffected offspring 62.5%<br>Affected offspring 73.7%<br>HC 64.5% |
| 10 | Mondelli et al. | 2008 | 29 BD wit psychosis<br>38 unaffected first-degree relatives of BD with psychosis<br>26 SCZ or schizoaffective disorder<br>44 unaffected first-degree relatives of SCZ or schizoaffective disorder<br>46 HC | BD 40.5±2.2<br>UAR of BD 42.2±2.6<br>SCZ 34.0±1.7<br>UAR of SCZ 49.7±2.1<br>HC 39.7±2.2 | BD 62.1%<br>UAR of BD 50.0%<br>SCZ 23.1%<br>UAR of SCZ 59.1%<br>HC 52.2% |

| Patients characteristics | Medicated | MRI | Measurement | Matter | Findings of BD |
|---|---|---|---|---|---|
| | All medicated<br>23 Li<br>13 LTG<br>12 CBZ<br>8 VPA<br>19 AP | 1.5T | Corpus callosum | WM | BD < HC and UAR<br>Mean callosal area<br><br>BD < HC<br>Thickness |
| | Affected offspring<br>2 Li<br>1 AD<br>1 AP<br>1 LTG<br>12 unmedicated | 1.5T | ROIs;<br>Caudate<br>Putamen | GM | Unaffected offspring > HC<br>Caudate |
| | Affected offspring<br>2 Li<br>1 AD<br>1 AP<br>1 LTG<br>12 unmedicated | 1.5T | ROIs;<br>Amygdala<br>Hippocampus | GM | N.S. |
| | Affected offspring<br>2 Li<br>1 AD<br>1 AP<br>1 LTG<br>12 unmedicated | 1.5T | ROI;<br>Pituitary | GM | N.S. |
| | | 1.5T | Pituitary | GM | N.S. |

(Continued)

TABLE 2.3 FAMILY STUDIES OF BIPOLAR DISORDER (CONTINUED)

| No | Study | Publication year | Subjects | Mean age | Female % |
|----|-------|------------------|----------|----------|----------|
| 11 | McDonald et al. | 2006 | 38 BD with familial BD<br>52 relatives of BD with familial BD<br>24 SCZ with familial SCZ<br>32 relatives of SCZ with familial SCZ<br>18 SCZ with nonfamilial SCZ<br>25 relatives of SCZ with nonfamilial SCZ<br>54 Controls, 5 with a history of MDD<br>('Familial' was defined as the index patient having other first- or second-degree relatives affected with a psychotic disorder) | BD with familial BD 41.0±11.7<br>Relatives of BD with familial BD<br>SCZ with familial SCZ 44.0±15.4<br>Relatives of SCZ with familial SCZ 47.1±13.1<br>SCZ with nonfamilial SCZ 32.8±5.0<br>Relatives of SCZ with nonfamilial SCZ 51.9±13.6<br>Controls 40.2±15.3 | BD with familial BD 60.5%<br>Relatives of BD with familial BD 51.9%<br>SCZ with familial SCZ 25%<br>Relatives of SCZ with familial SCZ 65.6%<br>SCZ with nonfamilial SCZ 27.8%<br>Relatives of SCZ with nonfamilial SCZ 60.0%<br>Controls 53.7% |
| 12 | McIntosh et al. | 2006 | 26 BD I with at least one first- and second degree relative with BD<br>22 unaffected first- and second degree relatives with at least two first- and second degree relatives with BD<br>19 BD with at least one first- and second degree relative with SCZ<br>26 unaffected first- and second degree relatives with at least one first- and second degree relative with SCZ and one with BD (mixed family)<br>26 SCZ with at least one first- and second degree relative with SCZ<br>24 unaffected first- and second degree relatives with at least two first- and second degree relatives with SCZ (mixed family)<br>49 HC | BD with BD family 40.5±12.1<br>UAR with BD family 34.7±12.6<br>BD with mixed family 39.7±9.2<br>UAR with mixed family 34.1±13.0<br>SCZ with SCZ family 36.9±13.7<br>UAR with SCZ family 38.9±12.9<br>HC 35.3±11.1 | BD with BD family 46.1%<br>UAR with BD family 59.1%<br>BD with mixed family 63.2%<br>UAR with mixed family 46.1%<br>SCZ with SCZ family 50%<br>UAR with SCZ family 54.2%<br>HC 53.1% |
| 13 | McIntosh et al. | 2005 | 26 BD I with at least one first- and second degree relative with BD<br>22 unaffected first- and second degree relatives with at least two first- and second degree relatives with BD<br>19 BD with at least one first- and second degree relative with SCZ<br>26 unaffected first- and second degree relatives with at least one first- and second degree relative with SCZ and one with BD (mixed family)<br>26 SCZ with at least one first- and second degree relative with SCZ<br>24 unaffected first- and second degree relatives with at least two first- and second degree relatives with SCZ (mixed family)<br>49 HC | BD with BD family 40.5±12.1<br>UAR with BD family 34.7±12.6<br>BD with mixed family 39.7±9.2<br>UAR with mixed family 34.1±13.0<br>SCZ with SCZ family 36.9±13.7<br>UAR with SCZ family 38.9±12.9<br>HC 35.3±11.1 | BD with BD family 46.1%<br>UAR with BD family 59.1%<br>BD with mixed family 63.2%<br>UAR with mixed family 46.1%<br>SCZ with SCZ family 50%<br>UAR with SCZ family 54.2%<br>HC 53.1% |

| Patients characteristics | Medicated | MRI | Measurement | Matter | Findings of BD |
|---|---|---|---|---|---|
| | BD<br>33 medicated<br>10 AP<br>4 unmedicated<br>41 medicated<br>SCZ | 1.5T | ROIs;<br>Cerebral<br>Lateral ventricle<br>Third ventricle<br>hippocampus | GM | SCZ < BD<br>Bilateral hippocampus |
| | | 1.5T | VBM in SPM99<br>(Different image analysis from the above studies) | GM and WM | N.S. |
| | | 1.5T | VBM in SPM99 | WM | BD with BD family < HC<br>Left anterior limb of the internal capsule<br><br>UAR with mixed family < HC<br>Right superior frontal subgyrus<br>Right medial frontal gyrus |

(Continued)

TABLE 2.3 FAMILY STUDIES OF BIPOLAR DISORDER (CONTINUED)

| No | Study | Publication year | Subjects | Mean age | Female % |
|----|-------|------------------|----------|----------|----------|
| 14 | McDonald et al. | 2004 | 37 BDI<br>50 their first-degree relatives without psychosis | BDI 40.7±11.6<br>Relatives 44.1±15.7 | BDI 59.5%<br>Relatives 52% |
| | | | 25 SCZ<br>36 their first-degree relatives without psychosis | SCZ 37.3±10.2<br>Relatives 48.5±13.0 | SCZ 28%<br>Relatives 61.1% |
| 15 | McIntosh et al. | 2004 | 26 BD I with at least one first- and second degree relative with BD<br>22 unaffected first- and second degree relatives with at least two first- and second degree relatives with BD<br>19 BD with at least one first- and second degree relative with SCZ<br>26 unaffected first- and second degree relatives with at least one first- and second degree relative with SCZ and one with BD (mixed family)<br>26 SCZ with at least one first- and second degree relative with SCZ<br>24 unaffected first- and second degree relatives with at least two first- and second degree relatives with SCZ (mixed family)<br>49 HC | BD with BD family 40.5±12.1<br>UAR with BD family 34.7±12.6<br>BD with mixed family 39.7±9.2<br>UAR with mixed family 34.1±13.0<br>SCZ with SCZ family 36.9±13.7<br>UAR with SCZ family 38.9±12.9<br>HC 35.3±11.1 | BD with BD family 46.1%<br>UAR with BD family 59.1%<br>BD with mixed family 63.2%<br>UAR with mixed family 46.1%<br>SCZ with SCZ family 50%<br>UAR with SCZ family 54.2%<br>HC 53.1% |

Abbreviations: BD = bipolar disorder; BDI = bipolar disorder type I; BDII = bipolar disorder type II; SCZ = schizophrenia; MDD = major depressive disorder; HC = healthy control subjects; MZ = monozygotes; DZ = dizygotes; UAR = unaffected relatives; VBM = voxel-based morphometry; GM = gray matter; WM = white matter; CSF = cerebrospinal fluid; ROI = region of interest; Li = lithium; VPA = valproate; MS = mood stabilizers; AP = antipsychotics; AD = antidepressants; AE = antiepileptics; SPM = statistical parametric mapping.

| Patients characteristics | Medicated | MRI | Measurement | Matter | Findings of BD |
|---|---|---|---|---|---|
| | BD 31 MS 1 Olanzapine 5 unmedicated  All SCZ medicated | 1.5T | Optimized VBM in SPM99 | GM and WM | Regions associated with genetic risk of BD GM, right medial frontal gyrus, right anterior cingulate gyrus, right caudate and anterior putamen  WM Right medial frontal lobe between the anterior cingulate/ medial frontal gyri and middle frontal gyrus, extending into the genu of the corpus callosum, left lateral frontal lobe between the inferior frontal gyrus, anterior insula, caudate nucleus, anterior cingulate gyrus, left temporal lobe between the superior/middle temporal gyri and hippocampus/parahippocampal gyrus, posterior cingulate gyrus, right parietal lobe between the lateral ventricle, posterior cingulate gyrus, precuneus and inferior parietal lobule, supramarginal/angular gyri, extending to the postcentral gyrus |
| | | 1.5T | VBM in SPM99 | GM | BD with mixed family < HC Right inferior frontal gyrus BD with BD family < HC Left anterior thalamus and body of caudate Right anterior thalamus and body of caudate  UAR with BD family < HC Left anterior thalamus and body of caudate  UAR with mixed family < HC Right anterior thalamus and body of caudate |

brain-derived neurotrophic factor (BDNF) (Chepenik et al., 2009; McIntosh et al., 2007; Matsuo et al., 2009), Interleukin-1 (IL-1) B (Papiol et al., 2008), the G72 gene (Zuliani et al., 2009) and the serotonin transporter (Scherk et al., 2009).

Carriers of the BDNF Met allele had smaller hippocampal volume than individuals homozygous for the Val allele, and Met carriers with bipolar disorder had the smallest hippocampal volumes compared with the other three groups (Chepenik et al., 2009). In another VBM study, BDNF gene polymorphisms were associated with smaller volumes of anterior cingulate and dorsolateral prefrontal cortex in patients with bipolar disorder (Matsuo et al., 2009). Similar results were found by McIntosh et al. (2007), in which smaller hippocampal volumes were associated with the BDNF Met allele among bipolar patients. In regard to the IL-1B gene, its allele 2 seems to be related to smaller whole brain gray matter volumes among bipolar patients (Papiol et al., 2008), whereas the TT genotype at the M23 loci in G72 is apparently associated with decreased gray-matter density of the left temporal pole and right amygdala in bipolar patients, but not healthy subjects (Zuliani et al., 2009). Finally, carriers of the short allele of the serotonin transporter gene had increased volume of the right amygdala compared with homozygous L-allele carriers in BD patients. However, this finding was also present among healthy subjects, and its potential relevance to the pathophysiology of bipolar disorder is still unclear (Scherk et al., 2009).

Together, these findings, although preliminary, support the well-known hypothesis that putative structural brain abnormalities involved in the pathogenesis of bipolar disorder are at least in part mediated by genetic factors.

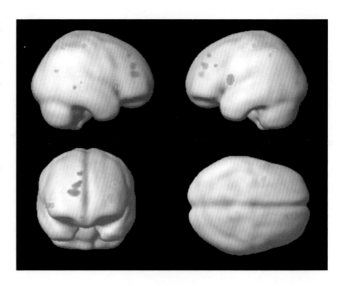

Figure 2.4 The regions showing significant gray (pink) and white matter (turquoise) difference between patients with bipolar disorder, unaffected first-degree relatives of bipolar disorder and healthy subjects. (Reprinted by permission from Macmillan Publishers Ltd: *Molecular Psychiatry*, Matsuo K, Kopecek M, Nicoletti MA, Hatch JP, Watanabe Y, et al., "New structural brain imaging endophenotype in bipolar disorder", Feb 15, 2011, copyright 2011.)

Additional structural imaging studies with other candidate genes will possibly bring about a better understanding of the relationship between gene variation and brain abnormality underlying the vulnerability to the disease and its manifestation, as well as a better characterization of endophenotypes in bipolar disorder. An example of these types of studies is provided in Figure 2.3.

## CONCLUSION: STRUCTURAL PATHOPHYSIOLOGY IN BIPOLAR DISORDER

Figure 2.5 contains a summary of this chapter and a systematization of the main brain structures apparently involved in the pathophysiology of bipolar disorder in light of available evidence. The proposed model comprises a neuronal circuit, which consists of four main parts: 1) the anterior medial frontal region including the subgenual, perigenual and rostral anterior cingulate, as well as the orbitofrontal cortex, inferior frontal and insular region; 2) the striatum, caudate, thalamus, putamen and globus pallidus; 3) the temporal cortex, including the hippocampus-amygdala complex; and 4) other areas including the dorsolateral prefrontal cortex and cerebellum. Whereas volumes of these structures are addressed in volumetric studies, the extensive inter-connections among them can be assessed through DTI studies.

Prior reviews of neuroimaging for mood disorders (Price & Drevets, 2010; Savitz & Drevets, 2009; Drevets, 2001; Adler et al., 2006; Strakowski et al., 2005; Soares & Mann,

**Neuroimaging Family and Genetic Studies in Bipolar Disorder**

- Found enlarged caudate, and decreased white matter volume and grey-matter density in medial frontal & precentral gyri, and insula in bipolar and healthy co-twins

- Found decreased hippocampal volumes and asymmetry and decreased total cortical volumes only in affected (bipolar) twins

- Found inconsistent white and gray matter abnormalities in unaffected relatives of bipolar probands

- Suggest some structural abnormalities observed in bipolar disorder may be linked to specific genetic alleles that may increase illness vulnerability

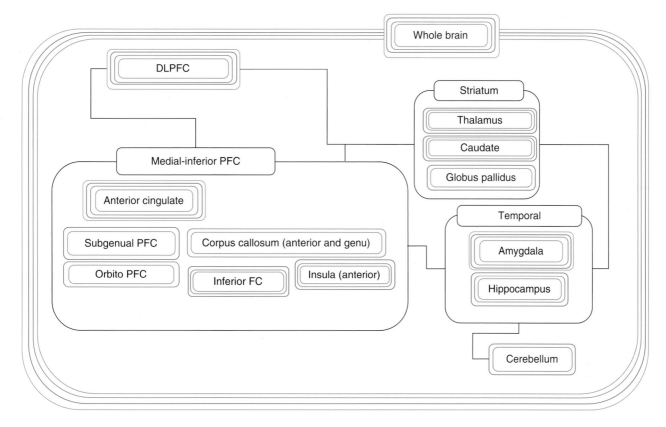

*Figure 2.5* An illustrated model of structural circuits for the pathophysiology in bipolar disorder. Color lines indicate the regions associated with evidence from structural imaging; gray, meta-analysis of bipolar disorder in comparison with healthy subjects; red, genetic; green, chronicity including duration of illness and number of episode; blue, first episode. DLPFC dorsolateral prefrontal cortex, PFC prefrontal cortex, FC frontal cortex.

1997; Phillips et al., 2008; Keener & Phillips, 2007) have proposed anatomical models of bipolar disorder and aberrant mood regulation in mood disorders based upon the evidence from neuropathological, neurocognitive and neuroimaging studies. The neural circuits in these models include regions known to play a crucial role in emotional regulation and cognitive processing. However, the brain mechanisms underpinning the abnormalities in bipolar disorder still remain unclear and the results of neuroimaging studies in bipolar disorder are often inconsistent. The variability of these findings may in part reflect different degrees of genetic loading among the subjects, as well as the clinical heterogeneity of samples. In addition, medications for bipolar disorder, in particular lithium, appear to have neurotrophic effects that might mitigate reduction of brain volume.

Future research using structural neuroimaging in bipolar disorder will face the challenge of combining different study designs and imaging techniques in order to contemplate changes in paradigms in regard to the focus on brain circuits rather than in brain structures. In addition, the multiplicity of etiological factors, with emphasis on the genetic components of bipolar disorder, will likely be integrated into neuroimaging investigations. Nonetheless, neuroimaging remains a powerful tool for clarifying the structural neuroanatomy of this important psychiatric illness.

## REFERENCES

Adler, C. M., DelBello M. P., & Strakowski, S. M. 2006. Brain network dysfunction in bipolar disorder. *CNS Spectrums,* 11(4): 312–320; quiz 323–324.

Adler, C. M., Holland, S. K., Schmithorst, V., Wilke, M., Weiss, K. L., Pan, H., & Strakowski, S. M. 2004. Abnormal frontal white matter tracts in bipolar disorder: a diffusion tensor imaging study. *Bipolar Disorders,* 6(3): 197–203.

Ahearn, E. P., Steffens, D. C., Cassidy, F., Van Meter, S. A., Provenzale, J. M., Seldin, M. F., . . . Krishnan, K. R. 1998. Familial leukoencephalopathy in bipolar disorder. *American Journal of Psychiatry,* 155(11): 1605–1607.

Altshuler, L. L., Curran, J. G., Hauser, P., Mintz, J., Denicoff, K., & Post, R. 1995. T2 hyperintensities in bipolar disorder: magnetic resonance imaging comparison and literature meta-analysis. *American Journal of Psychiatry,* 152(8): 1139–1144.

Arnone, D., Cavanagh, J., Gerber, D., Lawrie, S. M., Ebmeier, K. P., & McIntosh, A. M. 2009. Magnetic resonance imaging studies in bipolar disorder and schizophrenia: meta-analysis. *British Journal of Psychiatry,* 195(3): 194–201.

Arnone, D., McIntosh, A. M., Chandra, P., & Ebmeier, K. P. 2008. Meta-analysis of magnetic resonance imaging studies of the corpus callosum in bipolar disorder. *Acta Psychiatrica Scandinavica,* (Nov.) 118(5): 357–362.

Atmaca, M., Ozdemir, H., Cetinkaya, S., Parmaksiz, S., Belli, H., Poyraz, A. K., . . . Ogur, E. 2007. Cingulate gyrus volumetry in drug free bipolar patients and patients treated with valproate or valproate and quetiapine. *Journal of Psychiatric Research,* 41(10): 821–827.

Aylward, E. H., Roberts-Twillie, J. V., Barta, P. E., Kumar, A. J., Harris, G. J., Geer, M., . . . Pearlson, G. D. 1994. Basal ganglia volumes and white matter hyperintensities in patients with bipolar disorder. *American Journal of Psychiatry,* 151(5): 687–693.

Bearden, C. E., Thompson, P.M., Dalwani, M., Hayashi, K. M., Lee, A. D., Nicoletti, M., . . . Soares JC. Greater cortical gray matter density in lithium-treated patients with bipolar disorder. *Biological Psychiatry,* 2007;62(1): 7–16.

Benedetti, F., Yeh, P. H., Bellani, M., Radaelli, D., Nicoletti, M. A., Poletti, S., . . . Brambilla, P. 2011. Disruption of White Matter Integrity in Bipolar Depression as a Possible Structural Marker of Illness. *Biological Psychiatry,* 69(4): 309–317.

Beyer, J. L.,Young, R., Kuchibhatla, M., & Krishnan, K. R. 2009. Hyperintense MRI lesions in bipolar disorder: A meta-analysis and review. *International Review of Psychiatry,* 21(4): 394–409.

Beyer, J. L., Taylor, W. D., MacFall, J. R., Kuchibhatla, M., Payne, M. E., Provenzale, J.M., . . . Krishnan, K. R. 2005. Cortical white matter microstructural abnormalities in bipolar disorder. *Neuropsychopharmacology,* 30(12): 2225–2229.

Boccardi, M., Almici, M., Bresciani, L., Caroli, A., Bonetti, M., Monchieri, S., . . . Frisoni, G. B. 2010. Clinical and medial temporal features in a family with mood disorders. *Neuroscience Letters,* 468(2): 93–97.

Bora, E., Fornito, A., Yucel, M., & Pantelis, C. 2010. Voxelwise meta-analysis of gray matter abnormalities in bipolar disorder. *Biolological Psychiatry,* 67(11): 1097–1105.

Bora, E., Vahip, S., Akdeniz, F., Ilerisoy, H., Aldemir, E., & Alkan, M. 2009. Executive and verbal working memory dysfunction in first-degree relatives of patients with bipolar disorder. *Psychiatry Research,* 16(3): 318–324.

Bora, E., Yucel, M., & Pantelis, C. 2009. Cognitive endophenotypes of bipolar disorder: a meta-analysis of neuropsychological deficits in euthymic patients and their first-degree relatives. *Journal of Affective Disorders,* 113(1–2): 1–20.

Brambilla, P., Bellani, M., Yeh, P. H., Soares, J. C., & Tansella, M. 2009. White matter connectivity in bipolar disorder. *Internaional Review of Psychiatry,* 21(4): 380–386.

Breeze, J. L., Hesdorffer, D. C., Hong, X., Frazier, J. A., & Renshaw, P. F. 2003. Clinical significance of brain white matter hyperintensities in young adults with psychiatric illness. *Harvard Review of Psychiatry,* 11(5): 269–283.

Bruno, S., Cercignani, M., & Ron, M. A. 2008. White matter abnormalities in bipolar disorder: a voxel-based diffusion tensor imaging study. *Bipolar Disorders,* 10(4): 460–468.

Chaddock, C. A., Barker, G. J., Marshall, N., Schulze, K., Hall, M. H., Fern, A., . . . McDonald, C. 2009. White matter microstructural impairments and genetic liability to familial bipolar I disorder. *British Journal of Psychiatry,* 194(6): 527–534.

Chan, W. Y., Yang, G. L., Chia, M. Y., Woon, P. S., Lee, J., Keefe, R., . . . Sim, K. 2010. Cortical and subcortical white matter abnormalities in adults with remitted first-episode mania revealed by Tract-Based Spatial Statistics. *Bipolar Disorders,* 12(4): 383–389.

Chepenik, L. G., Fredericks, C., Papademetris, X., Spencer, L., Lacadie, C., Wang, F., . . . Blumberg, H. P. 2009. Effects of the brain-derived neurotrophic growth factor val66met variation on hippocampus morphology in bipolar disorder. *Neuropsychopharmacol,* 34(4): 944–951.

Chuang, D. M., & Manji, H. K. 2007. In search of the Holy Grail for the treatment of neurodegenerative disorders: has a simple cation been overlooked? *Biological Psychiatry,* 62(1): 4–6.

Cousins, D. A., Moore, P. B., Watson, S., Harrison, L., Ferrier, I. N., Young, A. H., & Lloyd, A. J. 2010. Pituitary volume and third ventricle width in euthymic patients with bipolar disorder. *Psychoneuroendocrinology,* 35(7): 1074–1081.

de Asis, J. M., Greenwald, B. S., Alexopoulos, G. S., Kiosses, D. N., Ashtari, M., Heo, M., & Young, R. C. 2006. Frontal signal hyperintensities in mania in old age. *American Journal of Geriatric Psychiatry,* 14(7): 598–604.

Drevets, W. C. 2001. Neuroimaging and neuropathological studies of depression: implications for the cognitive-emotional features of mood disorders. *Current Opinion in Neurobiology,* 11(2): 240–249.

Drevets, W. C., Price, J. L., Simpson, Jr. J. R., Todd, R. D., Reich. T., Vannier, M., & Raichle, M. E. 1997. Subgenual prefrontal cortex abnormalities in mood disorders. *Nature,* 386(6627): 824–827.

Drevets, W. C., Savitz, J., & Trimble, M. 2008. The subgenual anterior cingulate cortex in mood disorders. *CNS Spectrum,* 13(8): 663–681.

Dupont, R. M., Butters, N., Schafer, K., Wilson, T., Hesselink, J., & Gillin, J. C. 1995. Diagnostic specificity of focal white matter abnormalities in bipolar and unipolar mood disorder. *Biol Psychiatry,* 38(7): 482–486.

Ekman, C. J., Lind, J., Ryden, E., Ingvar, M., & Landen, M. 2010. Manic episodes are associated with grey matter volume reduction—a voxel-based morphometry brain analysis. *Acta Psychiatrica Scandinavica,* 122(6): 507–515.

Ellison-Wright, I., & Bullmore, E. 2010. Anatomy of bipolar disorder and schizophrenia: a meta-analysis. *Schizophrenia Research,* 117(1): 1–12.

Farrow, T. F., Whitford, T. J., Williams, L. M., Gomes, L., & Harris, A. W. 2005. Diagnosis-related regional gray matter loss over two years in first episode schizophrenia and bipolar disorder. *Biol Psychiatry,* 58(9): 713–723.

Figiel, G. S., Krishnan, K. R., Rao, V. P., Doraiswamy, M., Ellinwood, E. H. Jr., Nemeroff, C. B., . . . Boyko, O. 1991. Subcortical hyperintensities on brain magnetic resonance imaging: a comparison of normal and bipolar subjects. *The Journal of Neuropsychiatry and Clinical Neurosciences,* 3(1): 18–22.

Foland, L. C., Altshuler, L. L., Sugar, C. A., Lee, A. D., Leow, A. D., Townsend, J., . . . Thompson, P. M. 2008. Increased volume of the amygdala and hippocampus in bipolar patients treated with lithium. *Neuroreport,* 19(2): 221–224.

Fornito, A., Yucel, M., Wood, S. J., Bechdolf, A., Carter, S., Adamson, C., . . . Pantelis, C. 2009. Anterior cingulate cortex abnormalities associated with a first psychotic episode in bipolar disorder. *British Journal of Psychiatry,* 194(5): 426–433.

Germana, C., Kempton, M. J., Sarnicola, A., Christodoulou, T., Haldane, M., Hadjulis, M., . . . Frangou, S. 2010. The effects of lithium and anticonvulsants on brain structure in bipolar disorder. *Acta Psychiatrica Scandinavica,* 122(6): 481–487.

Goodwin, F. K., & Jamison, K. R. 2007. *Manic-Depressive Illness. Bipolar Disorders and Recurrent Depression.* Second Edition ed. New York: Oxford University Press.

Gottesman, I. I., & Shields, J. 1973. Genetic theorizing and schizophrenia. *British Journal of Psychiatry,* 122(566): 15–30.

Gulseren, S., Gurcan, M., Gulseren, L., Gelal, F., & Erol, A. 2006. T2 hyperintensities in bipolar patients and their healthy siblings. *Archives of Medical Research,* 37(1): 79–85.

Gunde, E., Novak, T., Kopecek, M., Schmidt, M., Propper, L., Stopkova, P., . . . Hajek, T. 2011. White matter hyperintensities in affected and unaffected late teenage and early adulthood offspring of bipolar parents: A two-center high-risk study. *Journal of Psychiatric Research,* 45(1): 76–82.

Ha, T. H., Ha, K., Kim, J. H., & Choi, J. E. 2009. Regional brain gray matter abnormalities in patients with bipolar II disorder:

a comparison study with bipolar I patients and healthy controls. *Neuroscience Letters*, 456(1): 44–48.

Hajek, T., Gunde, E., Slaney, C., Propper, L., MacQueen, G., Duffy, A., & Alda, M. 2009. Amygdala and hippocampal volumes in relatives of patients with bipolar disorder: a high-risk study. *Canadian Journal of Psychiatry*, 54(11): 726–733.

Hajek, T., Gunde, E., Slaney, C., Propper, L., MacQueen, G., Duffy, A., & Alda, M. 2009. Striatal volumes in affected and unaffected relatives of bipolar patients—high-risk study. *Journal of Psychiatric Research*, 43(7): 724–729.

Hajek, T., Kopecek, M., Kozeny, J., Gunde, E., Alda, M., & Hoschl, C. 2009. Amygdala volumes in mood disorders—meta-analysis of magnetic resonance volumetry studies. *Journal of Affective Disorders*, 115(3): 395–410.

Hajek, T., Kozeny, J., Kopecek, M., Alda, M., & Hoschl, C. 2008. Reduced subgenual cingulate volumes in mood disorders: a meta-analysis. *Journal of Psychiatry and Neuroscience*, 33(2): 91–99.

Hallahan, B., Newell, J., Soares, J. C., Brambilla, P., Strakowski, S. M., Fleck, D. E., . . . McDonald, C. 2011. Structural magnetic resonance imaging in bipolar disorder: an international collaborative mega-analysis of individual adult patient data. *Biological Psychiatry*, 69(4): 326–335.

Hasler, G., Drevets, W. C., Gould, T. D., Gottesman, I. I., & Manji, H. K. 2006. Toward constructing an endophenotype strategy for bipolar disorders. *Biological Psychiatry*, 60(2): 93–105.

Haznedar, M. M., Roversi, F., Pallanti, S., Baldini-Rossi, N., Schnur, D. B., Licalzi, E. M., . . . Buchsbaum, M. S. 2005. Fronto-thalamo-striatal gray and white matter volumes and anisotropy of their connections in bipolar spectrum illnesses. *Biological Psychiatry*, 57(7): 733–742.

Hoge, E. A., Friedman, L., & Schulz, S. C. 1999. Meta-analysis of brain size in bipolar disorder. *Schizophrenia Res*, 37(2): 177–181.

Houenou, J., Wessa, M., Douaud, G., Leboyer, M., Chanraud, S., Perrin, M., . . . Paillere-Martinot, M. L. 2007. Increased white matter connectivity in euthymic bipolar patients: diffusion tensor tractography between the subgenual cingulate and the amygdalo-hippocampal complex. *Molecular Psychiatry*, 12(11): 1001–1010.

Javadapour, A., Malhi, G. S., Ivanovski, B., Chen, X., Wen, W., & Sachdev, P. 2010. Hippocampal volumes in adults with bipolar disorder. *Journal of Neuropsychiatry and Clinical Neuroscience*, 22(1): 55–62.

Jones, L. D., Payne, M. E., Messer, D. F., Beyer, J. L., MacFall, J. R., Krishnan, K. R., & Taylor, W. D. 2009. Temporal lobe volume in bipolar disorder: relationship with diagnosis and antipsychotic medication use. *Journal of Affective Disorders*, 114(1–3): 50–57.

Kalmar, J. H., Wang, F., Spencer, L., Edmiston, E., Lacadie, C. M., Martin, A., . . . Blumberg, H. P. 2009. Preliminary evidence for progressive prefrontal abnormalities in adolescents and young adults with bipolar disorder. *Journal of the International Neuropsychological Society*, 15(3): 476–481.

Keener, M. T., & Phillips, M. L. 2007. Neuroimaging in bipolar disorder: a critical review of current findings. *Current Psychiatry Reports*, 9(6): 512–520.

Kempton, M. J., Geddes, J. R., Ettinger, U., Williams, S. C., & Grasby, P. M. 2008. Meta-analysis, database, and meta-regression of 98 structural imaging studies in bipolar disorder. *Archives of General Psychiatry*, 65(9): 1017–1032.

Kempton, M. J., Haldane, M., Jogia, J., Grasby, P. M., Collier, D., & Frangou, S. 2009. Dissociable brain structural changes associated with predisposition, resilience, and disease expression in bipolar disorder. *The Journal of Neuroscience*, 29(35): 10863–10868.

Kieseppa, T., van Erp, T. G., Haukka, J., Partonen, T., Cannon, T. D., Poutanen, V. P., . . . Lonnqvist J. Reduced left hemispheric white matter volume in twins with bipolar I disorder. *Biological Psychiatry*, 54(9): 896–905.

Koo, M. S., Levitt, J. J., Salisbury, D. F., Nakamura, M., Shenton, M. E., & McCarley, R. W. 2008. A cross-sectional and longitudinal magnetic resonance imaging study of cingulate gyrus gray matter volume

abnormalities in first-episode schizophrenia and first-episode affective psychosis. *Archives of General Psychiatry*, 65(7): 746–760.

Lin, F., Weng, S., Xie, B., Wu, G., & Lei, H. 2011. Abnormal frontal cortex white matter connections in bipolar disorder: A DTI tractography study. *Journal of Affective Disorders*, 131(1–3): 299–306.

Lloyd, A. J., Moore, P. B., Cousins, D. A., Thompson, J. M., McAllister, V. L., Hughes, J. H., . . . Young, A. H. 2009. White matter lesions in euthymic patients with bipolar disorder. *ACTA Psychiatrica Scandinavica*, 120(6): 481–491.

Lohoff, F. W., & Berrettini, W. H. 2010. Genetics of bipolar disorder. In Yatham LN, Maj M., eds., *Bipolar disorder: Clinical and Neurobiological Foundations*, (pp. 110–123). Chichester, UK: John Wiley & Sons.

Lyoo, I. K., Dager, S. R., Kim, J. E.,Yoon, S. J., Friedman, S. D., Dunner, D. L., & Renshaw, P. F. 2010. Lithium-induced gray matter volume increase as a neural correlate of treatment response in bipolar disorder: a longitudinal brain imaging study. *Neuropsychopharmacology*, 35(8): 1743–1750.

Lyoo, I. K., Lee, H. K., Jung, J. H., Noam, G. G., & Renshaw, P. F. 2002. White matter hyperintensities on magnetic resonance imaging of the brain in children with psychiatric disorders. *Comprehensive Psychiatry*, 43(5): 361–368.

Macritchie, K. A., Lloyd, A. J., Bastin, M. E., Vasudev, K., Gallagher, P., Eyre, R., . . . Young, A. H. 2010. White matter microstructural abnormalities in euthymic bipolar disorder. *British Journal of Psychiatry*, 196(1): 52–58.

Mahon, K., Wu, J., Malhotra, A. K., Burdick, K. E., DeRosse, P., Ardekani, B. A., & Szeszko, P. R. 2009. A voxel-based diffusion tensor imaging study of white matter in bipolar disorder. *Neuropsychopharmacology*, 34(6): 1590–1600.

Manji, H. K., Moore, G. J., & Chen, G. 2000. Clinical and preclinical evidence for the neurotrophic effects of mood stabilizers: implications for the pathophysiology and treatment of manic-depressive illness. *Biological Psychiatry*, 48(8): 740–754.

Matsuo, K., Kopecek, M., Nicoletti, M. A., Hatch, J. P., Watanabe, Y., Nery, F. G., . . . Soares, J. C. 2011. New structural brain imaging endophenotype in bipolar disorder. *Molecular Psychiatry*, Feb 15. [Epub ahead of print]

Matsuo, K., Walss-Bass, C., Nery, F. G., Nicoletti, M. A., Hatch, J. P., Frey, B. N., . . . Soares, J. C. 2009. Neuronal correlates of brain-derived neurotrophic factor Val66Met polymorphism and morphometric abnormalities in bipolar disorder. *Neuropsychopharmacology*, 34(8): 1904–1913.

McDonald, C., Bullmore, E. T., Sham, P. C., Chitnis, X., Wickham, H., Bramon, E., & Murray, R. M. 2004. Association of genetic risks for schizophrenia and bipolar disorder with specific and generic brain structural endophenotypes. *Archives of General Psychiatry*, 61(10): 974–984.

McDonald, C., Marshall, N., Sham, P. C., Bullmore, E. T., Schulze, K., Chapple, B., . . . Murray, R. M. 2006. Regional brain morphometry in patients with schizophrenia or bipolar disorder and their unaffected relatives. *American Journal of Psychiatry*, 163(3): 478–487.

McDonald, C., Zanelli, J., Rabe-Hesketh, S., Ellison-Wright, I., Sham, P., Kalidindi, S., . . . Kennedy, N. 2004. Meta-analysis of magnetic resonance imaging brain morphometry studies in bipolar disorder. *Biological Psychiatry*, 56(6): 411–417.

McDonald, W. M., Krishnan, K. R., Doraiswamy, P. M., & Blazer, D. G. 1991. Occurrence of subcortical hyperintensities in elderly subjects with mania. *Psychiatry Research*, 40(4): 211–220.

McDonald, W. M., Tupler, L. A., Marsteller, F. A., Figiel, G. S., DiSouza, S., Nemeroff, C. B., & Krishnan, K. R. 1999. Hyperintense lesions on magnetic resonance images in bipolar disorder. *Biological Psychiatry*, 45(8): 965–971.

McIntosh, A. M., Job, D. E., Moorhead, T. W., Harrison, L. K., Forrester, K., Lawrie, S. M., Johnstone, E. C. 2004. Voxel-based morphometry of patients with schizophrenia or bipolar disorder and their unaffected relatives. *Biological Psychiatry*, 56(8): 544–552.

McIntosh, A. M., Job, D. E., Moorhead, T. W., Harrison, L. K., Lawrie, S. M., & Johnstone, E. C. 2005. White matter density in patients with schizophrenia, bipolar disorder and their unaffected relatives. *Biological Psychiatry*, 58(3): 254–257.

McIntosh, A. M., Job, D. E., Moorhead, W. J., Harrison, L. K., Whalley, H. C., Johnstone, E. C., & Lawrie, S. M. 2006. Genetic liability to schizophrenia or bipolar disorder and its relationship to brain structure. *American Journal of Medical Genetics Part B: Neuropsychiatric Genetics*, 141(1): 76–83.

McIntosh, A. M., Moorhead, T. W., McKirdy, J., Sussmann, J. E., Hall, J., Johnstone, E. C., & Lawrie, S. M. 2007. Temporal grey matter reductions in bipolar disorder are associated with the BDNF Val66Met polymorphism. *Molecular Psychiatry*, 12(10): 902–903.

McIntosh, A. M., Munoz Maniega, S., Lymer, G. K., McKirdy, J., Hall, J., Sussmann, J. E., . . . Lawrie, S. M. 2008. White matter tractography in bipolar disorder and schizophrenia. *Biological Psychiatry*, 64(12): 1088–1092.

Mondelli, V., Dazzan, P., Gabilondo, A., Tournikioti, K., Walshe, M., Marshall, N., . . . Pariante, C. M. 2008. Pituitary volume in unaffected relatives of patients with schizophrenia and bipolar disorder. *Psychoneuroendocrinology*, 33(7): 1004–1012.

Monkul, E. S., Matsuo, K., Nicoletti, M. A., Dierschke, N., Hatch, J. P., Dalwani, M., . . . Soares, J. C. 2007. Prefrontal gray matter increases in healthy individuals after lithium treatment: a voxel-based morphometry study. *Neuroscience Letters*, 429(1): 7–11.

Moore, G. J., Bebchuk, J. M., Wilds, I. B., Chen, G., & Manji, H. K. 2000. Lithium-induced increase in human brain grey matter. *Lancet*, 356(9237): 1241–1242.

Moore, G. J., Cortese, B. M., Glitz, D. A., Zajac-Benitez, C., Quiroz, J. A., Uhde, T. W., . . . Manji, H. K. 2009. A longitudinal study of the effects of lithium treatment on prefrontal and subgenual prefrontal gray matter volume in treatment-responsive bipolar disorder patients. *Journal of Clinical Psychiatry*, 70(5): 699–705.

Moore, P. B., Shepherd, D. J., Eccleston, D., Macmillan, I. C., Goswami, U., McAllister, V. L., & Ferrier, I. N. 2001. Cerebral white matter lesions in bipolar affective disorder: relationship to outcome. *British Journal of Psychiatry*, 178: 172–176.

Moorhead, T. W., McKirdy, J., Sussmann, J. E., Hall, J., Lawrie, S. M., Johnstone, E. C., & McIntosh, A. M. 2007. Progressive gray matter loss in patients with bipolar disorder. *Bioogicall Psychiatry*, 62(8): 894–900.

Nasrallah, H. A., Jacoby, C. G., & McCalley-Whitters, M. 1981. Cerebellar atrophy in schizophrenia and mania. *Lancet*, 1(8229): 1102.

Nery, F. G., Chen, H. H., Hatch, J. P., Nicoletti, M. A., Brambilla, P., Sassi, R. B., . . . Soares, J. C. 2009. Orbitofrontal cortex gray matter volumes in bipolar disorder patients: a region-of-interest MRI study. *Bipolar Disorders*, 11(2): 145–153.

Neves-Pereira, M., Mundo, E., Muglia, P., King, N., Macciardi, F., & Kennedy, J. L. 2002. The brain-derived neurotrophic factor gene confers susceptibility to bipolar disorder: evidence from a family-based association study. *American Journal of Human Genetics*, 71(3): 651–655.

Noga, J. T., Vladar, K., & Torrey, E. F. 2001. A volumetric magnetic resonance imaging study of monozygotic twins discordant for bipolar disorder. *Psychiatry Research*. 106(1): 25–34.

Papiol, S., Molina, V., Desco, M., Rosa, A., Reig, S., Sanz, J., . . . Fananas, L. 2008. Gray matter deficits in bipolar disorder are associated with genetic variability at interleukin-1 beta gene (2q13). *Genes, Brain and Behavior*, 7(7): 796–801.

Penttila, J., Cachia, A., Martinot, J. L., Ringuenet, D., Wessa, M., Houenou, J., . . . & Paillere-Martinot, M. L. 2009. Cortical folding difference between patients with early-onset and patients with intermediate-onset bipolar disorder. *Bipolar Disorders*. 11(4): 361–370.

Persaud, R., Russow, H., Harvey, I., Lewis, S. W., Ron, M., Murray, R. M., & du Boulay, G. 1997. Focal signal hyperintensities in schizophrenia. *Schizophr Research*, 27(1): 55–64.

Phiel, C. J., & Klein, P. S. 2001. Molecular targets of lithium action. *Annual Review of Pharmacology and Toxicology*, 41: 789–813.

Phillips, M. L., Ladouceur, C. D., & Drevets, W. C. 2008. A neural model of voluntary and automatic emotion regulation: implications for understanding the pathophysiology and neurodevelopment of bipolar disorder. *Molecular Psychiatry*, 13(9): 829, 833–857.

Phillips, M. L., Travis, M. J., Fagiolini, A., & Kupfer, D. J. 2008. Medication effects in neuroimaging studies of bipolar disorder. *American Journal of Psychiatry*, 165(3): 313–320.

Pillai, J. J., Friedman, L., Stuve, T. A., Trinidad, S., Jesberger, J. A., Lewin, J. S., . . . Schulz, S. C. 2002. Increased presence of white matter hyperintensities in adolescent patients with bipolar disorder. *Psychiatry Research*, 114(1): 51–56.

Price, J. L., & Drevets, W. C. 2010. Neurocircuitry of mood disorders. *Neuropsychopharmacology*. 35(1): 192–216.

Rimol, L. M., Hartberg, C. B., Nesvag, R., Fennema-Notestine, C., Hagler, D. J., Jr., Pung, C. J., . . . Agartz, I. 2010. Cortical thickness and subcortical volumes in schizophrenia and bipolar disorder. *Biological Psychiatry*, 68(1): 41–50.

Rosso, I. M., Killgore, W. D., Cintron, C. M., Gruber, S. A., Tohen, M., & Yurgelun-Todd, D. A. 2007. Reduced amygdala volumes in first-episode bipolar disorder and correlation with cerebral white matter. *Biological Psychiatry*, 61(6): 743–749.

Rothschild, A. J., Benes, F., Hebben, N., Woods, B., Luciana, M., Bakanas, E., . . . Schatzberg, A. F. 1989. Relationships between brain CT scan findings and cortisol in psychotic and nonpsychotic depressed patients. *Biological Psychiatry*, 26(6): 565–575.

Sachdev, P. S., Wen, W., Christensen, H., & Jorm, A. F. 2005. White matter hyperintensities are related to physical disability and poor motor function. *Journal of Neurology, Neurosurgery and Psychiatry*, 76(3): 362–367.

Sanches, M., Keshavan, M.S., Brambilla, P., & Soares, J.C. 2008. Neurodevelopmental basis of bipolar disorder: a critical appraisal. *Progress in Neuro-Psychopharmacology and Biological Psychiatry*, 32(7): 1617–1627.

Sassi, R. B., Nicoletti, M., Brambilla, P., Mallinger, A. G., Frank, E., Kupfer, D. J., . . . Soares, J. C. 2002. Increased gray matter volume in lithium-treated bipolar disorder patients. *Neuroscience Letters*, 329(2): 243–245.

Savitz, J., & Drevets, W. C. 2009. Bipolar and major depressive disorder: neuroimaging the developmental-degenerative divide. *Neuroscience & Biobehavioral Reviews*, 33(5): 699–771.

Savitz, J., Nugent, A. C., Bogers, W., Liu, A., Sills, R., Luckenbaugh, D. A., . . . Drevets, W. C. 2010. Amygdala volume in depressed patients with bipolar disorder assessed using high resolution 3T MRI: the impact of medication. *Neuroimage*, 49(4): 2966–2976.

Scherk, H., Gruber, O., Menzel, P., Schneider-Axmann, T., Kemmer, C., Usher, J., . . . Falkai, P. 2009. 5-HTTLPR genotype influences amygdala volume. *European Archives of Psychiatry and Clinical Neuroscice*, 259(4): 212–217.

Soares, J. C., & Mann, J. J. 1997. The anatomy of mood disorders—review of structural neuroimaging studies. *Biological Psychiatry*, 41(1): 86–106.

Soares, J. C., & Mann, J. J. 1997. The functional neuroanatomy of mood disorders. *Journal of Psychiatric Research*, 31(4): 393–432.

Strakowski, S. M., DelBello, M. P., & Adler, C. M. 2005. The functional neuroanatomy of bipolar disorder: a review of neuroimaging findings. *Molecular Psychiatry*, 10(1): 105–116.

Sussmann, J. E., Lymer, G. K., McKirdy, J., Moorhead, T. W., Munoz Maniega, S., Job, D., . . . McIntosh, A. M. 2009. White matter abnormalities in bipolar disorder and schizophrenia detected using diffusion tensor magnetic resonance imaging. *Bipolar Disorders*, 11(1): 11–18.

Takahashi, T., Malhi, G. S., Wood, S. J., Yucel, M., Walterfang, M., Kawasaki, Y., . . . Pantelis, C. 2010. Gray matter reduction of the superior temporal gyrus in patients with established bipolar I disorder. *Journal of Affective Disorders*, 123(1–3): 276–282.

Takahashi, T., Walterfang, M., Wood, S. J., Kempton, M. J., Jogia, J., Lorenzetti, V., . . . Frangou, S,. 2010. Pituitary volume in patients with bipolar disorder and their first-degree relatives. *Journal of Affective Disorders*, 124(3): 256–261.

van der Schot, A. C., Vonk, R., Brans, R. G., van Haren, N. E., Koolschijn, P. C., Nuboer, V., . . . Kahn, R. S. 2009. Influence of genes and environment on brain volumes in twin pairs concordant and discordant for bipolar disorder. *Archives of General Psychiatry,* 66(2): 142–151.

van der Schot, A. C., Vonk, R., Brouwer, R. M., van Baal, G. C., Brans, R. G., van Haren, N. E., . . . Kahn, R. S. 2010. Genetic and environmental influences on focal brain density in bipolar disorder. *Brain,* 133 (10): 3080–3092.

Vederine, F. E., Wessa, M., Leboyer, M., Houenou, J. 2011. A meta-analysis of whole-brain diffusion tensor imaging studies in bipolar disorder. *Progress in Neuro-Psychopharmacology and Biological Psychiatry*, 35(8): 1820–1826.

Versace, A., Almeida, J. R., Hassel, S., Walsh, N. D., Novelli, M., Klein, C. R., . . . Phillips, M. L. 2008. Elevated left and reduced right orbitomedial prefrontal fractional anisotropy in adults with bipolar disorder revealed by tract-based spatial statistics. *Archives of General Psychiatry,* 65(9): 1041–1052.

Vita, A., De Peri, L., & Sacchetti, E. 2009. Gray matter, white matter, brain, and intracranial volumes in first-episode bipolar disorder: a meta-analysis of magnetic resonance imaging studies. *Bipolar Disorders,* 11(8): 807–814.

Walterfang, M.A., Wood, G., Barton, S., Velakoulis, D., Chen, J., Reutens, D. C., . . . Frangou, S. 2009. Corpus callosum size and shape alterations in individuals with bipolar disorder and their first-degree relatives. *Progress in Neuro-psychopharmacology and Biological Psychiatry*, 33(6): 1050–1057.

Wang, F., Jackowski, M., Kalmar, J. H., Chepenik, L. G., Tie, K., Qiu, M., . . . Blumberg, H. P. 2008. Abnormal anterior cingulum integrity in bipolar disorder determined through diffusion tensor imaging. *British Journal of Psychiatry,* 193(2): 126–129.

Wang, F. J., Kalmar, H., Edmiston, E., Chepenik, L. G., Bhagwagar, Z., Spencer, L., . . . Blumberg, H. P. 2008. Abnormal corpus callosum integrity in bipolar disorder: a diffusion tensor imaging study. *Biological Psychiatry,* 64(8): 730–733.

Wen, W., & Sachdev, P. 2004. The topography of white matter hyperintensities on brain MRI in healthy 60- to 64-year-old individuals. *Neuroimage,* 22(1): 144–154.

Womer, F. Y., Wang, F., Chepenik, L. G., Kalmar, J. H., Spencer, L., Edmiston, E., . . . Blumberg, H. P. 2009. Sexually dimorphic features of vermis morphology in bipolar disorder. *Bipolar Disorders,* 11(7): 753–758.

Yates, W. R., Jacoby, C. G., & Andreasen, N. C. 1987. Cerebellar atrophy in schizophrenia and affective disorder. *American Journal of Psychiatry,* 144(4): 465–467.

Yucel, K., Taylor, V. H., McKinnon, M. C., Macdonald, K., Alda, M., Young, L. T., & MacQueen, G. M. 2008. Bilateral hippocampal volume increase in patients with bipolar disorder and short-term lithium treatment. *Neuropsychopharmacology,* 33(2): 361–367.

Yurgelun-Todd, D. A., Silveri, M. M., Gruber, S. A., Rohan, M. L., & Pimentel, P. J. 2007. White matter abnormalities observed in bipolar disorder: a diffusion tensor imaging study. *Bipolar Disorders,* 9(5): 504–512.

Zanetti, M. V., Jackowski, M. P., Versace, A., Almeida, J. R., Hassel, S., Duran, F. L., . . . Phillips, M. L. 2009. State-dependent microstructural white matter changes in bipolar I depression. *European Archives of Psychiatry and Clinical Neuroscience*, 259(6): 316–328.

Zanetti, M. V., Schaufelberger, M. S., de Castro, C. C., Menezes, P. R., Scazufca, M., McGuire, P. K.,. . . Busatto, G. F. 2008. White-matter hyperintensities in first-episode psychosis. *British Journal of Psychiatry,* 193(1): 25–30.

Zuliani, R., Moorhead, T. W., Job, D., McKirdy, J., Sussmann, J. E., Johnstone, E. C., . . . McIntosh, A. M. 2009. Genetic variation in the G72 (DAOA) gene affects temporal lobe and amygdala structure in subjects affected by bipolar disorder. *Bipolar Disorders,* 11(6): 621–627.

# 3.

# FUNCTIONAL BRAIN IMAGING IN BIPOLAR DISORDER

## Lori L. Altshuler and Jennifer D. Townsend

## INTRODUCTION

Bipolar disorder is a chronic and severe mental illness with widespread effects. In the United States, the lifetime prevalence for bipolar disorder in the general population is estimated at around 3% (Grant et al., 2005), although these rates can vary depending on the methodology used and whether subtypes are delineated such as bipolar I, II, and NOS (Sherazi et al., 2006). Bipolar disorder exacts a tremendous cost not only on the patient, family and friends, but also on society. The World Health Organization regards bipolar disorder as one of the leading causes of disability worldwide (Murray & Lopez, 1996). The financial costs directly associated with bipolar disorder are from $24 to $30 billion dollars during a one-year period in the United States (Simon, 2003), although the total including indirect costs is surely higher.

As bipolar disorder is primarily a disorder of mood, many fMRI studies investigating bipolar disorder have focused on tasks involving emotion processing and emotion regulation. Using a variety of paradigms, these studies have specifically investigated the amygdala, a structure within the limbic system known to be critical for emotion, and the prefrontal cortex, a region known to have a regulatory function over the limbic system. The first section of this chapter therefore focuses on studies of emotion processing. Subsequent sections will explore findings in other cognitive domains, including reward, executive function, and response inhibition. In each domain, we summarize findings for each of the three mood states in bipolar disorder: mania/hypomania, euthymia, and depression. We identify the functional abnormalities present in specific mood states in an attempt to tease apart abnormalities that are specific to an acute mood state (i.e., "state related" abnormalities) versus those that persist across the different mood states (i.e., "trait related" illness abnormalities); the latter may represent a more enduring disability related to the underlying disorder.

The hallmark feature of bipolar disorder is an episode of mania. Key symptoms of mania include hyperactivity, impulsivity, and excessive involvement in pleasurable activities that have a high potential for painful consequences. These symptoms suggest that in addition to changes in mood or emotion, during mania there may be differences in functioning of the neural systems involved in reward. A number of studies of with bipolar disorder therefore focused on reward tasks in an effort to investigate these neural systems, which, as we know from studies of healthy populations, include cortical and subcortical pathways (Lawrence et al., 2009). The second section of this chapter will focus on reward systems and how they are impaired across mood states.

Subjects with bipolar disorder have also been reported to demonstrate impairment in executive functioning, a broad cognitive domain that includes attention, response inhibition, and working memory. A number of neurocognitive studies of bipolar disorder demonstrate these impairments (Bearden, Hoffman, & Cannon, 2001), and a number of fMRI studies have investigated the underlying neural mechanisms associated with performing these neurocognitive tasks. One of the symptoms of mania is distractibility, or an inability to maintain attention on important or relevant stimuli, and depressive episodes are often characterized by a diminished ability to think or concentrate. Consequently, these symptoms suggest impairment in brain regions underlying attention, such as the anterior cingulate cortex. A related area of research is response inhibition. Subjects with bipolar disorder demonstrate impairment in response inhibition not only while manic, as described previously (Dickerson et al., 2004; Martinez-Aran et al., 2004), but also demonstrate increased impulsivity while euthymic (Swann et al., 2001). The regions most often associated with response inhibition include the inferior frontal cortex (IFC), the striatum, and to a lesser extent, the anterior cingulate. Therefore, the third section of this chapter will focus on the broad domain of executive function and focus on studies in the specific areas of attention, response inhibition, interference, working memory and fluency. This section will discuss the dorsolateral prefrontal cortex (dlPFC), inferior frontal cortex (IFC), anterior cingulate, and striatum, as these regions have been implicated in numerous execution function studies in normal control populations.

Finally, a small number of studies are looking at neurofunctional differences in subjects with bipolar disorder compared to healthy populations during the resting state. These studies focus primarily on the default network, a network that is considered task-independent and may correspond to self-referential thought (Cole, Smith, & Beckmann, 2010). We will discuss these findings and the brain regions involved in these studies, particularly the posterior cingulate, medial prefrontal cortex and parietal cortex.

## EMOTION PROCESSING AND REGULATION

Bipolar disorder is characterized by a dysfunction of mood, alternating between mood states of mania (bipolar I) or hypomania (bipolar II), and depression. Thus, the primary abnormality appears to be an inability to regulate emotion, the result of which is the development of emotional extremes. Using tasks that assess neural functioning during emotion processing and emotion regulation, many fMRI studies have examined subjects with bipolar disorder during euthymia and depression. Fewer fMRI studies have been conducted on subjects during mania and fewer still included the same subjects in multiple mood states. Despite these limitations, both structural and functional imaging studies have demonstrated specific abnormalities in frontal-limbic regions.

Emotional dysregulation and lability in mania and depression may reflect disruption of a functional neuroanatomic network. Both structural and functional brain imaging studies suggest that abnormalities in frontal-limbic circuits may result in the emergence of both the manic and depressive symptoms seen in bipolar disorder (Bearden et al., 2001; Strakowski, DelBello, & Adler, 2005).

## EMOTION: HEALTHY FUNCTIONING

Functional neuroimaging studies in healthy subjects using neuropsychological paradigms that involve processing of emotional facial expressions reliably demonstrate specificity for activation of orbitolateral prefrontal cortex and amygdala (Adolphs, 2008; Breiter et al., 1996; Hariri, Bookheimer, & Mazziotta, 2000). The orbitofrontal cortex (OFC) plays a role in integrating emotional information

and regulating the intensity of emotional response (Cabeza & Nyberg, 2000; Fuster, 2001). Dysfunction in this region may provide a mechanism for understanding the failure of the OFC to modulate other limbic regions and may correlate with the mood shifts characteristic of bipolar disorder. Studies demonstrate that emotion processing and emotion regulation recruit activation in frontal and limbic brain regions. The orbitofrontal brain region has been implicated in processing emotional salience (Cabeza & Nyberg, 2000) and motivation (Tucker, Luu, & Pribram, 1995). Neuroimaging studies have demonstrated a role for the amygdala and insula in healthy emotion processing, and for the medial and lateral regions of the OFC in mood regulation (Baker, Frith, & Dolan, 1997; Northoff et al., 2000) and in associative emotional memory functions (Bookheimer, 2002; Price, 2003). Most studies of healthy subjects use emotional faces as stimuli and demonstrate robust amygdala activation in response to faces with both positive and negative valence (for review see Fusar-Polie et al., 2009) with the strongest amygdala activation occurring when viewing fearful faces. See Figure 3.1.

## EMOTION AND MANIA

Functional imaging studies during mania have been limited, no doubt because of the perceived difficulties in having

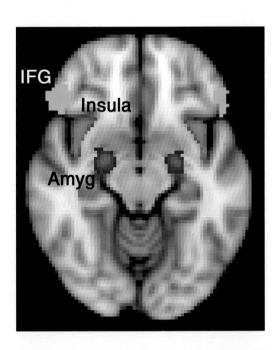

Figure 3.1 The inferior frontal gyrus (blue), insula (green) and amygdala (red), shown based on the Harvard-Oxford cortical and subcortical probability atlas (distributed with FSL; http://www.fmrib.ox.ac.uk/fsl/), are robustly activated in emotional tasks in normal control populations. Abnormal activation in these regions have been shown in subjects with bipolar disorder across a variety of studies.

manic subjects remain still during scanning. As amygdala enlargement (Altshuler et al., 1998; Brambilla et al., 2003; Strakowski et al., 1999) and heightened activation (Yurgelun-Todd et al., 2000) have been reported in bipolar disorder, most studies utilized tasks known to activate the amygdala in healthy individuals (Hariri et al., 2000) in order to assess amygdala reactivity and frontal-amygdala circuitry during mania (Blumberg et al., 2003; Blumberg et al., 1999; Hariri et al., 2000; Rubinsztein et al., 2001). One of the most consistent findings in mania is heightened limbic activation in response to emotional faces. A number of studies specifically found increased left amygdala activation compared to healthy subjects during simple emotion processing (i.e., viewing of emotional faces) (Altshuler et al., 2005), the viewing of positive pictures (Bermpohl et al., 2009), and during implicit, but not explicit, emotion processing (Chen et al., 2006). Another study, involving subjects in a variety of mood states, also found increased left amygdala activation in response to fearful faces (Yurgelun-Todd et al., 2000). This increased left amygdala response during mania correlated positively with YMRS scores (Bermpohl et al., 2009). These studies are interesting in light of several structural MRI studies that reported enlarged amygdala in subjects with bipolar disorder (Altshuler et al., 1998 Brambilla; et al., 2003; Strakowski et al., 1999). Although there is considerable convergence in amygdala findings, particularly in the left amygdala, at least one study (n = 10) found no significant differences in overall amygdala activation between manic and healthy subjects (Lennox et al., 2004). This finding may have been due to the relatively small sample size or the use of sad-only faces. However, subjects in the manic state exhibited a decreased load response in bilateral amygdala when examining sad faces of increasing intensity (Lennox et al., 2004).

Several fMRI studies of subjects with bipolar disorder during the manic state, including work from our group, demonstrated either attenuated orbitofrontal cortex (OFC) function or heightened amygdala activation compared to healthy subjects (Altshuler et al., 2005; Chen et al., 2006; Elliott et al., 2004; Lawrence et al., 2004). The amygdala has extensive reciprocal connection with the frontal cortex, including direct connection to the medial prefrontal cortex and the OFC (Van Hoesen, Pandya, & Butters, 1972). There is a striking convergence of studies using different paradigms suggesting attenuation of OFC function during mania (Elliott et al., 2004; Rubinsztein et al., 2001); (see the section on response inhibition and interference in this chapter for further discussion). A number of fMRI studies of mania specifically probing emotion processing demonstrated hypoactivation of the OFC during the processing of

negative faces (Altshuler et al., 2005), fear perception (Killgore, Gruber, & Yurgelun-Todd, 2008), and negatively captioned pictures (Malhi et al., 2004). Furthermore, hypo-activation of other frontal regions, including dorsolateral and medial prefrontal cortices, were also reported during mania (Killgore et al., 2008; Yurgelun-Todd et al., 2000). Animal work in monkeys revealed that the OFC serves to modulate the amygdala, as it has inhibitory GABAergic connections. Additionally, the orbitofrontal brain region has been implicated in processing emotional salience (Cabeza & Nyberg, 2000) and motivation (Tucker et al., 1995). The OFC is involved in regulating the highest level of control of behavior, especially in relation to emotion, through pathways between the OFC and autonomic systems that govern visceral responses associated with affective stimuli (Morris & Dolan, 2004). There is extensive anatomical connectivity between OFC, amygdala, and cingulate (Fuster, 2001; Morris & Dolan, 2004; Price, Carmichael, & Drevets, 1996). Orbital prefrontal areas are also connected with temporal polar and entorhinal temporal cortex and so have connections with the limbic cortex (Markowitsch et al., 1985; Van Hoesen et al., 1972). Neuroimaging studies have demonstrated a role for medial and lateral regions of the OFC in mood regulation (Baker et al., 1997; Northoff et al., 2000) and in associative emotional memory functions (Bookheimer, 2002; Cabeza & Nyberg, 2000; Price, 2003). Contrary to the above findings, which utilized negative emotional stimuli, one study of mania (n = 12) found increased OFC activation using both positive and negative emotional faces (Chen et al., 2010). This result is of interest because studies of healthy comparison subjects found engagement of the OFC during the processing of negative (i.e., fearful and angry) but not positive (happy) faces (Fusar-Poli et al., 2009).

Another region implicated in emotion processing is the insula, which has extensive connections with the amygdala, anterior cingulate, and OFC, among other regions (Augustine, 1996; Nagai, Kishi, & Kato, 2007). Sad and disgusted faces are known to preferentially activate insula in healthy subjects (Fusar-Poli et al., 2009), and may be recruited during the emotional response to potentially distressing interoceptive stimuli (Husted, Shapira, & Goodman, 2006). One study of manic subjects found increased left insular activation in response to sad faces (Lennox et al., 2004). The presence of an attenuated OFC response and a heightened amygdala or insula response in mania suggests an alteration in prefrontal-limbic circuits. Decreased negative connectivity between the amygdala and OFC (Foland et al., 2008) and between the amygdala and anterior cingulate (Wang et al., 2009) has been reported during mania. Studies of healthy subjects reported significant effective connectivity between the amygdala, insula, anterior cingulate, and OFC (Stein et al., 2007). The OFC has been purported to play a role in the integration of emotional information and the regulation of intensity of emotional response (Cabeza & Nyberg, 2000; Fuster, 2001). Dysfunction in this area could help explain a failure to appropriately modulate other limbic brain regions and perhaps result in a range of intensity of mood shifts in hypomania and mania in people with bipolar disorder.

## EMOTION AND DEPRESSION

Subjects with bipolar disorder spend the majority of their time in episodes of depression, not mania (Judd et al., 2005; Judd et al., 2002; Keller et al., 1993). As bipolar depression is associated with high levels of morbidity and mortality across the life span; efforts aimed at identifying biological mechanisms that contribute to this phase of the illness are imperative. Functional neuroimaging studies of subjects with unipolar depressive disorder have begun to reveal dysregulated neuroanatomic circuits associated with this syndrome (Drevets, 2000; Phillips et al., 2003). Similar studies in subjects with bipolar depression are more limited.

To our knowledge, only seven fMRI studies have been performed in subjects with bipolar disorder during the depressed phase using emotion processing paradigms known to activate limbic structures (Almeida et al., 2010; Altshuler et al., 2008; Chen et al., 2006; Lawrence et al., 2004; Malhi et al., 2004; Versace et al., 2010; Wang et al., 2009). Unlike the studies in mania, there was a much greater variability in the paradigms used and the activation patterns reported in bipolar depressed versus healthy samples. Several studies observed increased limbic function during bipolar depression. In one study in which subjects observed emotional expressions, subjects with bipolar depression demonstrated increased subcortical (left amygdala, caudate, putamen, thalamus, right globus pallidus) and prefrontal responses to both positive (happy) and negative (fearful) expressions compared to the healthy group (Lawrence et al., 2004). This pattern of overactivation in the left amygdala was also observed in another study using sad faces as stimuli, but was not seen for other emotions (Almeida et al., 2010). In another study involving the cognitive generation of affect, distinct patterns of regional activation were found with bipolar depressed subjects generating increased right-sided subcortical activation (basal ganglia, thalamus, hypothalamus, and amygdala) compared with healthy subjects

(Malhi et al., 2004). Using a paradigm to assess implicit versus explicit facial emotion recognition, one study found that bipolar depressed subjects tended to over-activate fronto-striato-thalamic regions in response to fearful faces (Chen et al., 2006).

Other studies suggest reduced activation of limbic system structures in bipolar depression. Work from our group demonstrated significant reductions in bilateral OFC (BA47) and right dlPFC and increased activation in medial PFC (BA10) (Altshuler et al., 2008) in bipolar depressed subjects in response to faces with negative emotions. Unlike the previous studies, hyperactivation of amygdala was not seen in our studies of bipolar depressed subjects while performing a face-matching task. In fact, there was less activation in the amygdala in the bipolar depressed versus healthy groups, although this did not obtain significant status compared to healthy subjects. Using functional connectivity techniques, Versace et al. (2010) found increased right and left amygdala-OFC connectivity in subjects with bipolar depression compared to healthy subjects while viewing sad faces, but decreased amygdala-OFC connectivity in response to happy faces. These results in conjunction with findings in mania that show reduced amygdala-OFC connectivity (Foland et al., 2008) suggest alterations in normal functional connectivity in both mania and depression. Another study, examining subjects with bipolar disorder in all three mood states, also found decreased frontal-limbic connectivity while viewing fearful and happy faces (Wang et al., 2009).

These studies suggest hypoactivation of the frontal lobe, abnormal connectivity between frontal and limbic structures, and abnormal amygdala activation that seem dependent on the specific stimuli used. Given the multiplicity of paradigms used and the heterogeneity of results, it is difficult at this time to discern a specific functional neuroanatomic circuit abnormality consistently demonstrated during bipolar depression. Clearly, more studies are needed.

## EMOTION AND EUTHYMIA

Impairments that persist into euthymia provide clues to the underlying brain regions involved in the primary pathology of bipolar disorder or impacted by the presence of the disorder. An enduring abnormality in a brain region may affect a brain circuit involved in homeostatic mood regulation. This abnormality could then, theoretically, predispose persons with bipolar disorder to relapse into acute mood episodes. Some studies suggest that subjects with bipolar disorder continue to display mood instability or increased mood reactivity even in the absence of an acute episode (Judd et al., 2005; Judd et al., 2002). This may represent an underlying neural vulnerability that could contribute to the triggering of new mood episodes.

Of the 10 studies examining emotion processing in euthymic subjects with bipolar disorder, the majority (6) found no significant differences in amygdala activation between healthy subjects and subjects with bipolar disorder during euthymia (Almeida, Mechelli et al., 2009; Almeida, Versace et al., 2009; Hassel et al., 2009; Hassel et al., 2008; Malhi et al., 2007; Robinson et al., 2008). It is interesting to note that all of the studies that found no group differences employed emotional faces as stimuli, using a variety of emotions. However, three studies found increased amygdala activation on the right using an emotional Stroop task (Lagopoulos & Malhi, 2007) and an emotional face task (Chen et al., 2010), and on the left (Surguladze et al., 2010) using emotional faces. Finally, one study using the emotional Stroop task actually found decreased left amygdala activation in a small sample (n = 10) of women with bipolar disorder during euthymia. From the literature, it appears that abnormalities of amygdala activation are more consistently found during acute mood states than during euthymia. Consequently, amygdala abnormalities may be state-related.

While amygdala function appears normal during euthymia, many of the previous studies reported abnormalities in OFC functioning during emotion processing even in euthymia. Two studies using emotional faces found increased activation in the right OFC (Chen et al., 2010; Robinson et al., 2008) in euthymic compared to healthy subjects. Two studies using the emotional Stroop task found decreased activation in left OFC (Lagopoulos & Malhi, 2007; Malhi et al., 2005), although it is interesting to note that both studies included only women. Decreased activation in OFC was also observed in a study that examined processing of sad faces by subjects with bipolar disorder in euthymic or depressed mood states (Jogia et al., 2008). Decreases in dorsolateral prefrontal activation were also reported in a number of these studies (Hassel et al., 2008; Lagopoulos & Malhi, 2007), perhaps suggesting impairment in frontal regions beyond those predictably activated in studies of emotion in healthy subjects. Imaging studies using affective induction and emotion regulation paradigms that are designed to identify regions most sensitive to provocation by external stressors may help elucidate the mechanisms mediating clinical relapse into mania or depression. Neural correlates of these clinical trait or disease diathesis markers are just beginning to be characterized.

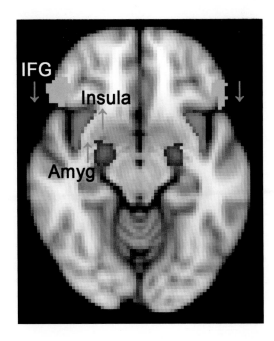

Figure 3.2 Many studies of emotion in mania show reduced activation bilaterally in the inferior frontal gyri and increased activation in the left insula and the left amygdala compared to normal comparison subjects.

## CONCLUSIONS OF EMOTION PROCESSING/ REGULATION

Despite the heterogeneity of the findings, most study findings converge with regard to amygdala and OFC (see Figure 3.2). In subjects with bipolar disorder, amygdala shows: *hyperactivation* in mania, *abnormal (decreased or, more commonly, increased) activation* during depression, and *normal activation* during euthymia when compared to healthy subjects. Amygdala changes may therefore be mood state-related. Conversely, orbitofrontal hypoactivation has been reported in the literature to be associated with manic, depressive and euthymic mood states (Angrilli et al., 1999; Grafman et al., 1986; Kruger et al., 2003), and may therefore be a trait-related characteristic that is present in all mood states. The OFC may be a brain region that

---

**fMRI of Emotion Processing in Bipolar Disorder Suggests:**

· Increased amygdala activation during mania and abnormal, often increased, amygdala activation during depression

· Normal amygdala activation during euthymia

· Orbitofrontal hypoactivation across all 3 mood states

· Impaired orbitofrontal control of limbic structures in mania

participates in aspects of emotional processing and expression that are not exclusively related to a specific valence of emotion. Lack of normal functioning in this region might result in dysregulation of mood to either pole. Dysfunction of an OFC-amygdala circuit might be a trait of bipolar disorder, rather than a state-dependent phenomenon.

## REWARD

The neural circuits that support motivation serve the purpose of regulating approach and avoidance behavior in response to anticipatory cues. The mesolimbic and neostriatal dopamine systems play a role in reward by mediating the incentive salience of rewards and modulating the motivational value (Berridge, 2007). In healthy subjects, tasks such as the IA gambling task and delayed monetary incentive task recruit this reward network. This network consists of nucleus accumbens, striato-thalamic regions, ventromedial PFC, and OFC, although other regions throughout the frontal lobe have also been implicated (Lawrence et al., 2009). The most studied brain substrates for reward are the dopamine projections from substantia nigra and ventral tegmentum to forebrain structures including nucleus accumbens and striatum, which in turn have connections to the frontal lobe (Cromwell, Hassani, & Schultz, 2005). This dopamine pathway is suggested to play a critical role in the incentive salience (i.e., "wanting") of a stimulus and is crucial to motivation (Berridge, 2007). See Figure 3.3.

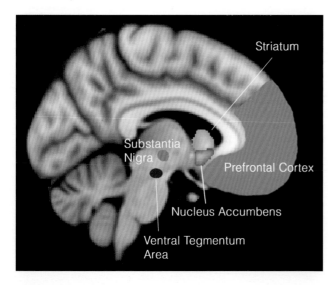

*Figure 3.3* Dopaminergic cell bodies of the mesocorticolimbic dopamine system originate in the ventral tegmental area. The VTA contains neurons that project to the substantia nigra, nucleus accumbens, striatum and prefrontal cortex, all of which comprise the reward circuitry.

Abnormal functioning of this system is implicated in bipolar disorder, as increased responsiveness to appetitive and reduced responsiveness to aversive cues are consistent with the symptoms of mania (i.e., the "excessive involvement in pleasurable activities that have a high potential for painful consequences," from DSM-IV). The symptoms of increased goal-directed activity during mania are also consistent with impairment in this reward network.

As these symptoms are specific to mania, the few studies of reward functioning in bipolar disorder are limited primarily to the manic mood state.

### REWARD AND MANIA

Two studies examined functioning of the reward system in bipolar disorder using fMRI (Abler et al., 2008; Bermpohl et al., 2009). One study used a monetary delayed incentive task known to activate ventral striatum and OFC in healthy subjects (Bermpohl et al., 2009). This study found that subjects with bipolar disorder scanned during mania showed increased left OFC (BA11/47) activation during the expectation of increasing gain and decreased left OFC activation during the expectation of increasing loss. This pattern is opposite to the pattern observed in healthy subjects, and when a subset of the subjects scanned during mania were scanned again while euthymic, they showed the same pattern as the healthy subjects. This finding suggests that some of the abnormalities observed in the OFC during mania may be specific to the manic mood state (i.e., state-related findings). Using a similar delayed monetary incentive task, Abler et al. (Abler et al., 2008) employed a region-of-interest approach and found that healthy subjects showed significantly greater nucleus accumbens activation upon the receipts vs. the omission of rewards compared to subjects with bipolar disorder during mania. These studies suggest impairment of the reward circuit during mania. More studies examining this network during mania may help to delineate the consistent abnormalities seen in mania.

### REWARD AND DEPRESSION

To our knowledge, no studies have been reported in Bipolar Depression.

### REWARD AND EUTHYMIA

As above, one more study using a reward task in euthymia also found reduced frontal activation in euthymic subjects with bipolar disorder compared to healthy subects (Frangou et al., 2008). Studies in euthymia and depression are needed to determine which of these findings are state-related and which are trait-related.

## EXECUTIVE FUNCTION

Executive function is a broad neurocognitive domain used to refer to the ability to conceptualize, plan, attend to, recall, and respond to relevant stimuli while ignoring irrelevant stimuli or inhibit undesired responses. Many studies have documented alterations in executive neurocognitive function in subjects with bipolar disorder during the manic and depressed mood states (Clark, Iversen, & Goodwin, 2001; Malhi et al., 2007; Martinez-Aran et al., 2004; Rubinsztein et al., 2000). Several studies additionally reported a persistence of neuropsychological dysfunction even in euthymia (Altshuler et al., 2004; Depp et al., 2007; Trivedi et al., 2008). Persistent neurocognitive abnormalities during euthymia in subjects with bipolar disorder, as well as abnormalities specific to the acute mood states, may provide clues to brain areas of underlying pathology in the disorder.

Executive function includes the integration of stimuli and production of behavioral responses that reflect the ability of a person to absorb, interpret and make decisions based upon relevant information. Deficits in executive function— that is, deficits in the ability to reason, anticipate, strategize, organize, and problem solve—are thought to exist in many psychiatric disorders. However, particular domains may be differentially affected in different psychiatric disorders and may therefore reflect different structural or functional underpinnings of each condition.

Executive cognitive functioning requires recruitment of brain regions throughout the frontal lobe, including regions of the prefrontal cortex (PFC) such as the dorsolateral PFC (BA46/9), ventrolateral PFC (BA47/44/45), medial PFC (BA6/8), and also the anterior cingulate (BA24/32) (Duncan & Owen, 2000). Functioning of the PFC depends on its functional and structural connections with a vast network of other structures beyond the frontal lobe (Fuster, 2001). Some of these other cortical and subcortical structures will be discussed in each of the relevant subsections of executive function, as there are striking similarities in functional activation in the parietal, temporal, and thalamus striatal structures across executive function tasks (Minzenberg et al., 2009).

Specific executive function domains that have been evaluated with fMRI include 1) sustained attention, 2) response inhibition, 3) interference, 4) working memory and 5) verbal fluency. Each of these will be discussed further below.

## SUSTAINED ATTENTION

Attention and concentration are essential for all domains of life, including emotion regulation, learning, memory, and social and occupational functioning. While some learning occurs outside of attention and conscious processing, most learning about the self, others, and the world depends on the integrity of attention processing. Impaired attention has been implicated in bipolar disorder and may be one of the reasons for the range of deficits seen (Czobor et al., 2007). Even in relatively simple tasks like performing a novel motor sequencing task, euthymic subjects with bipolar disorder show differences in attention from healthy subjects (Berns, Martin, & Proper, 2002). In contrast to the notion that these problems are state dependent, a misconception in some of the earlier literature, recent well-replicated studies have found such attentional disturbances in euthymic subjects with bipolar disorder (Bearden et al., 2001; Martinez-Aran et al., 2004).

### SUSTAINED ATTENTION: HEALTHY FUNCTIONING

One of the most common tests of attention is the continuous performance task (CPT). However, perhaps because there are many variations of the CPT task that also tap other realms of executive function, such as working memory and affective processing, relatively few imaging studies of bipolar disorder have utilized CPT tasks despite the fact that attentional problems are defining symptoms of both mania and depression (reviewed by Bearden et al., 2001). In healthy populations, focused attention is associated with increased activation throughout the frontal lobe including anterior cingulate, bilateral dorsolateral prefrontal cortex (BA46/9), bilateral orbitofrontal cortex (BA47) and medial frontal gyrus (BA11/10) (Nebel et al., 2005). In a meta-analysis of attention studies, which included both fMRI and PET studies, other areas involved in attention included left occipital (BA19) and bilateral inferior parietal cortex

(BA40/7) (Wager, Jonides, & Reading, 2004). Neuropsychological studies have found significant impairment in measures of attention in subjects with bipolar disorder while manic (Gruber et al., 2007; Malhi et al., 2007), depressed (Malhi, et al., 2007) and euthymic (Depp et al., 2007). The fMRI studies of attention are currently limited to mania and euthymia.

## SUSTAINED ATTENTION: MANIA

There are only two fMRI studies using paradigms of attention in subjects with bipolar disorder during mania. Both used the CPT, but with different variations. One used the identical-pairs form of the task (CPT-IP), which uses numbers as stimuli and, as such, is perhaps a more pure form of an attention task. In this study, manic subjects showed significant reductions in regions known to be involved in attention in healthy populations. Specifically, manic subjects (n = 50) demonstrated significantly less activation in the left striatum, left thalamus, and bilateral IFG over time compared to healthy subjects (Fleck et al., 2010). Interesting, even while using numbers as a nonemotional stimuli, manic subjects showed significant hyperactivation of the left amygdala. This finding is consistent with reports of left amygdala hyperactivation during mania while performing tasks of emotion processing (discussed above). The second study of attention in mania used the both neutral and emotional distracters (CPT-END). Using an ROI approach, manic subjects again showed blunted activation across bilateral ventrolateral and dorsolateral prefrontal cortex when responding to emotional and neutral images; blunted responses in anterior cingulate were also observed to neutral images (Strakowski et al., 2011). This finding suggests that manic subjects show impairment in engaging both the ventral (emotional) and dorsal (cognitive) neural processing regions. This finding was true even after accounting for medication exposure and alcohol and drug abuse history (Strakowski et al., 2011).

## SUSTAINED ATTENTION: DEPRESSION

There are currently no fMRI studies of attention in depressed subjects with bipolar disorder.

## SUSTAINED ATTENTION: EUTHYMIA

The study of attention in euthymia is limited to one relatively small preliminary study that used the CPT-IP. In this study, researchers found that unmedicated euthymic subjects with bipolar disorder have significantly less activation in the left medial frontal gyrus, consistent with findings in subjects during mania (Strakowski et al., 2004) (Figure 3.4). However, unlike manic subjects, there was significantly greater activation in bilateral ventral PFC (BA10/47) in euthymic compared to healthy subjects. Euthymic bipolar disorder subjects also had significantly greater activation in the left amygdala and parahippocampal regions, consistent with findings from the CPT-IP study of mania, despite the fact that the stimuli were numbers. This observation suggests that during a cognitive task, subjects with bipolar disorder continue to engage affective networks. This finding is consistent with studies that show strong emotional states interfere with attention (Yamasaki, LaBar, & McCarthy, 2002) and that processing of emotion requires attention resources (Pessoa, Kastner, & Ungerleider, 2002). This engagement of affective networks during a nonemotional task may explain the impairments in attention reported across mood states in bipolar disorder.

## SUSTAINED ATTENTION: CONCLUSIONS

Hypoactivation of brain regions implicated in attention has been seen in a very small number of studies in both manic and euthymic subjects with bipolar disorder. This finding is consistent with the neurocognitive literature showing functional impairments in attention during mania and euthymia. One potential confound when examining attention problems in bipolar disorder is comorbidity with attention-deficit hyperactivity disorder (ADHD), which occurs in 9.5%–19.4% of subjects with bipolar disorder (Kessler et al., 2006; Nierenberg et al., 2005). This confound is especially problematic since ADHD is not diagnosed as part of the Structured Clinical Interview for DSM-IV [SCID] (First MB, 2002), the most frequently used diagnostic tool for assessment. Moreover, attentional problems in childhood interact with the later development of bipolar disorder, since early attention problems that preceded unipolar depression or no mood disorder were not associated

---

**fMRI of Sustained Attention in Bipolar Disorder Suggests:**

- Ventrolateral prefrontal cortical hypofunction during mania and euthymia

- Amygdala hyperactivation to nonemotional cues during mania

- No studies during bipolar depression

- More studies are needed across all three mood states

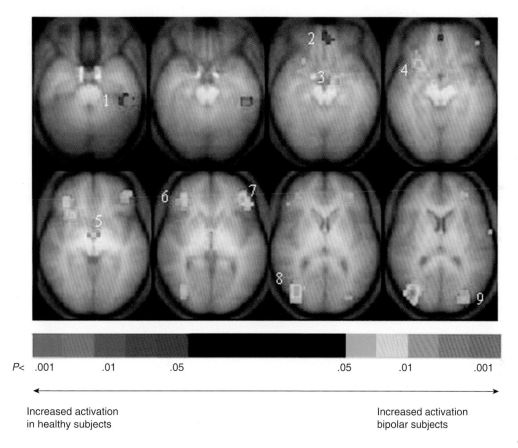

P< .001 .01 .05 .05 .01 .001

Increased activation
in healthy subjects

Increased activation
bipolar subjects

*Figure 3.4* Difference images displaying differences in brain activation between healthy subjects and euthymic subjects with bipolar disorder while performing an attentional task (CPT-IP). Areas in which healthy subjects exhibited greater activation are in blue tones and include: (1) left fusiform gyrus (BA 20) and (2) left medial frontal cortex (BA 11). Areas in which subjects with bipolar disorder exhibited greater activation are in yellow/green/ red hues and include: (3) left parahippocampus/amygdala (BA 34), (4) right inferior frontal cortex/insula (BA 13, 47), (5) hypothalamus, (6 and 7) bilateral ventral prefrontal cortex (BA 10, 47), and (8 and 9) bilateral mid-occipital/mid-temporal cortex (BA 18, 19, 39). Images are in radiological convention. (Source: Strakowski et al. 2004).

with executive dysfunction (Meyer et al., 2004). This observation also highlights that problems in attention are frequently associated with problems in other areas of executive function in euthymic bipolar disorder subjects.

## RESPONSE INHIBITION

The inferior frontal cortex (IFC) is involved in the modulation or inhibition of a range of impulsive behaviors. The IFC consists of the pars opercularis (Brodmann's Area (BA) 44), pars triangularis (BA45), and pars orbitalis (BA47). Animal studies demonstrated that lesions to the IFC resulted in increased perseverative interference motor activity, supporting a role for this region in the inhibition of movement (Iversen & Mishkin, 1970). Furthermore, lesions to this area in human subjects may result in dramatic behavioral changes resembling mania, including hyperactivity, elevated mood, disinhibition and reckless behavior (Starkstein et al., 1991).

## RESPONSE INHIBITION: HEALTHY FUNCTIONING

Impulsivity in healthy subjects is modulated by IFC, with greater impulsivity associated with attenuated IFC activity (Horn et al., 2003). The IFC, anterior cingulate, and striatal structures are part of the frontostrial network that has been shown to be activated in fMRI studies of motor and inhibition in healthy subjects (Cabeza & Nyberg, 2000; Horn et al., 2003).

Previous fMRI studies in healthy subjects using response inhibition paradigms like the GoNoGo and Stop Signal task have shown activation primarily in the right IFC, subthalamic nucleus (STN) and pre-supplementary motor area (pre-SMA) (Simmonds et al., 2008). Results of such studies and more recent connectivity studies (Aron, 2007) led to the proposal that the response inhibition results from interactions between the IFC, STN and pre-SMA. That is, activation of this fronto-basal-ganglia circuitry acts to facilitate inhibition of responses that have already been initiated, such as in the "NoGo" condition. Specifically, the right IFC

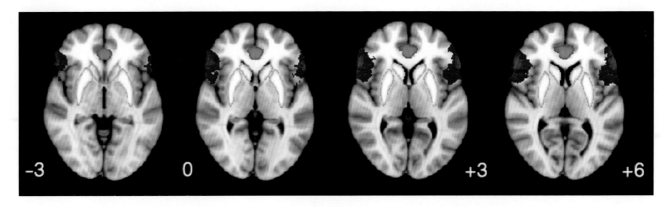

Figure 3.5 The inferior frontal cortex (blue), anterior cingulate (green) and striatum (pink), shown based on the Harvard-Oxford cortical and subcortical probabilistic atlas, are consistently activated in response inhibition studies of healthy populations.

has been posited to block execution of a "Go" response via the basal ganglia. Activation of the STN activates globus pallidus. This leads to response suppression, through increasing GABAergic (inhibitory) effects of pallidal neurons on the thalamus. Suppression of thalamic response, in turn, leads to a suppression (or lack of stimulation) of motor cortex, which is necessary to block the "Go" response (Aron, 2007). Figure 3.5 illustrates these considerations.

Studies suggest that even when subjects with bipolar disorder are euthymic, trait impulsivity remains elevated (Strakowski et al., 2010; Swann et al., 2001). Whether this may be associated with continued neural impairment in IFC function has been examined by a number of neuroimaging studies in subjects with bipolar disorder in all three mood states.

## RESPONSE INHIBITION: MANIA

One of the central features of mania is an inability to modulate or inhibit undesired responses, even in the face of negative consequences (DSM-IV) (First MB, 2002). Several studies have shown blunted IFC activation in subjects with bipolar disorder during mania (Altshuler et al., 2005; Blumberg et al., 2003; Blumberg et al., 1999; Mazzola-Pomietto et al., 2009). Two of these studies used a GoNoGo task and both found significantly decreased activation of bilateral IFC (BA47) in subjects during mania regardless of whether the paradigm design was block (Altshuler et al., 2005) or event-related (Mazzola-Pomietto et al., 2009). In the latter study, this hypoactivation of IFC persisted even while controlling for medication status. Another study also found significant reduction in bilateral IFC during an emotional GoNoGo task (Elliott et al., 2004). Attenuated activation in this frontal region that is

responsible for motor response and inhibition may help to explain the increased motor activity and reduced inhibition of mania, which is consistent with the reports of hypoactivation of the IFC in mania across a range of executive function tasks.

The IFC has extensive connections with other regions important for response inhibition such as anterior cingulate, striatum and motor/somatosensory cortex, and each of these regions has demonstrated abnormal activation during mania. One study using the GoNoGo task found reduced activation in subjects during mania in bilateral putamen compared to healthy subjects; this hypoactivation of putamen resolved once these subjects were remitted and evaluated while euthymic (Kaladjian, Jeanningros, Azorin, Nazarian, Roth, Anton et al., 2009). This finding provides some evidence that abnormalities seen in the striatum during mania may be state-related. Using the Stop Signal task, another study found reduced activation in bilateral thalamus and anterior cingulate in first-episode mania subjects, suggesting that this hypoactivation is not due to length of illness or prior number of episodes (Strakowski et al., 2008). This finding of reduced activation in the anterior cingulate during mania has been reported now in two studies of response inhibition (Altshuler et al., 2005; Strakowski et al., 2008) and one study of attention (Strakowski et al., 2011). All six studies of motor and response inhibition in mania found dysfunction of the frontostriatal circuit. It is interesting to note that a few studies of response inhibition in mania have found significantly increased amygdala activation compared to euthymic subjects (Kaladjian, Jeanningros, Azorin, Nazarian, Roth, Anton et al., 2009) and in unmedicated compared to medicated subjects during mania (Strakowski et al., 2008), despite the fact that the amygdala is not normally activated in motor or response inhibition tasks. This finding is consistent with the suggestion that the hypoactivation of the frontal lobe, in particular the OFC, may lead to overactive limbic structures such as amygdala, even in the absence of emotion processing.

## RESPONSE INHIBITION: DEPRESSION

Only three studies of motor and response inhibition have been conducted with depressed subjects with bipolar disorder, and they suffer collectively from additional confounds that are not present in the mania literature. Two of the three studies include both bipolar disorder type I and type II subjects (Caligiuri et al., 2003; Chen et al., 2006), and the third study included only men (Marchand et al., 2007). Nevertheless, these studies provided evidence of dysfunction in the frontostriatal circuit as well. Both Caligiuri et al. (2003) and Marchand et al. (2007), using motor tasks, found hyperactivation of the motor/somatosensory cortex in bipolar depressed compared to healthy subjects. This observation was consistent with the findings during mania (Caligiuri et al., 2003). Unlike during mania, though, subjects with bipolar depression showed increased (rather than decreased) activation in bilateral striatum, centered on caudate and anterior cingulate (Marchand et al., 2007). This observation suggests that increased activation in striatum and anterior cingulate may be state-related to bipolar depression, while other findings, such as increased motor and somatosensory cortex activation, may be associated with both acute mood states.

## RESPONSE INHIBITION: EUTHYMIA

Three studies examined response inhibition in subjects with bipolar disorder while euthymic, two using a basic GoNoGo task (Kaladjian, Jeanningros, Azorin, Nazarian, Roth, Anton et al., 2009; Kaladjian Jeanningros, Azorin, Nazarian, Roth, & Mazzola-Pomietto et al., 2009) and the third using both nonemotional and emotional GoNoGo tasks (Wessa et al., 2007). Consistent with findings in subjects during mania, Kaladijian et al. (2009) found reduced activation in bilateral striatum, specifically in putamen, in euthymic subjects with bipolar disorder compared to healthy subjects. In a larger sample of euthymic subjects with bipolar disorder, Kaladijian et al. (2009) found reduced left frontal activation (BA10). This BA10 region is part of the network activated during tasks requiring inhibition including the GoNoGo (Kelly et al., 2004) and the Stop Signal (Li et al., 2008) and has been shown to be important for the ability to hold in mind primary goals while processing secondary goals or response selection demands (Badre

& Wagner, 2004; Petrides, 2005). The authors interpreted hypoactivation of this frontopolar region during the GoNoGo task as euthymic subjects with bipolar disorder showing less efficiency in response inhibition (Sakai & Passingham, 2006). The third study of euthymic subjects bipolar disorder, combining both bipolar disorder I and II subjects, found no significant differences between euthymic and healthy subjects when including all GoNoGo vs. rest conditions (Wessa et al., 2007). However, during the emotional GoNoGo component, which required both response inhibition and emotion processing, euthymic bipolar disorder subjects showed significantly greater activation in bilateral frontopolar regions, anterior cingulate, left insula, and bilateral caudate than did healthy subjects. The conflicting frontopolar cortex results, with both decreases (Kaladjian Jeanningros, Azorin, Nazarian, Roth, & Mazzola-Pomietto et al., 2009) and increases (Wessa et al., 2007) being reported, may be due to different task demands with an additional emotion processing component or to the more heterogeneous patient population in the latter study. Wessa et al.'s (2007) findings of increased anterior cingulate and bilateral caudate activation during euthymia are consistent with findings during bipolar depression (Marchand et al., 2007), suggesting that some of these neural abnormalities do not completely resolve during euthymia. Furthermore, frontostriatal dysfunction seen in euthymia may provide a neural explanation for the continued problems in response inhibition even in the absence of an acute mood state (Strakowski et al., 2010; Swann et al., 2001).

---

**fMRI of Response Inhibition in Bipolar Disorder Suggests:**

· Reduced ventrolateral prefrontal activation during mania

· Variable findings in the striatum, with decreased caudate activation reported in both mania and euthymia

· Increased motor/pre-motor activity in mania and depression

· State-dependent findings in the anterior cingulate with decreased activation during mania and increased activation during depression

---

## INTERFERENCE

Cognitive interference tasks, such as the Stroop, have been used to measure executive function, specifically selective attention and inhibition of automatic responses. During the classic Stroop task, there are conflicts between the meaning of words and the color of the ink (i.e., the word "blue" is written in red ink). The Stroop task is used widely as an index of executive control and attention since subjects must actively inhibit the automatic response (word reading) to engage a more controlled, conscious response (color naming). As subjects with bipolar disorder show impaired function in measures of both attention and inhibition (Bearden et al., 2001 for review), many neuroimaging studies used various permutations of the Stroop task to evaluate the possible neural underpinnings of the neurocognitive deficits reported.

## INTERFERENCE: HEALTHY FUNCTIONING

In healthy populations, the classic color-word Stroop task robustly activates the anterior cingulate (BA24/32) and dorsolateral prefrontal cortex (DLPFC; BA46/9) (Bush et al., 1998; Gruber et al., 2002; Peterson et al., 1999). A meta-analysis of Stroop tasks showed significant activation in the anterior cingulate, premotor cortex, left middle temporal gyrus, right supramarginal gyrus and precuneous (Minzenberg et al., 2009), with especially consistent activations being reported in the anterior cingulate and parietal cortex (Cabeza & Nyberg, 2000). The anterior cingulate has a role in emotional and cognitive processing, and the cognitive subdivision has strong reciprocal connections between the DLPFC, parietal cortex and premotor and supplementary motor areas (Carter et al., 1998; Devinsky, Morrell, & Vogt, 1995). The cognitive anterior cingulate appears to activate during cognitive conflict resolution.

## INTERFERENCE: MANIA

Despite the fact that subjects during mania show significant impairments in attention and inhibition, and they perform worse than healthy subjects on the Stroop task (Clark et al., 2001), only one study to date examined subjects during mania using fMRI and the Stroop task. Using the classic color-word Stroop task, these subjects showed significantly less activation in the right ventral prefrontal cortex (BA47) compared to euthymic subjects with bipolar disorder and significantly less activation in the left ventral prefrontal cortex (BA47/10) compared to healthy subjects (Blumberg et al., 2003). This reduced activation in the left ventral prefrontal cortex was trait-related and present in subjects with bipolar disorder across all three mood states. This finding suggests that neurocognitive deficits seen during interferences tasks may be caused by this deficit.

## INTERFERENCE: DEPRESSION

Two studies examined performance on the classic color-naming Stroop task in depressed subjects with bipolar disorder (Blumberg et al., 2003; Marchand et al., 2007). Consistent with findings in mania, subjects with bipolar depression showed reduced activation in left ventral prefrontal cortex (BA47/19) compared to healthy subjects. In comparison to subjects with bipolar disorder during mania and euthymia, the subjects with bipolar depression showed increased activation in the left OFC (BA11) (Blumberg et al., 2003). The second study, using only men, found reduced activation in the posterior cingulate and in the occipital lobe (Marchand et al., 2007) in subjects with bipolar depression compared to healthy subjects. As these regions are not the primary regions engaged during an interference task like the Stroop and because the study included only males, it is more difficult to interpret these results. However, decreased activation in the posterior cingulate and occipital lobe is consistent with another study using the counting Stroop task to examine group differences between subjects with bipolar disorder, irrespective of mood state, and healthy subjects (Roth et al., 2006). The authors suggested that these findings may represent a failure to activate brain regions needed for cognitive interference tasks (Marchand et al., 2007), and this hypothesis is consistent with hypoactivation of brain regions implicated in this task and others.

## INTERFERENCE: EUTHYMIA

Most studies of interference have examined subjects with bipolar disorder during euthymia to investigate the neural underpinnings of attention and inhibition problems associated with the trait of bipolar disorder rather than acute mood states, since neuropsychological studies show persistent deficits in the Stroop task during euthymia (Bearden et al., 2001). Of the seven studies using interference tasks in subjects with bipolar disorder, the most consistent finding is reduced activation in the ventral prefrontal cortex in the subjects with bipolar disorder compared to healthy subjects. Four of the seven studies, using emotional, counting, and color-word Stroop tasks, found hypoactivation of the left (Blumberg et al., 2003; Kronhaus et al., 2006; Lagopoulos & Malhi, 2007) and right ventral prefrontal cortex (Strakowski et al., 2005). One of the studies examined structural correlates of these neurocognitive deficits and found that healthy subjects showed a positive correlation in grey matter density in the dorsal and ventral prefrontal cortex with performance on the Stroop task that did not occur in euthymic subjects with bipolar disorder (Haldane et al., 2008). Subjects with bipolar disorder had reduced grey matter density in bilateral ventral prefrontal cortex (Haldane et al., 2008), which may explain the functional hypoactivation in this region reported in the majority of these fMRI studies.

In the dorsolateral prefrontal cortex, studies are inconsistent, with two studies finding reduced activation in subjects with bipolar disorder (Kronhaus et al., 2006; Lagopoulos & Malhi, 2007), one study finding increased activation (Gruber, Rogowska, & Yurgelun-Todd, 2004) and three finding no difference between subjects with bipolar disorder and healthy subjects (Blumberg et al., 2003; Malhi et al., 2005; Strakowski et al., 2005). Some of these differences may be explained by the variety of stimuli used (i.e., emotional vs. nonemotional), the small sample sizes (i.e., most used 12 or fewer subjects), and the effects of medication. One study that specifically looked at the difference between medicated and unmedicated euthymic subjects with bipolar disorder found that medicated subjects had greater activation than unmedicated in dorsolateral prefrontal cortex (Strakowski et al., 2005).

Euthymic subjects with bipolar disorder demonstrated hypoactivation in the anterior cingulate, which is normally activated in interference tasks (Gruber et al., 2002) and plays a role in conflict monitoring (Botvinick, Cohen, & Carter, 2004). Gruber et al. (2004) found reduced activation specifically in the attention to action area (AAA), but not the more rostral vocalization area (VOA), of the anterior cingulate. The anterior cingulate can be subdivided between the affective (more rostral-ventral), and the cognitive (more dorsal), with the cognitive division being activated by Stroop tasks and deactivated during emotional tasks in healthy subjects (Bush et al., 1998; Devinsky et al., 1995). Gruber et al. (2004) found reduced activation in this cognitive division and Kronhaus et al. (2006) found increased activation in the affective division in euthymic

subjects with bipolar disorder. These observations suggest that the typical engagement of the cognitive division of the anterior cingulate is compromised by increased engagements of the affective division in subjects with bipolar disorder during a nonemotional Stroop task.

Finally, there is evidence of increased striatal activation in subjects with bipolar disorder. Two studies report significantly increased activation in the left (Strakowski et al., 2005) and right (Malhi et al., 2005; Strakowski et al., 2005) putamen, using two different versions of the Stroop task. Strakowski et al. (Strakowski et al., 2005) also found increased activation in the right caudate and right thalamus in euthymic subjects with bipolar disorder compared with healthy subjects, perhaps due to increased engagement of the motor network. However, four of the Stroop studies did not find evidence of differential striatal activation between healthy and euthymic subjects with bipolar disorder (Blumberg et al., 2003; Gruber et al., 2004; Kronhaus et al., 2006; Lagopoulos & Malhi, 2007), suggesting that these functional abnormalities warrant further study.

## WORKING MEMORY

### WORKING MEMORY: HEALTHY FUNCTIONING

Two consistent functional neuroimaging findings of working memory in healthy populations are activation of the dorsolateral prefrontal cortex (dlPFC) (BA9/46) and of the inferior, posterior parietal cortex (BA 39/40); the inferior frontal gyrus is also often involved (IFG; BA 47/44) (Belger et al., 1998; Cohen et al., 1997; Curtis, 2006; Smith & Jonides, 1998). These areas are part of the cognitive control network, defined by functional connectivity and described by Cole and Schneider (2007).

### WORKING MEMORY: MANIA

Many neuropsychological studies have documented working memory impairments in subjects with bipolar disorder during manic and depressed states (Bearden et al., 2001; Clark et al., 2001). It is possible that the working memory deficits in subjects with bipolar disorder implicate dysfunction in the dlPFC or posterior parietal cortex in these subjects. Despite the fact that subjects with bipolar disorder show significant impairment in working memory during mania (Martinez-Aran et al., 2004), only one fMRI study to date examined subjects during mania performing a working memory task. This study used the classic n-back task and found reduced activation in right dlPFC (BA46/9)

---

**fMRI of Interference Tasks (e.g., Stroop) in Bipolar Disorder Suggests:**

- Increased striatal activation during euthymia, typically left putamen

- Trait ventrolateral prefrontal hypoactivation, especially in the left hemisphere, across mood states

- More studies are needed during mania and bipolar depression

---

and right parietal cortex (BA40) in subjects during mania compared with healthy subjects (Townsend at al., 2010). Hypoactivation of these areas implicated in working memory was seen in subjects with bipolar disorder across all three mood states, which suggests a trait deficit in these areas (Townsend et al., 2010).

## WORKING MEMORY: DEPRESSION

Similar to mania, there have been few fMRI studies of working memory in bipolar depression. Townsend et al. (2010) found reduced activation in right dlPFC and right parietal cortex in subjects with bipolar depression and found that these abnormalities were seen in subjects with bipolar disorder during mania, depression, and euthymia; there were no significant differences among the three mood states. The other study of working memory in subjects with bipolar depression also used an n-back task, but added the component of sad, neutral or no mood induction. The authors found no significant differences in dlPFC activation in the no mood induction condition and increased left dlPFC and anterior cingulate activation in subjects with bipolar depression only during sad mood induction (Deckersbach et al., 2008). The age differences of subjects in these two studies, with decreased dlPFC observed using older subjects (average age in late thirties) and no significant difference seen in relatively younger subjects (average age late twenties) may explain some of the inconsistencies of these findings. In healthy populations, older subjects show less dlPFC activation than younger subjects during higher memory load (Cappell, Gmeindl, & Reuter-Lorenz, 2010). It is also possible that the latter study suffered from a lack of power to detect significant findings in either the dlPFC or parietal cortex. Further studies are needed to investigate these possibilities.

## WORKING MEMORY: EUTHYMIA

Euthymic subjects with bipolar disorder have been reported to perform significantly worse than healthy subjects on measures of executive function, including working memory (Altshuler et al., 2004; Depp et al., 2007; Trivedi et al., 2008). Persistent neurocognitive abnormalities in euthymic subjects may provide clues to brain areas underlying trait pathology in the illness. In contract to the paucity of studies investigating working memory during the acute mood states, there have been nine studies of euthymic subjects with bipolar disorder. Of these nine studies, three found significantly decreased activation in right dlPFC (Lagopoulos, Ivanovski, & Malhi, 2007; Monks et al., 2004;

Townsend et al., 2010), one found a trend of less activation in right dlPFC (Hamilton et al., 2009) and one found less activation in right dlPFC during the recall portion of a working memory task (Glahn et al., 2010). The remaining four found no significant differences in dlPFC, but two of these studies included bipolar disorder I and II subjects (Adler, Holland, Schmithorst, Tuchfarber et al., 2004; Gruber et al., 2010) and a third used only seven subjects, and as such, may have been underpowered (Frangou et al., 2008). Reduction in right dlPFC activation was the most consistent finding. Working memory tasks activate bilateral frontal and parietal regions, yet there is a laterality effect with the right hemisphere as predominant regardless of stimulus type (Nystrom et al., 2000). In this regard, it is interesting that the major differences between subjects with bipolar disorder and healthy subjects were found in the right hemisphere. The abnormal neurophysiologic pattern in this region, specifically the less robust right-sided dorsal frontal activation in bipolar disorder, may relate to the working memory impairment previously reported (Altshuler et al., 2004; Clark et al., 2001; Depp et al., 2007; Rubinsztein et al., 2006).

The findings in parietal cortex are less consistent in euthymia. Studies found increased left (Monks et al., 2004), decreased right (Townsend et al., 2010), and no significant differences in inferior parietal cortex (BA39/40) (Adler, Holland, Schmithorst, Tuchfarber et al., 2004; Drapier et al., 2008; Glahn et al., 2010; Gruber et al., 2010; Hamilton et al., 2009; Lagopoulos et al., 2007). One study found a unique effect of increased memory load in BA40/39 in euthymic subjects with bipolar disorder (Frangou et al., 2008), suggesting that some of the discrepancies in the literature might be explained by differences in task design and difficulty. In the posterior parietal lobe, consisting of the lingual gyrus and precuneous, the results are also inconsistent. Most studies did find significant differences in the posterior parietal lobe, but differed on the direction of the findings. Studies found both hyperactivation (Adler, Holland, Schmithorst, Tuchfarber et al., 2004; Drapier et al., 2008; Gruber et al., 2010) and hypoactivation (Hamilton et al., 2009; Lagopoulos et al., 2007; Monks et al., 2004) in euthymic subjects with bipolar disorder, utilizing a variety of working memory tasks including the N-back, Sternberg and delayed matched to sample tasks.

Decreased activation in the cingulate was also reported consistently, both in anterior (Lagopoulos et al., 2007; Monks et al., 2004) and posterior regions (Adler, Holland, Schmithorst, Tuchfarber et al., 2004). Decreased activation in euthymic subjects with bipolar disorder was also seen in the hippocampus and parahippocampus during both the delay (Lagopoulos et al., 2007) and recall (Glahn et al., 2010) processes of working memory. The cingulate and hippocampus/parahippocampus have functional interconnections (Stein et al., 2007) and have been implicated in a variety of working memory studies (for review, see (Wager & Smith, 2003).

Heightened activation in temporal lobe structures was observed in subjects with bipolar disorder that was not observed in the healthy group while performing this task (Townsend et al., 2010). Lagopoulos et al. (2007) and Adler et al. (Adler, Holland, Schmithorst, Tuchfarber et al., 2004) similarly found engagement of temporal lobe activation in the subjects with bipolar disorder when performing the working memory task. Thus, three studies that used fMRI to assess frontal lobe activation during a working memory task found that limbic/temporal lobe structures are activated in subjects with bipolar disorder during a task that does not normally activate these brain regions. Euthymic subjects with bipolar disorder show impairment on tests of visuospatial recognition memory, which implicates temporal lobe dysfunction (Rubinsztein et al., 2000), and temporal lobe hyperactivity may explain these neurocognitive deficits in verbal memory. Other imaging studies in subjects with bipolar disorder suggested limbic hyperactivity even during euthymia (Gruber et al., 2010; Lawrence et al., 2004; Yurgelun-Todd et al., 2000) across a variety of tasks. Whether this represents a compensatory mechanism or a chronically hyperactive brain region in bipolar illness remains to be further studied.

---

**fMRI of Working Memory in Bipolar Disorder Suggests:**

- Increased frontopolar activation and decreased hippocampus/parahippocampus in euthymia

- Trait dlPFC hypofunction, with right lateralization most commonly reported, across all three mood states

- Trait parietal hypoactivation across all three mood states

- More studies are needed during mania and depression

---

## FLUENCY

### FLUENCY: HEALTHY FUNCTIONING

Neuropsychological tasks, such as verbal fluency, provide another means by which to measure frontal lobe function. Such tasks, which typically use semantic or phonetic fluency, robustly activate frontal regions including Broca's area (BA44/45) in the left inferior frontal gyrus, as well as a more distributed network that includes dorsolateral prefrontal cortex (BA46/9), inferior frontal gyrus (BA47), supplemental motor area (BA6), and medial prefrontal cortex (BA10/6/8) in healthy populations (Amunts, Schleicher, & Zilles, 2004; Fu et al., 2002; Schlosser et al., 1998). Verbal fluency is used as a sensitive indicator of frontal lobe function (Schlosser et al., 1998). In one meta-analysis of studies involving subjects with bipolar disorder, impairments in executive function and verbal memory were proposed as endophenotypes for bipolar disorder, as abnormalities in these measures were seen in euthymic subjects across a range of studies and were also seen in first-degree relatives that are likely carrying susceptibility genes (Arts et al., 2008). Arts et al. (2008) found that verbal fluency has a relatively large effect size, and therefore investigating functional neural abnormalities using verbal fluency tasks may provide additional insight into regions of the brain that are implicated in bipolar disorder. Another review (Balanza-Martinez et al., 2008) also concluded that deficits in verbal learning and working memory were the most consistently reported neurocognitive abnormalities in bipolar disorder across mood states. These neurocognitive abnormalities may be due to underlying neurofunctional deficits in brain regions that serve these functions.

### FLUENCY: MANIA AND DEPRESSION

Despite the fact that persons in acute mood states frequently present with abnormalities in verbal fluency, including alteration in the speed, flow and content of their speech, there have been no fMRI studies of verbal fluency in subjects with bipolar disorder while either manic or depressed. This area needs future study.

### FLUENCY: EUTHYMIA

Three studies used fMRI to investigate verbal performance in euthymic subjects with bipolar disorder. One study of euthymic men with bipolar I disorder examined verbal decision making and fluency across phonetic and semantic domains and found widespread hyperactivation in both left ventromedial and dorsolateral prefrontal cortex (dlPFC) and in bilateral lingual gyri of the occipital lobe (Curtis et al., 2001). Hyperactivation of the left inferior frontal gyrus (IFG) in subjects with bipolar disorder was consistent with an earlier study that looked at a smaller sample of men with bipolar disorder, but did not report their mood state (Curtis et al., 2001). Another study using the Hayling Sentence Completion Test also found increased activation in the left IFG and left dlPFC in euthymic subjects with bipolar disorder compared to healthy subjects as task difficulty increased (McIntosh et al., 2008). However, a third study of verbal fluency in euthymic subjects with bipolar disorder, using a word generation task, found decreased activation in the left IFG compared to healthy subjects in the easy, but not difficult condition (Allin et al., 2010). These results suggest that, depending on the task design and difficulty, the direction of differences in activation may vary. Yet it is interesting to note that all three studies of verbal fluency in euthymic subjects with bipolar disorder showed abnormal activation in left IFG (Allin et al., 2010; V. A. Curtis et al., 2007; McIntosh et al., 2008). One study of verbal fluency using a combined group of depressed and euthymic subjects with bipolar disorder found decreased activation of left IFG, left precentral gyrus, and supplemental motor areas after treatment with lithium (Silverstone et al., 2005), suggesting that medications may affect these regions and may explain the discrepancies in the literature.

---

**fMRI of Verbal Fluency in Bipolar Disorder Suggests:**

- Hyperactivation of dlPFC and lingual gyrus during euthymia

- Hyperactivation of IFG during euthymia and depression, with left lateralization most commonly reported

- No studies have been performed during mania

- More studies are needed, especially in the acute mood states

---

## EXECUTIVE FUNCTION CONCLUSION

Deficits in executive function have been reported across mood states and are present in unaffected relatives who are likely carrying genes rendering susceptibility for the disorder. As such, it has been suggested that executive function deficits may represent an endophenotype for bipolar disorder (Arts et al., 2008). Bora, Yucel and Pantelis (2009) concluded from a meta-analysis that executive function deficits are consistently reported in remitted subjects with bipolar disorder and their first-degree relatives, and that response inhibition deficits show the largest effect size.

Understanding the neural correlates of diminished executive function is important, as these deficits in the cognitive domain have been associated with impaired overall psychosocial functioning (Martinez-Aran et al., 2004). Executive function impairments, though, are not specific to bipolar disorder. Subjects with bipolar disorder have demonstrated significantly better performance than individuals with schizophrenia on measures of executive function, but significantly worse than healthy subjects (Altshuler et al., 2004; Dickerson et al., 2004). Supporting the idea that executive functioning impairment is trait- rather than state-dependent, studies found that subjects with bipolar disorder across mood states showed cognitive dysfunction in frontal executive tasks compared to healthy subjects (Goswami et al., 2006; Martinez-Aran et al., 2004). While first-episode bipolar disorder subjects show this impairment, it is positively correlated with the number of mood episodes (Nehra et al., 2006). These deficits in executive function have been shown to be negatively correlated with the number of mood episodes, suggesting declining executive function during the course of bipolar disorder (Goswami et al., 2006). The cross-sectional nature of these studies, though, precludes determination of causality.

Neuroimaging studies of executive function suggest that impairment in executive function may be associated with abnormal neural activation of the frontal lobe. Studies of attention and response inhibition found decreased activation in inferior frontal regions across mood states, again suggesting a neural trait-related finding. Results in anterior cingulate, however, appear to depend on mood state, with heightened activation reported during euthymia or depression and attenuated activation associated with mania. Striatal results are more ambiguous and appear to depend on both mood state and task. Consistent with hypoactivation in the frontal lobe, many studies using interference tasks like the Stroop found decreased activation in ventrolateral prefrontal cortex (BA44/45/47) across mood states. Hypoactivation of this region was the most consistent abnormality seen in subjects with bipolar disorder across mood states and tasks, as it was seen in attention, response inhibition, and interference tasks. Decreases in dorsolateral prefrontal function were also widely reported across mood states in studies of executive function, particularly in studies of attention and working memory. Other regional activations associated with executive function were either less consistent across studies or changed in direction depending on mood state. Finally, subjects with bipolar disorder showed hyperactivation of limbic structures during executive function tasks. This abnormality was seen in studies of attention and response inhibition, in which there is usually not a significant recruitment of these structures in healthy subjects. This finding may represent an abnormal recruitment of or interference from affective regions during cognitive tasks.

## RESTING STATE

Some recent fMRI studies of bipolar disorder have focused on imaging the brain during the resting state, without any mental or emotional task. During such scanning sessions, subjects are asked to remain awake, but are otherwise given no explicit task to perform. The benefit of these task-independent studies is that they do not suffer from the same difficulties with design and task performance as most of the current fMRI literature of bipolar disorder.

## RESTING STATE: HEALTHY FUNCTIONING

The spontaneous neural or "default" activity of the brain at rest in healthy populations has been extensively studied. Most studies used either a hypothesis driven regions of interest analysis (seed-based correlation) or a model-free analysis (independent component analysis) to look at patterns of connectivity. There are eight common resting-state networks (RSN) that have been identified in healthy populations, and they are: 1) primary visual, 2) extrastriate visual, 3) auditory and other sensory association cortex, 4) somato-motor cortex, 5) default-mode network (deactivation during cognitive tasks), 6) executive control and salience processing, 7) left-lateralized frontal-parietal, and 8) right lateralized frontal-parietal RSNs (see D. M. Cole et al., 2010 for review). The executive control and salience processing and left-lateralized and right-lateralized frontal-parietal RSNs are particularly interesting as they consist of regions in the frontal and parietal lobes that have been implicated as functioning abnormally in studies of subjects with bipolar disorder using various cognitive tasks.

## RESTING STATE: BIPOLAR DISORDER AND MANIA, DEPRESSION, EUTHYMIA

To date, only three resting state studies have been performed in subjects with bipolar disorder and none have selectively involved subjects in only one mood state. Two used traditional fMRI BOLD sequences to look at the default mode in subjects with bipolar disorder (Anand et al., 2009; Chepenik et al., 2010) and one used a perfusion-weighted imaging sequence to calculate cerebral blood volume (Agarwal et al., 2008). All three studies utilized region-of-interest or seed-based methods, rather than independent component analysis, and included subjects in a variety of mood states (i.e., depressed, mixed, manic/hypomanic, and euthymic). Anand et al. (2009) found that subjects with bipolar disorder (including both manic and depressed subjects) had significantly less functional connectivity than

healthy subjects during resting state between the pregenual anterior cingulate (pgACC) and bilateral dorsomedial thalamus, bilateral amygdala, and left pallidostriatum. This study provided additional evidence of decreased corticolimbic functional connectivity, even in the absence of acute emotional or cognitive demands. Similarly, evidence for decreased corticolimbic connectivity was also reported by Chepenik et al. (2010). Using low frequency resting state fMRI, the authors found reduced functional connectivity between the left ventral prefrontal cortex and left amygdala in five manic, two depressed, and eight euthymic subjects with bipolar disorder (Chepenik et al., 2010). These findings are consistent with prior findings from our group using an activation task (affective faces) that demonstrated reduced connectivity in left ventral prefrontal cortex and left amygdala (Foland et al., 2008).

Subjects with bipolar disorder also showed reduced connectivity between left ventral and dorsal prefrontal corices and parietal cortex compared to healthy subjects (Chepenik et al., 2010)and increased interhemispheric connectivity between the left and right ventral prefrontal cortex, including regions of the anterior cingulate and ventral striatum (Chepenik et al., 2010). The final study of resting state in bipolar disorder used perfusion weighted imaging with a contrast agent (gadolinium-DTPA) to measure cerebral blood volume (CBV) differences in left and right frontal, temporal and parietal lobes (Agarwal et al., 2008). This study involved four manic, three depressed and seven euthymic subjects. Subjects with bipolar disorder showed significantly increased CBV in the left frontal and left temporal lobe and had significantly inverse laterality index for the frontal lobe (Agarwal et al., 2008).

These resting state data are interesting as they implicated brain regions that show abnormal functioning even in the absence of task demands. However, they are more difficult to interpret as manic, depressed and euthymic subjects were combined. Additionally, the number of subjects studied was very small, significantly impacting both statistical power and the risk of spurious results dominating the findings. Future studies that separate subjects by mood state will be

---

**fMRI of Resting State in Bipolar Disorder Suggests:**

- Frontal lobe abnormalities in samples in varied mood states

- Future analyses that separate subjects by mood state are needed.

- More studies are needed before conclusions can be drawn

---

able to shed some light on which of these findings are state=related and which are trait-related.

## fMRI STUDIES IN BIPOLAR DISORDER: CONCLUSION

Dysregulation in emotion processing in bipolar disorder reflects a vast neuroanatomic network. Both structural and functional brain-imaging studies suggest specific frontal and limbic regions in which abnormalities are associated with symptoms of bipolar disorder. Executive functioning and verbal memory deficits described previously implicate the prefrontal cortex, anterior cingulate and temporolimbic structures, especially ventromedial areas and parahippocampus/hippocampus.

Studies have focused largely on frontal-limbic circuitry as this network is suggested to be a key anatomical substrate for the emergence of both manic and depressive symptoms seen in bipolar disorder. In particular, fMRI studies consistently demonstrate increased amygdala and decreased orbitofrontal prefrontal activation in subjects with bipolar disorder during mania compared to healthy subjects during emotion processing tasks, suggesting dysfunction of the prefrontal-amygdala circuit during mania.

Dysfunction of this circuit appears to be a trait of bipolar disorder, rather than a state-dependent phenomenon. Evidence of this comes from a variety of fMRI studies in euthymic subjects with bipolar disorder that report reduced activation in ventrolateral prefrontal cortex using paradigms that activate this region (Strakowski et al., 2005; Lagopoulos & Malhi 2007; Malhi et al., 2005). Furthermore, subjects with bipolar disorder demonstrate reduced activation in left ventral prefrontal cortex that was independent of mood state (Blumberg et al., 2003). Increased amygdala activation has also been observed in some studies of euthymic subjects with bipolar disorder using paradigms known to activate the amygdala (Chen et al., 2010; Surguladze et al., 2010, Lagopoulos & Malhi 2007), but not all studies find significant differences in the amygdala during euthymia compared with healthy subjects (Almeida, Mechelli et al., 2009; Hassel et al., 2009; Malhi et al., 2007; Robinson et al., 2008). Again, the amygdala results are mixed during the depressive phase with some studies finding no significant differences from healthy subjects (Altshuler et al., 2008; Chen et al., 2006) and another finding increased amygdala activation (Malhi et al., 2004). These results suggest that increased amygdala activation during mania is the most consistent finding and as such, may be a state-related finding. Future studies that look at the same subjects across mania, depression and euthymia should be able to clarify this issue.

The orbitofrontal cortex (OFC) plays a role in integrating emotional information and regulating the intensity of emotional response (Cabeza & Nyberg, 2000; Fuster, 2001). Dysfunction in this region may provide a mechanism for understanding the failure to modulate other regions and may correlate with the mood shifts characteristic of bipolar disorder. Functional neuroimaging studies involving the processing of emotional faces reliably demonstrate specificity for activation of OFC and amygdala in healthy subjects (Adolphs et al., 1995; Breiter et al., 1996; Hariri et al., 2000). Previous work demonstrated significantly greater activation in this region in healthy compared with manic (Altshuler et al., 2005; Killgore et al., 2008), euthymic (Lagopoulos & Malhi, 2007; Malhi et al., 2005) and depressed subjects with bipolar disorder (Altshuler et al., 2008; Malhi et al., 2004). These observations suggests that hypoactivation of the OFC during emotion processing tasks may be a bipolar disorder trait. This hypothesis is further supported by the executive function literature that also finds significantly reduced activation in the OFC during attention (Fleck et al., 2010; Strakowski et al., 2011), response inhibition (Altshuler et al., 2005; Elliott et al., 2004; Mazzola-Pomietto et al., 2009), interference (Blumberg et al., 2003; Kronhaus et al., 2006; Roth et al., 2006) and working memory tasks (Lagopoulos & Malhi, 2007; Monks et al., 2004).

Positron emission tomography (PET) studies replicated the frontal-limbic circuit abnormalities seen in euthymic subjects with bipolar disorder using fMRI. One study measured regional blood flow while euthymic subjects completed a novel motor sequence task (Berns et al., 2002). Subjects with bipolar disorder displayed a unique pattern of widespread limbic network activity in response to the new sequence, while healthy subjects activated a spatial attention circuit. Bipolar disorder subjects failed to allocate attentional resources and instead utilized limbic circuitry (i.e., suggesting arousal rather than attention) to alter their performance on a nonemotional task. This pattern of subjects with bipolar disorder showing significantly greater engagement of limbic regions in response to cognitive tasks has been seen in a number of fMRI studies (Adler, Holland, Schmithorst, Wilke et al., 2004; Gruber et al., 2010; Thermenos et al., 2010). This finding has been confirmed in an fMRI study using medication-free euthymic subjects (Strakowski et al., 2004), suggesting it is not solely due to a confound of medication status. These common abnormalities, of increased limbic activation and decreased OFC activation, point to enduring trait deficits of bipolar disorder.

In general, studies report abnormalities in prefrontal cortical areas, striatum and amygdala early in the course of the illness that may predate illness onset (Strakowski et al., 2005). This set of abnormalities is seen not only functionally, but also structurally since some studies have found significant abnormalities in amygdala volume even in first-episode patients (Rosso et al., 2007). Other abnormalities may develop with repeated mood episodes and represent the effects of illness progression, although future studies are warranted to determine which of these functional abnormalities pre-date the illness onset and which may be caused by illness progression. These studies together suggest that there may be diminished prefrontal modulation of subcortical and medial temporal structures within the anterior limbic network that results in mood dysregulation.

## BIPOLAR I DISORDER VS. BIPOLAR II DISORDER AND THE BIPOLAR SPECTRUM

Only a few studies have directly examined the differences between bipolar I and II disorders in various domains. Likewise, few studies have tried to answer the question of whether differences in severity of manic symptoms reflect different neuroanatomy, neurofunctioning, and etiology, or how the differential time spent in depression affects these populations. Although bipolar I disorder is seen as the more severe form, bipolar II disorder is not simply the lesser of the bipolar disorders. Rather, it is a serious, chronic illness with predominantly depressive episodes that affect social and occupational functioning (Judd et al., 2003). Subjects with bipolar II disorder showed poorer quality of life measurements than those with bipolar I disorder, again even after controlling for age, age at onset, and length of illness (Maina et al., 2007). This may be due to the longer time spent depressed in bipolar II disorder. Consequently, this study suggests that, despite the view of bipolar I disorder as the more severe variant of bipolar disorder, bipolar II disorder, with its persistent depressive features, appears to have a larger impact on subjects' perceived quality of life, even during euthymia.

Studies have found that subjects with bipolar I disorder show more verbal memory impairment than subjects with bipolar II disorder. This may be related to the greater degree of psychotic symptoms in bipolar I disorder and the negative impact of the number of manic episodes (Martinez-Aran et al., 2004). These neurocognitive differences between bipolar disorder I and II subjects strongly suggest that future neurocognitive and neuroimaging studies separately analyze these groups, rather than combining them as many studies have done previously (Agarwal et al., 2008; Anand et al., 2009; Caligiuri et al., 2006; Caligiuri et al., 2003; Wessa et al., 2007).

In addition to the two defined bipolar disorder subtypes, many investigators suggest that bipolar disorder ought to be viewed as a broader bipolar spectrum, with some authors suggesting prevalence rates of bipolar disorder as high as 5% if "softer" clinical expressions are included (Akiskal et al., 2000). Some persons with the "softer expression" subtypes might demonstrate some of the same deficits as persons with bipolar I and II disorders. Further research may help elucidate the nature of the bipolar spectrum and how euthymia is characterized throughout it.

## LIMITATIONS

Some of the limitations of the bipolar neuroimaging literature are general to neuroimaging while others are specific to this patient population. Problems with neuroimaging reports, particularly with psychiatric populations, include relatively small sample sizes. Also, neuroimaging is a relatively new science and uses techniques not yet perfected, leading to interpretations of data that are not yet fully understood (Stern & Silbersweig, 2001). As such, careful attention is needed to the design of studies, with the limitation of each specific neuroimaging method in mind (i.e., PET studies have poor spatial resolution, while fMRI studies have poor temporal resolution). For example, the use of global signal scaling in many studies has been called into question, since use of such a statistical method may greatly distort findings in structures related to emotion processing. These limitations may contribute to conflicting findings (Junghofer et al., 2006).

Other limitations are inherent in working with this population. The first and perhaps most pertinent is the effect of medication on both the neuroimaging data itself and on interpretation of the findings. Virtually all studies using bipolar disorder populations include subjects on a variety of psychotropic medications, which limits the ability to compare groups. Studies that try to avoid this complication by using unmedicated populations (Strakowski et al., 2004) also limit the ability to generalize their findings, since these unmedicated subjects are likely an unrepresentative subset of individuals with bipolar disorder. The ethics of stopping or delaying medication for research make it difficult to design a controlled, double blind study that could provide more conclusive results. However, it is possible that future studies could recruit subjects as soon as they present in acute mood states and carefully monitor the effects of medication on both mood state and neural functioning.

Also, certain medications may affect blood flow, which is indirectly measured in fMRI studies (Loeber et al., 2002), may affect activation only in select regions (Strakowski et al., 2005), and might change grey matter volume in subjects with bipolar disorder (Gould & Manji, 2002). Consequently, medication issues must be considered when reviewing, interpreting and generalizing findings from studies.

Another problem, not specific to neuroimaging, is the use of heterogeneous populations by including multiple mood states in a single study without accounting for state differences (Lawrence et al., 2004; Mitchell et al., 2004; Roth et al., 2006; Silverstone et al., 2005) or failing to report the mood state (Adler, Holland, Schmithorst, Wilke et al., 2004). A similar confound arises from combining bipolar I and II disorder subjects, as noted previously (Caligiuri et al., 2003). These confounds make it difficult to differentiate trait and subtype differences in fMRI activation patterns. Nevertheless, neuroimaging provides a useful and powerful tool to extend the existing psychological literature and is essential for linking underlying anatomical and functional changes to those seen behaviorally.

## FUTURE AIMS

As previously noted, few existing studies involved medication-free subjects. Consequently, future studies are needed to specifically clarify the effects of medication on the various neurocognitive domains measured. Questions also remain as to what extent cognitive dysfunction is present before illness onset. Longitudinal studies following at-risk subjects might help answer not only these questions, but also can address whether cognitive impairments are stable or progressive. fMRI will continue to shed light on trait deficits in bipolar disorder and help us define the functional neuroanantomic underpinnings of this complex condition.

## REFERENCES

Abler, B., Greenhouse, I., Ongur, D., Walter, H., & Heckers, S. 2008. Abnormal reward system activation in mania. *Neuropsychopharmacology*, 33(9): 2217–2227.

Adler, C. M., Holland, S. K., Schmithorst, V., Tuchfarber, M. J., & Strakowski, S. M. 2004. Changes in neuronal activation in patients with bipolar disorder during performance of a working memory task. *Bipolar Disorders*, 6(6): 540–549.

Adler, C. M., Holland, S. K., Schmithorst, V., Wilke, M., Weiss, K. L., Pan, H., & Strakowski, S. M. . 2004. Abnormal frontal white matter tracts in bipolar disorder: a diffusion tensor imaging study. *Bipolar Disorders*, 6(3): 197–203.

Adolphs, R. 2008. Fear, faces, and the human amygdala. *Current Opinion in Neurobiology*, 18(2): 166–172.

Adolphs, R., Tranel, D., Damasio, H., & Damasio, A. R. 1995. Fear and the human amygdala. *Journal of Neuroscience.*, 15(9), 5879–5891.

Agarwal, N., Bellani, M., Perlini, C., Rambaldelli, G., Atzori, M., Cerini, R., . . . Brambilla, P. 2008. Increased fronto-temporal perfusion in bipolar disorder. *Journal of Affective Disorders*, 110(1–2): 106–114.

Akiskal, H. S., Bourgeois, M. L., Angst, J., Post, R., Moller, H., & Hirschfeld, R. 2000. Re-evaluating the prevalence of and diagnostic composition within the broad clinical spectrum of bipolar disorders. *Journal of Affective Disorders*, 59 Suppl 1: S5–S30.

Allin, M. P., Marshall, N., Schulze, K., Walshe, M., Hall, M. H., Picchioni, M., . . . McDonald, C. 2010. A functional MRI study of verbal fluency in adults with bipolar disorder and their unaffected relatives. *Psychological Medicine*, 40(12): 2025–2035.

Almeida, J. R., Mechelli, A., Hassel, S., Versace, A., Kupfer, D. J., & Phillips, M. L. 2009. Abnormally increased effective connectivity between parahippocampal gyrus and ventromedial prefrontal regions during emotion labeling in bipolar disorder. *Psychiatry Research*, 174(3): 195–201.

Almeida, J. R., Versace, A., Hassel, S., Kupfer, D. J., & Phillips, M. L. 2010. Elevated amygdala activity to sad facial expressions: a state marker of bipolar but not unipolar depression. *Biological Psychiatry*, 67(5): 414–421.

Almeida, J. R., Versace, A., Mechelli, A., Hassel, S., Quevedo, K., Kupfer, D. J., & Phillips, M. L. 2009. Abnormal amygdala-prefrontal effective connectivity to happy faces differentiates bipolar from major depression. *Biological Psychiatry*, 66(5): 451–459.

Altshuler, L., Bartzokis, G., Grieder, T., Curran, J., & Mintz, J. 1998. Amygdala enlargement in bipolar disorder and hippocampal reduction in schizophrenia: an MRI study demonstrating neuroanatomic specificity. *Archives of General Psychiatry*, 55(7): 663–664.

Altshuler, L., Bookheimer, S., Proenza, M. A., Townsend, J., Sabb, F., Firestine, A., . . . Cohen, M.S. 2005. Increased amygdala activation during mania: a functional magnetic resonance imaging study. *American Journal of Psychiatry*, 162(6): 1211–1213.

Altshuler, L., Bookheimer, S., Townsend, J., Proenza, M. A., Sabb, F., Mintz, J., & Cohen, M.S. 2008. Regional brain changes in bipolar I depression: a functional magnetic resonance imaging study. *Bipolar Disorders*, 10(6): 708–717.

Altshuler, L., Ventura, J., van Gorp, W. G., Green, M. F., Theberge, D. C., & Mintz, J. 2004. Neurocognitive function in clinically stable men with bipolar I disorder or schizophrenia and normal control subjects. *Biological Psychiatry*, 56(8): 560–569.

Amunts, K., Schleicher, A., & Zilles, K. 2004. Outstanding language competence and cytoarchitecture in Broca's speech region. *Brain and Language*, 89(2): 346–353.

Anand, A., Li, Y., Wang, Y., Lowe, M. J., & Dzemidzic, M. 2009. Resting state corticolimbic connectivity abnormalities in unmedicated bipolar disorder and unipolar depression. *Psychiatry Research*, 171(3): 189–198.

Angrilli, A., Palomba, D., Cantagallo, A., Maietti, A., & Stegagno, L. 1999. Emotional impairment after right orbitofrontal lesion in a patient without cognitive deficits. *Neuroreport*, 10(8): 1741–1746.

Aron, A. R. 2007. The neural basis of inhibition in cognitive control. *Neuroscientist*, 13(3): 214–228.

Arts, B., Jabben, N., Krabbendam, L., & van Os, J. 2008. Meta-analyses of cognitive functioning in euthymic bipolar patients and their first-degree relatives. *Psychological Medicine*, 38(6): 771–785.

Augustine, J. R. 1996. Circuitry and functional aspects of the insular lobe in primates including humans. *Brain Research. Brain Research Reviews*, 22(3): 229–244.

Badre, D., & Wagner, A. D. 2004. Selection, integration, and conflict monitoring; assessing the nature and generality of prefrontal cognitive control mechanisms. *Neuron*, 41(3): 473–487.

Baker, S. C., Frith, C. D., & Dolan, R. J. 1997. The interaction between mood and cognitive function studied with PET. *Psychological Medicine*, 27(3): 565–578.

Balanza-Martinez, V., Rubio, C., Selva-Vera, G., Martinez-Aran, A., Sanchez-Moreno, J., Salazar-Fraile, J., . . . Tabarés-Seisdedos, R. 2008. Neurocognitive endophenotypes (endophenocognitypes) from studies of relatives of bipolar disorder subjects: a systematic review. *Neuroscience and Biobehavioral Reviews*, 32(8): 1426–1438.

Bearden, C. E., Hoffman, K. M., & Cannon, T. D. 2001. The neuropsychology and neuroanatomy of bipolar affective disorder: a critical review. *Bipolar Disorders*, 3(3): 106–150; discussion 151–103.

Belger, A., Puce, A., Krystal, J. H., Gore, J. C., Goldman-Rakic, P., & McCarthy, G. 1998. Dissociation of mnemonic and perceptual processes during spatial and nonspatial working memory using fMRI. *Human Brain Mapping*, 6(1): 14–32.

Bermpohl, F., Dalanay, U., Kahnt, T., Sajonz, B., Heimann, H., Ricken, R., . . . Bauer, M. 2009. A preliminary study of increased amygdala activation to positive affective stimuli in mania. *Bipolar Disorders*, 11(1): 70–75.

Bermpohl, F., Kahnt, T., Dalanay, U., Hägele, C., Sajonz, B., Wegner, T., . . . Heinz, A. 2009. Altered representation of expected value in the orbitofrontal cortex in mania. *Human Brain Mapping*, Jul;31(7): 958–69.

Berns, G. S., Martin, M., & Proper, S. M. 2002. Limbic hyperreactivity in bipolar II disorder. *American Journal of Psychiatry*, 159(2): 304–306.

Berridge, K. C. 2007. The debate over dopamine's role in reward: the case for incentive salience. *Psychopharmacology (Berl)*, 191(3): 391–431.

Blumberg, H. P., Leung, H. C., Skudlarski, P., Lacadie, C. M., Fredericks, C. A., Harris, B. C., . . . Peterson, B.S. 2003. A functional magnetic resonance imaging study of bipolar disorder: state- and trait-related dysfunction in ventral prefrontal cortices. *Archives of General Psychiatry*, 60(6): 601–609.

Blumberg, H. P., Stern, E., Ricketts, S., Martinez, D., de Asis, J., White, T., . . . Silbersweig, D.A. 1999. Rostral and orbital prefrontal cortex dysfunction in the manic state of bipolar disorder. *American Journal of Psychiatry*, 156(12): 1986–1988.

Bookheimer, S. 2002. Functional MRI of language: new approaches to understanding the cortical organization of semantic processing. *Annual Review of Neuroscience*, 25: 151–188.

Bora, E., Yucel, M., & Pantelis, C. 2009. Cognitive endophenotypes of bipolar disorder: a meta-analysis of neuropsychological deficits in euthymic patients and their first-degree relatives. *Journal of Affective Disorders*, 113(1–2): 1–20.

Botvinick, M. M., Cohen, J. D., & Carter, C. S. 2004. Conflict monitoring and anterior cingulate cortex: an update. *Trends in Cognitive Sciences*, 8(12): 539–546.

Brambilla, P., Harenski, K., Nicoletti, M., Sassi, R. B., Mallinger, A. G., Frank, E., . . . Soares, J. C. 2003. MRI investigation of temporal lobe structures in bipolar patients. *Journal of Psychiatric Research*, 37(4): 287–295.

Breiter, H. C., Etcoff, N. L., Whalen, P. J., Kennedy, W. A., Rauch, S. L., Buckner, R. L., . . . Rosen, B.R. 1996. Response and habituation of the human amygdala during visual processing of facial expression. *Neuron*, 17(5): 875–887.

Bush, G., Whalen, P. J., Rosen, B. R., Jenike, M. A., McInerney, S. C., & Rauch, S. L. 1998. The counting Stroop: an interference task specialized for functional neuroimaging—validation study with functional MRI. *Human Brain Mapping*, 6(4): 270–282.

Cabeza, R., & Nyberg, L. 2000. Imaging cognition II: An empirical review of 275 PET and fMRI studies. *Journal of Cognitive Neuroscience*, 12(1): 1–47.

Caligiuri, M. P., Brown, G. G., Meloy, M. J., Eberson, S. C., Kindermann, S. S., Frank, L. R., . . . Lohr, J. B. 2003. An fMRI study of affective state and medication on cortical and subcortical brain regions during motor performance in bipolar disorder. *Psychiatry Research*, 123(3): 171–182.

Caligiuri, M. P., Brown, G. G., Meloy, M. J., Eberson, S., Niculescu, A. B., & Lohr, J. B. 2006. Striatopallidal regulation of affect in bipolar disorder. *Journal of Affective Disorders*, 91(2–3): 235–242.

Cappell, K. A., Gmeindl, L., & Reuter-Lorenz, P. A. 2010. Age differences in prefontal recruitment during verbal working memory maintenance depend on memory load. *Cortex*, 46(4): 462–473.

Carter, C. S., Braver, T. S., Barch, D. M., Botvinick, M. M., Noll, D., & Cohen, J. D. 1998. Anterior cingulate cortex, error detection, and the online monitoring of performance. *Science*, 280(5364): 747–749.

Chen, C. H., Lennox, B., Jacob, R., Calder, A., Lupson, V., Bisbrown-Chippendale, R., . . . Bullmore, E. 2006. Explicit and implicit facial affect recognition in manic and depressed States of bipolar disorder: a functional magnetic resonance imaging study. *Biological Psychiatry*, 59(1): 31–39.

Chen, C. H., Suckling, J., Ooi, C., Jacob, R., Lupson, V., Bullmore, E. T., & Lennox, B. R. 2010. A longitudinal fMRI study of the manic and euthymic states of bipolar disorder. *Bipolar Disorders*, 12(3): 344–347.

Chepenik, L. G., Raffo, M., Hampson, M., Lacadie, C., Wang, F., Jones, M. M., Blumberg, H. P. 2010. Functional connectivity between ventral prefrontal cortex and amygdala at low frequency in the resting state in bipolar disorder. *Psychiatry Research*, 182(3): 207–210.

Clark, L., Iversen, S. D., & Goodwin, G. M. 2001. A neuropsychological investigation of prefrontal cortex involvement in acute mania. *American Journal of Psychiatry*, 158(10): 1605–1611.

Cohen, J. D., Perlstein, W. M., Braver, T. S., Nystrom, L. E., Noll, D. C., Jonides, J., Smith, E. E. 1997. Temporal dynamics of brain activation during a working memory task. *Nature*, 386(6625): 604–608.

Cole, D. M., Smith, S. M., & Beckmann, C. F. 2010. Advances and pitfalls in the analysis and interpretation of resting-state FMRI data. *Frontiers in Systems Neuroscience*, 4:8. doi: 10.3389/fnsys.2010.00008

Cole, M. W., & Schneider, W. 2007. The cognitive control network: Integrated cortical regions with dissociable functions. *Neuroimage*, 37(1): 343–360.

Cromwell, H. C., Hassani, O. K., & Schultz, W. 2005. Relative reward processing in primate striatum. *Experimental Brain Research*, 162(4): 520–525.

Curtis, C. E. 2006. Prefrontal and parietal contributions to spatial working memory. *Neuroscience*, 139(1): 173–180.

Curtis, V. A., Dixon, T. A., Morris, R. G., Bullmore, E. T., Brammer, M. J., Williams, S. C., . . . McGuire, P.K. 2001. Differential frontal activation in schizophrenia and bipolar illness during verbal fluency. *Journal of Affective Disorders*, 66(2–3): 111–121.

Curtis, V. A., Thompson, J. M., Seal, M. L., Monks, P. J., Lloyd, A. J., Harrison, L., . . . Ferrier, I. N. 2007. The nature of abnormal language processing in euthymic bipolar I disorder: evidence for a relationship between task demand and prefrontal function. *Bipolar Disorders*, 9(4): 358–369.

Czobor, P., Jaeger, J., Berns, S. M., Gonzalez, C., & Loftus, S. 2007. Neuropsychological symptom dimensions in bipolar disorder and schizophrenia. *Bipolar Disorders*, 9(1–2): 71–92.

Deckersbach, T., Rauch, S. L., Buhlmann, U., Ostacher, M. J., Beucke, J. C., Nierenberg, A. A., . . . Dougherty, D. D. 2008. An fMRI investigation of working memory and sadness in females with bipolar disorder: a brief report. *Bipolar Disorders*, 10(8): 928–942.

Depp, C. A., Moore, D. J., Sitzer, D., Palmer, B. W., Eyler, L. T., Roesch, S., . . . Jeste, D. V. 2007. Neurocognitive impairment in middle-aged and older adults with bipolar disorder: comparison to schizophrenia and normal comparison subjects. *Journal of Affective Disorders*, 101(1–3): 201–209.

Devinsky, O., Morrell, M. J., & Vogt, B. A. 1995. Contributions of anterior cingulate cortex to behaviour. *Brain*, 118 (Pt 1): 279–306.

Dickerson, F., Boronow, J. J., Stallings, C., Origoni, A. E., Cole, S. K., & Yolken, R. H. 2004. Cognitive functioning in schizophrenia and bipolar disorder: comparison of performance on the Repeatable Battery for the Assessment of Neuropsychological Status. *Psychiatry Research*, 129(1): 45–53.

Drapier, D., Surguladze, S., Marshall, N., Schulze, K., Fern, A., Hall, M. H., . . . McDonald, C. 2008. Genetic liability for bipolar disorder is characterized by excess frontal activation in response to a working memory task. *Biological Psychiatry*, 64(6): 513–520.

Drevets, W. C. 2000. Neuroimaging studies of mood disorders. *Biological Psychiatry*, 48(8): 813–829.

Duncan, J., & Owen, A. M. 2000. Common regions of the human frontal lobe recruited by diverse cognitive demands. *Trends in Neurosciences*, 23(10): 475–483.

Elliott, R., Ogilvie, A., Rubinsztein, J. S., Calderon, G., Dolan, R. J., & Sahakian, B. J. 2004. Abnormal ventral frontal response during performance of an affective go/no go task in patients with mania. *Biological Psychiatry*, 55(12): 1163–1170.

First, M. B., S. R., Gibbon M, & Williams, J.B.W. 2002. *Structured Clinical Interview for DSM-IV-TR Axis I Disorders, Research Version, Patient Edition. (SCID-I/P).* New York: Biometrics Research, New York State Psychiatric Institute.

Fleck, D. E., Eliassen, J. C., Durling, M., Lamy, M., Adler, C. M., DelBello, M. P., . . . Strakowski, S. M. 2010 Oct 26. Functional MRI of sustained attention in bipolar mania. *Molecular Psychiatry advance online publication.* doi:10.1038/mp.2010.108

Foland, L. C., Altshuler, L. L., Bookheimer, S. Y., Eisenberger, N., Townsend, J., & Thompson, P. M. 2008. Evidence for deficient modulation of amygdala response by prefrontal cortex in bipolar mania. *Psychiatry Research*, 162(1): 27–37.

Frangou, S., Kington, J., Raymont, V., & Shergill, S. S. 2008. Examining ventral and dorsal prefrontal function in bipolar disorder: a functional magnetic resonance imaging study. *European Psychiatry*, 23(4): 300–308.

Fu, C. H., Morgan, K., Suckling, J., Williams, S. C., Andrew, C., Vythelingum, G. N., . . . McGuire, P. K. 2002. A functional magnetic resonance imaging study of overt letter verbal fluency using a clustered acquisition sequence: greater anterior cingulate activation with increased task demand. *Neuroimage*, 17(2): 871–879.

Fusar-Poli, P., Placentino, A., Carletti, F., Landi, P., Allen, P., Surguladze, S., . . . Politi, P. 2009. Functional atlas of emotional faces processing: a voxel-based meta-analysis of 105 functional magnetic resonance imaging studies. *Journal of Psychiatry and Neuroscience*, 34(6): 418–432.

Fuster, J. M. (2001). The prefrontal cortex—an update: time is of the essence. *Neuron*, 30(2): 319–333.

Glahn, D. C., Robinson, J. L., Tordesillas-Gutierrez, D., Monkul, E. S., Holmes, M. K., Green, M. J., . . . Bearden, C. E. 2010. Fronto-temporal dysregulation in asymptomatic bipolar I patients: a paired associate functional MRI study. *Human Brain Mapping*, 31(7): 1041–1051.

Goswami, U., Sharma, A., Khastigir, U., Ferrier, I. N., Young, A. H., Gallagher, P., . . . Moore, P. B. 2006. Neuropsychological dysfunction, soft neurological signs and social disability in euthymic patients with bipolar disorder. *British Journal of Psychiatry*, 188 (Apr): 366–373.

Gould, T. D., & Manji, H. K. 2002. Signaling networks in the pathophysiology and treatment of mood disorders. *Journal of Psychosomatic Research*, 53(2): 687–697.

Grafman, J., Vance, S. C., Weingartner, H., Salazar, A. M., & Amin, D. 1986. The effects of lateralized frontal lesions on mood regulation. *Brain*, 109 (Pt 6): 1127–1148.

Grant, B. F., Stinson, F. S., Hasin, D. S., Dawson, D. A., Chou, S. P., Ruan, W. J., . . . Huang, B. 2005. Prevalence, correlates, and comorbidity of bipolar I disorder and axis I and II disorders: results from the National Epidemiologic Survey on Alcohol and Related Conditions. *Journal of Clinical Psychiatry*, 66(10): 1205–1215.

Gruber, O., Tost, H., Henseler, I., Schmael, C., Scherk, H., Ende, G., . . . Rietschel, M 2010. Pathological amygdala activation during working memory performance: Evidence for a pathophysiological trait marker in bipolar affective disorder. *Human Brain Mapping*, 31(1): 115–125.

Gruber, S. A., Rogowska, J., & Yurgelun-Todd, D. A. 2004. Decreased activation of the anterior cingulate in bipolar patients: an fMRI study. *Journal of Affective Disorders*, 82(2): 191–201.

Gruber, S. A., Rogowska, J., Holcomb, P., Soraci, S., & Yurgelun-Todd, D. 2002. Stroop performance in normal control subjects: an fMRI study. *Neuroimage*, 16(2): 349–360.

Gruber, S., Rathgeber, K., Braunig, P., & Gauggel, S. 2007. Stability and course of neuropsychological deficits in manic and depressed bipolar patients compared to patients with Major Depression. *Journal of Affective Disorders*, 104(1–3): 61–71.

Haldane, M., Cunningham, G., Androutsos, C., & Frangou, S. 2008. Structural brain correlates of response inhibition in Bipolar Disorder I. *Journal of Psychopharmacology*, 22(2): 138–143.

Hamilton, L. S., Altshuler, L. L., Townsend, J., Bookheimer, S. Y., Phillips, O. R., Fischer, J., . . . Narr, K. L. 2009. Alterations in functional activation in euthymic bipolar disorder and schizophrenia during a working memory task. *Human Brain Mapping*, 30(12): 3958–3969.

Hariri, A. R., Bookheimer, S. Y., & Mazziotta, J. C. 2000. Modulating emotional responses: effects of a neocortical network on the limbic system. *Neuroreport*, 11(1): 43–48.

Hassel, S., Almeida, J. R., Frank, E., Versace, A., Nau, S. A., Klein, C. R., . . . Phillips, M. L. 2009. Prefrontal cortical and striatal activity to happy and fear faces in bipolar disorder is associated with comorbid substance abuse and eating disorder. *Journal of Affective Disorders*, 118(1–3): 19–27.

Hassel, S., Almeida, J. R., Kerr, N., Nau, S., Ladouceur, C. D., Fissell, K., . . . Phillips, M. L. 2008. Elevated striatal and decreased dorsolateral prefrontal cortical activity in response to emotional stimuli in euthymic bipolar disorder: no associations with psychotropic medication load. *Bipolar Disorders*, 10(8): 916–927.

Horn, N. R., Dolan, M., Elliott, R., Deakin, J. F., & Woodruff, P. W. 2003. Response inhibition and impulsivity: an fMRI study. *Neuropsychologia*, 41(14): 1959–1966.

Husted, D. S., Shapira, N. A., & Goodman, W. K. 2006. The neuro-circuitry of obsessive-compulsive disorder and disgust. *Progress in Neuro-psychopharmacol and Biological Psychiatry*, 30(3): 389–399.

Iversen, S. D., & Mishkin, M. 1970. Perseverative interference in monkeys following selective lesions of the inferior prefrontal convexity. *Experimental Brain Research*, 11(4): 376–386.

Jogia, J., Haldane, M., Cobb, A., Kumari, V., & Frangou, S. 2008. Pilot investigation of the changes in cortical activation during facial affect recognition with lamotrigine monotherapy in bipolar disorder. *British Journal of Psychiatry*, 192(3): 197–201.

Judd, L. L., Akiskal, H. S., Schettler, P. J., Endicott, J., Leon, A. C., Solomon, D. A., . . . Keller, M. B. 2005. Psychosocial disability in the course of bipolar I and II disorders: a prospective, comparative, longitudinal study. *Archives of General Psychiatry*, 62(12): 1322–1330.

Judd, L. L., Akiskal, H. S., Schettler, P. J., Endicott, J., Maser, J., Solomon, D. A., . . . Keller, M. B. 2002. The long-term natural history of the weekly symptomatic status of bipolar I disorder. *Archives of General Psychiatry*, 59(6): 530–537.

Judd, L. L., Schettler, P. J., Akiskal, H. S., Maser, J., Coryell, W., Solomon, D., . . . Keller, M. 2003. Long-term symptomatic status of bipolar I vs. bipolar II disorders. The *International Journal of Neuropsychopharmacology*, 6(2): 127–137.

Junghofer, M., Peyk, P., Flaisch, T., & Schupp, H. T. 2006. Neuroimaging methods in affective neuroscience: selected methodological issues. *Progress in Brain Research*, 156: 123–143.

Kaladjian, A., Jeanningros, R., Azorin, J. M., Nazarian, B., Roth, M., & Mazzola-Pomietto, P. 2009. Reduced brain activation in euthymic bipolar patients during response inhibition: an event-related fMRI study. *Psychiatry Research*, 173(1): 45–51.

Kaladjian, A., Jeanningros, R., Azorin, J. M., Nazarian, B., Roth, M., Anton, J. L., . . . Mazzola-Pomietto, P. 2009. Remission from mania is associated with a decrease in amygdala activation during motor response inhibition. *Bipolar Disorders*, 11(5): 530–538.

Keller, M. B., Lavori, P. W., Coryell, W., Endicott, J., & Mueller, T. I. 1993. Bipolar I: a five-year prospective follow-up. *Journal of Nervous and Mental Disease*, 181(4): 238–245.

Kelly, A. M., Hester, R., Murphy, K., Javitt, D. C., Foxe, J. J., & Garavan, H. 2004. Prefrontal-subcortical dissociations underlying inhibitory control revealed by event-related fMRI. *European Journal of Neuroscience*, 19(11): 3105–3112.

Kessler, R. C., Adler, L., Barkley, R., Biederman, J., Conners, C. K., Demler, O., . . . Zaslavsky, A. M. 2006. The prevalence and correlates of adult ADHD in the United States: results from the National Comorbidity Survey Replication. *American Journal of Psychiatry*, 163(4): 716–723.

Killgore, W. D., Gruber, S. A., & Yurgelun-Todd, D. A. 2008. Abnormal corticostriatal activity during fear perception in bipolar disorder. *Neuroreport*, 19(15): 1523–1527.

Kronhaus, D. M., Lawrence, N. S., Williams, A. M., Frangou, S., Brammer, M. J., Williams, S. C., . . . Phillips, M. L. 2006. Stroop performance in bipolar disorder: further evidence for abnormalities in the ventral prefrontal cortex. *Bipolar Disorders*, 8(1)L 28–39.

Kruger, S., Seminowicz, D., Goldapple, K., Kennedy, S. H., & Mayberg, H. S. 2003. State and trait influences on mood regulation in bipolar disorder: blood flow differences with an acute mood challenge. *Biological Psychiatry*, 54(11): 1274–1283.

Lagopoulos, J., & Malhi, G. S. 2007. A functional magnetic resonance imaging study of emotional Stroop in euthymic bipolar disorder. *Neuroreport*, 18(15): 1583–1587.

Lagopoulos, J., Ivanovski, B., & Malhi, G. S. 2007. An event-related functional MRI study of working memory in euthymic bipolar disorder. *Journal of Psychiatry and Neuroscience*, 32(3): 174–184.

Lawrence, N. S., Jollant, F., O'Daly, O., Zelaya, F., & Phillips, M. L. 2009. Distinct roles of prefrontal cortical subregions in the IA Gambling Task. *Cerebral Cortex*, 19(5): 1134–1143.

Lawrence, N. S., Williams, A. M., Surguladze, S., Giampietro, V., Brammer, M. J., Andrew, C., . . . Phillips, M. L. 2004. Subcortical and ventral prefrontal cortical neural responses to facial expressions distinguish patients with bipolar disorder and major depression. *Biological Psychiatry*, 55(6): 578–587.

Lennox, B. R., Jacob, R., Calder, A. J., Lupson, V., & Bullmore, E. T. 2004. Behavioural and neurocognitive responses to sad facial affect are attenuated in patients with mania. *Psychological Medicine*, 34(5): 795–802.

Li, C. S., Yan, P., Sinha, R., & Lee, T. W. (2008). Subcortical processes of motor response inhibition during a stop signal task. *Neuroimage*, 41(4): 1352–1363.

Loeber, R. T., Gruber, S. A., Cohen, B. M., Renshaw, P. F., Sherwood, A. R., & Yurgelun-Todd, D. A. 2002. Cerebellar blood volume in bipolar patients correlates with medication. *Biological Psychiatry*, 51(5): 370–376.

Maina, G., Albert, U., Bellodi, L., Colombo, C., Faravelli, C., Monteleone, P., . . . Maj, M. 2007. Health-related quality of life in euthymic bipolar disorder patients: differences between bipolar I and II subtypes. *Journal of Clinical Psychiatry*, 68(2): 207–212.

Malhi, G. S., Lagopoulos, J., Sachdev, P. S., Ivanovski, B., & Shnier, R. 2005. An emotional Stroop functional MRI study of euthymic bipolar disorder. *Bipolar Disorders*, 7 (Suppl 5): 58–69.

Malhi, G. S., Lagopoulos, J., Sachdev, P. S., Ivanovski, B., Shnier, R., & Ketter, T. 2007. Is a lack of disgust something to fear? A functional magnetic resonance imaging facial emotion recognition study in euthymic bipolar disorder patients. *Bipolar Disorders*, 9(4): 345–357.

Malhi, G. S., Lagopoulos, J., Ward, P. B., Kumari, V., Mitchell, P. B., Parker, G. B., . . . Sachdev, P. 2004. Cognitive generation of affect in bipolar depression: an fMRI study. *European Journal of Neuroscience*, 19(3): 741–754.

Marchand, W. R., Lee, J. N., Thatcher, G. W., Jensen, C., Stewart, D., Dilda, V., . . . Creem-Regehr, S. H. 2007. A functional MRI study of a paced motor activation task to evaluate frontal-subcortical circuit function in bipolar depression. *Psychiatry Research*, 155(3): 221–230.

Markowitsch, H. J., Emmans, D., Irle, E., Streicher, M., & Preilowski, B. 1985. Cortical and subcortical afferent connections of the primate's temporal pole: a study of rhesus monkeys, squirrel monkeys, and marmosets. *Journal of Comparative Neurology*, 242(3): 425–458.

Martinez-Aran, A., Vieta, E., Reinares, M., Colom, F., Torrent, C., Sanchez-Moreno, J., . . . Salamero, M. 2004. Cognitive function across manic or hypomanic, depressed, and euthymic states in bipolar disorder. *American Journal of Psychiatry*, 161(2): 262–270.

Mazzola-Pomietto, P., Kaladjian, A., Azorin, J. M., Anton, J. L., & Jeanningros, R. 2009. Bilateral decrease in ventrolateral prefrontal cortex activation during motor response inhibition in mania. *Journal of Psychiatry Research*, 43(4): 432–441.

McIntosh, A. M., Whalley, H. C., McKirdy, J., Hall, J., Sussmann, J. E., Shankar, P., . . . Lawrie, S. M. 2008. Prefrontal function and activation in bipolar disorder and schizophrenia. *American Journal of Psychiatry*, 165(3): 378–384.

Meyer, S. E., Carlson, G. A., Wiggs, E. A., Martinez, P. E., Ronsaville, D. S., Klimes-Dougan, B., . . . Yarrow, M. 2004. A prospective study of the association among impaired executive functioning, childhood attentional problems, and the development of bipolar disorder. *Development and Psychopathology*, 16(2): 461–476.

Minzenberg, M. J., Laird, A. R., Thelen, S., Carter, C. S., & Glahn, D. C. 2009. Meta-analysis of 41 functional neuroimaging studies of executive function in schizophrenia. *Archives of General Psychiatry*, 66(8): 811–822.

Mitchell, R. L., Elliott, R., Barry, M., Cruttenden, A., & Woodruff, P. W. 2004. Neural response to emotional prosody in schizophrenia and in bipolar affective disorder. *British Journal of Psychiatry*, 184(Mar): 223–230.

Monks, P. J., Thompson, J. M., Bullmore, E. T., Suckling, J., Brammer, M. J., Williams, S. C., . . . Curtis, V. A. 2004. A functional MRI study of working memory task in euthymic bipolar disorder: evidence for task-specific dysfunction. *Bipolar Disorders*, 6(6): 550–564.

Morris, J. S., & Dolan, R. J. 2004. Dissociable amygdala and orbitofrontal responses during reversal fear conditioning. *Neuroimage*, 22(1): 372–380.

Murray, C. J., & Lopez, A. D. 1996. Evidence-based health policy—lessons from the Global Burden of Disease Study. *Science*, 274(5288): 740–743.

Nagai, M., Kishi, K., & Kato, S. 2007. Insular cortex and neuropsychiatric disorders: a review of recent literature. *European Psychiatry*, 22(6): 387–394.

Nebel, K., Wiese, H., Stude, P., de Greiff, A., Diener, H. C., & Keidel, M. 2005. On the neural basis of focused and divided attention. *Brain Research. Cognitive Brain Research*, 25(3): 760–776.

Nehra, R., Chakrabarti, S., Pradhan, B. K., & Khehra, N. 2006. Comparison of cognitive functions between first- and multi-episode bipolar affective disorders. *Journal of Affective Disorders*, 93(1–3): 185–192.

Nierenberg, A. A., Miyahara, S., Spencer, T., Wisniewski, S. R., Otto, M. W., Simon, N., . . . Sachs, G. S. 2005. Clinical and diagnostic implications of lifetime attention-deficit/hyperactivity disorder comorbidity in adults with bipolar disorder: data from the first 1000 STEP-BD participants. *Biological Psychiatry*, 57(11): 1467–1473.

Northoff, G., Richter, A., Gessner, M., Schlagenhauf, F., Fell, J., Baumgart, F., . . . Heinz, H. J. 2000. Functional dissociation between medial and lateral prefrontal cortical spatiotemporal activation in negative and positive emotions: a combined fMRI/MEG study. *Cerebral Cortex*, 10(1): 93–107.

Nystrom, L. E., Braver, T. S., Sabb, F. W., Delgado, M. R., Noll, D. C., & Cohen, J. D. 2000. Working memory for letters, shapes, and locations: fMRI evidence against stimulus-based regional organization in human prefrontal cortex. *Neuroimage*, 11(5 Pt 1): 424–446.

Pessoa, L., Kastner, S., & Ungerleider, L. G. 2002. Attentional control of the processing of neural and emotional stimuli. *Brain Research. Cognitive Brain Research*, 15(1): 31–45.

Peterson, B. S., Skudlarski, P., Gatenby, J. C., Zhang, H., Anderson, A. W., & Gore, J. C. 1999. An fMRI study of Stroop word-color interference: evidence for cingulate subregions subserving multiple distributed attentional systems. *Biological Psychiatry*, 45(10): 1237–1258.

Petrides, M. 2005. Lateral prefrontal cortex: architectonic and functional organization. *Philosophical Transactions of the Royal Society of London. Series B, Biological Sciences*, 360(1456): 781–795.

Phillips, M. L., Drevets, W. C., Rauch, S. L., & Lane, R. 2003. Neurobiology of emotion perception II: Implications for major psychiatric disorders. *Biological Psychiatry*, 54(5): 515–528.

Price, J. L. 2003. Comparative aspects of amygdala connectivity. *Annals of the New York Academy of Sciences*, 985(Apr): 50–58.

Price, J. L., Carmichael, S. T., & Drevets, W. C. 1996. Networks related to the orbital and medial prefrontal cortex; a substrate for emotional behavior? *Progress in Brain Research*, 107: 523–536.

Robinson, J. L., Monkul, E. S., Tordesillas-Gutierrez, D., Franklin, C., Bearden, C. E., Fox, P. T., & Glahn, D. C. 2008. Fronto-limbic circuitry in euthymic bipolar disorder: evidence for prefrontal hyperactivation. *Psychiatry Research*, 164(2): 106–113.

Rosso, I. M., Killgore, W. D., Cintron, C. M., Gruber, S. A., Tohen, M., & Yurgelun-Todd, D. A. 2007. Reduced amygdala volumes in first-episode bipolar disorder and correlation with cerebral white matter. *Biological Psychiatry*, 61(6): 743–749.

Roth, R. M., Koven, N. S., Randolph, J. J., Flashman, L. A., Pixley, H. S., Ricketts, S. M., . . . Saykin, A. J. 2006. Functional magnetic resonance imaging of executive control in bipolar disorder. *Neuroreport*, 17(11): 1085–1089.

Rubinsztein, J. S., Fletcher, P. C., Rogers, R. D., Ho, L. W., Aigbirhio, F. I., Paykel, E. S., . . . Sahakian, B. J. 2001. Decision-making in mania: a PET study. *Brain*, 124 (Pt 12): 2550–2563.

Rubinsztein, J. S., Michael, A., Paykel, E. S., & Sahakian, B. J. 2000. Cognitive impairment in remission in bipolar affective disorder. *Psychological Medicine*, 30(5): 1025–1036.

Rubinsztein, J. S., Michael, A., Underwood, B. R., Tempest, M., & Sahakian, B. J. 2006. Impaired cognition and decision-making in bipolar depression but no "affective bias" evident. *Psychological Medicine*, 36(5): 629–639.

Sakai, K., & Passingham, R. E. 2006. Prefrontal set activity predicts rule-specific neural processing during subsequent cognitive performance. *Journal of Neuroscience*, 26(4): 1211–1218.

Schlosser, R., Hutchinson, M., Joseffer, S., Rusinek, H., Saarimaki, A., Stevenson, J., . . . Brodie, J. D. 1998. Functional magnetic resonance imaging of human brain activity in a verbal fluency task. *Journal of Neurology, Neurosurgery, and Psychiatry*, 64(4): 492–498.

Sherazi, R., McKeon, P., McDonough, M., Daly, I., & Kennedy, N. 2006. What's new? The clinical epidemiology of bipolar I disorder. *Harvard Review of Psychiatry*, 14(6): 273–284.

Silverstone, P. H., Bell, E. C., Willson, M. C., Dave, S., & Wilman, A. H. 2005. Lithium alters brain activation in bipolar disorder in a task- and state-dependent manner: an fMRI study. *Annals of General Psychiatry*, 4:14.

Simmonds, D. J., Pekar, J. J., & Mostofsky, S. H. 2008 Meta-analysis of Go/No-go tasks demonstrating that fMRI activation associated with response inhibition is task-dependent. *Neuropsychologia,* Jan 15;46(1):224–32. Epub 2007 Jul 28.

Simon, G. E. 2003. Social and economic burden of mood disorders. *Biological Psychiatry*, 54(3): 208–215.

Smith, E. E., & Jonides, J. 1998. Neuroimaging analyses of human working memory. *Proceedings of the National Academy of Sciences of the United States of America*, 95(20): 12061–12068.

Starkstein, S. E., Fedoroff, P., Berthier, M. L., & Robinson, R. G. 1991. Manic-depressive and pure manic states after brain lesions. *Biological Psychiatry*, 29(2): 149–158.

Stein, J. L., Wiedholz, L. M., Bassett, D. S., Weinberger, D. R., Zink, C. F., Mattay, V. S., & Meyer-Lindenberg, A. 2007. A validated network of effective amygdala connectivity. *Neuroimage*, 36(3): 736–745.

Stern, E., & Silbersweig, D. A. 2001. Advances in functional neuroimaging methodology for the study of brain systems underlying human neuropsychological function and dysfunction. *Journal of Clinical and Experimental Neuropsychology*, 23(1): 3–18.

Strakowski, S. M., Adler, C. M., Cerullo, M. A., Eliassen, J. C., Lamy, M., Fleck, D. E., . . . Delbello, M. P. 2008. Magnetic resonance imaging brain activation in first-episode bipolar mania during a response inhibition task. *Early Intervention in Psychiatry*, 2(4): 225–233.

Strakowski, S. M., Adler, C. M., Holland, S. K., Mills, N., & DelBello, M. P. 2004. A preliminary FMRI study of sustained attention in euthymic, unmedicated bipolar disorder. *Neuropsychopharmacology*, 29(9): 1734–1740.

Strakowski, S. M., Adler, C. M., Holland, S. K., Mills, N. P., DelBello, M. P., & Eliassen, J. C. 2005. Abnormal FMRI brain activation in euthymic bipolar disorder patients during a counting Stroop interference task. *American Journal of Psychiatry*, 162(9): 1697–1705.

Strakowski, S. M., DelBello, M. P., Sax, K. W., Zimmerman, M. E., Shear, P. K., Hawkins, J. M., . . . & Larson, E. R. 1999. Brain magnetic resonance imaging of structural abnormalities in bipolar disorder. *Archives of General Psychiatry*, 56(3): 254–260.

Strakowski, S. M., DelBello, M. P., & Adler, C. M. 2005. The functional neuroanatomy of bipolar disorder: a review of neuroimaging findings. *Molecular Psychiatry*, 10(1): 105–116.

Strakowski, S. M., Eliassen, J. C., Lamy, M., Cerullo, M. A., Allendorfer, J. B., Madore, M., . . . Adler, C. M. 2011. Functional magnetic resonance imaging brain activation in bipolar mania: evidence for disruption of the ventrolateral prefrontal-amygdala emotional pathway. *Biological Psychiatry*, 69(4): 381–388.

Strakowski, S. M., Fleck, D. E., DelBello, M. P., Adler, C. M., Shear, P. K., Kotwal, R., . . . Arndt, S. 2010. Impulsivity across the course of bipolar disorder. *Bipolar Disorders*, 12(3): 285–297.

Surguladze, S. A., Marshall, N., Schulze, K., Hall, M. H., Walshe, M., Bramon, E., . . . McDonald, C. 2010. Exaggerated neural response to emotional faces in patients with bipolar disorder and their first-degree relatives. *Neuroimage*, 53(1): 58–64.

Swann, A. C., Anderson, J. C., Dougherty, D. M., & Moeller, F. G. 2001. Measurement of inter-episode impulsivity in bipolar disorder. *Psychiatry Research*, 101(2): 195–197.

Thermenos, H. W., Goldstein, J. M., Milanovic, S. M., Whitfield-Gabrieli, S., Makris, N., Laviolette, P., . . . Seidman, L. J. 2010. An fMRI study of working memory in persons with bipolar disorder or at genetic risk for bipolar disorder. *American Journal of Medical Genetics. Part B, Neuropsychiatric Genetics*, 153B(1): 120–131.

Townsend, J., Bookheimer, S. Y., Foland-Ross, L. C., Sugar, C. A., & Altshuler, L. L. 2010. fMRI abnormalities in dorsolateral prefrontal cortex during a working memory task in manic, euthymic and depressed bipolar subjects. *Psychiatry Research*, 182(1): 22–29.

Trivedi, J. K., Dhyani, M., Sharma, S., Sinha, P. K., Singh, A. P., & Tandon, R. 2008. Cognitive functions in euthymic state of bipolar disorder: an Indian study. *Cognitive Neuropsychiatry*, 13(2): 135–147.

Tucker, D. M., Luu, P., & Pribram, K. H. 1995. Social and emotional self-regulation. *Annals of the New York Academy of Sciences*, 769(Dec 15): 213–239.

Van Hoesen, G. W., Pandya, D. N., & Butters, N. 1972. Cortical afferents to the entorhinal cortex of the Rhesus monkey. *Science*, 175(29): 1471–1473.

Versace, A., Thompson, W. K., Zhou, D., Almeida, J. R., Hassel, S., Klein, C. R., . . . Phillips, M. L. 2010. Abnormal left and right amygdala-orbitofrontal cortical functional connectivity to emotional faces: state versus trait vulnerability markers of depression in bipolar disorder. *Biological Psychiatry*, 67(5): 422–431.

Wager, T. D., & Smith, E. E. 2003. Neuroimaging studies of working memory: a meta-analysis. *Cognitive, Affectective, and Behavioral Neuroscience*, 3(4): 255–274.

Wager, T. D., Jonides, J., & Reading, S. 2004. Neuroimaging studies of shifting attention: a meta-analysis. *Neuroimage*, 22(4): 1679–1693.

Wang, F., Kalmar, J. H., He, Y., Jackowski, M., Chepenik, L. G., Edmiston, E. E., . . . Blumberg, H. P. 2009. Functional and structural connectivity between the perigenual anterior cingulate and amygdala in bipolar disorder. *Biological Psychiatry*, 66(5): 516–521.

Wessa, M., Houenou, J., Paillere-Martinot, M. L., Berthoz, S., Artiges, E., Leboyer, M., & Martinot, J. L. 2007. Fronto-striatal overactivation in euthymic bipolar patients during an emotional go/nogo task. *American Journal of Psychiatry*, 164(4): 638–646.

Yamasaki, H., LaBar, K. S., & McCarthy, G. 2002. Dissociable prefrontal brain systems for attention and emotion. *Proceedings of the National Academy of Sciences of the United States of America*, 99(17): 11447–11451.

Yurgelun-Todd, D. A., Gruber, S. A., Kanayama, G., Killgore, W. D., Baird, A. A., & Young, A. D. 2000. fMRI during affect discrimination in bipolar affective disorder. *Bipolar Disorders*, 2 (3 Pt 2): 237–248.

# 4.

# NEUROCHEMICAL AND METABOLIC IMAGING IN BIPOLAR DISORDER

Jieun E. Kim, In Kyoon Lyoo, and Perry F. Renshaw

Bipolar disorder is a common and potentially debilitating disorder that appears to have neurobiological underpinnings (Manji et al., 2000; Muller-Oerlinghausen et al., 2002; Belmaker 2004; Merikangas et al., 2007). Brain mechanisms that underlie the etiology of bipolar disorder are not yet completely understood, which may be, in part, a reason why a singularly effective treatment has not emerged. Pervasive alterations in neurotransmitter or signal transduction systems in bipolar disorder have been reported from extensive research conducted for several decades (Manji et al., 2000). A line of preclinical studies also suggests a crucial role of mitochondrial impairment in the pathophysiology of bipolar disorder (Konradi et al., 2004; Kasahara et al., 2006). Recent findings from *in vivo* magnetic resonance spectroscopy (MRS) studies in humans suggest that these mitochondrial abnormalities might represent a central biochemical pathology of bipolar disorder (Stork et al., 2005) (Figure 4.1).

As a noninvasive technique that affords a window into brain chemistry and function of patients with bipolar disorder, MRS has provided opportunities to look into the biochemical processes in the brains of patients with bipolar disorder. Proton ($^1$H) MRS can measure cerebral concentrations of *N*-acetyl aspartate (NAA), choline (Cho)-containing compounds, glutamate/glutamine (Glx), myo-inositol (mI), and lactate, all of which are important neurometabolites reflecting key mitochondrial functions (Dager et al., 2008) (Figure 4.2). Phosphorus ($^{31}$P) MRS studies in bipolar disorder patients also identified alterations in intracellular pH (pHi) and the levels of phosphocreatine (PCr) and phosphomonoesters (PMEs), which may demonstrate the level of efficiency in energy production and metabolism.

In this chapter, we propose a unifying hypothesis of mitochondrial dysfunction for the pathophysiology of bipolar disorder that integrates findings from MRS studies.

Based on this hypothesis, researchers may be inspired to develop new diagnostic techniques or innovative treatments (Stork et al., 2005). Considering recent reports which suggest limited efficacy of currently available treatments that are mostly based on neurotransmitter-related strategies (Sachs et al., 2007; Ghaemi 2008), this new understanding of the pathogenesis of bipolar disorder may lead to novel treatments that can be complementary, and hopefully superior in terms of efficacy and safety, to current ones (Stork et al., 2005).

## DECREASED LEVELS OF *N*-ACETYL ASPARTATE IN BIPOLAR DISORDER AS A MARKER FOR MITOCHONDRIAL DYSFUNCTION

*N*-acetyl aspartate (NAA), the second most prevalent amino acid in the central nervous system (CNS), has been thought to originate from mitochondria (Truckenmiller et al., 1985). Synthesis of NAA requires energy consumption, which is demonstrated by the stimulation of its production by adenosine diphosphate (ADP) from adenosine triphosphate (ATP) (Patel et al., 1979). The mitochondrial membrane-bound enzyme, *L*-aspartate *N*-acetyltransferase, which is found only in the CNS, is essential for producing NAA. Concentrations of this amino acid may therefore reflect the intactness of mitochondrial structure and function, in that its production depends on the energy produced by the mitochondria (Patel et al., 1979) and the enzyme that is bound to the mitochondrial membrane (Truckenmiller et al., 1985).

Furthermore, investigators have proposed that the process for NAA biosynthesis is closely coupled with energy production in the mitochondria of neurons, called the "mini citric acid cycle" (Madhavarao et al., 2003) (Figure 4.3). Extraordinarily high-energy demands in neurons have

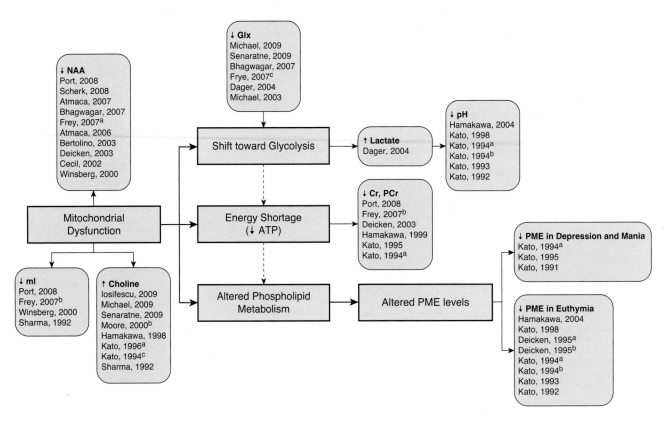

*Figure 4.1* A schematic presentation of the mitochondrial dysfunction hypothesis as one of the etiologies of bipolar disorder and recent magnetic resonance spectroscopy studies which support this hypothesis for each metabolite. *Abbreviations:* ATP, Adenosine triphosphate; Cr, Creatine + phosphocreatine; Glx, Glutamate + glutamine; mI, Myo-inositol; NAA, N-acetyl aspartate; PCr, Phosphocreatine; PME, Phosphomonoester. (Source: Adapted from Stork et al. 2005.)

been reported to be largely met by the oxidation of glutamate, which produces α-ketoglutarate within the mitochondria (Erecinska et al., 1988; Yudkoff et al., 1994). Alpha-ketoglutarate is an important intermediate in the Krebs cycle and is generated via either glutamate dehydrogenase pathway or aspartate aminotransferase pathway (Madhavarao et al., 2003). In order to produce α-ketoglutarate, neurons use the mini citric acid cycle, instead of the glutamate dehydrogenase reaction to avoid ammonia toxicity that results from the inefficient urea cycle in neurons (Madhavarao et al., 2003). Glutamate is converted to ammonia and α-ketoglutarate by glutamate dehydrogenase. Normally, ammonia, which can be toxic by raising the pH level within the cell, is converted into urea, a nontoxic compound. Since there is not an effective urea cycle system in the neuronal mitochondria, it appears that α-ketoglutarate is produced by the mini citric acid cycle, in an effort to avoid producing ammonia and subsequent neurotoxicity (Moffett et al., 2006). NAA biosynthesis plays a role in facilitating this mini citric acid cycle by removing the excess aspartate, so that this cycle could be steered toward

producing α-ketoglutarate and aspartate from glutamate (Madhavarao et al., 2003; Moffett et al., 2006).

Abundantly produced NAA is taken up and transported to the cytosol of the oligodendrocyte and degraded into acetate and *L*-aspartate, compensating for the citrate shortage during the mini citric acid cycle (Chakraborty et al., 2001). This step in the cycle demonstrates that NAA may be a marker that the integral process of normal energy production in the mitochondria is intact. Since traumatic brain injury-produced neuronal death has been shown to result in decreased NAA levels (Signoretti et al., 2001), NAA has long been considered a neuronal marker. However, based on the considerations we discussed here, investigators suggest that NAA is more accurately a marker of energy production within mitochondria (Clark et al., 1998; De Stefano et al., 1995). This consideration provides an important context for interpretation of MRS studies that have investigated abnormalities or changes in NAA concentrations.

In this context, reduced NAA levels (and perhaps NAA/ [PCr + Cr] levels) in bipolar relative to healthy subjects

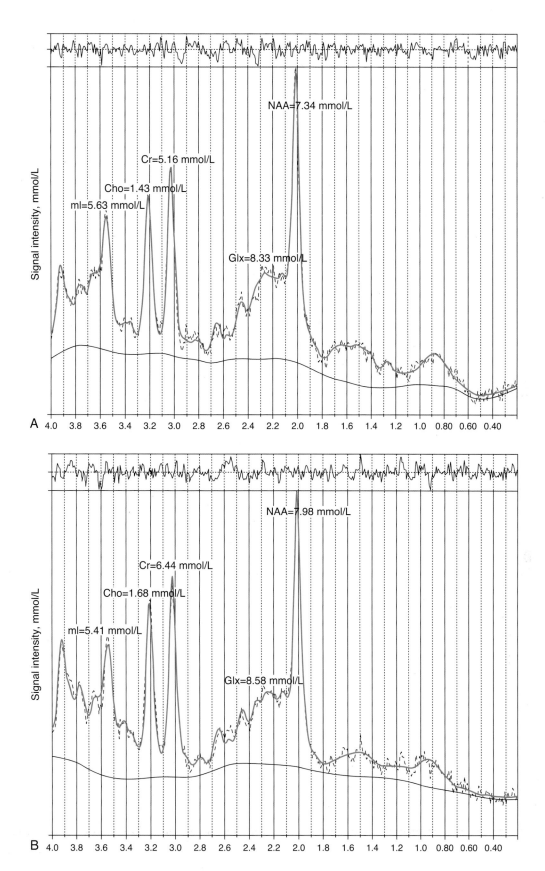

*Figure 4.2* Sample proton magnetic resonance spectroscopy spectra from a patient with bipolar disorder (A) and from a healthy individual (B).

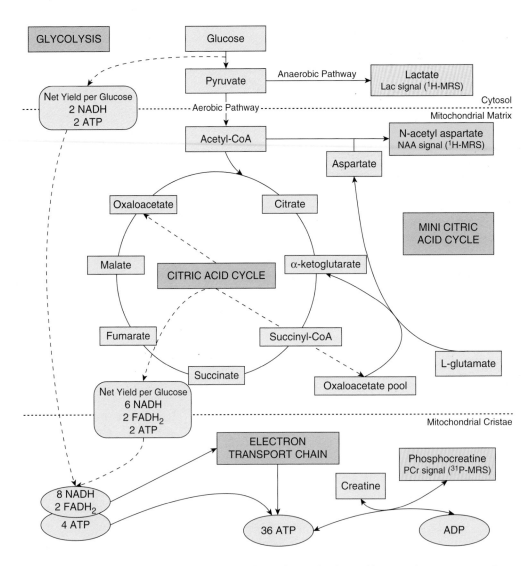

*Figure 4.3* A portrayal of mitochondrial function in the neuron and related signals that can be detected by magnetic resonance spectroscopy. Compounds in the colored boxes denote those visible by magnetic resonance spectroscopy. *Abbreviations:* ADP, Adenosine diphosphate; ATP, Adenosine triphosphate; FADH$_2$, Flavin adenine dinucleotide; Lac, Lactate; NAA, N-acetyl aspartate; NADH, Nicotinamide adenine dinucleotide; PCr, Phosphocreatine. (Source: Adapted from Stork et al. 2005.)

support the hypothesis that mitochondrial dysfunction may underlie the expression of bipolar disorder (Stork et al., 2005) (Table 4.1; Figure 4.4). Although there have been studies that reported increased NAA levels in bipolar disorder patients, studies conducted in drug-free or drug-naive adult bipolar disorder patients have consistently demonstrated reduced levels of NAA compared with healthy subjects (Winsberg et al., 2000; Atmaca et al., 2006; Atmaca et al., 2007; Bhagwagar et al., 2007; Port et al., 2008). Findings summarized in Table 4.1 suggest that mood state may not be an important moderator for this discrepancy. Reports which demonstrate that pharmacological treatment, including lithium, increases the level of NAA in bipolar disorder patients (Sharma et al., 1992; Moore et al.,

2000; Silverstone et al., 2003; Iosifescu et al., 2009; Brennan et al., 2010) suggest that confounding effects of pharmacological treatment on cerebral NAA levels may be responsible for the inconsistency of findings (Stork et al., 2005; Phillips et al., 2008). These reports also suggest that effective treatments may correct the underlying metabolic abnormality.

**Brain NAA Levels:**

- Reflect mitochondrial function and neuronal metabolism
- Are decreased in bipolar disorder
- Suggest mitochondrial abnormalities in bipolar disorder

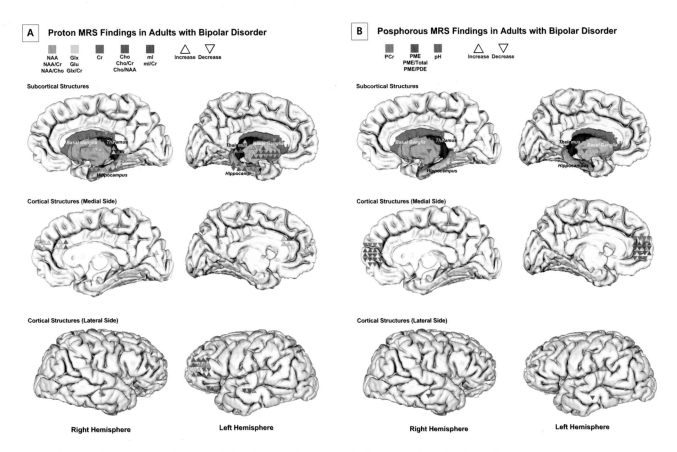

**A** Proton MRS Findings in Adults with Bipolar Disorder

NAA / NAA/Cr / NAA/Cho | Glx Glu Glx/Cr | Cr | Cho Cho/Cr Cho/NAA | ml ml/Cr | △ Increase ▽ Decrease

Subcortical Structures

Cortical Structures (Medial Side)

Cortical Structures (Lateral Side)

Right Hemisphere | Left Hemisphere

**B** Posphorous MRS Findings in Adults with Bipolar Disorder

PCr | PME PME/Total PME/PDE | pH | △ Increase ▽ Decrease

Subcortical Structures

Cortical Structures (Medial Side)

Cortical Structures (Lateral Side)

Right Hemisphere | Left Hemisphere

*Figure 4.4* A schematic presentation of proton and phosphorus MRS regional brain findings in adults with bipolar disorder.

## EVIDENCE FOR A GLYCOLYTIC SHIFT AWAY FROM OXIDATIVE PHOSPHORYLATION SUGGESTING MITOCHONDRIAL DYSFUNCTION

Findings from MRS research conducted over a couple of decades have demonstrated increased levels of lactate and glutamate + glutamine along with lower pHi in bipolar disorder patients compared with healthy subjects, which indicates a shift toward glycolysis for energy production in the mitochondria (Figure 4.3). Anaerobic glycolytic energy production occurs when the respiratory chain for cellular metabolism in the mitochondria is not available (Stork et al., 2005). Energy production by glycolysis is significantly less efficient compared to that by oxidative phosphorylation (Figure 4.3), which may contribute to neural malfunction. For each glucose molecule, a maximum of 34 ATPs could be produced in neurons via the aerobic pathway that includes the citric acid cycle and electron transport chain, while only two ATPs could be produced during the anaerobic glycolysis (Figure 4.3) (Berg et al., 2010).

Dager and colleagues (2004) reported increased levels of Glx (glutamate + glutamine), and lactate in bipolar disorder patients. Alterations in the Glx level may indicate changes in the glutamate/glutamine cycle, which is the recycling system of glutamate through transportation of glutamine between neurons and glial cells (Figure 4.5). Since glutamate is the most abundant amino acid in the brain and primarily has excitatory effects, a rise in the Glx level, which indicates an overall increase in glutamate and glutamine, would put large metabolic demands on brain cells. If neuronal mitochondria cannot fully respond to these demands with the normal oxidative phosphorylation process, glycolysis will occur. Glycolysis is an inefficient means of energy production, and provides relatively less cellular energy (i.e., ATP) compared to oxidative phosphorylation (Yuksel et al., 2010). As illustrated in Figure 4.3, reflecting this process, pyruvate, which receives hydrogen from NADH to make NAD, converts to lactate during glycolysis. This process results in an increase in the level of lactate (Figure 4.3), which may thereby explain the findings of Dager et al. (2004) in depressed bipolar disorder patients.

Increased Glx is among the most consistent MRS findings in bipolar disorder research. Table 4.1 shows that all currently available studies except a study by Port et al.

**TABLE 4.1 PROTON MRS FINDINGS IN ADULTS WITH BIPOLAR DISORDER**

## DEPRESSED STATE

| Study | Subjects | No. of subjects | Mean Age (SD) | Medication Status |
|---|---|---|---|---|
| Frye, 2007[b] | BD I, II | 23 | 35.6 (11.2) | 5 Li |
| | HC | 12 | 32.8 (10.9) | |
| Moore, 2000[b] | BD I | 9 | 37.9 (9.7) | 5 Li, 4 Valp, 5 AD |
| | HC | 14 | 36.1 (10.5) | |
| Hamakawa, 1998 | BC I, II, NOS | 11 | 48.3 (13.4) | 9 medication (3 Li, 3 AP, 3 others) |
| | HC | 20 | 43.7 (9.5) | |
| Kato, 1994[c] | BD I, II, NOS | 11 | N/A | 11 medication |
| | HC | 22 | 37.9 (8.4) | |
| Michael, 2009 | BD II RC | 6 | 53.5 (8.3) | 2 drug free, 4 MS |
| | BD non RC | 6 | 51.6 (10.4) | 1 drug free, 5 PT |
| | HC | 6 | 51.5 (7.1) | |
| Hamakawa, 1999 | BD I, II | 8 | N/A | 2 Li, 4 AP, 2 drug free (1 wk) |
| | HC | 20 | 37.0 (10.0) | |

## MANIC STATE

| Study | Subjects | No. of subjects | Mean Age (SD) | Medication Status |
|---|---|---|---|---|
| Öngür, 2008 | BD I | 15 | 36.3 (11.6) | 9 Li, 8 AC, 15 AP, 7 AX |
| | HC | 21 | 34.3 (10.0) | |
| Frye, 2007[a] | BD I | 16 | 37.5 (11.5) | 5 Li, 5 AP, 7 Valp |
| | HC | 17 | 32.9 (11.5) | |
| Sharma, 1992 | BD I | 4 | N/A | 4 Li |
| | HC | 9 | 31 (4.8) | |
| Michael, 2003[a] | BD I | 8 | 40.1 (13.9) | 1 Li, 6 drug naïve |
| | HC | 8 | 40.7 (14.7) | |
| Atmaca, 2007 | BD I | 10 | 23.4 (5.6) | 10 drug naïve (First episode) |
| | HC | 10 | 24.3 (4.3) | |
| Atmaca, 2006 | BD I | 12 | 28.2 (6.5) | 12 drug free (2 wks) |
| | HC | 12 | 26.8 (7.6) | |

## EUTHYMIC STATE

| Study | Subjects | No. of subjects | Mean Age (SD) | Medication Status |
|---|---|---|---|---|
| Hamakawa, 1998 | BD I, II, NOS | 16 | 44.4 (10.9) | 14 medication (6 Li, 6 AP) |
| | HC | 20 | 43.7 (9.5) | |

| T | ROI | NAA | Glx | Cr | Cho | ml |
|---|---|---|---|---|---|---|
| 1.5 | ACC+MPFC | | ▲<br>Glu▲ | ▲ | | |
| 1.5 | (R) ACC | | | | /Cr▲ | |
| 1.5 | (L) Basal ganglia | | | | ▲<br>/Cr▲<br>/NAA▲ | |
| 1.5 | (L) Basal ganglia | | | | /Cr ▲<br>/NAA▲ | |
| 1.5 | (L) DLPFC | ▲ | ▲ | ▲ | ▲ | |
| | (L) DLPFC | ▲ | | ▲ | ▲ | |
| 1.5 | (L) Frontal cortex | | | ▼ | | |
| 4 | ACC | | Gln/Glu▲ | | | |
| | POC | | Gln/Glu▲ | | | |
| 3 | (R) Basal ganglia | ▼<br>/Cr▼ | | | | |
| 1.5 | (L) Basal ganglia | /Cr▲ | | | /Cr▲ | /Cr▲ |
| 1.5 | DLPFC | | ▲ | | | |
| 1.5 | Hippocampus | /Cr▼<br>/Cho▼ | | | | |
| 1.5 | Hippocampus | /Cr▼<br>/Cho▼ | | | | |
| 1.5 | (L) Basal ganglia | | | | /Cr▲<br>/NAA▲ | |

(Continued)

## EUTHYMIC STATE

| Study | Subjects | No. of subjects | Mean Age (SD) | Medication Status |
|---|---|---|---|---|
| Kato, 1996[a] | BD I, II | 19 | 41.6 (9.4) | 10 (Li + PT)<br>9 (Li free + PT) |
| | HC | 19 | 40.3 (6.3) | |
| Michael, 2009 | BD II RC | 8 | 53.5 (8.3) | 2 drug free, 4 MS |
| | HC | 6 | 51.5 (7.1) | |
| Molina, 2007 | BD I | 13 | 37.8 (6.7) | 10 Li, 3 Valp, 5 PT |
| | HC | 10 | 27.2 (4.9) | |
| Winsberg, 2000 | BD I, II | 20 | 37.9 (13.8) | 16 drug free (2 wks) |
| | HC | 20 | 33.5 (13.9) | |
| Iosifescu, 2009 | BD | 20 | 40.7 (11.9) | 20 medication |
| | HC | 10 | 38.9 (10.1) | |
| Colla, 2009 | BD I | 21 | 54.2 (1.9) | 21 Li |
| | HC | 19 | 54.6 (2.1) | |
| Scherk, 2008 | BD I | 13 | 31.5(6.23) | 12 MS<br>(3 Li, 5 Valp, 7 others),<br>5 AD, 6 AP |
| | HC | 13 | 31.5 (6.26) | |
| Deicken, 2003 | BD I | 15 | 39.3 (10.3) | 12 medication<br>(4 Li, 3AP) |
| | HC | 20 | 36.0 (10.7) | |
| Senaratne, 2009 | BD I, II | 12 | 42.1 (12.8) | 8 Li, 6 AP, 13 PT |
| | HC | 12 | 37.9 (13.4) | |
| Bhagwagar, 2007 | BD I | 16 | 37.0 (13.8) | 16 drug free ( > 3 mo) |
| | HC | 18 | 37.6 (14.0) | |
| Wu, 2004 | BD I, II | 14 Li | 40.4 (3.0) | 14 Li (7 AX, 5AD, 2AP),<br>11 Valp (5 AX, 5AD, 4AP) |
| | | 11 Valp | 35.5 (2.3) | |
| | HC | 18 | 31.4 (2.9) | |

| T | ROI | NAA | Glx | Cr | Cho | ml |
|---|---|---|---|---|---|---|
| 1.5 | (L) Basal ganglia | | | | /Cr▲ <br><br> /Cr▲ (Li free) <br><br> /NAA▲ (Li free) | |
| 1.5 | (L) DLPFC | ▲ | ▲ | ▲ | ▲ | |
| 1.5 | (L) DLPFC | /Cr ▲ | | | | |
| 1.5 | (R) DLPFC | /Cr▼ <br> /Cho▼ | | | | /Cr▲* |
| | (L) DLPFC | /Cr▼ <br> /Cho▼ | | | | |
| 4 | (R) Hippocampus | ▲ | | ▲ | ▲ | |
| | (L) Hippocampus | | | ▲ | ▲ | |
| 3 | (L) Hippocampus | | Glu▲ | | | |
| 1.5 | (L) Hippocampus | /Cr▼ | | | | |
| 1.5 | (R) Hippocampus | ▼ | | ▼ | | |
| | (L) Hippocampus | ▼ | | ▼ | | |
| 3 | (L) Hippocampus | | | | ▲ | |
| | (L) OFC | | | | ▲ | |
| | (L) Occipital cortex | | ▲ | | | |
| 1.5 | Occipital cortex | /Cr▼ | /Cr▲ | | | |
| 3 | (L) Temporal lobe | | | | /Cr▼ (14 Li) <br><br> /Cr▼ (11 Valp) | |

(Continued)

**EUTHYMIC STATE**

| Study | Subjects | No. of subjects | Mean Age (SD) | Medication Status |
|---|---|---|---|---|
| Silverstone, 2003 | BD I, II | 25 | N/A | 14 Li, 11 Valp 22 other PT |
|  | HC | 18 | 31.4 (2.9 |  |
| Deicken, 2001 | BD I | 15 | 41.1 (10.6) | 13 medication (5 Li, 2 AP) |
|  | HC | 15 | 37.5 (11.1) |  |

**VARIOUS STATE**

| Study | Subjects | No. of subjects | Mean Age (SD) | Medication Status |
|---|---|---|---|---|
| Port, 2008 | BD I, II, NOS | 21 (10 manic, 5 depressed, 6 euthymic) | 30.8 | 21 drug free |
|  | HC | 21 | 31.1 |  |
| Frey, 2007 | BD I, II | 32 (7 manic, 17 depressed, 7 euthymic, 1 mixed) | 33.8 (10.2) | 32 drug free |
|  | HC | 32 | 33.8 (9.0) |  |
| Dager, 2004 | BD I, II | 32 (mixed, depressed) | 30.3 (10.8) | 32 drug free ( > 8 wks) |
|  | HC | 23 | 31.9 (7.7) |  |
| Bertolino, 2003 | BD I | 17 (4 manic, 7 depressed, 6 euthymic) | 40.1 (12.9) | 11 medication (6 Li, 2 Valp, 10 PT) |
|  | HC | 17 | 37.6 (10.3) |  |
| Cecil, 2002 | BD I | 17 (9 manic, 8 mixed) | 22.3 (7.3) | 17 medication (2Li, 13 AP) |
|  | HC | 21 | 21.7 (5.2) |  |

Proton MRS Findings in Adults with Bipolar Disorder. *Abbreviations*: ACC, Anterior cingulate cortex; AC, Anticonvulsant; AD, Antidepressants; AP Antipsychotics; AX, Anxiolytics; BD, Bipolar disorder; Cho, Choline; Cr, Creatine; DLPFC, Dorsolateral prefrontal cortex; Gln, Glutamine; Glu, Glutamate; Glx, Glutamate + Glutamine; HC, Healthy comparison subjects; (L), Left; Li, Lithium; ml, myo-Inositol; MPFC, Medial prefrontal cortex; MS, Mood stabilizer; N/A, Not applicable; NAA, N-acetyl aspartate; NOS, Not otherwise specified; OFC, Orbitofrontal cortex; POC, Parieto-occipital cortex; PT, Psychotropics; (R), Right; RC, Rapid cycling; ROI, Region of interest; SD, Standard deviation; T, Tesla; Valp, Valproate; WM, White matter.

\* p = 0.06.

Among studies reporting MRS findings in adult patients with bipolar disorder, those reported nonsignificant results (Amaral, 2006; Brambilla, 2005; Bruhn, 1993; Deicken, 1995a; Deicken, 1995b; Frey, 2005; Michael, 2003b; Ohara, 1998; Öngür, 2009; Sarramea-Crespo, 2008; Scherk, 2009; Silverstone, 2002; Stoll, 1992) are not included in this table.

| T | ROI | NAA | Glx | Cr | Cho | ml |
|---|---|---|---|---|---|---|
| 3 | Temporal lobe | /Cr ▲ | | | | |
| 1.5 | (R) Thalamus | ▲ | | ▲ | | |
| | (L) Thalamus | ▲ | | ▲ | | |
| 3 | (R) Caudate head | ▼ | | ▼ | ▼ | |
| | (L) Caudate head | ▼ | | | | ▲ |
| | Frontal WM | | ▼ | | | |
| | (R) Lentiform | | ▼ | | | |
| | (L) Lentiform | ▼ | | | | |
| 1.5 | (L) DLPFC | | | ▼ | ▼ | ▲* |
| 1.5 | Frontal WM, Parietal WM, Cingulate, Caudate, Putamen, Thalamus, Occiput, Insula | | ▲ | | | |
| 1.5 | Hippocampus | /Cr▼ /Cho▼ | | | | |
| 1.5 | Medial OFC | ▼ | | | ▼ | |

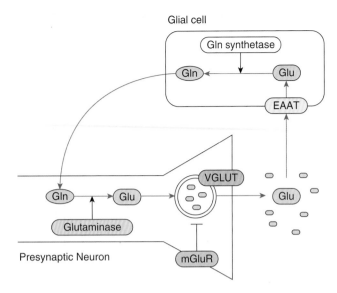

Glial cell

*Figure 4.5* A schematic presentation of the glutamate/glutamine cycle. *Abbreviations:* Gln, Glutamine; Glu, Glutamate; EAAT, Excitatory amino-acid transporter; VGLUT, Vesicular glutamate transporter; mGluR, Metabotropic glutamate receptor. (Source: Adapted from Sanacora et al. 2008.)

(2008) documented increased Glx level in bipolar disorder compared to healthy subjects (see also Figure 4.4). In a recent study by Port et al. (2008), the authors reported decreased levels of Glx in white matter voxels of the brain and in the right lentiform nucleus. Studies that report increased Glx level primarily placed MRS voxels within gray matter. In Dager and colleagues' report, averaged Glx values from bilateral frontal and parietal white matter voxels were not different between patients with bipolar disorder and healthy subjects, although patients with bipolar disorder type II demonstrated increased levels of Glx compared to healthy participants. Studies that examined basal ganglia regions including the lentiform nucleus reported no differences in the levels of Glx between bipolar and healthy subjects (Frye et al., 2007a) or did not report the level of Glx (Sharma et al., 1992; Kato et al., 1994c; Kato et al., 1996a; Hamakawa et al., 1998). Taken together, disparity among studies may have arisen from voxel position differences considering that alterations of Glx can be region-specific.

Few studies have reported lactate levels in bipolar disorder (Dager et al., 2004). This may be due to difficulties in measuring lactate levels using MRS techniques, since the lactate peak tends to overlap with the peaks of macromolecules and lipids (Moore et al., 2002). Proton echo-planar spectroscopic imaging (PEPSI) sequences could provide a more adequate way to measure cerebral lactate levels (Corrigan et al., 2010). PEPSI sequences provide additional spectral information that is unavailable with long echo time sequences due to T2 relaxation and J coupling (Posse et al., 1994), increase the signal-to-noise ratio (Dager et al., 1999) and adopt appropriate lipid suppression to avoid contamination from extracranial fat (Posse et al., 1997), enabling more sensitive and reliable measurement of lactate levels.

Elevated cerebral lactate is also closely coupled with decreased pHi (Clausen et al., 2001). A logarithmic relationship of the two measures has been suggested as follows: (pH = 7.949–0.138(ln[Lac]), $p(b_0) = 0.0258$, $p(b_1) = 0.1921$). Dager et al. reported that differences of lactate of 0.22mM between bipolar disorder patients (mM) and healthy subjects (mM) led to the decrease of pH by 0.016, acidifying the cells (Dager et al., 2004). This equation shows that lactate concentrations have a logarithmic relationship with brain tissue pH. Studies in which cerebral pHi was evaluated using [31]P MRS have demonstrated reduced levels of pHi in bipolar disorder (Kato et al., 1992; Kato et al., 1993; Kato et al., 1994b; Kato et al., 1998; Hamakawa et al., 2004) (Table 4.2, Figure 4.4). Additionally, Clausen et al. (2001) found that isolated mitochondrial failure in the feline brain induces both an increase in lactate and a decrease in pHi levels, which corroborates the suggestion that mitochondrial dysfunction underlies the expression of bipolar disorder.

In accordance with this hypothesis, successful pharmacological treatment has been associated with normalization of the increased Glx (Brennan et al., 2010, Yoon et al., 2009), decreased lactate (Kim et al., 2007) and increased NAA levels (Moore, G.J. et al., 2000; Iosifescu et al., 2009; Brennan et al., 2010). This observation suggests that the therapeutic mechanism of effective treatments in bipolar disorder is associated with normalization of the glycolytic shift in energy production, possibly with the restoration of mitochondrial function.

**Studies of Glycolysis and Oxidative Phosphorylation in the Bipolar Brain Suggest:**

- Increases in brain glutamate + glutamine levels in bipolar disorder would cause a rise in energy demand, altering metabolic processes

- Increased brain lactate levels and the decreased pHi in bipolar disorder reflect a shift toward glycolysis which is substantially inefficient in energy production

- Insufficient energy supply from mitochondria may lead to neuronal malfunction

## IMPAIRED ENERGY PRODUCTION AS EVIDENCED BY DECREASED LEVELS OF HIGH-ENERGY COMPOUNDS IN BIPOLAR DISORDER

Decreases in the level of high-energy compounds such as PCr have been repeatedly reported in bipolar disorder. Table 4.2 and Figure 4.4 provide a summary of findings from phosphorus MRS studies, which shows decreased PCr levels in bipolar disorder patients compared to healthy subjects. Synthesized from Cr within mitochondria with the help of creatine kinase (CK), PCr is a reservoir energy compound that can be degraded to produce ATP in response to neuronal energy demands (Frey et al., 2007b). While short-term decreases in PCr reflect neuronal activity, long-term reduction in the level of PCr is associated with mitochondrial dysfunction, such as in mitochondrial encephalomyopathy, lactic acidosis, and stroke-like episodes (MELAS). In animal MRS studies, both lithium and valproic acid administration decreased levels of Cr and PCr, suggesting the possibility that decreased PCr observed in bipolar disorder patients may be caused by treatment with lithium and mood stabilizing agents (O'Donnell et al., 2000). However, in a study by Friedman et al. (2004) in which 21 drug-free bipolar disorder patients, most of whom had never been treated with either mood stabilizing agents or antipsychotics, were randomized to lithium (n = 12) or valproic acid treatment (n = 9), changes in Cr levels were not noted while changes in mI and Glx levels occurred in the lithium-treatment group.

Decreased PCr levels demonstrate impaired functioning of the mitochondria in producing high-energy compounds, although further *in vivo* human studies are needed to investigate whether the reduction in PCr is due to the confounding effects of treatment. Such studies might identify new avenues of research that identify more specific treatment interventions than are currently available.

---

**Studies of High Energy Phosphorus Compounds in the Bipolar Brain Suggest:**

· Brain levels of high-energy compounds, such as PCr, are decreased

· Long-term reduction in PCr levels is associated with mitochondrial dysfunction

· Further investigations on the cause of the reduction in PCr levels are needed

---

## IMPAIRED PHOSPHOLIPID METABOLISM AS EVIDENCED BY ELEVATED CHOLINE AND MYO-INOSITOL LEVELS IN BIPOLAR DISORDER

One of the major functions of the mitochondria is the metabolism of membrane lipids (Stork et al., 2005). The MRS literature has provided support for impaired phospholipid metabolism in bipolar disorder (Figure 4.6). *De novo* biosynthesis of phospholipids requires a sizeable portion of ATP produced in brain cells (Purdon et al., 1998). Mitochondrial dysfunction, therefore, affects the metabolism of phospholipids in that energy production would be limited and therefore be unable to maintain normal membrane lipid turnover and function.

As shown in the Figure 4.6, increased levels of mI and Cho indicate altered phospholipid metabolism (Table 4.2). Since the steps that convert choline to phosphocholine, ethanolamine to phosphoethanolamine, and mI to CDP-diacylglycerol are ATP dependent, energy shortages would result in increased concentrations of the precursors to membrane compounds, such as choline and mI. Additionally, the PME signal in $^{31}P$ MRS would be decreased because it reflects the combined level of phosphocholine and phosphoethanolamine, which are synthesized using ATP from choline and ethanolamine, respectively (Stork et al., 2005).

Although there have been only a few reports (Kato et al., 1991, 1994a, and 1995), thereby requiring replication, a pattern of PME level increase in depressed or manic states and PME level decrease in euthymic state is identifiable (Table 4.2). As was stated, the PME signal is primarily from phosphocholine and phosphoethanolamine, but it also contains various compounds of sugar, inositol phosphates, even Cho and mI (Gyulai et al., 1984; Pettegrew et al., 1987; Stork et al., 2005). These molecules can be increased in concentration during active turnover of membranes, and therefore the transient high levels of PME during active illness phases of manic or depressed states may reflect active degradation and the brain's attempts to normalize membrane metabolism (Stork et al., 2005). Further studies to elucidate the mood state-dependent PME level alterations are needed.

In an effort to reduce the energy requirements for the synthesis of phosphocholine in bipolar disorder (Hurtado et al., 2005; Mir et al., 2003; Radad et al., 2007), cytidine has been orally administered to patients with bipolar disorder (Yoon et al., 2009). Since synthesis of cytidine, that builds components of RNA and DNA, requires energy consumption, exogenous cytidine supplementation would reduce brain energy requirements. Patients who were

## TABLE 4.2 PHOSPHORUS MRS FINDINGS IN ADULTS WITH BIPOLAR DISORDER

### DEPRESSED STATE

| Study | Subjects | No. of subjects | Mean Age (SD) | Medication Status |
|---|---|---|---|---|
| Kato, 1994[a] | BD I, II | 12 BD II | 39.3 (12.6) | 4 drug free, 1 drug naïve, 7 medication |
|  | HC | 59 | 38.1 (12.6) | |
| Kato, 1995 | BD | 11 | 38.6 (10.0) | 3 drug free, 1 drug naïve, 6 medication |
|  | HC | 21 | 42.5 (10.2) | |

### MANIC STATE

| Study | Subjects | No. of subjects | Mean Age (SD) | Medication Status |
|---|---|---|---|---|
| Kato, 1995 | BD | 12 | 39.5 (7.4) | 2 drug free, 10 medication |
|  | HC | 21 | 42.5 (10.2) | |
| Kato, 1994[a] | BD I, II | 10 BD II | 43.8 (14.9) | 2 drug free, 1 drug naïve, 7 medication |
|  | HC | 59 | 38.1 (12.6) | |
| Kato 1991 | BD | 11 | 40.8 (11.0) | 11 medication (11 Li, 7 others) |
|  | HC | 9 | 39.8 (10.9) | |

### EUTHYMIC STATE

| Study | Subjects | No. of subjects | Mean Age (SD) | Medication Status |
|---|---|---|---|---|
| Hamakawa, 2004 | BD | 13 | 49.4 (12.1) | 8 Li, 1 Valp, 2AD, 12AX, 10AP, 5AC |
|  | HC | 10 | 43.2 (13.7) | |
| Kato, 1998 | BD I | 7 | 44.1 (16.9) | 7 drug free ( > 10 days) |
|  | HC | 60 | 39.6 (13.9) | |
| Deicken, 1995[a] | BD | 12 | 40.3 (8.7) | 12 drug free (1 wk) |
|  | HC | 16 | 39.9 (11.1) | |
| Kato, 1995 | BD | 17 | 40.4 (9.2) | 3 drug free, 14 medication |
|  | HC | 21 | 42.5 (10.2) | |
| Kato, 1994[a] | BD I, II | 12 BD I | 44.0 (9.7) | 2 drug free, 1 drug naïve, 7 medication |
|  |  | 9 BD II | 46.7 (17.3) | 1 drug free, 8 medication |
|  | HC | 59 | 38.1 (12.6) | |
| Kato, 1994[b] | BD I, NOS | 40 | 42.0 (12.4) | 40 Li, 11 AP, 6 AD |
|  | HC | 60 | 39.6 (13.9) | |

| T | ROI | PCr | PME | pH |
|---|---|---|---|---|
| 1.5 | Frontal lobe | ▼ | ▲ | |
| 1.5 | (L) Frontal lobe | ▼ | ▲ | |
| 1.5 | (R) Frontal lobe | ▼ | | |
| 1.5 | Frontal lobe | ▼ | ▲ | |
| 1.5 | Frontal lobe (9 vs. 9) | | PME/total▲<br><br>PME/PDE▲ | |
| 1.5 | Basal ganglia (12 vs. 8) | | | ▼ |
| | Non-localized (11 vs. 10) | | | ▼ |
| 1.5 | Frontal lobe | | | ▼ |
| 2 | (R) Frontal lobe | | ▼ | |
| | (L) Frontal lobe | | ▼ | |
| 1.5 | (R) Frontal lobe | ▼ | | |
| 1.5 | Frontal lobe | | ▼ | ▼ |
| | Frontal lobe | ▼ | | |
| 1.5 | Frontal lobe | | ▼ | ▼ |

(Continued)

**EUTHYMIC STATE**

| Study | Subjects | No. of subjects | Mean Age (SD) | Medication Status |
|---|---|---|---|---|
| Kato, 1993 | BD | 17 | 40.1 (10.8) | 17 medication |
| | HC | 17 | 39.1 (10.1) | |
| Kato, 1992 | BD | 10 | 42.0 (8.6) | 10 medication |
| | HC | 10 | 40.8 (9.1) | |
| Deicken, 1995[b] | BD | 10 | 40.1 (8.3) | 10 medication |
| | HC | 10 | 40.8 (9.1) | |

Phosphorus MRS Findings in Adults with Bipolar Disorder. *Abbreviations:* AC, Anticonvulsant; AD, Antidepressants; AP, Antipsychotics; AX, Anxiolytics; BD, Bipolar disorder; DRESS, Depth-resolved surface coil spectroscopy; HC, Healthy comparison subjects; (L), Left; Li, Lithium; NOS, Not otherwise specified; PDE, Phosphodiester; PME, Phosphomonoester; (R), Right; ROI, Region of interest; SD, Standard deviation; T, Tesla; Valp, Valproate.

Among studies reporting MRS findings in adult patients with bipolar disorder, those reported nonsignificant results (Jensen, 2008; Murashita, 2000; Silverstone, 2002) are not included in this table. ROIs for which non-significant results were reported are not included in this table.

randomized to cytidine, in addition to standard treatment with valproic acid, showed earlier symptom improvement and greater Glx normalization (Yoon et al., 2009), consistent with the hypothesis of mitochondrial dysfunction in bipolar disorder (Table 4.3 summarizes treatment-induced changes in neurometabolites).

> **Studies of Neuronal Membrane Synthesis in Bipolar Disorder Suggest:**
>
> · Insufficient supply of energy due to mitochondrial dysfunction disturbs the metabolism of membrane lipids
>
> · Increased brain levels of mI and Cho imply accumulation of precursors of membrane compounds
>
> · PME levels in bipolar disorder are state dependent

## MITOCHONDRIAL DYSFUNCTION IN BIPOLAR DISORDER AND POTENTIALLY ASSOCIATED CLINICAL FEATURES

Clinical cases have been reported of patients with mitochondrial disorders who also demonstrated features of bipolar disorder (Stewart et al., 1990; Ciafaloni et al., 1991; Suomalainen et al., 1992; Kato et al., 1996b; Miyaoka et al., 1997; Siciliano et al., 2003), consistent with the mitochondrial dysfunction hypothesis of bipolar disorder. Common manifestations of mitochondrial disorders, such as retarded behavior and slowed thoughts, are more frequently observed in patients with bipolar depression than in those with unipolar depression (Mitchell et al., 2004). In a cross-national population-based study, patients who had experienced a manic episode had a higher prevalence of chronic fatigue

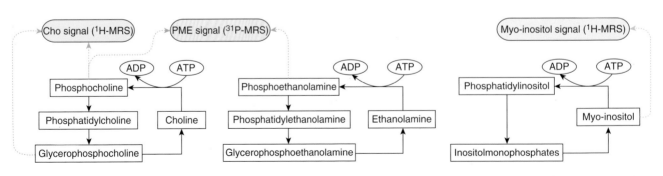

*Figure 4.6* A partial portrayal of phospholipid metabolism in the neuron and related signals that can be detected by magnetic resonance spectroscopy. Compounds in the colored boxes denote those visible by magnetic resonance spectroscopy. *Abbreviations*: ADP, Adenosine diphosphate; ATP, Adenosine triphosphate; Cho, Choline; PME, Phosphomonoester. (Source: Adapted from Stork et al. 2005.)

| T | ROI | PCr | PME | pH |
|---|---|---|---|---|
| 1.5 | Frontal lobe | | ▼ | ▼ |
| 1.5 | Frontal lobe | | ▼ | ▼ |
| 2 | (R) Temporal lobe | | ▼ | |
| | (L) Temporal lobe | | ▼ | |

syndrome by over 3 fold than individuals without histories of mania (McIntyre et al., 2006). Considering that brain and muscle tissues require high mitochondrial function in order to meet high and fluctuating energy demands, if mitochondrial dysfunction is present in bipolar disorder it is not surprising that chronic fatigue syndrome, whose core symptoms include muscle pain and post-exertional malaise, is prevalent in individuals with a history of manic episodes and that patients with bipolar disorder experience psychomotor retardation.

Mood swings, a core feature of bipolar disorder, may also be explained in view of mitochondrial impairment (Chen et al., 2010). Mice with mutant *POLG* show altered rhythms and magnitudes of activity levels, which worsens with the administration of tricyclic antidepressants and stabilizes with lithium treatment (Kasahara et al., 2006). Considering that a mutation (D181A) of mitochondrial DNA polymerase-γ (POLG) leads to mitochondrial DNA deletion, and mice with mutant *POLG* show robust activity swings that are translated into human mood swings, mitochondrial dysfunction may be related to the core feature, mood swings, of the bipolar disorder (Chen et al., 2010).

## MITOCHONDRIAL DYSFUNCTION IN BIPOLAR DISORDER AND IMPLICATIONS FOR INNOVATIVE TREATMENT STRATEGIES

A line of evidence suggests that the efficacy of mood stabilizers may be provided by enhancing the mitochondrial function (Quiroz et al., 2008). Various pharmacological treatments that may be relevant to mitochondrial function have shown promising effects. Glutamatergic modulators like riluzole, memantine, and ketamine may reduce excessive energy demands that may result in death of brain cells with dysfunctional mitochondria (Zarate et al., 2009). Glutamate, a major excitatory neurotransmitter in the brain, excites the neuronal cells, and the energy demands substantially increases in cases of excessive glutamate production (Schurr et al., 1999). The antiglutamatergic effects of riluzole, memantine, and ketamine may reduce the excessive energy demands and diminish the possibility of excitotoxicity.

Cytidine supplementation has shown antidepressant-like effects in patients with bipolar disorder and animal models of depression (Carlezon et al., 2002; Yoon et al., 2009). Exogenous provision of cytidine may reduce the burden of mitochondria from producing the pyrimidines, resulting in improved glia-neuronal glutamate/glutamine recycling, which is an energy-requiring step (Yoon et al., 2009) (Figure 4.5).

By reducing oxidative stress with *N*-acetyl cysteine (Berk et al., 2008), the vicious cycle from mitochondrial dysfunction through increased oxidative stress to cellular death may be damped down (Kato et al., 2010). *N*-acetyl cysteine is thought to work through its numerous molecular modes of action, which include inhibition of activation of c-Jun N-terminal kinase, redox-sensitive activating protein-1 and p38 MAP kinase (Zafarullah et al., 2003).

Adjunctive use of omega-3 fatty acids has shown efficacy in reducing depressive symptoms in patients with bipolar disorder (Montgomery et al., 2008). This may be

**TABLE 4.3 TREATMENT-INDUCED CHANGES IN NEUROMETABOLITES MEASURED BY MRS IN ADULTS WITH BIPOLAR DISORDER**

| Study | Treatment | Subjects | No. of subjects | Mean Age (SD) |
|---|---|---|---|---|
| Friedman, 2004 | Li or Valp | BD I, II | 12 Li, 9 Valp | Li : 31.3 (9.6) Valp : 28.4 (8.5) |
| | | HC | 12 | 30.6 (5.5) |
| Moore, 2000[a] | Lithium | BD I, II (depressed) | 12 | 36.3 |
| | | HC | 9 | 27.1 |
| Moore, 1999 | Lithium | BD I, II (depressed) | 12 → 10 | 36.3 |
| Brennan, 2010 | Riluzole | BD I, II (depressed) | 14 | 44.5 (12.0) |
| Frye, 2007[b] | Lamotrigine | BD I, II (depressed) | 23 → 17 | 35.6 (11.2) |
| | | HC | 12 → 10 | 32.8 (10.9) |
| Iosifescu, 2009 | Glutamine-ER | BD (euthymic) | 8 | 40.7 (11.9) |
| Yoon, 2009 | Valp+Cytidine or Valp+Placebo | BD I, II (depressed) | 18 Cytidine | 33.5 (7.7) |
| | | | 17 Placebo | 36.8 (10.7) |
| Kim, 2007 | Quetiapine | BD RC | 42 | 31.6 (7.3) |
| Jensen, 2008 | TAU | BD I, II (depressed) | 11 → 9 | 46.2 (11.8) |

Treatment-induced Changes in Neurometabolites Measured by MRS in Adults with Bipolar Disorder. *Abbreviations*: ACC, Anterior cingulate cortex; AP, Antipsychotics; AX, Anxiolytics; BD, Bipolar disorder; Cho, Choline; Cr, Creatine; Gln, Glutamine; Glu, Glutamate; Glx, Glutamate + glutamine; GM, Gray matter; HC, Healthy comparison subjects; (L), Left; Li, Lithium; ml, Myo-inositol; MPFC, Medial prefrontal cortex; NAA, N-acetyl aspartate; No diff., No difference; POC, Parieto-occipital cortex; PT, Psychotropics; (R), Right; RC, Rapid cycling; ROI, Region of interest; SD, Standard deviation; T, Tesla; TAU, Triacetyluridine; Valp, Valproate.

| Follow-up Period & Medication Status | T | ROI | Quantification | Result |
|---|---|---|---|---|
| 2 mths washout, Li : 3.6 (1.9) mths Valp : 1.4 (1.7) mths | 1.5 | Caudate, Cingulate, Occiput, Putamen, Thalamus | ΔGlx (GM) | ▼ (Li) |
| | | | Δml (GM) | ▼ (Li) |
| 2 wks washout, Li : 4 wks | 1.5 | (R) Frontal lobe (L) Temporal lobe (L) Parietal lo be Occipital lobe | NAA | No diff. →▲ |
| | | | NAA | No diff. →▲ |
| 2 wks washout, Li : 4 wks | | | NAA | No diff. →▲ |
| | | | NAA | No diff. →▲ |
| 2 wks washout, Li : 3~4 wks | 1.5 | (R) Frontal lobe | ml | ▼ |
| Riluzole : 2 days → 6 wks (9 medication) | 4 | ACC | Gln/Glu | ▲→No diff. |
| | | | NAA | No diff. →▲ |
| | | POC | Gln/Glu | ▲→No diff. |
| | | | NAA | No diff. →▲ |
| AP free 4 wks, Lamotrigine : 12 wks | 1.5 | ACC+MPFC | Glx | ▲→No diff. |
| | | | Glu | ▲→No diff. |
| | | | Gln | No diff. →▲ |
| | | | Cr | ▲→No diff. |
| | | | NAA/Cr | No diff. →▼ |
| Glutamine-ER : 16 wks (19 medicaiton) | 4 | (L) Hippocampus | NAA | ▲ |
| | | | Cho | ▼ |
| 1wk washout, Valp+Cytidine :12 wks | 3 | Midfrontal cortex | Glu/Gln | Faster ▼ in cytidine group |
| Valp+Placebo : 12 wks | | | | |
| > 2 days washout, Quetiapine : 12 wks (AX was allowed.) | 3 | Midfrontal cortex (n=30) | Lactate | ▼ |
| No washout, TAU : 6 wks (1 drug free, 10 medication) | 4 | Non-localized (6 Responders) | pH | ▲ |

mediated by the effects of omega-3 fatty acids on increasing membrane fluidity that can modulate mitochondrial function (Hirashima et al., 2004). Choline administration may also be beneficial for membrane phospholipid synthesis in patients with bipolar disorder (Lyoo et al., 2003).

Uridine and triacetyluridine (TAU) are also synthesized *de novo*, and exogenous administration of these drugs in bipolar disorder improved depressive symptoms along with the bioenergetics indices showing the recovery of the mitochondrial impairment (Carlezon et al., 2005; Jensen et al., 2008; Zarate et al., 2009). Patients with bipolar disorder in depressed episodes may benefit from treatment with creatine monohydrate (Lyoo et al., 2003; Roitman et al., 2007), or S-adenosyl-L-methionine, which may modulate high-energy phosphate metabolism, although further clinical studies are warranted. A previous $^{31}$P-MRS study in healthy volunteers has suggested that the Cr supplementation increases the high-energy phosphate pool as well as produces ATP from PCr (Lyoo et al., 2003).

## SUMMARY AND CONCLUSIONS

There are limitations to MRS research, potentially due to the diverse clinical characteristics, mood states, and pharmacological treatment histories of subjects as well as the current limitations of MRS techniques. However, many of the existing findings support a mitochondrial dysfunction hypothesis in bipolar disorder. In chapter 5 (see the section titled *Magnetic Resonance Spectroscopy (MRS)*), MRS findings from children and adolescents with bipolar disorder are reviewed. Decreased levels of NAA and increased levels of mI, Glx, and Cho have also been reported in patients with bipolar disorder in these age groups (Castillo et al., 2000; Cecil et al., 2003; Chang et al., 2003; Davanzo et al., 2003; Sassi et al., 2005; DelBello et al., 2006; Olvera et al., 2007), corroborating the mitochondrial dysfunction hypothesis in bipolar disorder, although there are some variable findings regarding these neurometabolites (Moore et al., 2007; Patel et al., 2008a; Patel et al., 2008b) reflecting the potential confounding effects of neurodevelopmental

processes (Patel et al., 2009). As demonstrated in chapter 11 (see the section titled *Altered mitochondrial gene and protein expression in bipolar disorder*), evidence from genetic studies also supports the hypothesis of mitochondrial dysfunction in bipolar disorder. Newer approaches with genetic and neuroimaging techniques and designs, including treatment trials combined with MRS evaluations, would provide additional insights. Together, these approaches might guide innovative lines of research to identify novel treatment interventions that provide greater efficacy and specificity to bipolar disorder patients. Such advances could revolutionize how bipolar disorder is managed and the impact it has on the lives of affected people.

## ACKNOWLEDGMENTS

We thank Hyeonseok S. Jeong, Kristen Delmastro, and Han Byul Cho for technical assistance. This work was in part supported by grants MH058681 (Dr. Renshaw), DA015116 (Dr. Renshaw), and DA024070 (Drs. Lyoo and Renshaw) from the National Institutes of Health; grant KRF-2008–220-#00021 (Dr. Lyoo) funded by the National Research Foundation of Korea.

## REFERENCES

Amaral, J. A., Tamada, R. S., Issler, C. K., Caetano, S. C., Cerri, G. G., de Castro, C. C., & Lafer, B. 2006. A 1HMRS study of the anterior cingulate gyrus in euthymic bipolar patients. *Human Psychopharmacology*, 21(4): 215–220.

Atmaca, M., Yildirim, H., Ozdemir, H., Poyraz, A. K., Tezcan, E., & Ogur, E. 2006. Hippocampal 1H MRS in first-episode bipolar I patients. *Progress in Neuro-Psychopharmacology & Biological Psychiatry*, 30(7): 1235–1239.

Atmaca, M., Yildirim, H., Ozdemir, H., Ogur, E., & Tezcan, E. 2007. Hippocampal 1H MRS in patients with bipolar disorder taking valproate versus valproate plus quetiapine. *Psychological Medicine*, 37(1): 121–129.

Berk, M., Copolov, D. L., Dean, O., Lu, K., Jeavons, S., Schapkaitz, I., . . . Bush, AI. 2008. N-acetyl cysteine for depressive symptoms in bipolar disorder: A double-blind randomized placebo-controlled trial. *Biological Psychiatry*, 64(6): 468–475.

Belmaker, R. H. 2004. Bipolar disorder. *New England Journal of Medicine*, 351(5): 476–486.

Berg, J. M., Tymoczko, J. L., & Stryer L. 2010. *Biochemistry*. 7th edition. New York: W H Freeman.

Bertolino, A., Frye, M., Callicott, J. H., Mattay, V. S., Rakow, R., Shelton-Repella, J., . . . Weinberger, D. R. 2003. Neuronal pathology in the hippocampal area of patients with bipolar disorder: a study with proton magnetic resonance spectroscopic imaging. *Biological Psychiatry*, 53(10): 906–913.

Bhagwagar, Z., Wylezinska, M., Jezzard, P., Evans, J., Ashworth, F., Sule, A., . . . Cowen, P. J. 2007. Reduction in occipital cortex gamma-aminobutyric acid concentrations in medication-free recovered unipolar depressed and bipolar subjects. *Biological Psychiatry*, 61(6): 806–812.

Brambilla, P., Stanley, J. A., Nicoletti, M. A., Sassi, R. B., Mallinger, A. G., Frank, E., . . . Soares. J. C. 2005. 1H magnetic resonance spectroscopy investigation of the dorsolateral prefrontal cortex in bipolar disorder patients. *Journal of Affective Disorders*, 86(1): 61–67.

Brennan, B. P., Hudson, J. I., Jensen, J. E., McCarthy, J., Roberts, J. L., Prescot, A. P., . . . Ongur, D. 2010. Rapid enhancement of glutamatergic neurotransmission in bipolar depression following treatment with riluzole. *Neuropsychopharmacology*, 35(3): 834–846.

Bruhn, H. S., Staedt, G., Merboldt, K. D., Hanicke, W., & Frahm, J. 1993. Quantitative proton MRS in vivo shows cerebral myo-inositol and cholines to be unchanged in manic-depressive patients treated with lithium. *Proceedings of the International Society for Magnetic Resonance in Medicine*, 1543.

Carlezon, W. A., Pilakas, A. M., Parow, A. M., Detke, M. J., Cohen, B. M., & Renshaw, P. F. 2002. Antidepressnat-like effects of cytidine in the forced swim test in rats. *Biological Psychiatry*, 51(11): 882–889.

Carlezon, W. A., Mague, S. D., Parow, A. M., Stoll, A. L., Cohen, B. M., & Renshaw, P. F. 2005. Antidepressnat-like effects of uridine and omega-3 fatty acids are potentiated by combined treatments in rats. *Biological Psychiatry*, 57(4): 343–350.

Castillo, M., Kwock, L., Courvoisie, H., & Hooper, S. R. 2000. Proton MR spectroscopy in children with bipolar affective disorder: Preliminary observations. *American Journal of Neuroradiology*, 21(5): 832–838.

Cecil, K. M., DelBello, M. P., Morey, R., & Strakowski, S. M. 2002. Frontal lobe differences in bipolar disorder as determined by proton MR spectroscopy. *Bipolar Disorders*,4(6): 357–365.

Cecil, K. M., DelBello, M. P., Sellars, M. C., & Strakowski, S. M. 2003. Proton magnetic resonance spectroscopy of the frontal lobe and cerebellar vermis in children with a mood disorder and a familial risk for bipolar disorders. *Journal of Child and Adolescent Psychopharmacology*,13(4): 545–555.

Chakraborty, G., Mekala, P., Yahya, D., Wu, G., & Ledeen, R. W. 2001. Intraneuronal N-acetylaspartate supplies acetyl groups for myelin lipid synthesis: evidence for myelin-associated aspartoacylase. *Journal of Neurochemistry*, 78(4): 736–745.

Chang, K., Adelman, N., Dienes, K., Barnea-Goraly, N., Reiss, A., & Ketter, T. 2003. Decreased N-acetylaspartate in children with familial bipolar disorder. *Biological Psychiatry*, 53(11): 1059–1065.

Chen, G., Henter, I. D., & Manji, H. K. 2010. Translational research in bipolar disorder: Emerging insights from genetically based models. *Molecular Psychiatry*, 15(9): 883–895.

Ciafaloni, E., Shanske, S., Apostolski, S., Griggs, R. L., Bird, T. D., Sumi, M., & Dimauro, S. 1991. Multiple deletions of mitochondrial DNA. *Neurology*, 41 (Suppl): 207.

Clark, J. B. 1998. N-acetyl aspartate: a marker for neuronal loss or mitochondrial dysfunction. *Developmental Neuroscience*, 20(4–5): 271–276.

Clausen, T., Zauner, A., Levasseur, J. E., Rice, A. C., & Bullock, R. 2001. Induced mitochondrial failure in the feline brain: implications for understanding acute post-traumatic metabolic events. *Brain Research*, 908(1): 35–48.

Colla, M., Schubert, F., Bubner, M., Heidenreich, J. O., Bajbouj, M., Seifert, F., . . . Kronenberg, G. 2009. Glutamate as a spectroscopic marker of hippocampal structural plasticity is elevated in long-term euthymic bipolar patients on chronic lithium therapy and correlates inversely with diurnal cortisol. *Molecular Psychiatry*, 14(7): 696–704, 647.

Corrigan, N. M., Richards, T. L., Friedman, S. D., Petropoulos, H., & Dager, S. R. 2010. Improving 1H MRSI measurement of cerebral lactate for clinical applications. *Psychiatry Research*, 182(1): 40–47.

Dager, S. R., Friedman, S. D., Heide, A., Layton, M. E., Richards, T., Artru, A., . . . Posse, S. 1999. Two-dimensional proton echo-planar spectroscopic imaging of brain metabolic changes during lactate-induced panic. *Archives of General Psychiatry*, 56(1): 70–77.

Dager, S. R., Friedman, S. D., Parow, A., Demopulos, C., Stoll, A. L., Lyoo, I. K., . . . Renshaw, P. F. 2004. Brain metabolic alterations in medication-free patients with bipolar disorder. *Archives of General Psychiatry*, 61(5): 450–458.

Dager, S. R., Corrigan, N. M., Richards, T. L., & Posse, S. 2008. Research applications of magnetic resonance spectroscopy to investigate psychiatric disorders. *Topics in Magnetic Resonance Imaging*, 19(2): 81–96.

Davanzo, P., Yue, K., Thomas, M. A., Belin, T., Mintz, J., Venkatraman, T. N., . . . McCracken, J. 2003. Proton magnetic resonance spectroscopy of bipolar disorder versus intermittent explosive disorder in children and adolescents. *American Journal of Psychiatry*, 160(8): 1442–1452.

De Stefano, N., Matthews, P. M., & Arnold, D. L. 1995. Reversible decreases in N-acetylaspartate after acute brain injury. *Magnetic Resonance in Medicine*, 34(5): 721–727.

Deicken, R. F., Fein, G., Weiner, M. W. 1995a. Abnormal frontal lobe phosphorus metabolism in bipolar disorder. *American Journal of Psychiatry*, 152(6): 915–918.

Deicken, R. F., Weiner, M. W., & Fein, G. 1995b. Decreased temporal lobe phosphomonoesters in bipolar disorder. *Journal of Affective Disorders*, 33(3): 195–199.

Deicken, R. F., Eliaz, Y., Feiwell, R., & Schuff, N. 2001. Increased thalamic N-acetylaspartate in male patients with familial bipolar I disorder. *Psychiatry Research*, 106(1): 35–45.

Deicken, R. F., Pegues, M. P., Anzalone, S., Feiwell, R., & Soher B. 2003. Lower concentration of hippocampal N-acetylaspartate in familial bipolar I disorder. *American Journal of Psychiatry*, 160(5): 873–882.

DelBello, M. P., Cecil, K. M., Adler, C. M., Daniels, J. P., & Strakowski, S. M. 2006. Neurochemical effects of olanzapine in first-hospitalization manic adolescents: A proton magnetic resonance spectroscopy study. *Neuropsychopharmacology*, 31:1264–1273.

Erecinska, M., Zaleska, M. M., Nissim, I., Nelson, D., Dagani, F., & Yudkoff, M. 1988. Glucose and synaptosomal glutamate metabolism: studies with [15N]glutamate. *Journal of Neurochemistry*, 51(3): 892–902.

Frey, B. N., Folgierini, M., Nicoletti, M., Machado-Vieira, R., Stanley, J. A., Soares, J. C., & Kapczinski, F. 2005. A proton magnetic resonance spectroscopy investigation of the dorsolateral prefrontal cortex in acute mania. *Human Psychopharmacology*, 20(2): 133–139.

Frey, B. N., Stanley, J. A., Nery, F. G., Monkul, E. S., Nicoletti, M. A., Chen, H. H., . . . Soares, J. C. 2007. Abnormal cellular energy and phospholipid metabolism in the left dorsolateral prefrontal cortex of medication-free individuals with bipolar disorder: an in vivo 1H MRS study. *Bipolar Disorders*, 9 (Suppl 1): 119–127.

Friedman, S. D., Dager, S. R., Parow, A., Hirashima, F., Demopulos, C., Stoll, A. L., . . . Renshaw, P. F. 2004. Lithium and valproic acid treatment effects on brain chemistry in bipolar disorder. *Biological Psychiatry*, 56(5): 340–348.

Frye, M. A., Thomas, M. A., Yue, K., Binesh, N., Davanzo, P., Ventura, J., . . . Mintz, J. 2007a. Reduced concentrations of N-acetylaspartate (NAA) and the NAA-creatine ratio in the basal ganglia in bipolar disorder: a study using 3-Tesla proton magnetic resonance spectroscopy. *Psychiatry Research*, 154(3): 259–265.

Frye, M. A., Watzl, J., Banakar, S., O'Neill, J., Mintz, J., Davanzo, P., . . . Thomas, M. A. 2007b. Increased anterior cingulate/medial prefrontal cortical glutamate and creatine in bipolar depression. *Neuropsychopharmacology*, 32(12): 2490–2499.

Ghaemi, S. N. 2008. Why antidepressants are not antidepressants: STEP-BD, STAR*D, and the return of neurotic depression. *Bipolar Disorders*, 10(8): 957–968.

Gyulai, L., Bolinger, L., Leigh, J. S. Jr., Barlow, C., & Chance, B. 1984. Phosphorylethanolamine-the major constituent of the phosphomonoester peak observed by 31P-NMR on developing dog brain. *FEBS Letters*, 178(1): 137–142.

Hamakawa, H., Kato, T., Murashita, J., & Kato, N. 1998. Quantitative proton magnetic resonance spectroscopy of the basal ganglia in patients with affective disorders. *European Archives of Psychiatry and Clinical Neuroscience,* 248(1): 53–58.

Hamakawa, H., Kato, T., Shiori, T., Inubushi, T., & Kato, N. 1999. Quantitative proton magnetic resonance spectroscopy of the bilateral frontal lobes in patients with bipolar disorder. *Psychological Medicine,* 29(3): 639–644.

Hamakawa, H., Murashita, J., Yamada, N., Inubushi, T., Kato, N., & Kato, T. 2004. Reduced intracellular pH in the basal ganglia and whole brain measured by 31P-MRS in bipolar disorder. *Psychiatry and Clinical Neurosciences,* 58(1): 82–88.

Hurtado O, Moro MA, Cardenas A, Sanchez V, Fernandez-Tome P., Leza JC, . . . Lizasoain I. 2005. Neuroprotection afforded by prior citicoline administration in experimental brain ischemia: effects on glutamate transport. *Neurobiology* of Disease, 18(2): 336–345.

Iosifescu DV, Moore CM, Deckersbach T, Tilley CA, Ostacher MJ, Sachs GS, Nierenberg AA. 2009. Galantamine-ER for cognitive dysfunction in bipolar disorder and correlation with hippocampal neuronal viability: a proof-of-concept study. *CNS Neuroscience & Therapeutics,* 15(4): 309–319.

Jensen JE, Daniels M, Haws C, Bolo NR, Lyoo IK, Yoon SJ, . . . Renshaw PF. 2008. Triacetyluridine (TAU) decreases depressive symptoms and increases brain pH in bipolar patients. *Experimental and Clinical Psychopharmacology,* 16(3): 199–206.

Kasahara T, Kubota M, Miyauchi T, Noda Y, Mouri A, Nabeshima T, Kato T. 2006. Mice with neuron-specific accumulation of mitochondrial DNA mutations show mood disorder-like phenotypes. *Molecular Psychiatry.* 11(6): 577–593, 523.

Kato T, Shiori T, Takahashi S, Inubushi T. 1991. Measurement of brain phosphoinositide metabolism in bipolar patients using in vivo 31P-MRS. *Journal of Affective Disorders,* 22(4): 185–190.

Kato T, Takahashi S, Shiori T, Inubushi T. 1992. Brain phosphorus metabolism in depressive disorders detected by phosphorus-31 magnetic resonance spectroscopy. *Journal of Affective Disorders,* 26(4): 223–230.

Kato T, Takahashi S, Shiori T, Inubushi T. 1993. Alterations in brain phosphorus metabolism in bipolar disorder detected by in vivo 31P. and 7Li magnetic resonance spectroscopy. *Journal of Affective Disorders,* 27(1): 53–59.

Kato T, Takahashi S, Shiori T, Murashita J, Hamakawa H, Inubushi T. 1994a. Reduction of brain phosphocreatine in bipolar II disorder detected by phosphorus-31 magnetic resonance spectroscopy. *Journal of Affective Disorders,* 31(2): 125–133.

Kato, T., Shiori, T., Murashita, J., Hamakawa, H., Inubushi, T., & Takahashi, S. 1994b. Phosphorus-31 magnetic resonance spectroscopy and ventricular enlargement in bipolar disorder. *Psychiatry Research,* 55(1): 41–50.

Kato, T., Hamakawa, H., Shiori, T., Murashita, J., Inubushi, T., & Takahashi S. 1994c. Proton MRS of the basal ganglia in patients with bipolar disorders. *Proceedings of the International Society for Magnetic Resonance in Medicine,* 605.

Kato, T., Shiori, T., Murashita, J., Hamakawa, H., Takahashi, Y., Inubushi, T., & Takahashi, S. 1995. Lateralized abnormality of high energy phosphate metabolism in the frontal lobes of patients with bipolar disorder detected by phase-encoded 31P-MRS. *Psychological Medicine,* 25(3): 557–566.

Kato, T., Hamakawa, H., Shiori, T., Murashita, J., Takahashi, Y., Takahashi, T., Inubushi, T. 1996a. Choline-containing compounds detected by proton magnetic resonance spectroscopy in the basal ganglia in bipolar disorder. *Journal of Psychiatry and Neuroscience,* 21(4): 248–254.

Kato, T., & Takahashi Y. 1996b. Deletion of leukocyte mitochondrial DNA in bipolar disorder. *Journal of Affective Disorders,* 37(2-3): 67–73.

Kato, T., Murashita, J., Kamiya, A., Shiori, T., Kato, N., & Inubushi T. 1998. Decreased brain intracellular pH measured by 31P-MRS in bipolar disorder: a confirmation in drug-free patients and correlation with white matter hyperintensity. *European Archives of Psychiatry and Clinical Neuroscience,* 248(6): 301–306.

Kato, T., Kapczinski, F., & Berk, M. 2010. Mitochondrial dysfunction and oxidative stress. In Yatham, L. N., & Maj, M, eds. *Bipolar Disorder: Clinical and Neurobiological Foundations,* (pp. 244–254). West Sussex, UK: Wiley-Blackwell Publishing.

Kim, D. J., Lyoo, I. K., Yoon, S. J., Choi, T., Lee, B., Kim, J. E., . . . Renshaw, P. F. 2007. Clinical response of quetiapine in rapid cycling manic bipolar patients and lactate level changes in proton magnetic resonance spectroscopy. *Progress in Neuro-Psychopharmacology and Biological Psychiatry,* 31(6): 1182–1188.

Konradi, C., Eaton, M., MacDonald, M. L., Walsh, J., Benes, F. M., & Heckers, S. 2004. Molecular evidence for mitochondrial dysfunction in bipolar disorder. *Archives of General Psychiatry,* 61(3): 300–308.

Lyoo, I. K., Kong, S. W., Sung, S. M., Hirashima, F., Parow, A., Hennen, J., . . . Renshaw, P. F. 2003. Multinuclear magnetic resonance spectroscopy of high-energy phosphate metabolites in human brain following oral supplementation of creatine-monohydrate. *Psychiatry Research,* 123: 87–100.

Madhavarao, C. N., Chinopoulos, C., Chandrasekaran, K., & Namboodiri, M. A. 2003. Characterization of the N-acetylaspartate biosynthetic enzyme from rat brain. *Journal of Neurochemistry,* 86(4): 824–835.

Manji, H. K., & Lenox, R. H. 2000. The nature of bipolar disorder. Journal of Clinical Psychiatry. 61 (Supp 13): 42–57.

McIntyre, R. S., Konarski, J. Z., Soczynska, J. K., Wilkins, K., Panjwani, G., Bouffard, B., . . . Kennedy, S. H. 2006. Medical comorbidity in bipolar disorder: Implications for functional outcomes and health service utilization. *Psychiatric Services,* 57(8): 1140–1144.

Merikangas, K. R., Akiskal, H. S., Angst, J., Greenberg, P. E., Hirschfeld, R. M., Petukhova, M., & Kessler, R. C. 2007. Lifetime and 12-month prevalence of bipolar spectrum disorder in the National Comorbidity Survey replication. *Archives of General Psychiatry,* 64(5): 543–552.

Michael, N., Erfurth, A., Ohrmann, P., Gossling, M., Arolt, V., Heindel, W., & Pfleidererm B. 2003a. Acute mania is accompanied by elevated glutamate/glutamine levels within the left dorsolateral prefrontal cortex. *Psychopharmacology,* 168(3): 344–346.

Michael, N., Erfurth, A., Ohrmann, P., Arolt, V., Heindel, W., & Pfleiderer, B. 2003b. Neurotrophic effects of electroconvulsive therapy: a proton magnetic resonance study of the left amygdalar region in patients with treatment-resistant depression. *Neuropsychopharmacology,* 28(4): 720–725.

Michael, N., Erfurth, A., & Pfleiderer, B. 2009. Elevated metabolites within dorsolateral prefrontal cortex in rapid cycling bipolar disorder. *Psychiatry Research,* 172(1): 78–81.

Mir, C., Clotet, J., Aledo, R., Durany, N., Argemi, J., Lozano, R., . . . Casals, N. 2003. CDP-choline prevents glutamate-mediated cell death in cerebellar granule neurons. *Journal of Molecular Neuroscience,* 20(1): 53–60.

Mitchell, P., & Malhi, GS. 2004. Bipolar depression: Phenomenological overview and clinical characteristics. *Bipolar Disorders,* 6(6): 530–539.

Miyaoka, H., Suzuki, Y., Taniyama, M., Miyaoka, Y., Shishikura, K., Kamijima, K., . . . Matsuoka, K. 1997. Mental disorders in diabetic patients with mitochondrial transfer RNALeu(UUR) mutation at position 3243. *Biological Psychiatry,* 42(6): 524–526.

Moffett, J. R., Tieman, S. B., Weinberger, D. R., Coyle, J. T., & Namboodiri, A. M. 2006. *N-acetylaspartate-A unique neuronal molecule in the central nervous system.* New York: Springer.

Molina, V., Sanchez, J., Sanz, J., Reig, S., Benito, C., Leal, I., . . . Desco, M. 2007. Dorsolateral prefrontal N-acetyl-aspartate concentration in male patients with chronic schizophrenia and with chronic bipolar disorder. *European Psychiatry,* 22(8): 505–512.

Moore, C. M., Breeze, J. L., Gruber, S. A., Babb, S. M., Frederick, B. B., Villafuerte, R. A., . . . Renshaw, P. F. 2000. Choline, myo-inositol and mood in bipolar disorder: a proton magnetic resonance spectroscopic imaging study of the anterior cingulate cortex. *Bipolar Disorders,* 2 (3 Pt 2): 207–216.

Moore, C. M., Frazier, J. A., Glod, C. A., Breeze, J. L., Dieterich, M., Finn, C. T., . . . Renshaw, P. F. 2007. Glutamine and glutamate levels in children and adolescents with bipolar disorder: A 4.0-T proton magnetic resonance spectroscopy study of the anterior cingulate cortex. *Journal of the American Academy of Child and Adolescent Psychiatry,* 46(4): 524–534.

Moore, G. J., Bebchuk, J. M., Parrish, J. K., Faulk, M. W., Arfken, C. L., Strahl-Bevacqua, J., Manji, H. K. 1999. Temporal dissociation between lithium-induced changes in frontal lobe myo-inositol and clinical response in manic-depressive illness. *American Journal of Psychiatry,* 156(12): 1902–1908.

Moore, G. J., Bebchuk, J. M., Hasanat, K., Chen, G., Seraji-Bozorgzad, N., Wilds, I. B., . . . Manji, H. K. 2000. Lithium increases N-acetyl-aspartate in the human brain: in vivo evidence in support of bcl-2's neurotrophic effects? *Biological Psychiatry,* 48(1): 1–8.

Moore, G. J., & Galloway, M. P. 2002. Magnetic resonance spectroscopy: neurochemistry and treatment effects in affective disorders. *Psychopharmacology Bulletin.* 36(2): 5–23.

Muller-Oerlinghausen B, Berghofer A, Bauer M. 2002. Bipolar disorder. *Lancet,* 359(9302): 241–247.

Murashita, J., Kato, T., Shioiri, T., Inubushi, T., & Kato, N. 2000. Altered brain energy metabolism in lithium-resistant bipolar disorder detected by photic stimulated 31P-MR spectroscopy. *Psychological Medicine,* 30(1): 107–115.

O'Donnell, T., Rotzinger, S., Nakashima, T. T., Hanstock, C. C., Ulrich, M., Silverstone, P. H. 2000. Chronic lithium and sodium valproate both decrease the concentration of myo-inositol and increase the concentration of inositol monophosphates in rat brain. *Brain Research,* 880(1–2): 84–91.

Ohara, K., Isoda, H., Suzuki, Y., Takehara, Y., Ochiai, M., Takeda, H., & Igarashi, Y. 1998. Proton magnetic resonance spectroscopy of the lenticular nuclei in bipolar I affective disorder. *Psychiatry Research,* 84(2–3): 55–60.

Olvera, R. L., Caetano, S. C., Fonseca, M., Nicoletti, M., Stanley, J. A., Chen, H. H., . . . Soares, J. C. 2007. Low levels of N-acetyl aspartate in the left dorsolateral prefrontal cortex of pediatric bipolar patients. *Journal of Child and Adolescent Psychopharmacology,* 17(4): 461–473.

Öngür, D., Jensen, J. E., Prescot, A. P., Stork, C., Lundy, M., Cohen, B. M., & Renshaw, P. F. 2008. Abnormal glutamatergic neurotransmission and neuronal-glial interactions in acute mania. *Biological Psychiatry,* 64(8): 718–726.

Öngür, D., Prescot, A. P., Jensen, J. E., Cohen, B. M., & Renshaw, P. F. 2009. Creatine abnormalities in schizophrenia and bipolar disorder. *Psychiatry Research,* 172(1): 44–48.

Patel, T. B., & Clark, J. B. 1979. Synthesis of N-acetyl-L-aspartate by rat brain mitochondria and its involvement in mitochondrial/cytosolic carbon transport. *Biochemical Journal,* 184(3): 539–546.

Patel, N. C., Cecil, K. M., Strakowski. S. M., Adler, C. M., & DelBello, M. P. 2008a. Neurochemical alterations in adolescent bipolar depression: A proton magnetic resonance spectroscopy pilot study of the prefrontal cortex. *Journal of Child and Adolescent Psychopharmacology,* 18(6): 623–627.

Patel, N. C., DelBello, M. P., Cecil, K. M., Stanford, K. E., Adler, C. M., & Strakowski, S. M. 2008b. Temporal changes in N-acetyl-aspartate concentrations in adolescents with bipolar depression treated with lithium *Journal of Child and Adolescent Psychopharmacology,* 18(2): 132–139.

Patel, N. C., Cerullo, M. A., Fleck, D. E., Nandagopal, J. J., Adler, C. M., Strakowski, S. M., & DelBello, M. P. 2009. Neuroimaging biomarkers for bipolar disorder across the lifespan. In Ritsner, M. S, ed. *The Handbook of Neuropsychiatric Biomarkers, Endophenotypes and Genes,* (pp. 171–199). New York: Springer.

Pettegrew, J. W., Kopp, S. J., Minshew, N. J., Glonek, T., Feliksik, J. M., Tow, J. P., & Cohen, M. M. 1987. 31P. nuclear magnetic resonance studies of phosphoglyceride metabolism in developing and degenerating brain: preliminary observations. *Journal of Neuropathology and Experimental Neurology,* 46(4): 419–430.

Phillips, M. L., Travis, M. J., Fagiolini, A., & Kupfer, D. J. 2008. Medication effects in neuroimaging studies of bipolar disorder. *American Journal of Psychiatry,* 165(3): 313–320.

Port, J. D., Unal, S. S., Mrazek, D. A., & Marcus, S. M. 2008. Metabolic alterations in medication-free patients with bipolar disorder: a 3T CSF-corrected magnetic resonance spectroscopic imaging study. *Psychiatry Research,* 162(2): 113–121.

Posse, S., DeCarli, C., & Le Bihan, D. 1994. Three-dimensional echo-planar MR spectroscopic imaging at short echo times in the human brain. *Radiology,* 192(3): 733–738.

Posse, S., Dager, S. R., Richards, T. L., Yuan, C., Ogg, R., & Artru, A. A., . . . Hayes, C. 1997. In vivo measurement of regional brain metabolic response to hyperventilation using magnetic resonance: proton echo planar spectroscopic imaging (PEPSI). *Magnetic Resonance in Medicine,* 37(6): 858–865.

Purdon, A. D., & Rapoport, S. I. 1998. Energy requirements for two aspects of phospholipid metabolism in mammalian brain. *Biochemical Journal,* 335 (Pt 2): 313–318.

Quiroz, J. A., Gray, N. A., Kato, T., & Manji, H. K. 2008. Mitochondrially mediated plasticity in the pathophysiology and treatment of bipolar disorder. *Neurospcyhopharmacology,* 33(11): 2551–2565.

Radad, K., Gille, G., Xiaojing, J., Durany, N., & Rausch, W. D. 2007. CDP-choline reduces dopaminergic cell loss induced by MPP(+) and glutamate in primary mesencephalic cell culture. *International Journal of Neuroscience,* 117(7): 985–998.

Sachs, G. S., Nierenberg, A. A., Calabrese, J. R., Marangell, L. B., Wisniewski, S. R., Gyulai, L., . . . Thase, M. E. 2007. Effectiveness of adjunctive antidepressant treatment for bipolar depression. *New England Journal of Medicine* 356(17): 1711–1722.

Sanacora, G., Zarate, C. A., Krystal, J. H., Manji, H. K. 2008. Targeting the glutamatergic system to develop novel, improved therapeutics for mood disorders. *Nature Reviews Drug Discovery* 7: 426–437.

Sarramea Crespo, F., Luque, R., Prieto, D., Sau, P., Albert, C., Leal, I., . . . Molina, V. 2008. Biochemical changes in the cingulum in patients with schizophrenia and chronic bipolar disorder. *European Archives of Psychiatry and Clinical Neuroscience,* 258(7): 394–401.

Sassi, R. B., Stanley, J. A., Axelson, D., Brambilla, P., Nicoletti, M. A., Keshavan, M. S., . . . Soares, J. C. 2005. Reduced NAA levels in the dorsolateral prefrontal cortex of young bipolar patients. *American Journal of Psychiatry,* 162(11): 2109–2115.

Scherk, H., Backens, M., Schneider-Axmann, T., Kemmer, C., Usher, J., Reith, W., . . . Gruber, O. 2008. Neurochemical pathology in hippocampus in euthymic patients with bipolar I disorder. *Acta Psychiatrica Scandinavica,* 117(4): 283–288.

Scherk, H., Backens, M., Schneider-Axmann, T., Usher, J., Kemmer, C., Reith, W., . . . Gruber, O. 2009. Cortical neurochemistry in euthymic patients with bipolar I disorder. *World Journal* of Biological Psychiatry, 10(4): 285–294.

Schurr, A., Miller, J. J., Payne, R. S., & Rigor, B. M. 1999. An increase in lactate output by brain tissue serves to meet the energy needs of glutamate-activated neurons. *Journal of Neuroscience,* 19(1): 34–39.

Senaratne, R., Milne, A. M., MacQueen, G. M., & Hall, G. B. 2009. Increased choline-containing compounds in the orbitofrontal cortex and hippocampus in euthymic patients with bipolar disorder: a proton magnetic resonance spectroscopy study. *Psychiatry Research,* 172(3): 205–209.

Sharma, R., Venkatasubramanian, P. N., Barany, M., & Davis JM. 1992. Proton magnetic resonance spectroscopy of the brain in schizophrenic and affective patients. *Schizophrenia Research,* 8(1): 43–49.

Siciliano, G., Tessa, A., Petrini, S., Mancuso, M., Bruno, C., Grieco, G. S., . . . Murrai, L. 2003. Autosomal dominant external ophthalmoplegia and bipolar affective disorder associated with a mutation in the ANT1 gene. *Neuromuscular Disorders,* 13(2): 162–165.

Signoretti, S., Marmarou, A., Tavazzi, B., Lazzarino, G., Beaumont, A., & Vagnozzi, R. 2001. N-Acetylaspartate reduction as a measure of injury severity and mitochondrial dysfunction following diffuse traumatic brain injury. *Journal of Neurotrauma,* 18(10): 977–991.

Silverstone, P. H., Wu, R. H., O'Donnell, T., Ulrich, M., Asghar, S. J., & Hanstock, C. C. 2002. Chronic treatment with both lithium and sodium valproate may normalize phosphoinositol cycle activity in bipolar patients. *Human Psychopharmacology*, 17(7): 321–327.

Silverstone, P. H., Wu, R. H., O'Donnell, T., Ulrich, M., Asghar, S. J., Hanstock, C. C. 2003. Chronic treatment with lithium, but not sodium valproate, increases cortical N-acetyl-aspartate concentrations in euthymic bipolar patients. *International Clinical Psychopharmacology*, 18(2): 73–79.

Stewart, J. B., & Naylor, G. J. 1990. Manic-depressive psychosis in a patient with mitochondrial myopathy—a case report. *Medical Science Research*, 18(7): 265–266.

Stoll, A. L., Renshaw, P. F., Sachs, G. S., Guimaraes, A. R., Miller, C., Cohen, B. M., . . . Gonzalez, R. G. 1992. The human brain resonance of choline-containing compounds is similar in patients receiving lithium treatment and controls: an in vivo proton magnetic resonance spectroscopy study. *Biolological Psychiatry*, 32(10): 944–949.

Stork, C., & Renshaw, P. F. 2005. Mitochondrial dysfunction in bipolar disorder: evidence from magnetic resonance spectroscopy research. *Molecular Psychiatry*, 10(10): 900–919.

Suomalainen, A., Majander, A., Haltia, M., Somer, H., Lonnqvist, J., Savontaus, M. L., & Peltonen, L. 1992. Multiple deletions of mitochondrial DNA in several tissues of a patient with severe retarded depression and familial progressive external ophthalmoplegia. *Journal of Clinical Investigation*, 90(1): 61–66.

Truckenmiller, M. E., Namboodiri, M. A., Brownstein, M. J., & Neale, J. H. 1985. N-Acetylation of L-aspartate in the nervous system: differential distribution of a specific enzyme. *Journal of Neurochemistry*, 45(5): 1658–1662.

Winsberg, M. E., Sachs, N., Tate, D. L., Adalsteinsson, E., Spielman, D., & Ketter, T. A. 2000. Decreased dorsolateral prefrontal N-acetyl aspartate in bipolar disorder. *Biological Psychiatry*, 47(6): 475–481.

Wu, R. H., O'Donnell, T., Ulrich, M., Asghar, S. J., Hanstock, C. C., Silverstone, P. H. 2004. Brain choline concentrations may not be altered in euthymic bipolar disorder patients chronically treated with either lithium or sodium valproate. *Annals of General Psychiatry*, 3(1): 13.

Yildiz-Yesiloglu, A., & Ankerst, D. P. 2006. Neurochemical alterations of the brain in bipolar disorder and their implications for pathophysiology: a systematic review of the in vivo proton magnetic resonance spectroscopy findings. *Progress in Neuro-Psychopharmacology and Biological Psychiatry*, 30(6): 969–995.

Yildiz, A., Sachs, G. S., Dorer, D. J., & Renshaw, P. F. 2001. 31P. Nuclear magnetic resonance spectroscopy findings in bipolar illness: a meta-analysis. *Psychiatry Research*, 106(3): 181–191.

Yoon, S. J., Lyoo, I. K., Haws, C., Kim, T. S., Cohen, B. M., & Renshaw, P. F. 2009. Decreased glutamate/glutamine levels may mediate cytidine's efficacy in treating bipolar depression: a longitudinal proton magnetic resonance spectroscopy study. *Neuropsychopharmacology*, 34(7): 1810–1818.

Yudkoff, M., Nelson, D., Daikhin, Y., & Ereci ska, M. 1994. Tricarboxylic acid cycle in rat brain synaptosomes. Fluxes and interactions with aspartate aminotransferase and malate/aspartate shuttle. *Journal of Biological Chemistry*, 269(44): 27414–27420.

Yuksel, C., & Ongur, D. 2010. Magnetic Resonance Spectroscopy Studies of Glutamate-Related Abnormalities in Mood Disorders. *Biological Psychiatry*, 68(9): 785–794.

Zafarullah, M., Li, W. Q., Sylvester, J., & Ahmad, M. 2003. Molecular mechanisms of N-acetylcysteine actions. *Cellular and Molecular Life Sciences*, 60(1): 6–20.

Zarate, Z. A., & Manji, H. K. 2009. Potential novel treatment for bipolar depression. In Zarate, C. A., & Manji, H. K, eds. *Bipolar Depression: Molecular Neurobiology, Clinical Diagnosis and Pharmacotherapy*, (pp. 191–209). Basel: Birhäuser Verlag.

# 5.

# NEUROIMAGING STUDIES OF BIPOLAR DISORDER IN YOUTH

## Manpreet K. Singh, Melissa P. DelBello, and Kiki D. Chang

## INTRODUCTION

Bipolar disorder is a common, serious, and recurrent psychiatric condition with an onset typically during adolescence. In youth, bipolar disorder is associated with a high risk of suicide attempts and self-injurious behaviors (Goldstein et al., 2005), co-occurring psychiatric disorders (Axelson et al., 2006), family dysfunction (Romero et al., 2005), academic problems (Pavuluri et al., 2006), and substance abuse (Wilens et al., 1999, 2004). While the occurrence of mania defines bipolar I disorder, episodes of depression often precede the onset of mania and predominate the course of illness. Numerous studies have demonstrated that despite advances in identifying cases of bipolar disorder in young people, as well as improvements in the pharmacological management of this illness, problems related to symptom relapse, medication nonadherence, and comorbid disorders such as substance abuse continue to affect the long-term morbidity and mortality associated with bipolar illness (Leverich et al., 2007; DelBello et al., 2007). Despite the established adverse impact of bipolar disorder on families and society, and its obvious significant public health relevance, research has still not clearly elucidated the neurophysiological basis of this disorder (DelBello et al., 2006).

Neuroimaging is a promising tool for uncovering the pathogenesis of bipolar disorder. Specifically, since neuroimaging studies have demonstrated that bipolar disorder is a brain-based disorder (see Martinowich et al., 2009 and Salvadore et al., 2010 for reviews), there are likely to be brain structural, functional, and chemical characteristics that are critical to its pathogenesis. Multi-modal magnetic resonance imaging (MRI) provides a safe, noninvasive tool that is ideally suited for simultaneously identifying aberrant brain structure, function, and neurochemistry in bipolar disorder. With *in vivo* MRI technology, we can bridge a clinical assessment of emotion dysregulation with biologically mediated brain abnormalities to advance our understanding of the pathophysiology of bipolar disorder.

Bipolar disorder is characterized by dysfunction in the regulation of emotion and cognition (Strakowski et al., 2005). Disturbances in core emotional and cognitive functions may provide a basis for understanding the origins of symptom manifestations associated with bipolar disorder. In addition, investigating the neural sources of these core features using neuroimaging may be more informative than basing paradigms on symptoms, particularly when controversies regarding diagnostic criteria of bipolar disorder in youth inevitably arise.

Although researchers may disagree about which brain regions are most relevant to the onset and maintenance of bipolar symptoms, most would agree that altered interactions between prefrontal and subcortical regions of the brain appear to contribute to dysfunctional regulation of emotion and cognitive processes (Blumberg et al., 2003, Chang et al., 2004, DelBello et al., 2004, Dickstein et al., 2006). Moreover, altered interactions among these regions may be a developmental phenomenon. For example, typically subcortical gray matter development precedes prefrontal development and pruning, and there appears to be a shift in functional dependence from subcortical to prefrontal structures around puberty (Thompson et al., 2000). Consequently, puberty may represent a critical period when such functional shifts are vulnerable to alterations and the development of psychopathology (Casey et al., 2008). It is therefore not surprising that the onset of bipolar disorder most commonly occurs in adolescence (Perlis et al., 2009).

Taking into account genetic and epigenetic factors, this review is guided by a theoretical model of processes underlying bipolar disorder onset and progression (Miklowitz & Chang, 2008) (Figure 5.1). Factors preceding or relating to illness onset may be considered etiological and should be differentiated from factors that are associated with the course of illness. For example, genetic, inflammatory, and stress diatheses of bipolar disorder may all be etiological and expressed phenotypically as dysregulation of emotion: hyperarousal, hypersensitivity, difficulty with

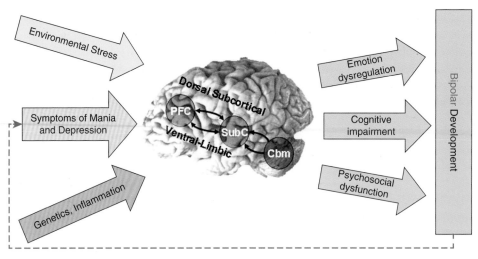

PFC = Prefrontal Cortex, SubC = Subcortical structures, Cbm = Cerebellum

*Figure 5.1* Factors contributing to the early development of bipolar disorder illustrating the interactions of environmental stress, genetics and recurrences of affective symptoms and episodes. *Abbreviations:* PFC = prefrontal cortex; SubC = subcortical structures (e.g., striatum, amygdala); Cbm = cerebellum.

affect decoding or labeling, or problems with "repair" of emotional responses (Chang et al., 2000; Shaw et al., 2005). With time, chronic illness-related stress may incite more stress and inflammatory states, which then may have a direct neurotoxic effect, contributing to the development and progression of mood episodes. Moreover, the combination of genetic vulnerability, inflammation, temperamental phenotypes, and disturbances in mood regulation converge in the expression of early subthreshold forms of bipolar disorder: persistent hypomania or depression, episodic irritability, rapid mood fluctuation, and low social functioning (Leibenluft et al., 2006; Correll, et al., 2007; Beesdo et al., 2009). These pathological processes, layered with a family history of bipolar disorder, may elevate the liability for progression to bipolar disorder and to neurobiological sequelae.

Over time, untreated or repeated mood episodes may place individuals with bipolar disorder at risk for neurobiological sequelae manifested as structural brain changes and increasing functional impairment. One neural model that may explain the onset of bipolar disorder in youth is an abnormality in prefrontal-subcortical connectivity that may result in failure of normal prefrontal regulation of subcortical processes associated with emotion. This failure may in turn result in the appearance of disease specific anatomic abnormalities that may be unique to youth with bipolar disorder, such as reductions in amygdala volumes (Pfeifer et al., 2008), thereby creating vulnerabilities in other brain regions involved in emotion including the ventrolateral prefrontal cortex (VLPFC), the anterior cingulate cortex (ACC),

thalamus, striatum, hippocampus, and the cerebellar vermis (Blumberg et al., 2003; Cecil et al., 2002 and 2003; Chang et al., 2004; Brambilla et al., 2005; Caetano et al., 2005; Frazier et al., 2005, Adler et al., 2006a, Monkul et al., 2008). Abnormal emotion regulation and cognition in bipolar disorder may arise from aberrant reciprocal connections between amygdala and dorsal and ventral prefrontal areas as described by others in mood disorders in general (Mayberg et al., 1999; Strakowski el al., 1999; Chang et al., 2004; DelBello et al., 2004). Comparisons of pediatric and adult bipolar studies of brain functional responses to stress add a developmental component to this model, suggesting that limbic hyperactivity (e.g., in the amygdala) may occur early in childhood (Chang et al., 2004), eventually becoming associated with decreased prefrontal activation (Malhi et al., 2007) and control over amygdala activity in adulthood (Foland et al., 2008) (e.g., in the ventrolateral and dorsolateral prefrontal cortex (VLPFC and DLPFC)). As bipolar disorder progresses, prefrontal abnormalities become more important, and neurodegenerative sequelae of the illness prevail (Monkul et al., 2005). In this context, the role of the prefrontal cortex may be what makes bipolar disorder unique and exclusive to humans and what precludes modeling in other animal species (Nesler & Hyman, 2010).

In this chapter, we review structural, functional, neurochemical, and other neuroimaging modalities used to study the neurophysiological alterations associated with bipolar disorder in youth. Additionally, we review neuroimaging studies of youth at familial risk for bipolar disorder (who are not yet ill) in an effort to explore potential endophenotypic markers of illness. After reviewing each modality as it applies to youth with and at familial risk for developing bipolar disorder, we will conclude by illustrating how, taken together, these studies suggest a model for bipolar disorder that is rooted in abnormalities in prefrontal-subcortical connectivity. Finally, we will propose areas of future study that will further explain the biological correlates of bipolar onset and progression.

## STRUCTURAL NEUROIMAGING STUDIES

Structural MRI studies have implicated abnormalities in selected brain regions in bipolar youth. Using tools such as manual volumetry and voxel-based morphometry (VBM), researchers have observed specific volumetric differences in youth with bipolar disorder relative to healthy children and adolescents. VBM is a boundary-free method of analysis that provides information about areas within brain regions that maximally differ between groups, whereas manual volumetry relies on sulcal-gyral and other anatomical landmarks to delineate brain regions that can then be compared. Findings to date have suggested that disruptions

in prefrontal-subcortical circuits in pediatric bipolar disorder may be caused, in part, by structural volumetric abnormalities within regions in these circuits, or as a result of longstanding network differences in bipolar disorder that may lead to less glial or neuronal support for certain brain structures. These interrelated functional and structural abnormalities may in turn lead to the development of bipolar illness. For example, the decreased volumes found in prefrontal cortex (Dickstein et al., 2005), amygdala (DelBello et al., 2004; Chang et al., 2005a), and hippocampus (Frazier et al., 2005) in youth with bipolar disorder relative to healthy subjects may represent neurotoxic effects leading to mood dysregulation. Alternatively, increased volumes in the striatum (Wilke et al., 2004; DelBello et al., 2006) may represent abnormal synaptic pruning, neuronal proliferation, or a compensatory response resulting from an illness-associated putative toxic event. Neuroanatomical measurements in youth experiencing their first mood episode, or in individuals who are at familial risk for bipolar disorder, might clarify whether structural abnormalities are etiologic or are a consequence of a mood disorder. To begin, we will review in detail volumetric abnormalities described in pediatric bipolar disorder in regions across the brain (Table 5.1, Figure 5.2).

**TABLE 5.1** REGIONAL STRUCTURAL BRAIN CHANGES IN PEDIATRIC BIPOLAR DISORDER VERSUS HEALTHY YOUTH

| Brain region | Findings in bipolar subjects | References |
|---|---|---|
| Whole Brain | Decreased<br>No differences | DelBello et al. 2004; Frazier et al. 2005<br>Chang et al. 2005 |
| Anterior cingulate cortex | Decreased | Wilke et al. 2004; Kaur et al. 2005; Chiu et al. 2008 |
| Prefrontal Cortex (PFC)<br>Dorsolateral PFC<br>Ventrolateral PFC<br>Orbitofrontal cortex | 1) Decreased; 2) no differences<br>Decreased with age<br>Decreased in males | 1) Dickstein et al 2005; 2)Sanches 2005<br>Blumberg et al. 2006<br>Najit et al. 2007 |
| Corpus Callosum | No differences | Yasar et al. 2006 |
| Striatum<br>Putamen<br>Caudate<br>Nucleus accumbens | No differences, structures combined<br>Increased<br>1) Increased; 2) No difference<br>Decreased<br>Increased with comorbid ADHD | Sanches et al. 2005<br>DelBello et al. 2004<br>1) Wilke et al. 2004; 2) Chang et al. 2005<br>Dickstein et al. 2005<br>DelBello et al. 2004 |
| Thalamus | No differences | DelBello et al. 2004; Chang et al. 2005; Frazier et al. 2005; Monkul et al. 2006 |
| Amygdala | Decreased | Chen et al. 2004c; DelBello et al. 2004; Wilke et al. 2004; Blumberg et al. 2005; Chang et al. 2005; Dickstein et al. 2005; Frazier et al. 2005 |
| Hippocampus | No differences<br>Decreased | DelBello et al. 2004; Chang et al. 2005;<br>Frazier et al. 2005; Bearden et al. 2008 |
| Superior temporal gyrus | Decreased | Chen et al. 2004a |

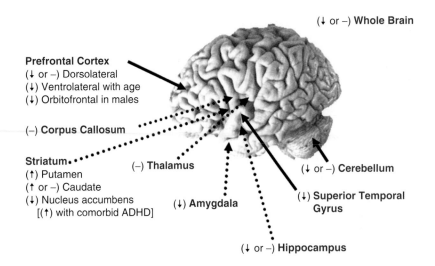

## WHOLE BRAIN AND LOBAR ANATOMY

Overall brain volume reductions were found in youth with bipolar disorder as compared to healthy subjects in at least two different studies (DelBello et al., 2004; Frazier et al., 2005a). These studies suggested that reductions in total cerebral volumes, inclusive of cerebral gray and white matter but not cerebrospinal fluid, may be due to early apoptotic pruning of neuronal circuits (Rajkowska et al., 2001; Frazier et al., 2005; Kim et al., 2010). However, not all structural neuroimaging studies in bipolar youth found differences from healthy subjects in this measure (Chang et al., 2005a). This variability among studies may be due to variations in how total brain volume was measured and nonuniform scaling across brain regions examined from study to study. This scaling is particularly important in pediatric neuroimaging studies, since, depending on the developmental stage of the child, there may be variations in head and brain size. To correct for this variation, most structural studies provide volumetric measurements as a ratio to overall brain volume. Variation in whole brain measurements between groups is therefore an important consideration when evaluating specific regions within the brain.

The next level of cortical organization is the lobes of the brain, including the frontal, parietal, temporal, and occipital regions. Since cortical gray matter volume deficits were previously reported in adults with bipolar disorder, Frazier et al. (2005b) performed an analysis comparing lobar (gray and white matter) volumes of 32 children (mean age = 11 years) with bipolar disorder and 15 age-matched healthy subjects. Parietal and temporal lobe deficits in regions associated with attentional control, face recognition, and

memory were observed in youth with bipolar disorder relative to healthy subjects (Frazier et al., 2005b). The superior temporal gyrus (STG) in the temporal lobe appears to be particularly affected, showing volumetric reductions in pediatric bipolar disorder (Chen et al., 2004a). Collectively, these studies demonstrate volumetric deficits in multiple cortical and subcortical brain regions that may lead to functional deficits at critical periods of neurodevelopment.

## PREFRONTAL CORTEX

The prefrontal cortex has been extensively studied in youth with bipolar disorder. Regions within prefrontal cortex are structurally and functionally distinct. Subregions of prefrontal cortex relevant to bipolar disorder include dorsolateral (DLPFC) and ventrolateral (VLPFC) prefrontal cortices, anterior (ACC) and subgenual (sgACC) cingulate cortices, and orbitofrontal cortex (OFC), all of which are involved in reasoning and other executive functions, regulation of emotion and attention, and processing of rewards and motivation. Reductions in DLPFC (Dickstein et al., 2005) and VLPFC (Blumberg et al., 2006) volumes have been reported in youth with bipolar disorder, with VLPFC reductions being inversely correlated with increasing age.

Three studies found reductions in ACC (Wilke et al., 2004; Kaur et al., 2005; Chiu et al., 2008), a region important for executive functioning and mood regulation. To further demonstrate that reductions in ACC may be related to pediatric-onset bipolar disorder, one study measured volumetric changes in youth before and after developing a diagnosis of bipolar disorder using dynamic mapping of cortical development and found decreased bilateral anterior and subgenual cingulate cortices (sgACC) in children particularly after illness onset (Gogtay et al., 2007). The sgACC, a region of particular interest in major depressive and other mood disorders, has shown mixed results. Sanches et al. (2005a) initially found no group differences in the sgACC volumes in children and adolescents with bipolar disorder compared to healthy subjects. In a recent larger follow-up study, it appeared that reductions in sgACC volumes were present in the left hemisphere particularly in youth with a family history of bipolar disorder (Baloch et al., 2010). However, in a study of 20 children and adolescents with familial bipolar disorder as compared to healthy subjects, no differences were found in sgACC volumes, but additional analyses suggested that bipolar disorder subjects with past mood stabilizer exposure had significantly increased bilateral posterior sgACC volumes compared to bipolar disorder subjects without mood stabilizer exposure and to healthy subjects (Mitsunaga et al., 2011).

Finally, findings in the OFC have suggested that sex may be a factor involved in illness pathophysiology among young bipolar patients. In one study in bipolar youth, girls showed increased gray matter volumes in the OFC, whereas boys had gray matter reductions in the OFC (Najt et al., 2007), compared with healthy subjects. Early volumetric changes in portions of prefrontal cortex may have a significant impact on cognitive development and the regulation of emotion, and suggest vulnerability factors for a chronic bipolar illness course.

## SUBCORTICAL REGIONS: STRIATUM, AMYGDALA, HIPPOCAMPUS

Volumetric changes have also been demonstrated in key subcortical brain regions in pediatric bipolar disorder. The striatum, including the collective structures of caudate, putamen, and nucleus accumbens, are involved in movement, perseverative behaviors, impulse control, reward processing, and decision-making. Prior studies in pediatric bipolar disorder demonstrated volumetric increases in putamen (DelBello et al., 2004) and caudate (Wilke et al., 2004), while others found no departures from healthy subjects in these structures (Chang et al., 2005a; Sanches et al., 2005b). However, in youth with bipolar disorder, bilateral caudate and left putamen volumes may be inversely related to age (Sanches et al., 2005b), demonstrating the importance of stratifying by age in pediatric structural neuroimaging analyses. Pubertal status is another variable that may influence volumetric differences in youth with bipolar disorder. In one study, trends for increased nucleus accumbens volumes became significant in prepubertal youth with bipolar disorder as compared to pubertal youth with bipolar disorder and healthy subjects (Ahn et al., 2007). A VBM study found a signal for left nucleus accumbens enlargement in youth with bipolar disorder relative to healthy subjects (Dickstein et al., 2005). In contrast, another study found smaller nucleus accumbens and amygdala volumes to be associated with greater numbers of independent life events, suggesting that important environmental stressors may impact neural structure in key subcortical regions (Geller et al., 2009). Given the small size and lack of distinct boundaries in humans of the nucleus accumbens, reliable measurements of this structure are difficult, limiting our interpretation of these conflicting findings.

Studies of children with attention deficit with hyperactivity disorder (ADHD) have demonstrated decreases in striatal volume (Castellanos et al., 2003) that may complicate interpretation of striatal volumes in pediatric bipolar disorder due to the common co-occurrence of these conditions. One recent study compared youth with bipolar disorder with and without ADHD to subjects with ADHD alone, and to healthy subjects, and found that the ADHD-only group had smaller caudate and putamen volumes compared with the other groups. The comorbid bipolar disorder and ADHD youth had moderately increased nucleus accumbens volumes relative to healthy subjects (Lopez-Larson et al., 2009). Interestingly, youth with bipolar disorder in this study with and without ADHD did not differ from one another, but did appear to differentiate from ADHD-only youth. In another study, caudate, putamen, and globus pallidus volumes were manually traced on high resolution anatomical MRI images from youth in four groups: bipolar disorder with comorbid ADHD (n = 17), bipolar disorder without comorbid ADHD (n = 12), ADHD alone (n = 11), and healthy subjects (n = 24); this study found that subjects with ADHD had significantly decreased caudate, putamen, and globus pallidus volumes compared to the bipolar disorder and healthy groups (Liu et al., 2011). Additionally, subjects with bipolar disorder without comorbid ADHD had increased caudate, putamen, and globus pallidus volumes compared with healthy subjects. The group with bipolar disorder without ADHD had significantly increased caudate volumes as compared to the bipolar disorder with ADHD group. Therefore, the presence or absence of comorbid ADHD in patients with bipolar disorder was associated with distinct alterations in caudate volumes, suggesting that these groups have different, but related, mechanisms of neuropathology. Additional studies with larger sample sizes accounting for age, puberty, other comorbidities, and environmental factors, along with improved measurements of small structures are warranted to clarify the role of the striatum in pediatric bipolar disorder.

Among the most consistent neuroanatomic findings in youth with bipolar disorder is a reduction in amygdala volume. The amygdala regulates emotional valence and perception and is involved in learning and memory. Several separate research groups have found reductions in amygdala volume in pediatric bipolar disorder (Chen et al., 2004c; DelBello et al., 2004; Wilke et al., 2004; Blumberg et al., 2005; Chang et al., 2005a; Dickstein et al., 2005; Frazier et al., 2005), making it the most replicated neuroanatomical finding in youth with bipolar disorder. As such, three meta-analyses or reviews examined this finding in the context of developing bipolar disorder over the lifespan, and suggested that reduced amygdala volumes may be a developmental finding unique to children and adolescents rather than adults with bipolar disorder (Pfeifer et al., 2008; Hajek et al., 2009; Usher et al., 2010). Interestingly, this finding has not been reported in youth at risk for bipolar disorder (Ladouceur et al., 2008; Singh et al., 2008; Karchemskiy et al., 2011) or in first episode mania samples, suggesting that reduced amygdala volumes may be a consequence of disease progression rather than representing an etiological abnormality per se. Alternatively, adolescents with mania may fail to show normal increases in amygdala volume that typically occur during healthy adolescent neurodevelopment (Bitter et al., 2011). Moreover, in contrast to adults with bipolar disorder, children are less exposed to factors such as chronic medication exposure, repeated mood episodes or substance abuse, which may have neuroregenerative or neurotoxic properties on the brain (Moore et al., 2009). Consequently, neuroimaging studies in youth may more accurately reflect neuroanatomical abnormalities that are associated with bipolar disorder rather than confounding factors associated with illness course.

Less consistently, reductions in hippocampal volumes have been observed in pediatric bipolar disorder samples. The hippocampus is involved in appraisal and regulation of stress and emotional responses through inhibitory connections with other subcortical structures, and therefore may be relevant for mood disorders. In pediatric bipolar disorder, two studies found reductions in hippocampal volume (Frazier et al., 2005; Bearden et al., 2008), one showed a statistical trend for reduction possibly due to combining adults and youth with bipolar disorder (Blumberg et al., 2003b), and two other studies found no difference between youth with bipolar disorder and healthy subjects in hippocampal volumes (DelBello et al., 2004; Chang et al.,

2005a). Variability across studies may be due to a variety of factors including the presence of other co-occurring psychiatric disorders. For example, in a familial bipolar disorder sample, one recent study demonstrated that hippocampal volume was negatively correlated with degree of comorbid anxiety (Simeonova et al., 2009). Comorbidites create heterogeneity in studies of individuals with bipolar disorder, which may affect neural structures and obfuscate or potentially create findings, just as the presence or absence of comorbid ADHD may affect striatal volumes as noted previously.

## THALAMUS AND OTHER REGIONS

The thalamus relays information selectively to various brain regions, and regulates states of sleep and wakefulness or arousal. To date, no pediatric bipolar disorder structural imaging study reported differences in thalamic volume in pediatric bipolar disorder versus healthy subjects (DelBello et al., 2004; Chang et al., 2005a; Frazier et al., 2005; Monkul et al., 2006). Other regions studied in bipolar youth, due to their relevance in adults with bipolar disorder, include the corpus callosum (Yasar et el., 2006), cerebellar vermis (Monkul et al., 2008), and pituitary gland (Chen et al., 2004b); no significant differences from healthy subjects were observed in these studies.

## AT-RISK STUDIES:

Most of the previous studies included youth who were already fully symptomatic with bipolar disorder. Researchers have speculated whether structural changes in these young people predated the onset of illness or if they were a consequence of illness burden. However, few studies have examined neurobiological endophenotypes associated with risk for bipolar disorder independent of common confounds associated with illness onset or precede illness onset, including comorbidities, medication exposure, or substance use. One way to address these issues is to evaluate offspring of parents with bipolar disorder. Studies of youth at risk for bipolar disorder not only identify potential endophenotypic neural abnormalities that may exist prior to illness onset, they also may be useful to identify factors associated with risk or resilience in youth, who may then be followed longitudinally to assess how these factors progress with illness development.

Studies in youth at risk for bipolar disorder may be categorized based on the level of symptoms present at the time of assessment. Some youth offspring of parents with bipolar disorder already show phenotypic expression of mood symptoms that may not meet duration or severity threshold criteria for fully syndromal bipolar disorder, while other youth at risk for bipolar disorder may be symptom free at the time of assessment. In one study, 22 youth of parents with bipolar disorder had amygdala, hippocampus, and thalamus volumes measured by manual tracing; of note, although they did not meet criteria for bipolar disorder, these young people exhibited ADHD and moderate mood symptoms at the time of assessment. No significant volumetric differences were found in any of these brain regions as compared to youth of healthy parents (Karchemskiy et al., 2011), suggesting that any morphometric abnormalities in these structures found in subjects with bipolar disorder may occur only after more prolonged illness rather than as a preexisting risk factor. This study may have been underpowered to differentiate at-risk youth most likely to progress to bipolar disorder from healthy subjects as conversion rates in at-risk youth are relatively low. Similarly, another structural neuroimaging study of at-risk youth found no structural abnormalities differentiating symptomatic high-risk offspring of parents with bipolar disorder from youth of healthy parents (Singh et al., 2008). However, asymptomatic or a healthy subset of offspring of parents with bipolar disorder in this study showed trends for increased prefrontal cortical volumes (Singh et al., 2008), suggesting an abnormality in typical neuronal proliferation, in pruning of prefrontal cortical circuits, or represent a compensatory neuroprotective effect. In another study, gray matter volume increases in the parahippocampal gyri were found in healthy offspring of parents with bipolar disorder compared to offspring of healthy parents (Ladouceur et al., 2008). These latter two studies suggested either the presence of trait-related structural changes predating illness onset, an abnormality in the healthy neuronal proliferation or pruning, or compensatory effects on neural circuits to prevent the onset of mood symptoms in youth at risk for bipolar disorder. Moreover, increases in prefrontal and parahippocampal regions and lack of structural differences in other regions from typically developing youth may represent features of resilience rather than risk in a subset of at-risk youth who do not develop symptoms. Longitudinal studies are needed to confirm whether volumetric changes represent risk or resilience factors (or neither) for the development of bipolar disorder.

Collectively, these studies demonstrate disruptions in key prefrontal and subcortical regions in youth with fully expressed bipolar symptoms that warrant further investigation with larger samples over time to address important demographic and developmental factors that may be contributing to volumetric results.

**Structural MRI Studies in Youth with or at Risk for Bipolar Disorder:**

- Suggest alterations in prefrontal, amygdala, and possibly striatal regions

- Suggest that brain abnormalities represent aspects of developmental alterations, sequelae of illness effects, and possibly etiological significance

- May reflect confounds in some instances, such as the presence of comorbidities like ADHD, the developmental stage at the time of assessment, variable exposure to unquantifiable environmental stressors, and treatment exposure

- Suggest that amygdala abnormalities may be developmental or progressive rather than etiologic

## DIFFUSION TENSOR IMAGING (DTI)

Imaging studies in adults with bipolar disorder suggest that dysfunction in prefrontal and subcortical regions may be related to abnormalities within white matter tracts connecting these brain regions. White matter hyperintensities (WMH), areas of increased signal intensity on T2 MRI images that may be indicative of neuropathological changes in white matter tracts, are more common in adults with bipolar I disorder than in healthy adults (Beyer et al., 2009). White matter hyperintensities may be early signs of demyelination (Hajek et al., 2005), but remain poorly understood and may be confused with vascular abnormalities such as Virchow-Robin spaces (Yetkin et al., 1992). Increased white matter hyperintensities have been found in some (Botteron et al., 1992; Lyoo et al., 2002) but not all (Chang et al., 2005b) pediatric bipolar disorder studies. In contrast to hyperintensities in white matter, decreased signal intensities in the corpus callosum in youth with bipolar disorder have suggested decreased myelination in callosal subregions (Caetano et al., 2008). However, from these techniques it is unclear if signal intensity differences reflect myelin changes, reduced axon density, or an entirely different process related to regional differences in vasculature. To further quantitatively characterize white matter tracts communicating between prefrontal and subcortical regions, alternative approaches, such as diffusion tensor imaging, need to be considered.

Diffusion tensor imaging (DTI) is a MRI technique that uses measurement of water diffusion to study white matter tracts *in vivo*. Water diffusion in white matter is highly anisotropic (i.e., not equal in all directions), as diffusion tends to be greater parallel to the fiber axis than perpendicular to it. Anisotropy within a given white matter voxel is determined mostly by microstructural features of the tissue, including fiber diameter and density, degree of myelination, and macrostructural features such as intravoxel fiber-tract coherence. Changes in these features as a result of disease states can be detected as changes in water diffusion. Three commonly used scalar measures of anisotropy in DTI research include fractional anisotropy (FA), trace apparent diffusion coefficient (TADC) that is a measure of mean intravoxel diffusivity derived from the diffusion tensor, and apparent diffusion coefficient (ADC) that is a measure of intravoxel diffusivity derived from diffusion weighted images.

Although there have been relatively few DTI studies of youth with bipolar disorder, the limited data available suggest abnormalities in white matter tracts connecting portions of the prefrontal cortex to subcortical structures. The first DTI study in adolescents with bipolar disorder investigated 11 first-episode manic or mixed adolescents and 17 typically developing healthy subjects (Adler et al., 2006b). FA and TADC values were measured in white matter tracts adjacent to the prefrontal and posterior cortex. FA values were reduced in the bipolar group only in the superior prefrontal region, and TADC values did not differ between the two groups, suggesting the presence of axonal disorganization in prefrontal white matter early in bipolar disorder. Reduced white matter integrity due to lower FA in the right orbital frontal lobe and higher ADC in the right and left subgenual region was recently demonstrated in adolescents with bipolar I disorder compared with healthy youth (Kafantaris et al., 2009). By using additional regions of interest (ROIs) or voxel-by-voxel analyses as well as fiber-tracking techniques, another DTI study examined adolescents with familial bipolar disorder relative to healthy subjects (Barnea-Goraly et al., 2009). This study showed lower FA values than healthy subjects in the fornix, the left mid-posterior cingulate gyrus, throughout the corpus callosum, in fibers extending from the fornix to the thalamus, and in parietal and occipital corona radiata bilaterally (Barnea-Goraly et al., 2009). In comparing youth with bipolar disorder to those with ADHD and healthy subjects, decreased FA has been shown in the anterior corona radiata fiber tract in both bipolar and ADHD samples, implying an impaired fiber density or reduced myelination in this prefrontal tract (Pavuluri et al., 2009). This latter study also showed increased ADC across multiple white matter tracts in ADHD youth indicating extensive cellular abnormalities with less diffusion restriction compared with youth with bipolar disorder. Finally, a recent study performed a

*post hoc* DTI analysis in children and adolescents with bipolar disorder who underwent transverse relaxation time (T2) imaging to examine membrane fluidity (Gönenç et al., 2010) in bilateral cingulate-paracingulate white matter. This study found FA reductions and trace and radial diffusivity increases in the left hemisphere, and increased trace diffusivity and decreased T2 in the right hemisphere in youth with bipolar disorder compared to healthy subjects. Taken together, these studies suggest impairments in prefrontal-subcortical white matter tracts early in bipolar disorder.

To explore white matter characteristics in youth at familial risk for bipolar disorder, a study compared white matter integrity in 10 children with bipolar disorder, seven children at risk for bipolar disorder, and eight healthy subjects (Frazier et al., 2007). This study found that the group with bipolar disorder had decreased FA in right and left superior frontal tracts, including the superior longitudinal fasciculus I (SLF I) and the cingulate-paracingulate white matter. In addition, the bipolar disorder group had reduced FA in left orbital frontal white matter and in the right corpus callosum body. Although children with bipolar disorder showed reduced FA in the right and left cingulate-paracingulate white matter (CG-PAC WM) relative to at-risk youth, both bipolar disorder and at-risk groups showed reduced FA in bilateral SLF I relative to healthy subjects. These findings suggest that SLF I deficits in bipolar disorder and at-risk youth might be trait-related while deficits in the CG-PAC WM in youth with bipolar disorder might be disease-state related. Another recent study performed DTI in 20 healthy offspring with a parent diagnosed with bipolar disorder and 25 healthy control offspring of healthy parents (Versace et al., 2010). Results from this cross-sectional study showed altered white matter

---

**Diffusion Tensor Imaging (DTI) Studies in Youth with or at-risk for Bipolar Disorder:**

- Suggest structural abnormalities including axonal disorganization and reduced integrity in prefrontal-subcortical white matter tracts

- Indicate that additional studies in youth at risk for bipolar disorder are warranted to determine when white matter impairments occur relative to bipolar illness onset

- In tandem with other imaging modalities will aid in elucidating the pathophysiological mechanisms associated with early onset bipolar disorder development in healthy offspring of a bipolar parent compared with healthy children of healthy parents in the corpus callosum and temporal associative tracts. Given that this sample was without any medical or psychiatric diagnosis, these findings may represent an endophenotype unrelated to bipolar disorder development or potential early resiliency markers or risk factors for future bipolar disorder development. Longitudinal DTI analyses are needed to understand these results in the context of bipolar risk.

## FUNCTIONAL NEUROIMAGING

Functional MRI (fMRI) provides data regarding brain activation as reflected in the levels of oxygenated versus de-oxygenated hemoglobin in a brain region, referred to as the blood oxygen level dependent (BOLD) signal. fMRI studies have examined BOLD signal changes, and consequently regional brain activation, in response to a variety of emotional and cognitive stimuli in youth with bipolar disorder (Chang et al., 2004; Rich et al., 2006). In adults with bipolar disorder, limbic hyperactivity appears to coincide with prefrontal hypoactivity (Foland et al., 2008; Yurgelun-Todd et al., 2000). In contrast, prefrontal activation appears to be relatively intact in bipolar youth, and euthymic children with bipolar disorder show prefrontal *over*activation during emotional tasks (Chang et al., 2004). Furthermore, amygdala hyperactivity appears to be inversely related to the reduced amygdala volume that was described previously (Kalmar et al., 2009). Activations also correlate with mood symptoms, as illustrated in the finding of increased left putamen activation correlating with depressive symptoms in youth with bipolar disorder during a Stroop task (Blumberg et al., 2003). More closely examining specific paradigms studied in pediatric bipolar disorder and organized by an evolution of foci from cognitive and emotional functions to the interplay between them will further illustrate the functional importance of prefrontal and subcortical regions highlighted in previous sections of this chapter.

## SELECTIVE ATTENTION USING STROOP PARADIGMS

Initial fMRI studies in pediatric bipolar disorder examined neural responses during color-naming Stroop paradigms with the prediction that mood symptoms of bipolar disorder would interfere with cognitive processing associated with these tasks. Blumberg and colleagues (2003a) observed significantly increased activation of the left putamen and thalamus in pediatric bipolar disorder during a

color-naming Stroop task. This study also showed a positive correlation between depressive symptoms and activation in a ventral striatal region of interest. Emotional stroop paradigms have been more recently employed, in which participants are required, for example, to match the color of an emotionally valenced word to the color of either of two adjacent circles. Relative to healthy subjects, euthymic youth with bipolar disorder demonstrated reduced ventrolateral prefrontal activation combined with amygdala hyperactivation in response to negative stimuli using this paradigm, suggesting disinhibition of emotional reactivity in the limbic system and reduced function in prefrontal systems that regulate those responses (Pavuluri et al., 2008). This interaction between affective and cognitive circuitry may contribute to the reduced capacity for affect regulation and behavioral self-control in pediatric bipolar disorder. In another study, during cognitive control of emotion processing, patients with bipolar disorder deployed the ventrolateral prefrontal cortex (VLPFC) to a greater extent than healthy subjects, whereas an ADHD comparison group showed decreased VLPFC engagement relative to both healthy and bipolar groups (Passarotti et al., 2010a). Consequently, youth with bipolar disorder appear to differentially activate VLPFC during periods when cognitive control and emotional processing intersect.

## WORKING MEMORY AND EMOTIONALLY VALENCED PICTURE STIMULI

Visuospatial working memory and exposure to affectively valenced visual stimuli have also been employed to further understand relationships between cognitive and emotional function. Chang et al. (2004) found that youth with bipolar disorder had greater activation in prefrontal-subcortical circuits, namely bilateral anterior cingulate, left putamen, left thalamus, left dorsolateral prefrontal cortex (DLPFC), and right inferior frontal gyrus during visuospatial working memory, whereas healthy youth exhibited greater activation in the cerebellar vermis. While viewing negatively valenced pictures, subjects with bipolar disorder had greater activation in the bilateral DLPFC, inferior frontal gyrus, and right insula whereas healthy subjects showed greater activation in the right posterior cingulate gyrus. For positively valenced pictures, subjects with bipolar disorder had greater activation in the bilateral caudate and thalamus, left middle/superior frontal gyrus, and left anterior cingulate, whereas healthy subjects had no areas of greater activation. These patterns of anomalous neural activation in bipolar children and adolescents were among the initial observations of prefrontal-subcortical dysfunction.

When compared to youth with ADHD, youth with bipolar disorder appeared to also show greater deployment of emotion-processing circuitry and reduced deployment of working memory circuitry while viewing angry, neutral, and happy faces (Passarotti et al., 2010b). All of these studies demonstrate the impact of emotion dysregulation on working memory.

## EMOTIONAL FACE PROCESSING

Neural responses to facial expressions have also been studied by contrasting emotional from nonemotional aspects of faces presented to youth with bipolar disorder and healthy subjects during fMRI. Rich et al. (2006) found that compared with healthy subjects, bipolar disorder youth perceived greater hostility in neutral faces and reported more fear when viewing them. These subjects also exhibited greater activation in left amygdala, accumbens, putamen, and ventral prefrontal cortex when rating face hostility, and in left amygdala and bilateral accumbens when rating fear. Authors of this study suggested that these findings demonstrate deficient emotion-attention interactions in bipolar disorder in youth. Other studies that examined emotional face processing found that compared with healthy subjects, youth with bipolar disorder show reduced activation of right rostral ventrolateral prefrontal cortex together with increased activity in right pregenual anterior cingulate, amygdala, and paralimbic cortex in response to angry and happy relative to neutral faces (Pavuluri et al., 2007). They also observed reduced connectivity between left amygdala and right posterior cingulate/precuneus and right fusiform gyrus/parahippocampal gyrus while viewing emotional versus nonemotional aspects of faces (Rich et al., 2008). Finally, bipolar compared with healthy subjects demonstrated reduced memory for emotional faces paired with increased activation in the striatum and anterior cingulate when successfully encoding happy faces and in the orbitofrontal cortex when successfully encoding angry faces (Dickstein et al., 2007).

Pavuluri et al. (2009) divided emotional processing into directed versus incidental conditions, in which subjects were asked to judge whether emotion in a facial expression was positive or negative (directed), and whether faces expressing similar affect were older or younger than 35 years (incidental). This study found increased amygdala activation in youth with bipolar disorder during incidental emotional processing relative to directed emotional processing suggesting more intense automatic emotional reactivity. In addition, the right prefrontal systems appeared less engaged in patients with bipolar disorder regardless of whether the emotion processing was incidental or directed, signifying possible reductions in top-down control of emotional reactivity in pediatric bipolar disorder (Pavuluri et al., 2009).

## RESPONSE INHIBITION AND SUSTAINED ATTENTION

Given the propensity for impulsivity, attentional dysfunction and motor hyperactivity in bipolar disorder, researchers have also examined patterns of motor or response inhibition in youth with bipolar disorder using paradigms such as the Go/NoGo task. In one study that posited that deficits in motor inhibition might contribute to impulsivity and irritability in children with bipolar disorder, youth with bipolar disorder and healthy subjects completed an event-related fMRI study while they performed a motor inhibition task (Leibenluft et al., 2007). During failed inhibitory trials, healthy subjects showed greater bilateral striatal and right ventral prefrontal cortex activation than did subjects with bipolar disorder, suggesting deficits in the ability of bipolar youth to engage these brain regions during unsuccessful inhibition. In a first episode mania sample of adolescents and young adults, successful response inhibition was associated with greater activation in anterior and posterior cingulate, medial dorsal thalamus, middle temporal gyrus and precuneus in the healthy subjects, whereas patients with bipolar disorder exhibited prefrontal activation (BA 10) that was not observed in healthy subjects (Strakowski et al., 2008). In another Go/NoGo study, bipolar relative to healthy youth showed increased recruitment of the right dorsolateral prefrontal cortex in order to successfully inhibit a motor response (Singh et al., 2010). Bipolar youth also showed behavioral evidence of deficits in sustained attention with fewer correct responses on Go and overall trials as compared to the healthy group. In this latter study, 81% of the bipolar disorder group exhibited co-occurring ADHD, but the independent effects of this comorbidity on task performance could not be evaluated in any of the studies described previously due to insufficient sample sizes of subgroups with either ADHD or bipolar disorder alone.

Eleven bipolar adolescents with comorbid ADHD and 15 bipolar adolescents without ADHD were recruited to participate in an fMRI examination while doing a single-digit continuous performance task alternating with a control task in a block-design paradigm (Adler et al., 2005). This study found that ADHD comorbidity was associated with less activation in the ventrolateral prefrontal cortex (Brodmann 10) and anterior cingulate, and greater activation in posterior parietal cortex and middle temporal gyrus.

To further evaluate the neurophysiological basis of bipolar disorder in contrast to ADHD, a study using a continuous performance task with a response inhibition component examined 11 adolescents with bipolar disorder during a manic episode, 10 adolescents with ADHD, and 13 healthy adolescents, and found that youth with ADHD showed increased activation in the superior temporal lobe during successful response inhibition, whereas increased left parahippocampal activation in the bipolar group was associated with increased manic symptoms (Cerullo et al., 2009). Another study using a response inhibition paradigm in youth with bipolar disorder in comparison to those with ADHD and healthy subjects characterized the bipolar group as showing decreased activation in left ventrolateral prefrontal cortex, at the junction of the inferior and middle frontal gyri, and in right anterior cingulate cortex relative to healthy subjects (Passarotti et al., 2010c). Prefrontal dysfunction was observed in both the ADHD and bipolar disorder groups relative to healthy youth, although it was more extensive and accompanied by subcortical over-activity in ADHD. Collectively, these studies suggest that youth with bipolar disorder demonstrate divergent patterns of neurophysiological dysfunction predominantly in the prefrontal cortex than youth with ADHD during response inhibition, and that the co-occurrence of these two disorders may result in even greater variation in patterns of prefrontal and subcortical activations than the individual disorders alone.

## COGNITIVE FLEXIBILITY

Response flexibility, reversal learning, and paradigms probing emotional reactivity have also been used to understand the pathophysiology of early onset bipolar disorder. On correctly-performed change trials relative to correctly-performed go trials, participants with bipolar disorder generated significantly more activity in the left DLPFC and in the primary motor cortex than did healthy subjects during a response flexibility task (Nelson et al., 2007). Activation of the DLPFC was considered a deficit in this study that may extend beyond the realm of motor control and also affect emotion regulation. Event-related fMRI during a probabilistic reversal task was the basis for evaluating how well individuals with bipolar disorder acquired a stimulus/response relationship through trial-and-error learning, and then discern when the stimulus/reward relationship reverses. During this reversal learning task, euthymic youth with bipolar disorder as compared to healthy subjects had significantly greater fronto-parietal activation in response to punished reversal errors (Dickstein et al., 2010a), demonstrating inefficient neural recruitment while processing

response conflict in the former group. Together, these findings suggest deficits in prefrontal, parietal, and subcortical brain regions relevant for cognitive flexibility and learning.

## fMRI RESPONSE TO A PHARMACOLOGICAL INTERVENTION

Many of the previous studies were confounded by youth with bipolar disorder receiving varying levels of exposure to psychotropic medications at the time of their fMRI scan. Recently, a few researchers have begun to directly examine the effects of pharmacological intervention in fMRI activation. In an open-label study, Chang and colleagues (2008) examined the neural effects of lamotrigine in adolescents with bipolar depression and found that adolescents with bipolar disorder treated with lamotrigine for 8 weeks demonstrated less amygdala activation when viewing negative stimuli as depressive symptoms improved; whether the changes in fMRI activation were due to lamotrigine exposure or improvements in depressive symptoms (as a consequence of lamotrigine treatment) could not be determined. In another multimodal neuroimaging study, Chang et al. (2009) examined the effect of divalproex on brain structure, chemistry, and function in symptomatic youth at high risk for bipolar disorder. Although there were no significant effects on brain structure or neurochemistry after 12 weeks of treatment with divalproex, decreases in prefrontal brain activation correlated with decreases in depressive symptom severity (Chang et al., 2009). This finding suggests that it is symptom change, rather than medication exposure *per se*, that impacts fMRI findings. A third study examined 17 youth with bipolar disorder after 14 weeks of treatment with a second-generation antipsychotic followed by lamotrigine monotherapy, and compared fMRI activation to that of healthy subjects. The investigators observed treatment related decreases in the ventromedial prefrontal cortex (VMPFC) and the dorsolateral prefrontal cortex (DLPFC) in the bipolar subjects (Pavuluri et al., 2010). Finally, in a recent intervention study in which an affective working memory task was presented before and after sequential treatment for 8 weeks with an atypical antipsychotic followed by 6 weeks of lamotrigine to previously unmedicated youth with bipolar disorder, pharmacotherapy resulted in normalization of symptoms and higher cortical and cognitive regional activation in youth with bipolar disorder versus healthy subjects, but did not normalize amygdala overactivation (Passarotti et al., 2011). Improvement on Young Mania Rating Scale (YMRS) score significantly correlated with decreased activity in ventromedial prefrontal cortex within the patient group, so again these observations may have reflected the therapeutic effects of treatment, rather than medication exposure *per se*, on fMRI activation. Larger controlled studies in individuals who were previously medication naïve would aid in understanding the specific effects of medication exposure on neural activation in bipolar disorder.

## RESTING STATE FUNCTIONAL CONNECTIVITY

All of the previous studies employed paradigms that targeted specific brain regions and functions associated with cognition and emotion. Task-independent spontaneous resting state functional connectivity (RSFC) has recently been employed to better understand brain activity and relationships among prefrontal and subcortical structures at rest. Unlike task-activation studies, RSFC can directly assess neural systems without contamination by differences in performance that might inflate individual variability across the study group. RSFC is determined by correlating this activity temporally and such patterns are believed to reflect synchronous interaction among brain regions. One particular resting-state network in healthy subjects is the default mode network (DMN), which collectively involves the anterior cingulate (ACC) and a large portion of medial prefrontal cortex (MPFC) extending inferiorly into orbitofrontal cortex (OFC). This network may be involved with internally generated thought and is inhibited when attending to external stimuli requiring attention and cognition. Younger children have weaker connectivity in these areas. It is likely that the default mode network becomes established during adolescence or young adulthood (Fair et al., 2008). In the only published RSFC analysis in pediatric bipolar disorder to date, Dickstein et al. (2010b) found that pediatric participants with bipolar disorder had significantly greater negative RSFC between the left dorsolateral prefrontal cortex and the right superior temporal gyrus than healthy subjects. These regions are important for working memory and learning, and appear consistent with the previous structural and functional findings. This study, however, was limited in sample size so could not evaluate the effects of age, gender, development, and treatment on this circuit in pediatric bipolar disorder. Future studies using this RSFC are needed to better characterize functional relations between prefrontal and subcortical neurocircuitry in the pediatric bipolar disorder brain at rest.

FMRI is limited by its relative sensitivity to state-dependent features of bipolar illness, which are consequently difficult to distinguish from trait-related phenomena (Frazier et al., 2005a). This complication is especially true when subjects are scanned during various mood states, but grouped together for analysis. Additionally, it can be challenging to select appropriate cognitive tasks and to standardize paradigms in children who are undergoing maturation in cognition and emotion. There are other cognitive domains that have not been explored in youth with bipolar disorder. For example, bipolar disorder is associated with risk-taking behaviors that may have rewarding or highly painful consequences, so anticipation and receipt of reward-related stimuli represents another paradigm that could be studied with fMRI in pediatric bipolar disorder. Future studies will benefit by carefully selecting paradigms and forming *a priori* hypotheses to advance our understanding of functional impairments in youth with bipolar disorder. In addition, more fMRI studies need to be performed in symptomatic and never-ill youth at familial risk for bipolar disorder to determine whether there is evidence of early functional impairment prior to the onset of bipolar disorder.

**fMRI Studies in Youth with or at-risk for Bipolar Disorder:**

- Suggest aberrant activation patterns in prefrontal and subcortical brain regions while performing certain cognitive and emotional tasks

- Show greater deployment of emotion-processing circuitry and reduced activation of cognition-related circuitry, suggesting disinhibition from reduced prefrontal modulation of emotional networks

- Show that increased prefrontal activation reflects inefficient use of neural resources during cognitive flexibility and motor response inhibition tasks

- Show normalization of aberrant prefrontal but not amygdala activation patterns with treatment that parallel symptom improvement

- Have found less amygdala activation abnormalities than adult studies

## MAGNETIC RESONANCE SPECTROSCOPY (MRS)

Data demonstrating macroscopic structural and functional changes in selective brain regions in bipolar disorder imply underlying cellular and molecular dysfunction. Magnetic resonance spectroscopy (MRS) is a noninvasive neuroimaging method that yields molecular level biochemical data to quantitatively examine neuronal function. Most MRS studies in youth with bipolar disorder have employed proton ($^1$H-MRS) acquisitions focused primarily on key prefrontal cortical regions. For example, studies of bipolar youth have shown altered medial and dorsolateral prefrontal concentrations of N-acetyl aspartate (NAA) and phosphocreatine/creatine (PCr/Cr), healthy nerve cell markers putatively involved in maintaining energy production and myelin formation in the brain (Chang et al., 2003). In addition, increases (Patel et al., 2008a) and decreases (Cecil et al., 2003) in prefrontal myo-inositol (mI) levels, a marker for cellular metabolism and second messenger signaling pathways, have also been found in youth with bipolar disorder. These neuronal markers appear to be sensitive to lithium treatment in children with bipolar disorder (Davanzo et al., 2001). Some, but not all, prior studies have demonstrated that alterations in neurometabolite concentrations may occur early in the development of bipolar disorder (Figure 5.3) and are described subsequently.

## PREFRONTAL CORTEX

N-Acetyl aspartate (NAA) decreases have been observed in pediatric bipolar disorder in prefrontal regions, including the dorsolateral prefrontal cortex (DLPFC) (Chang et al., 2003, Olvera et al., 2007; Caetano et al., 2011) and medial prefrontal cortex (Caetano et al., 2011). Explanations for these changes include abnormal dendridic arborization and neuropil in the neurodevelopmental milieu of mania, loss of neuronal matter due to age-dependent processes (Brooks et al., 2001), or disease related fluid shifts in prefrontal regions of the brain (Winsberg et al., 2000). In youth with bipolar depression, increases in NAA, myo-inositol (mI), and creatine were found in anterior cingulate and bilateral

ventrolateral prefrontal cortex (Patel et al., 2008a), suggesting the possibility of decreased prefrontal metabolism; this decrease in metabolism may result in additional energy sources available to synthesize NAA, leading to increased NAA concentrations (Stork and Renshaw 2005). Increased orbitofrontal mI has also been demonstrated in offspring of parents with bipolar disorder who were scanned while they had moderate mood symptoms not meeting criteria for bipolar I or II disorder (Cecil et al., 2003). However, further comparisons of NAA levels in bilateral dorsolateral prefrontal cortex in high-risk offspring with and without mania found no statistically significant decrements in NAA, suggesting that decrements of NAA may not be seen until the development of fully syndromal mania or longer duration of bipolar illness (Gallelli et al., 2005).

Another neurometabolite measurable by [1]H-MRS in the prefrontal cortex that may be associated with abnormal mood regulation is the excitatory neurotransmitter glutamate. Castillo et al. (2000) used [1]H-MRS and found increased levels of glutamate, its precursor and storage form glutamine, or a combined contribution of glutamate and glutamine (Glx) in the frontal lobes in children 6 to 12 years old with bipolar disorder. Similar findings were observed in children with co-occurring bipolar disorder and attention deficit with hyperactivity disorder (ADHD) (Moore et al., 2006), and in the anterior cingulate (ACC) in risperidone-medicated (Moore et al., 2007a) and unmedicated (Moore et al., 2007b) children and adolescents with bipolar disorder. In a recent study of offspring of parents

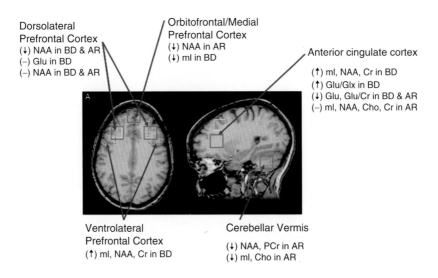

**Dorsolateral Prefrontal Cortex**
(↓) NAA in BD & AR
(–) Glu in BD
(–) NAA in BD & AR

**Orbitofrontal/Medial Prefrontal Cortex**
(↓) NAA in AR
(↓) mI in BD

**Anterior cingulate cortex**
(↑) mI, NAA, Cr in BD
(↑) Glu/Glx in BD
(↓) Glu, Glu/Cr in BD & AR
(–) mI, NAA, Cho, Cr in AR

**Ventrolateral Prefrontal Cortex**
(↑) mI, NAA, Cr in BD

**Cerebellar Vermis**
(↓) NAA, PCr in AR
(↓) mI, Cho in AR

*Figure 5.3* Selected magnetic resonance spectroscopy findings in youth with bipolar disorder (BD) or youth at risk for bipolar disorder, that is, with bipolar parents (AR), compared respectively to healthy youth, or healthy youth not at risk for bipolar disorder, that is, with healthy parents. *Abbreviations*: NAA = n-acetyl aspartate; mI = myo-inositol; Cr = creatine; Glu = glutamate; glx = glutamate/glutamine/GABA MRS peak; Cho = choline; PCr = phosphocreatine; BD = bipolar disorder; AR = at-risk. (up arrow) = increased volume; (down arrow) = decreased volume; (–) no difference.

with bipolar disorder, decreases in ACC glutamate concentrations and trends for decreases in glutamate levels relative to creatine concentrations were found, but only in a subset of youth who had developed syndromal mania (Singh et al., 2010). This latter observation suggests that for high-risk offspring, altered glutamatergic functioning may represent a marker for a more fully symptomatic clinical course of mania rather than for familial risk alone. Other studies have shown no differences in glutamatergic neurochemistry in pediatric patients with bipolar disorder compared with healthy or clinical comparison groups in prefrontal regions (Davanzo et al., 2003; Olvera et al., 2007). This discrepancy could be due to different sampling criteria, varying field strengths, non-uniform protocols for spectral acquisition and voxel placement, or variable levels of medication exposure that create variability across studies.

## BASAL GANGLIA

Increases in combined glutamate and glutamine (Glx) have also been reported in the basal ganglia of children six to 12 years old with bipolar disorder shortly after a one-week drug washout (Castillo et al., 2000). This study suggested that dysregulated excitatory neurotransmitter activity might explain why bipolar disorder is challenging to treat pharmacologically. Yet elevations in basal ganglia Glx appear to be responsive to two weeks of lithium treatment in healthy adult bipolar men (Shibuya-Tayoshi et al., 2008), suggesting that lithium might normalize this neurochemical abnormality. A study in adults with bipolar disorder has demonstrated that decreases in NAA in the basal ganglia were associated with acute mania (Frye et al., 2007), emphasizing the importance of examining this region further for potential neurochemical abnormalities in bipolar disorder.

## CEREBELLAR VERMIS

Studies on the neural aspects of emotion have discovered that, in addition to regulating motor coordination, balance, and speech, the cerebellum may play an important role in regulating emotion. The cerebellum has rich bidirectional connections to key regions in the cerebral cortex that modulate emotion. Symptomatic offspring of parents with bipolar disorder who themselves have mood disorders other than bipolar I or II disorder have demonstrated decreased concentrations of N-Acetyl aspartate (NAA) and phosphocreatine/creatine (PCr/Cr) in the cerebellar vermis (Cecil et al., 2003). Cerebellar vermis myo-inositol (mI) and choline deficits were also recently observed in youth at familial risk for bipolar disorder that had a nonbipolar mood disorder compared with healthy subjects (Singh et al., 2011). Myo-inositol reductions in this latter study may be associated with altered cellular signaling via second messenger pathways, regulation of neuronal osmolarity, and metabolism of membrane-bound phospholipids. Similarly, reductions in choline could reflect disruption in cell membrane synthesis, maintenance, and repair. As these two studies sampled youth at risk for bipolar disorder who did not meet criteria for bipolar I or II disorder, these findings suggest that metabolite alterations in the cerebellum may be occurring even prior to the development of a fully symptomatic clinical course of bipolar disorder.

## MRS CHANGES IN RESPONSE TO PHARMACOLOGICAL INTERVENTION

Both N-Acetyl aspartate (NAA) and myo-inositol (mI) demonstrated changes in concentrations in response to lithium treatment in pediatric populations (Davanzo et al., 2003; Patel et al., 2008b). Specifically, Davanzo et al. (2003) found that after 1 week of acute lithium treatment, baseline elevations of mI/creatine ratios (mI/Cr) in the anterior cingulate cortex in 11 youth with bipolar disorder decreased, and this decrement was significant for lithium responders versus non-responders. However, Patel and colleagues (2006) observed that in 12–18 year old youth with bipolar depression, lithium did not have any acute (1 week) or chronic (42 days) effects in changing myo-inositol levels in the medial and lateral prefrontal cortices. In a different study, Patel and colleagues (2008b) did find that after 42 days of lithium administration, a sample of 12- to 18-year-old youth with bipolar disorder demonstrated reductions in NAA concentration in the ventral but not lateral prefrontal cortex. In this study, there was a time-by-remission-status interaction of NAA concentrations in the right ventrolateral prefrontal cortex, such that youth who remitted developed decreased mean NAA concentration from day seven to day 42 whereas nonremitters showed an increase in mean NAA concentration during that same time period. The authors speculated that higher lithium levels earlier in the treatment course might have resulted in lithium-induced increases in prefrontal metabolism (Patel et al., 2008b). In adults, chronic lithium exposure has been shown to nonselectively increase NAA concentrations in prefrontal, temporal, parietal, and occipital regions (Moore et al., 2000), thereby perhaps increasing neuronal viability and function. Some of these findings suggest that by modulating neurometabolites involved in neuronal cell fluid balance and the second-messenger related neurometabolite myo-inositol, lithium exerts its action either by fluid shifts or through intracellular calcium signaling pathways.

The effects of neurometabolite changes in the prefrontal cortex were also examined after treatment with divalproex (Chang et al., 2009) and the atypical antipsychotic olanzapine (DelBello et al., 2006). Although there were no statistically significant differences in pre- or post- divalproex NAA to Cr (NAA/Cr) ratios, there was a large effect size (d = 0.94) for a decrease in right dorsolateral prefrontal NAA/Cr after treatment with divalproex. First hospitalized adolescents with bipolar I disorder, manic or mixed, who achieved remission with olanzapine demonstrated increases in ventral prefrontal NAA as compared to nonremitting patients, who showed decreases in prefrontal NAA concentrations. Given the potential neurogenic effects of these medications in rat brains and neural stem cells (Hashimoto et al., 2003; Laeng et al., 2004), additional studies examining *in vivo* effects of these medications in individuals with bipolar disorder are needed to clarify their role in reversing the pathophysiological effects of this disorder.

Changes in metabolite concentrations have not been replicated in other studies of offspring at high-risk for bipolar disorder (Gallelli et al., 2005; Hajek et al., 2008) or in youth with severe mood dysregulation (Dickstein et al., 2008). Diagnostic and developmental heterogeneity, mood state at the time of scan, partial volumes of gray and white matter in the regions of interest, and other demographic variables may account for differences across studies. Nevertheless, MRS studies provide an important window for understanding the molecular pathophysiology of bipolar disorder. Additional opportunities to examine underlying disease mechanisms using this technology include a more precise examination of energy metabolism using phosphorus MRS (Kato et al., 2005). It should be noted that there is debate as to whether it is more informative to measure and report metabolite ratios versus absolute concentrations. Given that different researchers report either ratios or absolute values, it is difficult to compare results from various studies. Similarly, our understanding of the relationship between specific neurometabolites and mood disorders has been complicated by incongruent findings of among MRS studies. These often contradictory findings may result from specific technological confounds such as the use of different voxel acquisitions (in different brain regions) across studies, as well as the use of different magnet strengths and software to measure and analyze metabolite levels. MRS is still an evolving technology that may require further refinement before more definitive conclusions regarding specific neurometabolite markers may be made.

**MRS Studies in Youth with or at-risk for Bipolar Disorder:**

· Suggest early N-acetyl aspartate, myo-inositol, glutamate, and choline neurometabolite changes in the prefrontal cortex, basal ganglia, and cerebellar vermis

· Suggest that these changes are state-dependent features of bipolar disorder

· Should in the future be applied in medication and symptom free populations to elucidate etiological mechanisms of bipolar illness onset

## NEURODEVELOPMENTAL MODEL OF BIPOLAR DISORDER

Based on the studies reviewed in this chapter, a neurobiological framework for the development of bipolar disorder may be postulated. Literature in adults with bipolar disorder points to a neurodegenerative model that has created an imperative for early intervention to prevent neuronal loss and to regenerate neural tissue to restore function. In youth with bipolar disorder, we have the capacity to lessen the impact of common confounds associated with chronic course of illness, including medication exposure and long-standing comorbidities such as substance dependence, and we can better examine etiological factors associated with the onset and progression of bipolar disorder. Based upon studies of youth with bipolar disorder, it appears that the prefrontal cortex, amygdala, and hippocampus are potentially vulnerable to volume loss, perhaps due to neurotoxic effects of mood dysregulation (e.g., excessive glutamate levels). Yet, other structures such as those within the striatum, may show increased volumes possibly associated with abnormal synaptic pruning or neuronal proliferation. Similarly, we see mixed results of over- and under-activation in fMRI studies in key prefrontal and subcortical regions that may have aberrant white matter connections as demonstrated by DTI. The structural and functional relationships among these regions require further examination by functional connectivity methods, so that activation patterns and the relations between structure and function may be clarified. Moreover, such studies would advance our understanding of the downstream effects of structural and functional deficits on other areas of brain function as bipolar illness progresses.

An illustration of postulated relationships among prefrontal and subcortical structures as bipolar disorder progresses over time is summarized in Figure 5.4. With poor coping skills/environmental stress and inborn genetic vulnerabilities, children may develop mood dysregulation and

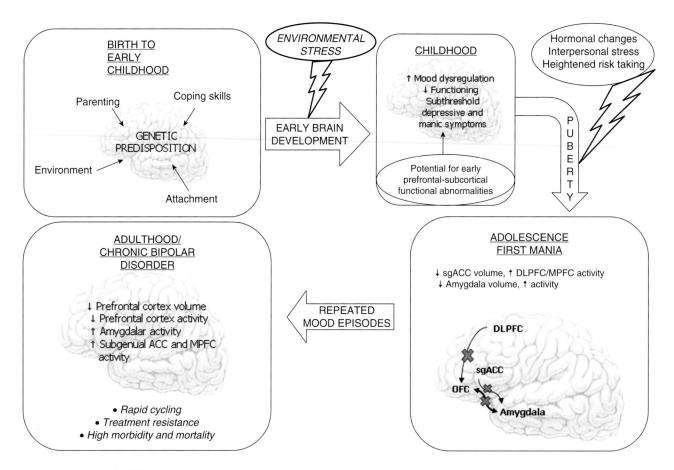

*Figure 5.4* Putative model of BD development. Environmental stress interacting genetic risk during the course of development leads to childhood mood dysregulation and psychosocial dysfunction. Pathological reactions to stress interrupt healthy development of brain networks required to regulate mood. These might include disrupted relationships between dorsal regulatory areas including dorsolateral prefrontal cortex (DLPFC), and ventral areas including the ventrolateral prefrontal cortex (VLPFC), amygdala, orbitofrontal cortex (OFC) and subgenual anterior cingulate cortex (sgACC). Without intervention, children eventually develop mania displaying further functional connectivity (FC) abnormalities among nodes in mood regulation networks. With repeated mood episodes into adulthood, rapid cycling and more severe episodes develop.

begin to exhibit dysfunction in cognitive, emotional, and psychosocial domains. Pathological reactions to stress can be detected acutely by clinical symptoms, and over time, by examining brain structural and functional changes, which interrupt healthy development of networks of brain structures that are important for mood regulation. Disrupted relationships among dorsal regulatory areas, including the dorsolateral prefrontal cortex (DLPFC) and dorsal anterior cingulate cortex (dACC), and ventral areas, including the amygdala and subgenual anterior cingulate cortex (sgACC) may lead to mood dysregulation or cognitive impairments. Without adequate intervention, children then eventually develop a full manic episode displaying further functional connectivity (FC) abnormalities between nodes in mood regulation networks; for example, inverse functional connectivity between amygdala and DLPFC is lost or task dependent excessive medial prefrontal (MPFC) activation is observed. With repeated mood episodes into

adulthood, further neurodegeneration of prefrontal areas might occur, leading to rapid cycling, treatment resistance, and more severe episodes causing increasing morbidity and mortality.

Studies in youth at risk for bipolar disorder indicate that most structural and neurochemical changes do not occur prior to the onset of syndromal mania, suggesting the possibility of preventing disease onset and progression if an underlying mechanism can be identified. Furthermore, a relative lack of morphometric abnormalities in symptomatic youth at high-risk for bipolar disorder points to the probability that structural effects are a consequence of illness. Studies in healthy offspring of parents with bipolar disorder suggest clues for resilience factors that may be important in preventing the onset of illness, including enlargement of prefrontal and parahippocampal structures. Therefore, MRI studies in youth with and at risk for bipolar disorder are identifying brain findings that may be amenable to early intervention to prevent or ameliorate the natural course of bipolar disorder. Larger studies are needed to test these suggestions.

## SUMMARY

Convergence in structural, functional, and neurochemical abnormalities early in bipolar illness course support the hypothesis that dysfunction in specific prefrontal and subcortical brain regions underlies the pathophysiology of bipolar disorder. Available studies to date, however, have been limited by confounding illness-related variables that make it difficult to elucidate the role of neurodevelopment in the pathogenesis of bipolar disorder (Brambilla et al., 2005; Chang et al., 2006). Other technologies such as magnetoencephalography (MEG), which provides worse spatial but better temporal resolution than fMRI, are being utilized in pediatric bipolar disorder (Rich et al., 2010) to better understand brain network function. Moreover, neuroimaging findings such as amygdala activation abnormalities in youth with bipolar disorder are being associated with specific genotypes (Liu et al., 2010). Advances in genetic and imaging technology may enable us to understand the role of genetics in creating brain abnormalities that then create risk for bipolar disorder development.

Other MRI techniques, such as cortical thickness measurements or advanced brain mapping approaches, have not yet been applied to youth with bipolar disorder. Additional functional and resting state connectivity studies are important to evaluate networks involved in clinical aspects of bipolar disorder, such as executive function, self-monitoring, and mood regulation. In addition, paradigms that highlight core symptoms of mania, such as increased goal directed behavior and disrupted motivation, could expand how we conceptualize youth with bipolar disorder. FMRI studies in healthy and subsyndromal youth at risk for bipolar disorder would aid in determining functional endophenotypes, and MRS studies using phosphorous and multivoxel approaches in regions other than the prefrontal cortex would elaborate on molecular mechanisms associated with bipolar disorder. Finally, it is crucial that we find systematic ways of integrating neuroimaging data across multiple modalities with the use of multivariate statistical approaches and conduct meaningful longitudinal neuroimaging studies in at-risk and fully bipolar populations.

Despite progress in understanding the neurobiological basis of bipolar disorder, future longitudinal controlled studies are needed to examine the effects of specific mood states on neuroimaging findings, to identify neurobiomark-

ers in order to establish rational treatment strategies in youth with and at-risk for developing bipolar disorder, and to determine the neurodevelopmental and genetic mechanisms that contribute to illness onset. With additional investigations the complex etiopathophysiology of bipolar disorder may be clarified so that young patients diagnosed with bipolar disorder may be more accurately diagnosed and effectively treated.

## REFERENCES

Adler, C. M., DelBello, M. P., Mills, N. P., Schmithorst, V., Holland, S., & Strakowski SM. 2005. Comorbid ADHD is associated with altered patterns of neuronal activation in adolescents with bipolar disorder performing a simple attention task. *Bipolar Disorders*, 7(6): 577–588.

Adler, C. M., DelBello, M. P., & Strakowski, S. M 2006. Brain dysfunction in bipolar disorder. *CNS Spectrums*, 11(4): 312–320.

Adler, C. M., Adams, J., DelBello, M. P., Holland, S. K., Schmithorst, V., Levine, A., . . . Strakowski, S. M. 2006. Evidence of white matter pathology in bipolar disorder adolescents experiencing their first episode of mania: a diffusion tensor imaging study. *American Journal of Psychiatry*, 163(2): 322–324.

Ahn, M.S., Breeze, J.L., Makris, N., Kennedy, D.N., Hodge, S.M., Herbert, M.R., . . . Frazier, J.A. 2007. Anatomic brain magnetic resonance imaging of the basal ganglia in pediatric bipolar disorder. *Journal of Affective Disorders*, 104(1-3): 147–54.

Axelson, D., Birmaher, B., Strober, M., Gill, M.K., Valeri, S., Chiappetta, L., . . . Keller, M. 2006. Phenomenology of children and adolescents with bipolar spectrum disorders. *Archives of General Psychiatry*, 63(10): 1139–1148.

Baloch, H. A., Hatch, J. P., Olvera, R. L., Nicoletti, M., Caetano, S. C., Zunta-Soares, G. B., & Soares, J. C. 2010. Morphology of the subgenual prefrontal cortex in pediatric bipolar disorder. *Journal of Psychiatric Research*, 44(15): 1106–1110.

Barnea-Goraly, N., Chang, K. D., Karchemskiy, A., Howe, M. E., & Reiss, AL. 2009. Limbic and corpus callosum aberrations in adolescents with bipolar disorder: a tract-based spatial statistics analysis. *Biological Psychiatry*, 66(3): 238–244.

Bearden, C. E., Soares, J. C., Klunder, A. D., Nicoletti, M., Dierschke, N., Hayashi, K. M., . . . Thompson, P. M. 2008. Three-dimensional mapping of hippocampal anatomy in adolescents with bipolar disorder. *Journal of American Academy of Child and Adolescent Psychiatry*, 47(5): 515–525.

Beesdom K., Höfler, M., Leibenluft, E., Lieb, R., Bauer, M., & Pfennig, A. 2009. Mood episodes and mood disorders: patterns of incidence and conversion in the first three decades of life. *Bipolar Disorders* 11(6): 637–649.

Beyer, J. L., Young, R., Kuchibhatla, M., & Krishnan, K. R. 2009. Hyperintense MRI lesions in bipolar disorder: A meta-analysis and review. *International Review of Psychiatry*, 21(4): 394–409.

Bitter, S.M., Mills, N.P., Adler, C.M., Strakowski, S.M., & DelBello, M.P. 2011. Progression of amygdala volumetric abnormalities in adolescents after their first manic episode. *Journal of the American Academy of Child and Adolescent Psychiatry*, 50(10): 1017–26.

Blumberg, H. P., Martin, A., Kaufman, J., Leung, H. C., Skudlarski, P., Lacadie, C., . . . Peterson, B. S 2003a. Frontostriatal abnormalities in adolescents with bipolar disorder: preliminary observations from functional MRI. *American Journal of Psychiatry*, 160(7): 1345–1347.

Blumberg, H. P., Kaufman, J., Martin, A., Whiteman, R., Zhang, J. H., Gore, J. C., . . . Peterson, B. S. 2003b. Amygdala and hippocampal volumes in adolescents and adults with bipolar disorder. *Archives of General Psychiatry*, 60(12): 1201–1208.

Blumberg, H.P., Fredericks, C., Wang, F., Kalmar, J.H., Spencer, L., Papademetris, X., . . . Krystal, J.H. 2005. Preliminary evidence for persistent abnormalities in amygdala volumes in adolescents and young adults with bipolar disorder. *Bipolar Disorders*, 7(6): 570–576.

Blumberg, H. P., Krystal, J. H., Bansal, R., Martin, A., Dziura, J., Durkin, K., . . . Peterson, B. S. 2006. Age, rapid-cycling, and pharmacotherapy effects on ventral prefrontal cortex in bipolar disorder: a cross-sectional study. *Biological Psychiatry*, 59(7): 611–618.

Botteronm K. N., Figiel, G. S., Wetzel, M. W., Hudziak, J., & VanEerdewegh, M. 1992. MRI abnormalities in adolescent bipolar affective disorder. *Journal of American Academy of Child and Adolescent Psychiatry*, 31(2):258–261.

Brambilla, P. 2005. Magnetic resonance findings in bipolar disorder. *Psychiatric Clinics of North America*, 28(2): 443–467.

Brooks, J. C., Roberts, N., Kemp, G. J., Gosney, M. A., Lye, M., & Whitehouse, G. H. 2001. A proton magnetic resonance spectroscopy study of age-related changes in frontal lobe metabolite concentrations. *Cerebral Cortex*, 11(7): 598–605.

Castellanos, F. X., Sharp, W. S., Gottesman, R. F., Greenstein, D. K., Giedd, J. N., & Rapoport, J. L. 2003. Anatomic brain abnormalities in monozygotic twins discordant for attention deficit hyperactivity disorder. *American Journal of Psychiatry*, 60(9): 1693–1696.

Caetano, S. C., Olvera, R. L., Glahn, D., Fonseca, M., Pliszka, S., & Soares, J. C 2005. Fronto-limbic brain abnormalities in juvenile onset bipolar disorder. *Biological Psychiatry*, 58(7): 525–531.

Caetano, S. C., Silveira, C. M., Kaur, S., Nicoletti, M., Hatch, J. P., Brambilla, P., . . . Soares, J. C. 2008. Abnormal corpus callosum myelination in pediatric bipolar patients. *Journal of Affective Disorders*, 108(3): 297–301.

Caetano, S. C., Olvera, R. L., Hatch, J. P., Sanches, M., Chen, H. H., Nicoletti, M., . . . Soares, J. C. 2011. Lower N-acetyl-aspartate levels in prefrontal cortices in pediatric bipolar disorder: a $^1$H magnetic resonance spectroscopy study. *Journal of American Academy of Child and Adolescent Psychiatry*, 50(1): 85–94.

Casey, B. J., Getz., S., & Galvan, A. 2008. The adolescent brain. *Developmental Review*, 28(1): 62–77.

Castillo, M., Kwock, L., Courvoisie, H., & Hooper, S. R. 2000. Proton MR spectroscopy in children with bipolar affective disorder: preliminary observations. *AJNR American Journal of Neuroradiology*, 21(5): 832–838.

Cecil, K. M., DelBello, M. P., Morey, R., & Strakowski, S. M 2002. Frontal lobe differences in bipolar disorder as determined by proton MR spectroscopy. *Bipolar Disorders*, 4(6): 357–365.

Cecil, K. M., DelBello, M. P., Sellars, M. C., & Strakowski, S. M 2003. Proton magnetic resonance spectroscopy of the frontal lobe and cerebellar vermis in children with a mood disorder and a familial risk for bipolar disorders. *Journal of Child and Adolescent Psychopharmacology*, 13(4): 545–555.

Cerullo, M. A., Adler, C. M., Lamy, M., Eliassen, J. C., Fleck, D. E., Strakowski, S. M., & DelBello, M. P. 2009. Differential brain activation during response inhibition in bipolar and attention-deficit hyperactivity disorders. *Early Intervention in Psychiatry*. 3(3): 189–197.

Chang, K. D., Steiner, H., & Ketter, T. A. 2000. Psychiatric phenomenology of child and adolescent bipolar offspring. *Journal of American Academy of Child and Adolescent Psychiatry*, 39(4): 453–460.

Chang, K., Adleman, N., Dienes, K., Barnea-Goraly, N., Reiss, A., Ketter, T. 2003. Decreased N-acetylaspartate in children with familial bipolar disorder. *Biological Psychiatry*, 53(11): 1059–1065.

Chang, K., Adleman, N. E., Dienes, K., Simeonova, D. I., Menon, V., & Reiss, A 2004. Anomalous prefrontal-subcortical activation in familial pediatric bipolar disorder: a functional magnetic resonance imaging investigation. *Archives of General Psychiatry*, 61(8): 781–792.

Chang, K., Karchemskiy, A., Barnea-Goraly, N., Garrett, A., Simeonova, D.I. & Reiss, A. 2005a. Reduced amygdalar grey matter volume in familial pediatric bipolar disorder. *Journal of American Academy of Child and Adolescent Psychiatry*, 44(6): 565–573.

Chang, K., Barnea-Goraly, N., Karchemskiy, A., Simeonova, D. I., Barnes, P., Ketter, T., Reiss, A. L. 2005b. Cortical magnetic resonance imaging findings in familial pediatric bipolar disorder. *Biological Psychiatry*, 58(3): 197–203.

Chang, K., Adleman, N., Wagner, C., Barnea-Goraly, N., & Garrett, A. 2006. Will neuroimaging ever be used to diagnose pediatric bipolar disorder? *Developmental Psychopathology*, 18(4): 1133–46.

Chang, K. D., Wagner, C., Garrett, A., Howe, M., & Reiss, A. 2008. A preliminary functional magnetic resonance imaging study of prefrontal-amygdalar activation changes in adolescents with bipolar depression treated with lamotrigine. *Bipolar Disorders*, 10(3): 426–431.

Chang, K., Karchemskiy, A., Kelley, R., Howe, M., Garrett, A., Adleman, N., & Reiss, A. 2009. Effect of divalproex on brain morphometry, chemistry, and function in youth at high-risk for bipolar disorder: a pilot study. *Journal of Child and Adolescent Psychopharmacology*, 19(1): 51–59.

Chen, H. H., Nicoletti, M. A., Hatch, J. P., Sassi, R. B., Axelson, D., Brambilla, P., . . . Soares, J. C 2004a. Abnormal left superior temporal gyrus volumes in children and adolescents with bipolar disorder: a magnetic resonance imaging study. *Neuroscience Letters*, 363(1): 65–68.

Chen, H. H., Nicoletti, M., Sanches, M., Hatch, J. P., Sassi, R. B., Axelson, D., . . . Soares, J. C. 2004b. Normal pituitary volumes in children and adolescents with bipolar disorder: a magnetic resonance imaging study. *Depression and Anxiety*, 20(4): 182–186.

Chen, B. K., Sassi, R., Axelson, D., Hatch, J. P., Sanches, M., Nicoletti, M., . . . Soares, J. C. 2004c. Cross-sectional study of abnormal amygdala development in adolescents and young adults with bipolar disorder. *Biological Psychiatry*, 56(6): 399–405.

Chiu, S., Widjaja, F., Bates, M. E., Voelbel, G. T., Pandina, G., Marble, J., . . . Hendren, R. L. 2008. Anterior cingulate volume in pediatric bipolar disorder and autism. *Journal of Affective Disorders*, 105(1-3): 93–99.

Correll, C. U., Penzner, J. B., Lencz, T., Auther, A., Smith, C. W., Malhotra, A. K., . . . Cornblatt, B. A. 2007. Early identification and high-risk strategies for bipolar disorder. *Bipolar Disorders*, 9(4): 324–338.

Davanzo, P., Thomas, M. A., Yue, K., Oshiro, T., Belin, T., Strober, M., & McCracken, J 2001. Decreased anterior cingulate myoinositol/creatine spectroscopy resonance with lithium treatment in children with bipolar disorder. *Neuropsychopharmacology*, 24(4): 359–369.

Davanzo, P., Yue, K., Thomas, M. A., Belin, T., Mintz, J., Venkatraman, T. N., . . . McCracken, J. 2003. Proton magnetic resonance spectroscopy of bipolar disorder versus intermittent explosive disorder in children and adolescents. *American Journal of Psychiatry*, 160(8): 1442–1452.

DelBello, M. P., Zimmerman, M. E., Mills, N. P., Getz, G. E., & Strakowski, S. M 2004. Magnetic resonance imaging analysis of amygdala and other subcortical brain regions in adolescents with bipolar disorder. *Bipolar Disorders*, 6(1): 143–152.

DelBello, M. P., Adler, C. M., & Strakowski, S. M 2006. The neurophysiology of childhood and adolescent bipolar disorder: A review of neuroimaging studies. *CNS Spectrums*, 11(4): 298–311.

DelBello, M. P., Cecil, K. M., Adler, C. M., Daniels, J. P., Strakowski, S. M. 2006. Neurochemical effects of olanzapine in first-hospitalization manic adolescents: a proton magnetic resonance spectroscopy study. *Neuropsychopharmacology*, 31(6): 1264–1273.

DelBello, M. P., Hanseman, D., Adler, C. M., Fleck, D. E., & Strakowski, S. M 2007. Twelve-month outcome of adolescents with bipolar disorder following first hospitalization for a manic or mixed episode. *American Journal of Psychiatry*, 164(4): 582–590.

Dickstein, D. P., Milham, M. P., Nugent, A. C., Drevets, W. C., Charney, D. S., Pine, D. S., & Leibenluft, E. 2005. Frontotemporal alterations in pediatric bipolar disorder: results of a voxel-based morphometry study. *Arch Gen Psychiatry*, 62(7): 734–741.

Dickstein, D. P., & Leibenluft, E 2006. Emotion regulation in children and adolescents: boundaries between normalcy and bipolar disorder. *Developmental Psychopathology*, 18(4): 1147–1168.

Dickstein, D. P., Rich, B. A., Roberson-Nay, R., Berghorst, L., Vinton, D., Pine, D. S., & Leibenluft, E. 2007. Neural activation during encoding of emotional faces in pediatric bipolar disorder. *Bipolar Disorders*, 9(7): 679–692.

Dickstein, D. P., van der Veen, J. W., Knopf, L., Towbin, K. E., Pine, D. S., & Leibenluft E. 2008. Proton magnetic resonance spectroscopy in youth with severe mood dysregulation. *Psychiatry Research*, 163(1): 30–39.

Dickstein, D. P., Gorrostieta, C., Ombao, H., Goldberg, L. D., Brazel, A. C., Gable, C. J., . . . Milham, M. P. 2010. Fronto-temporal spontaneous resting state functional connectivity in pediatric bipolar disorder. *Biological Psychiatry*, 68(9): 839–846.

Dickstein, D. P., Finger, E. C., Skup, M., Pine, D. S., Blair, J. R., & Leibenluft, E. 2010. Altered neural function in pediatric bipolar disorder during reversal learning. *Bipolar Disorders*, 12(7): 707–719.

Fair, D. A., Cohen, A. L., Dosenbach, N. U., Church, J. A., Miezin, F. M., Barch, D. M., . . . Schlaggar, B. L. 2008. The maturing architecture of the brain's default network. *Proceedings of the National Academy of Sciences of the United States of America*, 105(10): 4028–4032.

Foland, L. C., Altshuler, L. L., Bookheimer, S. Y., Eisenberger, N., Townsend, J., & Thompson, P. M. 2008. Evidence for deficient modulation of amygdala response by prefrontal cortex in bipolar mania. *Psychiatry Research*, 162(1): 27–37.

Frazier, J. A., Breeze, J. L., Makris, N., Giuliano, A. S., Herbert, M. R., Seidman, L., . . . Caviness, VS. 2005. Cortical gray matter differences identified by structural magnetic resonance imaging in pediatric bipolar disorder. *Bipolar Disorders*, 7(6): 555–569.

Frazier, J. A., Chiu, S., Breeze, J. L., Makris, N., Lange, N., Kennedy, D.N., . . . Biederman, J. 2005b. Structural brain magnetic resonance imaging of limbic and thalamic volumes in pediatric bipolar disorder. *American Journal of Psychiatry*, 162(7): 1256–1265.

Frazier, J. A., Breeze, J. L., Papadimitriou, G., Kennedy, D. N., Hodge, S. M., Moore, C. M., . . . Makris, N. 2007. White matter abnormalities in children with and at risk for bipolar disorder. *Bipolar Disorders*, 9(8): 799–809.

Frye, M. A., Thomas, M. A., Yue, K., Binesh, N., Davanzo, P., Ventura, J., . . . Mintz, J. 2007. Reduced concentrations of N-acetylaspartate (NAA) and the NAA-creatine ratio in the basal ganglia in bipolar disorder: a study using 3-Tesla proton magnetic resonance spectroscopy. *Psychiatry Research*, 154(3): 259–265.

Gallelli, K. A., Wagner, C. M., Karchemskiy, A., Howe, M., Spielman, D., Reiss, A., & Chang, K. D. 2005. N-acetylaspartate levels in bipolar offspring with and at high-risk for bipolar disorder. *Bipolar Disorders*, 7(6): 589–597.

Geller, B., Harms, M. P., Wang, L., Tillman, R., DelBello, M. P., Bolhofner, K., & Csernansky, J.G. 2009. Effects of age, sex, and independent life events on amygdala and nucleus accumbens volumes in child bipolar I disorder. *Biological Psychiatry*, 65(5): 432–437.

Gogtay, N., Ordonez, A., Herman, D. H., Hayashi, K. M., Greenstein, D., Vaituzis, C., . . . Rapoport J. L. 2007. Dynamic mapping of cortical development before and after the onset of pediatric bipolar illness. *Journal of Child Psychology and Psychiatry*, 48(9): 852–862.

Goldstein, T. R., Birmaher, B., Axelson, D., Ryan, N. D., Strober, M. A., Gill, M. K., . . . Keller, M. 2005. History of suicide attempts in pediatric bipolar disorder: factors associated with increased risk. *Bipolar Disorders*, 7(6): 525–535.

Gönenç, A., Frazier, J. A., Crowley, D. J., & Moore, C. M. 2010. Combined diffusion tensor imaging and transverse relaxometry in early-onset bipolar disorder. *Journal of American Academy of Child and Adolescent Psychiatry*, 49(12): 1260–1268.

Hajek, T., Carrey, N., & Alda, M. 2005. Neuroanatomical abnormalities as risk factors for bipolar disorder. *Bipolar Disorders*, 7(5): 393–403.

Hajek, T., Kopecek, M., Kozeny, J., Gunde, E., Alda, M., & Höschl, C. 2009. Amygdala volumes in mood disorders–meta-analysis of magnetic resonance volumetry studies. *Journal of Affective Disorders*, 115(3): 395–410.

Hajek, T., Bernier, D., Slaney, C., Propper, L., Schmidt, M., Carrey, N., . . . Alda, M. 2008. A comparison of affected and unaffected relatives of patients with bipolar disorder using proton magnetic resonance spectroscopy. *Journal of Psychiatry and Neuroscience*, 33(6): 531–540.

Hashimoto, R., Senatorov, V., Kanai, H., Leeds, P., & Chuang DM: 2003. Lithium stimulates progenitor proliferation in cultured brain neurons. *Neuroscience*, 117(1): 55–61.

Kafantaris, V., Kingsley, P., Ardekani, B., Saito, E., Lencz, T., Lim, K., & Szeszko, P. 2009. Lower orbital frontal white matter integrity in adolescents with bipolar I disorder. *Journal of American Academy of Child and Adolescent Psychiatry*, 48(1): 79–86.

Kalmar, J. H., Wang, F., Chepenik, L. G., Womer, F. Y., Jones, M. M., Pittman, B., . . . Blumberg, H. P. 2009. Relation between amygdala structure and function in adolescents with bipolar disorder. *Journal of American Academy of Child and Adolescent Psychiatry*, 48(6): 636–642.

Karchemskiy, A., Garrett, A., Howe, M. E., Adleman, N., Simeonova, D. I., Alegria, D., . . . Chang, K. D. 2011. Amygdalar, hippocampal, and thalamic volumes in youth at high risk for development of bipolar disorder, *Psychiatry Research*, 194(3): 319-25.

Kato, T. 2005. Mitochondrial dysfunction in bipolar disorder: from 31P-magnetic resonance spectroscopic findings to their molecular mechanisms. *International Review of Neurobiology*, 63: 21–40.

Kaur, S., Sassi, R. B., Axelson, D., Nicoletti, M., Brambilla, P., Monkul, E. S., . . . Soares, J. C. 2005. Cingulate cortex anatomical abnormalities in children and adolescents with bipolar disorder. *American Journal of Psychiatry*, 162(9): 1637–1643.

Kim, H. W., Rapoport, S. I., & Rao, J. S. 2010. Altered expression of apoptotic factors and synaptic markers in postmortem brain from bipolar disorder patients. *Neurobiology of Disease*, 37(3): 596–603.

Ladouceur, C. D., Almeida, J. R., Birmaher, B., Axelson, D. A., Nau, S., Kalas, C., . . . Phillips, M. L. 2008. Subcortical gray matter volume abnormalities in healthy bipolar offspring: potential neuroanatomical risk marker for bipolar disorder? *Journal of American Academy of Child and Adolescent Psychiatry*, 47(5): 532–539.

Laeng, P., Pitts, R. L., Lemire, A. L., Drabik, C. E., Weiner, A., Tang, H., . . . Altar, C. A. 2004. The mood stabilizer valproic acid stimulates GABA neurogenesis from rat forebrain stem cells. *Journal of Neurochemistry*, 91(1): 238–251.

Leibenluft, E., Cohen, P., Gorrindo, T., Brook, J.S., & Pine, D. S. 2006. Chronic versus episodic irritability in youth: a community-based, longitudinal study of clinical and diagnostic associations. *Journal of Child and Adolescent Psychopharmacology*, 16(4): 456–466.

Leibenluft, E., Rich, B. A., Vinton, D. T., Nelson, E. E., Fromm, S. J., Berghorst, L. H., . . . Pine, D. S. 2007. Neural circuitry engaged during unsuccessful motor inhibition in pediatric bipolar disorder. *American Journal of Psychiatry*, 164(1): 52–60.

Leverich, G. S., Post, R. M., Keck, P. E. Jr., Altshuler, L.L., Frye, M.A., Kupka, R.W., . . . Luckenbaugh, D. 2007. The poor prognosis of childhood-onset bipolar disorder. *Journal of Pediatrics*, 150: 485–490.

Liu, I.Y., Howe, M., Garrett, A., Karchemskiy, A., Kelley, R., Alegria, D., . . . Chang, K. 2011. Striatal Volumes in Pediatric Bipolar Patients with and without Comorbid ADHD. *Psychiatry Research*, 194(1): 14–20.

Liu, X., Akula, N., Skup, M., Brotman, M. A., Leibenluft, E., & McMahon, F. J. 2010. A genome-wide association study of amygdala activation in youths with and without bipolar disorder. *Journal of American Academy of Child and Adolescent Psychiatry*, 49(1): 33–41.

Lopez-Larson, M., Michael, E. S., Terry, J. E., Breeze, J. L., Hodge, S. M., Tang, L., . . . Frazier, J. A. 2009. Subcortical differences among youths with attention-deficit/hyperactivity disorder compared to those with bipolar disorder with and without attention-deficit/hyperactivity disorder. *Journal of Child and Adolescent Psychopharmacology*, 19(1): 31–39.

Lyoo, I. K., Lee, H. K., Jung, J. H., Noam, G. G., & Renshaw, P. F. 2002. White matter hyperintensities on magnetic resonance imaging of the brain in children with psychiatric disorders. *Comprehensive Psychiatry*, 43(5): 361–368.

Malhi, G. S., Lagopoulos, J., Owen, A. M., Ivanovski, B., Shnier, R., & Sachdev, P. 2007. Reduced activation to implicit affect induction in euthymic bipolar patients: an fMRI study. *Journal of Affective Disorders*, 97(1–3): 109–122.

Martinowich, K., Schloesser, R. J., & Manji, H. K. 2009. Bipolar disorder: from genes to behavior pathways. *The Journal of Clinical Investigation*, 119(4): 726–736.

Mayberg, H. S., Liotti, M., Brannan, S. K., McGinnis, S., Mahurin, R.K., Jerabek, P.A.,...Fox, P.T. 1999. Reciprocal limbic-cortical function and negative mood: converging PET findings in depression and normal sadness. *American Journal of Psychiatry*, 156(5): 675–682.

Miklowitz, D. J., & Chang, K. D. 2008. Prevention of bipolar disorder in at-risk children: theoretical assumptions and empirical foundations. *Developmental Psychopathology*, 20(3): 881–897.

Mitsunaga, M. M., Garrett, A., Howe, M. E., Karchemskiy, A., Reiss, A. L., & Chang, K. 2011. Increased subgenual cortex volume in pediatric bipolar disorder associated with mood stabilizer exposure, *Journal of Child and Adolescent Psychopharmacology*, 21(2): 149–55.

Monkul, E. S., Malhi, G. S., & Soares, J. C. 2005. Anatomical MRI abnormalities in bipolar disorder: do they exist and do they progress? *Australian and New Zealand Journal of Psychiatry*, 39(4): 222–226.

Monkul, E. S., Nicoletti, M. A., Spence, D., Sassi, R. B., Axelson, D., Brambilla, P.,...Soares JC. 2006. MRI study of thalamus volumes in juvenile patients with bipolar disorder. *Depression and Anxiety*, 23(6): 347–352.

Monkul, E. S., Hatch, J. P., Sassi, R. B., Axelson, D., Brambilla, P., Nicoletti, M. A.,...Soares, J. C. 2008. MRI study of the cerebellum in young bipolar patients. *Prog Neuropsychopharmacol Biological Psychiatry*, 32(3): 613–619.

Moore, G. J., Bebchuk, J. M., Hasanat, K., Chen, G., Seraji-Bozorgzad, N., Wilds, I. B.,...Manji, H. K. 2000. Lithium increases N-acetyl-aspartate in the human brain: in vivo evidence in support of bcl-2's neurotrophic effects? *Biological Psychiatry*, 48(1): 1–8.

Moore, C. M., Biederman, J., Wozniak, J., Mick, E., Aleardi, M., Wardrop, M.,...Renshaw, P.F. 2006. Differences in brain chemistry in children and adolescents with attention deficit hyperactivity disorder with and without comorbid bipolar disorder: a proton magnetic resonance spectroscopy study. *American Journal of Psychiatry*, 163(2): 316–318.

Moore, C. M., Biederman, J., Wozniak, J., Mick, E., Aleardi, M., Wardrop, M.,...Renshaw, P. F. 2007a. Mania, glutamate/glutamine and risperidone in pediatric bipolar disorder: a proton magnetic resonance spectroscopy study of the anterior cingulate cortex. *Journal of Affective Disorders*, 99(1–3): 19–25.

Moore, C. M., Frazier, J. A., Glod, C. A., Breeze, J. L., Dieterich, M., Finn, C. T.,...Renshaw, P. F. 2007b. Glutamine and glutamate levels in children and adolescents with bipolar disorder: a 4.0-T proton magnetic resonance spectroscopy study of the anterior cingulate cortex. *Journal of American Academy of Child and Adolescent Psychiatry*, (4): 524–534.

Moore, G. J., Cortese, B. M., Glitz, D. A., Zajac-Benitez, C., Quiroz, J. A., Uhde, T. W.,...Manji, H. K. 2009. A longitudinal study of the effects of lithium treatment on prefrontal and subgenual prefrontal gray matter volume in treatment-responsive bipolar disorder patients. *Journal of Clinical Psychiatry*, 70(5): 699–705.

Najt, P., Nicoletti, M., Chen, H. H., Hatch, J. P., Caetano, S. C., Sassi, R. B.,...Soares, J. C. 2007. Anatomical measurements of the orbitofrontal cortex in child and adolescent patients with bipolar disorder. *Neuroscience Letters*, 413(3): 183–186.

Nelson, E. E., Vinton, D. T., Berghorst, L., Towbin, K. E., Hommer, R. E., Dickstein, D. P.,...Leibenluft, E. 2007. Brain systems underlying response flexibility in healthy and bipolar adolescents: an event-related fMRI study. *Bipolar Disorders*, 9(8): 810–819.

Nestler, E. J., & Hyman, S. E. 2010. Animal models of neuropsychiatric disorders. *Nature Neuroscience*, 13(10): 1161–1169.

Olvera, R. L., Caetano, S. C., Fonseca, M., Nicoletti, M., Stanley, J. A., Chen, H. H.,...Soares, J. C. 2007. Low levels of N-acetyl aspartate in the left dorsolateral prefrontal cortex of pediatric bipolar patients. *Journal of Child and Adolescent Psychopharmacology*, 17(4): 461–473.

Passarotti, A. M., Sweeney, J. A., & Pavuluri, M. N. 2010a. Differential engagement of cognitive and affective neural systems in pediatric bipolar disorder and attention deficit hyperactivity disorder. *Journal of the International Neuropsychological Society*, 16(1): 106–117.

Passarotti, A. M., Sweeney, J. A., & Pavuluri, M. N. 2010b. Emotion processing influences working memory circuits in pediatric bipolar disorder and attention-deficit/hyperactivity disorder. *Journal of American Academy of Child and Adolescent Psychiatry*, 49(10): 1064–1080.

Passarotti, A. M., Sweeney, J. A., & Pavuluri, M. N. 2010c. Neural correlates of response inhibition in pediatric bipolar disorder and attention deficit hyperactivity disorder. *Psychiatry Research*, 181(1): 36–43.

Passarotti, A. M., Sweeney, J. A., & Pavuluri, M. N. 2011. Fronto-limbic dysfunction in mania pre-treatment and persistent amygdala over-activity post-treatment in pediatric bipolar disorder. *Psychopharmacology*, 216(4): 485–99.

Patel, N. C., DelBello, M. P., Cecil, K. M., Adler, C. M., Bryan, H. S., Stanford, K. E., & Strakowski, S. M. 2006. Lithium treatment effects on Myo-inositol in adolescents with bipolar depression. *Biological Psychiatry*, 60(9): 998–1004.

Patel, N. C., Cecil, K. M., Strakowski, S. M., Adler, C. M., & DelBello, M. P. 2008a. Neurochemical alterations in adolescent bipolar depression: a proton magnetic resonance spectroscopy pilot study of the prefrontal cortex. *Journal of Child and Adolescent Psychopharmacology*, 18(6): 623–627.

Patel, N. C., DelBello, M. P., Cecil, K. M., Stanford, K. E., Adler, C. M., & Strakowski, S. M. 2008b. Temporal change in N-acetyl-aspartate concentrations in adolescents with bipolar depression treated with lithium. *Journal of Child and Adolescent Psychopharmacology*, 18(2): 132–139.

Pavuluri, M. N., O'Connor, M. M., Harral, E. M., Moss, M., Sweeney, J.A. 2006. Impact of neurocognitive function on academic difficulties in pediatric bipolar disorder: a clinical translation. *Biological Psychiatry* 60(9): 951–956.

Pavuluri, M. N., O'Connor, M. M., Harral, E., & Sweeney, J. A. 2007. Affective neural circuitry during facial emotion processing in pediatric bipolar disorder. *Biological Psychiatry*, 62(2): 158–167.

Pavuluri, M. N., O'Connor, M. M., Harral, E. M., & Sweeney, J. A. 2008. An fMRI study of the interface between affective and cognitive neural circuitry in pediatric bipolar disorder. *Psychiatry Research*, 162(3): 244–255.

Pavuluri, M. N., Yang, S., Kamineni, K., Passarotti, A. M., Srinivasan, G., Harral, E. M.,...Zhou, X. J. 2009. Diffusion tensor imaging study of white matter fiber tracts in pediatric bipolar disorder and attention-deficit/hyperactivity disorder. *Biological Psychiatry*, 65(7): 586–593.

Pavuluri, M. N., Passarotti, A. M., Harral, E. M., & Sweeney, J. A. 2009. An fMRI study of the neural correlates of incidental versus directed emotion processing in pediatric bipolar disorder. *Journal of American Academy of Child and Adolescent Psychiatry*, 48(3): 308–319.

Pavuluri, M. N., Passarotti, A. M., Parnes, S. A., Fitzgerald, J. M., & Sweeney, J. A. 2010. A pharmacological functional magnetic resonance imaging study probing the interface of cognitive and emotional brain systems in pediatric bipolar disorder. *Journal of Child and Adolescent Psychopharmacology*, 20(5): 395–406.

Perlis, R. H., Dennehy, E. B., Miklowitz, D. J., DelBello, M. P., Ostacher, M., Calabrese, J. R., . . . Sachs, G 2009. Retrospective age at onset of bipolar disorder and outcome during two-year follow-up: results from the STEP-BD study. *Bipolar Disorders*, 11(4): 391–400.

Pfeifer, J. C., Welge, J., Strakowski, S. M., Adler, C. M., & DelBello, MP. 2008. Meta-analysis of amygdala volumes in children and adolescents with bipolar disorder. *Journal of American Academy of Child and Adolescent Psychiatry*, 47(11): 1289–1298.

Rajkowska, G., Halaris, A., & Selemon, L. D. 2001. Reductions in neuronal and glial density characterize the dorsolateral prefrontal cortex in bipolar disorder. *Biological Psychiatry*, 49(9): 741–752.

Rich, B. A., Vinton, D. T., Roberson-Nay, R., Hommer, R.E., Berghorst, L.H., McClure, E.B., . . . Leibenluft, E. 2006. Limbic hyperactivation during processing of neutral facial expressions in children with bipolar disorder. *Proceedings of the National Academy of Sciences of the United States of America.* 103(23): 8900–8905.

Rich, B. A., Fromm, S. J., Berghorst, L. H., Dickstein, D.P., Brotman, M.A., Pine, D.S., & Leibenluft, E. 2008. Neural connectivity in children with bipolar disorder: impairment in the face emotion processing circuit. *Journal of Child Psychology and Psychiatry.* 49(1): 88–96.

Rich, B. A., Holroyd, T., Carver, F. W., Onelio, L. M., Mendoza, J. K., Cornwell, B. R., . . . Leibenluft, E. 2010. A preliminary study of the neural mechanisms of frustration in pediatric bipolar disorder using magnetoencephalography. *Depression and Anxiety*, 27(3): 276–286.

Romero, S., DelBello, M. P., Soutullo, C. A., Stanford, K., & Strakowski, S. M. 2005. Family environment in families with versus families without parental bipolar disorder: a preliminary comparison study. *Bipolar Disorders*, 7(6): 617–622.

Salvadore, G., Quiroz, J. A., Machado-Vieira, R., Henter, I. D., Manji, H. K., & Zarate, C. A. Jr. 2010. The neurobiology of the switch process in bipolar disorder: a review. *Journal of Clinical Psychiatry*, 71(11): 1488–1501.

Sanches, M., Roberts, R. L., Sassi, R. B., Axelson, D., Nicoletti, M., Brambilla, P., . . . Soares, J. C. 2005a. Developmental abnormalities in striatum in young bipolar patients: a preliminary study. *Bipolar Disorders*, 7(2): 153–158.

Sanches, M., Roberts, R. L., Sassi. R. B., Axelson, D., Nicoletti, M., Brambilla, P., . . . Soares, J. C. 2005b. Developmental abnormalities in striatum in young bipolar patients: a preliminary study. *Bipolar Disorders*, 7(2): 153–158.

Shaw, J. A., Egeland, J. A., Endicott, J., Allen, C. R., & Hostetter, A. M. 2005. A 10-year prospective study of prodromal patterns for bipolar disorder among Amish youth. *Journal of American Academy of Child and Adolescent Psychiatry*, 44(11): 1104–1111.

Shibuya-Tayoshi S, Tayoshi S, Sumitani S, Ueno S, Harada M, & Ohmori T. 2008. Lithium effects on brain glutamatergic and GABAergic systems of healthy volunteers as measured by proton magnetic resonance spectroscopy. *Progress in Neuropsychopharmacology and Biological Psychiatry*, 32(1): 249–256.

Simeonova, D. I., Jackson, V., Attalla, A., Karchemskiy, A., Howe, M., Adleman, N., & Chang, K. 2009. Subcortical volumetric correlates of anxiety in familial pediatric bipolar disorder: a preliminary investigation. *Psychiatry Research*, 173(2): 113–120.

Singh, M. K., DelBello, M. P., Stanford, K., & Strakowski, S. M. 2008. Neuroanatomical Characterization of Child Offspring of Parents with Bipolar Disorder. *Journal of American Academy of Child and Adolescent Psychiatry*, 47(5): 526–531.

Singh, M. K., Chang, K. D., Mazaika, P., Garrett, A., Adleman, N., Kelley, R., . . . Reiss, A. 2010. Neural correlates of response inhibition in pediatric bipolar disorder. *Journal of Child and Adolescent Psychopharmacology*, 20(1): 15–24.

Singh, M., Spielman, D., Adleman, N., Alegria, D., Howe, M., Reiss, A., & Chang, K. 2010. Brain glutamatergic characteristics of pediatric offspring of parents with bipolar disorder. *Psychiatry Research*, 182(2): 165–171.

Singh, M. K., Spielman, D., Libby, A., Adams, E., Acquaye, T., Howe, M., . . . Chang, K. 2011. Neurochemical Deficits in the Cerebellar Vermis in Child Offspring of Parents with Bipolar Disorder. *Bipolar Disorders*, 13(2): 189–197.

Stork, C., & Renshaw, P. F. 2005. Mitochondrial dysfunction in bipolar disorder: evidence from magnetic resonance spectroscopy research. *Molecular Psychiatry*, (10): 900–919.

Strakowski, S. M., DelBello, M. P., Sax, K. W., Zimmerman, M. E., Shear, P. K., Hawkins, J. M., & Larson, E. R. 1999. Brain magnetic resonance imaging of structural abnormalities in bipolar disorder. *Archives of General Psychiatry*, 56(3): 254–260.

Strakowski, S. M., DelBello, M. P., & Adler, C. M. 2005. The functional neuroanatomy of bipolar disorder: a review of neuroimaging findings. *Molecular Psychiatry*, 10(1): 105–116.

Strakowski, S. M., Adler, C. M., Cerullo, M. A., Eliassen, J. C., Lamy, M., Fleck, D. E., . . . DelBello, M. P. 2008. MRI brain activation in first-episode bipolar mania during a response inhibition task. *Early Intervention in Psychiatry*, 2(4): 225–233.

Thompson, P. M., Giedd, J. N., Woods, R. P., MacDonald, D., Evans, A. C., & Toga, A. W. 2000. Growth patterns in the developing brain detected by using continuum mechanical tensor maps. *Nature*, 404(6774): 190–193.

Usher, J., Leucht, S., Falkai, P., & Scherk, H. 2010. Correlation between amygdala volume and age in bipolar disorder—a systematic review and meta-analysis of structural MRI studies. *Psychiatry Research*, 182(1): 1–8.

Versace, A., Ladouceur, C. D., Romero, S., Birmaher, B., Axelson, D. A., Kupfer, D. J., & Phillips, M. L. 2010. Altered development of white matter in youth at high familial risk for bipolar disorder: a diffusion tensor imaging study. *Journal of American Academy of Child and Adolescent Psychiatry*, 49(12): 1249–1259.

Wilens, T. E., Biederman, J., Millstein, R. B., Wozniak, J., Hahesy, A. L., & Spencer, T. J. 1999. Risk for substance use disorders in youths with child- and adolescent-onset bipolar disorder. *Journal of American Academy of Child and Adolescent Psychiatry*, 38(6): 680–685.

Wilens, T. E., Biederman, J., Kwon, A., Ditterline, J., Forkner, P., Moore, H., . . . Faraone, S. V. 2004. Risk of substance use disorders in adolescents with bipolar disorder. *Journal of American Academy of Child and Adolescent Psychiatry*, 43(11): 1380–1386.

Wilke, M., Kowatch, R. A., DelBello, M. P., Mills, N. P., & Holland, S. K. 2004. Voxel-based morphometry in adolescents with bipolar disorder: first results. *Psychiatry Research*, 131(1): 57–69.

Winsberg, M. E., Sachs, N., & Tate, D. L. Adalsteinsson E. Spielman D. Ketter TA. 2000. Decreased dorsolateral prefrontal N-acetyl aspartate in bipolar disorder. *Biological Psychiatry*, 47(6): 475–481.

Yasar, A. S., Monkul, E. S., Sassi, R. B., Axelson, D., Brambilla, P., Nicoletti, M. A., . . . Soares, J. C. 2006. MRI study of corpus callosum in children and adolescents with bipolar disorder. *Psychiatry Research*, 146(1): 83–5.

Yetkin, F. Z., Haughton, V. M., Fischer, M. E., Papke, R. A., Daniels, D. L., Mark, L. P., . . . Johansen, J. 1992. High-signal foci on MR images of the brain: observer variability in their quantification. *AJR American Journal of Roentgenology*, 159(1): 185–188.

Yurgelun-Todd, D. A., Gruber, S. A., Kanayama, G., Killgore, W. D., Baird, A. A., & Young, A. D. 2000. fMRI during affect discrimination in bipolar affective disorder. *Bipolar Disorders*, 2 (3 Pt 2): 237–248.

# 6.

# NEUROIMAGING STUDIES OF BIPOLAR AND UNIPOLAR DEPRESSION

Amelia Versace, Jorge R. C. Almeida, and Mary L. Phillips

## INTRODUCTION

Bipolar disorder is one of the ten most debilitating of all illnesses, with a 15% suicide rate, and direct annual costs in the United States of $7.6 billion (Kleinman et al., 2003). Nonetheless, the absence of biologically-relevant diagnostic markers of bipolar disorder results in its misdiagnosis as recurrent unipolar depression in 60% of treatment seeking individuals. Misdiagnosis leads to inadequate treatment that promotes switching to mania and worsens illness outcome illnesses (Hirschfeld et al., 2003). Indeed, only 20% of patients with bipolar disorder are correctly diagnosed within the first year of seeking treatment (Hirschfeld 2003), indicating a strong bias away from diagnosing bipolar disorder in patients presenting in a depressed episode. It is therefore crucial to society and the well-being of individuals with bipolar disorder that objective markers are identified to help distinguish bipolar from unipolar disorder as early as possible in the lifetime of these individuals. A first stage toward this ultimate goal is identifying objective biological markers reflecting pathophysiological processes that may differ between bipolar and unipolar depression.

One promising approach is to use structural and functional measures of neural circuitry supporting emotion processing and regulation (e.g., magnetic resonance imaging, MRI) in order to examine both bipolar and unipolar individuals concurrently. The extent to which these measures may distinguish bipolar from unipolar depression has potential to increase understanding of pathophysiological processes that may differ between these conditions.

In this chapter, we therefore describe extant findings from neuroimaging studies of individuals with bipolar disorder and individuals with a history of unipolar depression, and focus in particular on studies that directly compared individuals with these two conditions. We reviewed studies that employed different structural and functional neuroimaging techniques including: studies using structural neuroimaging of gray matter volumes, studies examining white matter connectivity using diffusion tensor imaging, and studies employing functional and effective connectivity techniques to assess the functional integrity of neural circuitry supporting emotion processing and emotion regulation (Phillips, Ladouceur et al., 2008).

## STRUCTURAL NEUROIMAGING STUDIES OF BIPOLAR AND UNIPOLAR DISORDER

Structural neuroimaging studies have consistently shown regional abnormalities in adults and youth with bipolar and unipolar disorders. While evidence suggests that individuals with these disorders do not significantly differ in whole brain gray matter volumes compared with healthy individuals, relative increases in ventricle to brain ratios, as well as decreases in regional gray matter volumes, have been reported in both adults and youth with bipolar and unipolar disorders (for a recent review see Konarski et al., 2008). Reduction of prefrontal gray matter volumes, particularly in anterior cingulate and orbitofrontal cortical regions, have been consistently reported in both adults with bipolar and unipolar disorders when directly compared with healthy adults (Bremner et al., 2002; Lopez-Larson et al., 2002; Ballmaier et al., 2004; Hastings et al., 2004; Lacerda et al., 2004; Lyoo et al., 2004; Sassi et al., 2004; Kaur et al., 2005; Caetano et al., 2006). The paucity of structural neuroimaging studies directly comparing adults with bipolar and unipolar disorders (Drevets et al., 1997; Brambilla et al., 2002), however, makes it difficult to draw definitive conclusions as to the nature of structural neuroimaging findings that may differentiate adults these two conditions. Nonetheless, studies reported independently increases in gray matter in adults with bipolar disorder and decreases in gray matter in adults with unipolar disorder relative to healthy adults, suggesting potential diagnostic group differences (Altshuler et al., 1998; Sheline et al., 1998; Bremner et al., 2000; Frodl et al., 2002; Brambilla et al., 2003; MacMillan et al., 2003; Ballmaier et al., 2004; Hastings et al., 2004; Caetano et al., 2006). Differential patterns of changes in gray matter (relative to healthy individuals) have also been observed in the hippocampus-amygdala complex: While decreased hippocampal gray matter volume, together with inconsistent findings regarding amygdala gray matter changes have been shown in adults with unipolar disorder (Sheline et al., 1998; Bremner et al., 2000; Frodl et al., 2002; MacMillan et al., 2003; Hastings et al., 2004; Caetano et al., 2006), increases in amygdala, but not hippocampal, gray matter have been more consistently reported in adults with bipolar disorder (Altshuler et al., 1998; Strakowski et al., 1999; Brambilla et al., 2003; Ballmaier et al., 2004). Recent findings in children and adolescents with bipolar disorder, however, indicate decreases (DelBello et al., 2004; Blumberg et al., 2005; Chang et al., 2005; Dickstein et al., 2005), rather than increases, in amygdala gray matter in these youth. These latter findings suggest a possible age effect upon patterns of abnormal amygdala gray matter in youth with bipolar disorder that in turn suggests abnormal developmental trajectories of amygdala gray matter in the illness that perhaps is not present in unipolar depression.

> **Structural Imaging of Gray Matter:**
>
> · Rarely compared unipolar and bipolar disorders directly
>
> · Suggests possible gray matter differences between the disorders within the amygdala-hippocampal complex
>
> · Suggests possible abnormal developmental trajectories of amygdala gray matter in bipolar disorder

## WHITE MATTER CONNECTIVITY STUDIES OF BIPOLAR AND UNIPOLAR DISORDERS

### STUDIES IN BIPOLAR DISORDER

Neuropathological studies reported cytoarchitectural and neurochemical abnormalities of neuronal and glial cells in adults with bipolar disorder (for reviews see Harrison 2002; Rajkowska 2002). To date, microstructural white matter abnormalities have been consistently reported *in vivo* by neuroimaging studies in youth and adults with bipolar disorder, using diffusion tensor imaging. Abnormalities in the corpus callosum and in the white matter of frontal and (anterior) cingulate cortices have also been reported in adults with bipolar disorder in *region-of-interest* (ROI) based analyses (Beyer et al., 2005; Haznedar et al., 2005; Adler et al., 2006; Yurgelun-Todd et al., 2007; Wang et al., 2009; Macritchie et al., 2010), *voxel-based* analyses (Bruno et al., 2008; Chaddock et al., 2009; Mahon et al., 2009; Sussmann et al., 2009; Wessa et al., 2009; Zanetti et al., 2009), *tract-based spatial statistics* analyses (Versace et al., 2008; Wessa et al., 2009), and *tractography-based* analyses (Lin et al.; Houenou et al., 2007; McIntosh et al., 2008; Mahon et al., 2009). Taken together, these findings suggest that abnormal white matter integrity may play an important role in the pathophysiology of bipolar disorder (for reviews see Heng et al., 2010; Mahon et al., 2010), and further suggest that a deficient frontal modulation of subcortical and limbic structures may underlie mood dysregulation in bipolar disorder (Phillips, Ladouceur et al., 2008) (Table 6.1).

Using diffusion tensor imaging and fractional anisotropy (FA), a measure of the structural integrity of brain white matter, in adults with bipolar disorder, we found abnormal fiber alignment in the right and left uncinate fasciculus, a key white matter tract connecting frontotemporal cortical areas that are thought to be involved in emotion processing and regulation (Phillips, Ladouceur et al., 2008). These findings in the uncinate fasciculus in adults with bipolar disorder parallel other reports of reduced FA in adults (McIntosh et al., 2008; Sussmann et al., 2009) and adolescents (Frazier et al., 2005; Kafantaris et al., 2009) with bipolar disorder, relative to their age-matched healthy counterparts (Table 6.1).

Understanding the meaning of FA changes in pathological groups can be challenging, because these changes can be interpreted several ways, including as alterations in longitudinally/obliquely-oriented fibers ratio, as changes in axonal integrity, as changes in tightness of axonal packing, as alterations in permeability of myelin sheaths, or as abnormalities of one set of fibers in a large group of intersecting fiber pathways. It has therefore been suggested that eigenvalues—measures of directional diffusivity—may provide more information regarding the nature of WM pathology in pathological groups. Radial diffusivity appears to reflect changes in myelin in white matter, whereas longitudinal diffusivity is more sensitive to axonal degeneration (Song, Sun et al., 2002; Hasan and Narayana 2006; Alexander et al., 2007). To date, there are few studies in adults and youth with bipolar disorder that have included measures of FA, together with measures of longitudinal (Versace et al., 2008; Mahon et al., 2009; Pavuluri et al., 2009; Versace

**TABLE 6.1** DIFFUSION NEUROIMAGING STUDIES IN BIPOLAR DISORDERS

| Study | Group (M/F) Age (yy) | Non-colinear directions | Main findings |
|---|---|---|---|
| **REGION OF INTEREST APPROACH** | | | |
| Adler et al. 2004 | 9 BDI (4/5) 32±8yy 9 HI (6/3) 31±7yy | 25 | The FA of ROIs 25 and 30 mm above the AC was significantly reduced in BDI; FA of all ROIs showed high-mediumto large effect sizes. No significant group differences were identified in trace ADC |
| Haznedar et al. 2005 | 17 BDI (n.a.) 39.8±13.4yy 7 BDII (n.a.) 43.8±6.7yy 16 cyclothymia (n.a.) 43.9±9.2yy 36 HI (n/a) 40.7±11.6yy | 6 | Bipolar spectrum patients as a single group did not differ from healthy adults in thalamus and the basal ganglia volumes, but the cyclothymia patients had reductions in the volumes of putamen and the thalamus compared with healthy adults. Bipolar spectrum patients had significantly reduced volume of the white and the gray matter of the frontal cortex. Furthermore, compared with healthy adults, Bipolar spectrum patients as a group showed alterations in anisotropy of the internal capsule adjacent to the striatum and thalamus and the frontal white matter. |
| Yurgelun-Todd et al. 2007 | 11 BDI (6/5) 32.9±10.5yy 10 HI (4/6) 32.4±9.1yy | 6 | BDI had significantly higher FA in the midline of the genu compared with healthy adults. Regional white matter differences were also observed, with significantly lower FA in the genu than forward projecting regions in both groups and lower FA in the genu than the splenium in healthy adults. |
| Wang et al. 2008 | 33 BD (19/11) 29.2±9.2yy 40 HI (30/10) 32±10.1yy | 32 | In ROI-based analyses, FA was significantly decreased in the anterior and middle corpus callosum in the BD group (p < 0.05). Voxel-based analyses similarly localized group differences to the genu, rostral body, and anterior mid body of corpus callosum (p < 0.05, corrected). |
| Wang et al., 2009 | 33 BD (10/13) 31.8±9.6yy 31 (14/17) 30.4±10.8yy | 32 | A significant positive association between pergenual anterior cingulate gyrus-amygdala functional coupling and FA in ventrofrontal WM, including the region of the uncinate fasciculus, was identified (p < 0.005). |
| Macritchie et al. 2010 | 28 BD (16/12) 43.0±11.5yy 28HI (16/12) 43.0±11.7yy | 6 | Comparing the whole data-sets using the sign test, in adults with BD, MD was greater at all 15 sites (P<0.001) and FA was reduced at 13 (P<0.01). The effect of diagnosis was significant for callosal MD and FA and for deep/periventricular MD. Comparing individual regions, prefrontal and periventricular MD were significantly increased; callosal and occipital FA were significantly reduced. Former substance use and lithium were possible confounding factors. Periventricular WM hyperintensities were associated with significantly increased periventricular MD in individuals with bipolar disorder. |
| Frazier et al. 2007 | 10 BD (4/6) 9.2±3.0yy 7 HR for BD (4/3) 8.9±3.0yy 8 HI (5/3) 9.2±2.4YY | 6 | Compared with healthy youth, youth with BD had decreased FA in right and left superior frontal tracts, including the superior longitudinal fasciculus I and the cingulate-paracingulate WM. In addition, youth with BD had reduced FA in left orbital frontal WM and the right corpus callosum body. Compared with youth at risk for BD, youth with BD showed reduced FA in the right and left cingulate-paracingulate WM. Both the BD and at risk-BD groups showed reduced FA relative to healthy youth in bilateral superior longitudinal fasciculus I. |
| Adler et al. 2006 | 11 BD (5/6) 17 HI (7/10) | n/a | Adolescents with BD in their 1st episode of mania and free of medications showed significantly decreased FA only in superior-frontal WM tracts. |
| Kafantaris et al. 2009 | 14±2yy (all sample) 26 BDI (12/14) 16.0 yy 26 HI (14/12) 15.3 yy | 6 | Compared with healthy youth, youth with BD demonstrated abnormalities in WM regions predicted to differ a priori between groups, including lower FA in the right orbital frontal lobe and higher ADC in the right and left subgenual region (p < 0.005, uncorrected; cluster size > = 100). There were no areas of higher FA or lower ADC in BD compared with healthy volunteers. Lower FA across regions that differed significantly between groups correlated significantly with slower visuomotor speed among BD. |

*(Continued)*

| Study | Group (M/F) Age (yy) | Non-colinear directions | Main findings |
|-------|----------------------|--------------------------|---------------|
| **VOXEL BASED MORPHOMETRY APPROACH** | | | |
| Bruno et al. 2008 | 36 BD (13/23) 39yy 28 HI (matched) | 6 | In the patient group, MD was increased in the right posterior frontal and bilateral prefrontal WM, while FA was decreased [corrected] in the inferior, middle temporal and middle occipital regions. |
| Chaddock et al. 2009 | 19 BD (9/10) 43.3±10.2yy 21 BD relatives (12/9) 42.5±13.6yy 18 HI (10/8) 41.7±12.2yy | | Adults with BD had decreased FA compared with healthy adults in the genu of the corpus callosum, right inferior longitudinal fasciculus and left superior longitudinal fasciculus. Increased genetic liability for bipolar disorder was associated with reduced FA across distributed regions of WM in adults with BD and their unaffected relatives. |
| Sussmann et al. 2009 | 42 BDI (22/20) 39.6±10.1yy 28 SCZ (15/13) 38.0±9.9yy 38 HI (19/19) 37.2±11.9yy | 51 | Reduced FA was found in the anterior limb of the internal capsule anterior thalamic radiation, and in the region of the uncinate fasciculus in adults with BD and those with schizophrenia compared with healthy adults. A direct comparison between patient groups found no significant differences in these regions. None of the findings were associated with psychotropic medication. Reduced integrity of the anterior limb of the internal capsule, uncinate fasciculus, and anterior thalamic radiation regions was common to both adults with schizophrenia and BD. |
| Mahon et al. 2009 | 30 BD (15/15) 33.4±8.7yy 38HI (22/16) 31.9±8.6yy | 25 | Relative to healthy volunteers, adults with BD demonstrated significantly (p<0.001; cluster size >/= 50) higher FA within the right and left frontal WM and lower FA within the left cerebellar WM. Examination of individual eigenvalues indicated that group differences in both axial diffusivity and radial diffusivity contributed to abnormal FA within these regions |
| Wessa et al. 2009 | 22 BD (11/11) 45.5±12.6yy 21 HI (12/9) 43.0±13.2yy | 41 | FA was significantly increased in adults with bipolar disorder relative to healthy adults in medial frontal, precentral, inferior parietal, and occipital white matter. No group differences in MD were found. |
| Zanetti et al. 2009 | 37 BDI (13/24) 34.1±9.0yy 26 HI (12/14) 28.8±9.5yy | 6 | Significantly decreased FA and increased MD in bilateral prefronto-limbic-striatal WM and right inferior fronto-occipital, superior and inferior longitudinal fasciculi were shown in all adults with BD versus healthy adults, as well as in depressed adults with BD versus both healthy adults and remitted adults with BD. Depressed adults with BD also exhibited increased FA in the ventromedial prefrontal cortex. Remitted adults with BD did not differ from healthy adults in FA or MD. |
| **TRACT BASED SPATIAL STATISTICS APPROACH** | | | |
| Versace et al. 2008 | 31 BDI (11/20) 35.9±8.9yy 25 HI (11/14) 29.5±9.4yy | 6 | Adults with BD vs healthy adults had significantly greater FA (t > 3.0, P <or = 0.05 corrected) in the left uncinate fasciculus (reduced radial diffusivity distally and increased longitudinal diffusivity centrally), left optic radiation (increased longitudinal diffusivity), and right anterior thalamic radiation (no significant diffusivity change). Adults with BD vs healthy adults had significantly reduced FA (t > 3.0, P <or = 0.05 corrected) in the right uncinate fasciculus (greater radial diffusivity). Among adults with BD, significant negative correlations (P < 0.01) were found between age and FA in bilateral uncinate fasciculi and in the right anterior thalamic radiation, as well as between medication load and FA in the left optic radiation. Decreased FA (P < 0.01) was observed in the left optic radiation and in the right anterior thalamic radiation among adults with BD taking vs those not taking mood stabilizers, as well as in the left optic radiation among depressed vs remitted adults with BD. |
| Barnea-Goraly et al. 2009 | 21 BD (15/6) 16.1±2.7yy 18 HI (14/4) 14.5±2.7yy | 6 | Youth with BD had lower FA values than healthy youth in the fornix, the left mid-posterior cingulate gyrus, throughout the corpus callosum, in fibers extending from the fornix to the thalamus, and in parietal and occipital corona radiata bilaterally. There were no significant between-group differences in trace or ADC values and no significant correlation between behavioral measures, medication exposure, and FA values. |

TABLE 6.1 (CONTINUED)

| Study | Group (M/F) Age (yy) | Non-colinear directions | Main findings |
|---|---|---|---|
| Pavuluri et al. 2009 | 13 BD (n/a) 14.8±2.5yy 13 ADHD (ns) 13.4±3.0yy 15 HI (ns) 13.7±2.7yy | 27 | Significantly lower FA was observed in anterior corona radiata in both youth with BD and ADHD relative to healthy youth. In addition, FA and r-FCI values were significantly lower in youth with ADHD relative to youth with BD and healthy youth in both the anterior limb of the internal capsule and the superior region of the internal capsule. Further, ADC was significantly greater in ADHD relative to both youth with BD and healthy youth in anterior corona radiata, anterior and posterior limb of the internal capsule, superior region of the internal capsule, cingulate gyrus, superior and inferior longitudinal fasciculi. |
| **TRACTOGRAPHY BASED APPROACH** | | | |
| McIntosh et al. 2008 | 40 BD (21/19) 39.9±10.1yy 25 SCZ (14/9) 37.2±9.2yy 49 HI (28/21) 35.3±11.0yy | 51 | Patients with schizophrenia or BD showed common reductions in the uncinate fasciculus and anterior thalamic radiation. These reductions were unrelated to age, duration of illness, current medication, or current psychiatric symptoms in all patients or the lifetime presence of psychotic symptoms in adults with BD. |
| Houenou et al. 2007 | 16 BD (8/8) 41.9±12.8yy 16 HI (9/7) 40.5±12.8yy | 41 | The tractography results revealed a significantly increased number of reconstructed fibers between the left subgenual cingulate and left amygdala-hippocampus in adults with BD as compared to healthy adults. FA and ADC of the reconstructed fiber tract did not differ significantly between the groups. Furthermore, no significant group differences were observed neither for reconstructed fiber tracts between the right subgenual cingulate and right amygdala-hippocampus nor between the regions |
| Mahon et al. 2009 | 30 BD (15/15) 33.4±8.7yy 38HI (22/16) 31.9±8.6yy | 25 | This was a voxel-based morphometric and tractography-based study. Please, for details see above. |
| Lin et al. 2011 | 18 BD (6/12) 28.5±11.1yy 16HI (4/12) 29.9±9.2yy | 13 | When compared with healthy, adults with BD showed significantly decreased FA in the anterior thalamic radiation and uncinate fasciculus, and a trend towards lower FA in the superior longitudinal fasciculus and cingulum. However, there were no FA differences between groups in the inferior fronto-occipital fasciculus |

ROIs = Regions of Interest; FA = Fractional Anisotropy; MD = Mean Diffusivity; ADC = Apparent Diffusion Coefficients; WM = White Matter; BD = Bipolar Disorder; BDI = Bipolar Disorder type-I; SCZ = Schizophrenia; ADHD = Attention Deficit Hyperactivity Disorder; HI = Healthy Individuals; ns = not specified.

et al., 2010) and radial (Versace et al., 2008; Versace et al., 2010) diffusivity. To better understand our FA findings (Versace et al., 2008), we included these latter measures and found that altered FA in right and left uncinate fasciculus in adults with bipolar disorder, relative to healthy adults, was associated with abnormal radial and longitudinal diffusivity, respectively, indicating abnormally increased proportions of left-sided longitudinally aligned, and right-sided obliquely aligned, myelinated fibers (Table 6.1).

Studies of youth with bipolar disorder have shown white matter abnormalities in temporal (Kafantaris et al., 2009) and occipital (Barnea-Goraly et al., 2009; Kafantaris et al., 2009) cortices, and in the corpus callosum (Frazier et al., 2007; Barnea-Goraly et al., 2009), suggesting white matter changes may occur early in development. More data are needed to better understand these developmental trajectories and how they might have gone awry in bipolar youth.

White matter abnormalities have also been reported in the corpus callosum of healthy relatives of adults with bipolar disorder, along with white matter abnormalities in the right inferior longitudinal fasciculus and in the left superior longitudinal fasciculus (Chaddock et al., 2009; Versace et al., 2010,). These findings further suggest that white matter abnormalities may underline potential vulnerability for future psychiatric disorders in healthy relatives of adults with bipolar disorder.

## STUDIES IN UNIPOLAR DEPRESSION

Neuropathological studies have reported cytoarchitectural abnormalities in neuronal/glial size and density in the left prefrontal cortex of brains form individuals with unipolar disorder (Rajkowska et al., 1999; Cotter et al., 2002; for reviews see Harrison 2002; Rajkowska 2002).

TABLE 6.2 DIFFUSION NEUROIMAGING STUDIES IN UNIPOLAR DISORDERS

| Study | Group (M/F) Age (yy) | Non-collinear directions | Main findings |
|---|---|---|---|
| **REGION OF INTEREST APPROACH** | | | |
| Taylor et al. (2001) | 14 UD (4/8) 19 HI 69 ± 1.66 yy | 7 | Hyperintensities showed higher ADC and lower anisotropy than normal regions. Gray matter exhibited similar trends. There was no significant difference in diffusion characteristics of hyperintensities between adults with UD and healthy adults |
| Alexopoulos et al. (2002) | 13 UD (n/a) (no healthy group) 60–77yy | 7 | Lower FA of the right and the left frontal WM regions 15mm above the AC–PC plane (approximately anterior cingulate) was associated with a low remission rate after age was considered. Remission was not significantly associated with FA of lower frontal regions or a temporal region |
| Nobuhara et al. (2004) | 8 UD (1/7) 12 HI 62.9 ± 5.8 yy | ns | Significant WM FA reduction in widespread frontal and temporal brain regions in patients with depression before electroconvulsive treatment compared with healthy adults. A significant increase in frontal WM FA was seen following electroconvulsive treatment. A course of bilateral electroconvulsive treatment ameliorated WM integrity in frontal brain regions. |
| Taylor et al. (2004) | 17 UD (7/10) 16 HI 67.5 ± 6.1 yy | 7 | Even after ling for age, sex, hypertension, and heart disease, the authors found significantly lower FA values in the right superior frontal gyrus WM of depressed adults with UD than comparison subjects |
| Steele et al. (2005) | 15 UD (4/11) 14 HI 45.9 yy | 7 | No reduced FA in the brainstem |
| Bae et al. (2006) | 106 UD (33/73) 84 HI 70.4 ± 6.4 yy | 7 | Depressed adults with UD had significantly lower FA values in WM of the right anterior cingulate gyrus, bilateral superior frontal gyri, and left middle frontal gyrus |
| Nobuhara et al. (2006) | 13 UD (4/9) 13 HI 62.8 ± 6.6 yy | 7 | Significant FA reduction in widespread frontal and temporal lobe of MDD patients. Evidence that WM FA in inferior frontal is inversely related MDD severity |
| Li et al. (2007) | 19 UD (4/15) 20 HI 28.1 ± 7.4 yy | 13 | Compared with healthy, young adults with UD showed significantly lower FA values in prefrontal WM at bilateral 20mm, right 16mm, and right 12mm above the AC–PC. Furthermore, there was no significant correlation between the FA value of any ROI and illness course as well as severity of depression |
| Xia et al. (2007) | 18 UD (10/8) 13 HI 36.08 ± 10.81 yy | 25 | Adults with UD who failed to respond to treatment had a significantly lower FA in frontal WM those successful responders, and healthy adults |
| Yang et al. (2007) | 31 UD (11/20) 15 HI 64.6 ± 5.21 yy | 25 | FA values were significantly decreased in the frontal (superior and middle frontal gyrus), and temporal (right parahippocampal gyrus) regions of elderly adults with UD compared with healthy adults |
| Alexopoulos et al. (2008) | 25 remitted UD (ns) 23 nonremitted UD 70.1 ± 5.5 yy | 8 | Adults with UD who failed to achieve remission (N = 23) had lower FA in multiple frontal limbic brain areas, including the rostral and dorsal anterior cingulate, dorsolateral prefrontal cortex, genu of the corpus callosum, WM adjacent to the hippocampus, multiple posterior cingulate cortex regions, and insular WM, relative to those who achieved remission (N = 25). In addition, lower FA was detected in the neostriatum and midbrain as well as select temporal and parietal regions |
| Hoptman et al. (2009) | 41 UD (16/25) (no healthy group) 70.1 ± 6.3 yy | 8 | High blood pressure is associated with microstructural WM abnormalities (lower FA) in the dorsal anterior cingulate and multiple frontostriatal and frontotemporal WM regions in geriatric adults with UD |
| Taylor et al. (2008) | 37 remitted UD (21/16) 65.8 ± 5.7 yy 37 nonremitted UD (19/18) 70.5 ± 8.0 yy | 7 | Adults with UD who did not remit to sertraline exhibited higher FA values in the superior frontal gyri and anterior cingulate cortices bilaterally |

TABLE 6.2 (CONTINUED)

| Study | Group (M/F) Age (yy) | Non-collinear directions | Main findings |
|-------|----------------------|--------------------------|---------------|
| **WHOLEBRAIN ANALYSIS** | | | |
| Ma (2007) | 14 treatment-naïve UD (2/12) 14 HI 28.9 ± 8.0 yy | 13 | Treatment-naïve young adults with UD exhibited significantly lower FA values than healthy comparison young adults in WM of the right middle frontal gyrus, the left lateral occipitotemporal gyrus, and the subgyral and angular gyri of the right parietal lobe |
| Yuan (2007) | 16 remitted UD (7/9) 14 HI 66.9 ± 7.0 yy | 25 | Adults with UD relative to healthy adults showed lower FA in WM at the right superior frontal gyrus, left inferior frontal gyrus, left middle temporal gyrus, right inferior parietal lobule, right middle occipital gyrus, left lingual gyrus, right putamen, and right caudate |
| Zou et al. (2008) | 45 UD (15/30) 45 HI 33.2 ± 8.9 yy | 15 | Significant decrease in FA in the left hemisphere, including the anterior limb of the internal capsule and the inferior parietal portion of the superior longitudinal fasciculus, in adults with UD compared with healthy adults. Diffusion tensor imaging measures in the left anterior limb of the internal capsule were negatively related to the severity of depressive symptoms (controlled for age and sex) |

ROIs = Regions of Interest; FA = Fractional Anisotropy; MD = Mean Diffusivity; ADC = Apparent Diffusion Coefficients; WM = White Matter; UD = Unipolar Disorder; HC = Healthy Control Individuals; ns = not specified.

Microstructural white matter abnormalities have been reported in vivo in neuroimaging studies in adults and youth with unipolar disorder, although the majority of these studies focused on late-life depression and employed a region of interest rather than a whole brain approach. Decreases in FA in frontal lobe have been reported in older adults with unipolar depression (Alexopoulos et al., 2002; Taylor et al., 2004; Bae et al., 2006; Nobuhara et al., 2006; Li et al., 2007; Yang et al., 2007) and in young (Li et al., 2007; Xia et al., 2007). Similarly, the small number of whole brain diffusion tensor imaging studies in unipolar depression reported decreased FA in prefrontal regions in older (Murphy, Gunning-Dixon et al., 2007; Yuan et al., 2007) and younger (Ma et al., 2007; Zou et al., 2008) adults with unipolar disorder relative to healthy adults. In one of these studies, FA abnormalities in the left anterior limb of the internal capsule were reported to be negatively associated with depression severity in adults with unipolar disorder relative to healthy adults (Zou et al., 2008). (Table 6.2).

There remains a lack of tractography-based studies in unipolar disorder. Furthermore, the extent to which patterns of white matter connectivity between prefrontal cortical and limbic regions can differentiate depressed adults with bipolar from those with unipolar disorder remains little studied.

In a recent study (Versace, Almeida et al., 2010), we therefore compared depressed adults with bipolar and unipolar depression using whole brain tract-based spatial statistics analyses as a first step toward identifying white matter connectivity abnormalities that may help differentiate these two conditions. Our previous findings in adults with bipolar disorder, and findings from other previous studies in adults with unipolar disorder (see the preceding section) allowed us to hypothesize that depressed adults with bipolar and unipolar disorder would be distinguished by patterns of amygdala-orbitomedial prefrontal structural connectivity, specifically with depressed bipolar adults showing abnormal bilateral, and depressed unipolar adults showing abnormal left-sided, structural connectivity between these regions. Our whole brain analytic approach also allowed us to examine the extent to which WM connectivity in other regions over the whole brain distinguished depression in bipolar disorder from unipolar disorder.

We compared depressed adults with bipolar and unipolar disorder who had a similar clinical presentation, in terms of illness duration, age at illness onset and depression severity. Our findings indicated a significant main effect of group in left-sided sensory and visuospatial information processing regions, namely in the region of left superior longitudinal fasciculus, in the inferior temporal and primary sensory cortices, and in the region of the left inferior longitudinal fasciculus in the lateral occipital cortex. Here, depressed adults with bipolar disorder showed significantly decreased FA in left superior longitudinal fasciculus in the region of inferior temporal cortex, relative to depressed adults with unipolar disorder, and in the region of primary sensory cortex relative to healthy adults. In contrast, depressed adults with unipolar disorder showed significantly decreased FA in the region of the left inferior longitudinal fasciculus relative to healthy adults. *Post-hoc* whole brain comparisons further revealed in depressed adults with bipolar disorder, significant differences in FA in the region of the right uncinate fasciculus relative to both depressed adults with unipolar disorder and healthy adults. Here, depressed adults with bipolar disorder showed significantly reduced FA in the right uncinate fasciculus in the region of orbitofrontal cortex relative to healthy adults, but significantly increased FA in the right uncinate fasciculus in the region of subgenual cortex relative to depressed adults with unipolar disorder. Furthermore, comparing only the women in the study, there was a significant main effect of group in the right uncinate fasciculus, in which depressed women with bipolar disorder showed significantly decreased FA relative to healthy women. These findings were in partial support of our main hypothesis of abnormal right-sided amygdala-orbitomedial prefrontal structural connectivity in depressed adults with bipolar disorder, but not unipolar disorder.

In the comparison between depressed adults with bipolar and unipolar disorder, we found that decreased FA was associated with decreased longitudinal diffusivity and greater radial diffusivity in the region of right uncinate fasciculus in orbitofrontal cortex in bipolar, but not unipolar, disorder, relative to healthy subjects. These findings also paralleled our previous findings of greater mean diffusivity, an indirect measure of radial diffusivity in right orbitomedial prefrontal cortex in depressed adults with bipolar disorder relative to healthy adults (Zanetti et al., 2009). Our findings therefore suggest that depressed adults with bipolar and unipolar disorder may be distinguished by FA in the right uncinate fasciculus in the region of subgenual cortex. The pattern of greater FA in this region in depressed adults with bipolar disorder relative to depressed adults with unipolar disorder may reflect greater white matter connectivity between amygdala and subgenual cingulate gyrus in depressed adults with bipolar disorder relative to depressed adults with unipolar disorder.

Our findings indicated that depression in bipolar and unipolar disorder may be distinguished by FA in right uncinate fasciculus that in turn may reflect different pathophysiological processes associated with emotion dysregulation in the two types of depression. Furthermore, diffusion tensor imaging findings in depressed adults with unipolar disorder (Zou et al., 2008) described previously are consistent with our finding of decreased FA in the region of left uncinate fasciculus in depressed adults with unipolar disorder relative to healthy adults, although our finding was specific to unipolar depressed women. These findings support our hypothesis that depressed adults with unipolar disorder show left- but not right-sided abnormalities in amygdala-orbitomedial prefrontal cortical structural connectivity, and further suggest that differential patterns of abnormal right and left orbitomedial prefrontal cortical-limbic structural connectivity may underlie the predisposition to depression in woman with depression, in both bipolar and unipolar disorders.

Our whole brain analyses allowed us to examine structural connectivity in regions other than orbitomedial prefrontal cortex. We showed a main effect of group in left superior longitudinal fasciculus in the region of inferior temporal and primary sensory cortices, resulting from depressed adults with bipolar disorder showing significantly decreased FA in these regions relative to depressed adults with unipolar disorder and healthy adults, respectively, and in left inferior longitudinal fasciculus in lateral occipital cortex, resulting from depressed adults with unipolar disorder showing significantly decreased FA in this region relative to healthy adults. Depressed adults with bipolar disorder also showed significantly decreased FA in right superior longitudinal fasciculus in the region of primary sensory cortex (Figure 6.1). Our findings in depressed adults with bipolar disorder are consistent with previous findings of decreased FA in left superior longitudinal fasciculus in adults with bipolar disorder (Chaddock et al., 2009), and of bilateral decreases in FA in superior longitudinal fasciculus in adolescents with, and those at high-risk of, bipolar disorder (Frazier et al., 2007). Our findings of decreased FA in left inferior longitudinal fasciculus in depressed adults with unipolar disorder relative to healthy adults, and of decreased left superior longitudinal fasciculus FA in depressed women with unipolar disorder relative to healthy women, support findings of previous diffusion tensor imaging studies showing decreased FA in depressed adults with unipolar disorder relative to healthy adults in temporal white matter (Nobuhara et al., 2006; Yang et al., 2007), as well as occipital and subcortical white matter (Yuan et al., 2007). Our specific finding of decreased left inferior longitudinal fasciculus FA in depressed adults with unipolar disorder relative to healthy adults supports that of a previous whole brain DTI study (Zou et al., 2008). This latter study reported decreased FA in depressed adults with unipolar disorder relative to healthy adults in a temporo-occipito-parietal region similar in location to the left inferior longitudinal fasciculus region in lateral occipital cortex

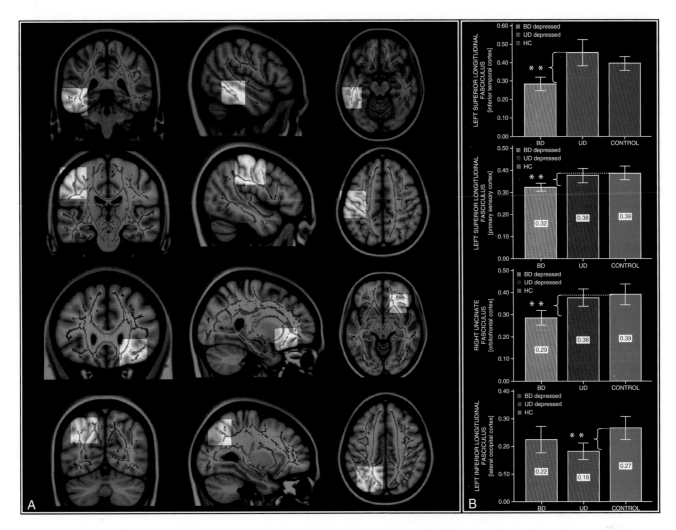

*Figure 6.1* Right Orbitofrontal Corticolimbic and Left Corticocortical White Matter Abnormalities in Bipolar and Unipolar Depression Panel A. FA maps showing three orthogonal (coronal, sagittal and axial) views of the main effect of group on FA in depressed adults with bipolar disorder, depressed adults with unipolar disorder and healthy adults (from top to bottom): left superior longitudinal fasciculus in inferior temporal cortex; left superior longitudinal fasciculus in primary sensory cortex; right uncinate fasciculus in orbitofrontal cortex, and left inferior longitudinal fasciculus in lateral occipital cortex. Background: MNI152 brain and WM skeleton used for Randomise analysis (in green). The images represent findings (in red-yellow) projected onto the WM skeleton. The red-yellow spectrum represents a significance range: 2<f<20. Monte Carlo simulation with the alphasim approach was conducted on uncorrected F and t statistical maps (p<0.001), obtaining a dual thresholding of both type I error (alpha; p<0.05) and cluster-size thresholding (CST). Panel B. Bar Graphs show mean FA values and 95% confidence intervals for each group for each of the above four regions in which there was a main effect of group on FA. Highlighted (**) is the significant pairwise between-group posthoc comparison that resulted in the main effect of group in each of these four regions. (Depressed adults with bipolar disorder in red, depressed adults with unipolar disorder in blue and healthy adults in green.) For each region, the third group that did not contribute to the main effect of group is also graphically represented (bar obscured) From top to bottom: pairwise comparison between depressed adults with bipolar disorder and depressed adults with unipolar disorder in the left superior longitudinal fasciculus in inferior temporal cortex [MNI x, y, z = -51, -38, -17]; pairwise comparison between depressed adults with bipolar disorder relative to healthy adults in the left superior longitudinal fasciculus in primary sensory cortex [MNI x, y, z = -40, -27, 50] and the right uncinate fasciculus in orbitofrontal cortex [MNI x, y, z = 26, 26, -11]; and pairwise comparison between depressed adults with unipolar disorder relative to healthy adults in the left inferior longitudinal fasciculus in lateral occipital cortex [MNI x, y, z = -28, -76, 40](Versace et al. 2010).

showing decreased FA in depressed adults with unipolar disorder relative to healthy adults in our study.

Some methodological considerations are needed when interpreting diffusion tensor imaging data (for a detailed review see Jones & Cercignani, 2010). Region-of-interest approaches circumvent the use of multiple comparisons, but are observer-dependent, and therefore subject to

reliability and reproducibility issues; they are also sensitive to partial volume effects. While voxel- and tract-based methods allow for between groups-comparisons, voxel-based approaches require multiple options in each stage of the processing pipeline (normalizing, smoothing, statistical analysis) that can have a profound influence on the outcome of the analysis (Jones & Cercignani, 2010). Tract-based spatial statistics (Smith et al., 2006) are based on a non-linear registration of FA images from multiple subjects, circumvent arbitrariness of the choice of smoothing factors (Jones et al., 2005), and increase statistical power by reducing the total number of voxels to be tested by deriving a white matter skeleton. It is noteworthy to mention here that none of these approaches can directly localize specific tracts or provide anatomical information on connectivity of fiber tracts. By reconstructing white matter pathways in vivo, these analyses offer alternative approaches (Conturo et al., 1999; Mori et al., 1999; Basser et al., 2000).

Overall, the paucity of structural and diffusion tensor imaging studies directly comparing individuals with bipolar and unipolar disorders, the methodological heterogeneity among studies, as well as relatively small sample sizes in many studies, are limitations that need to be addressed in the future. Methodological advances in magnetic resonance magnetic field strengths, tissue segmentation techniques, and employment of sophisticated algorithms of surface and fiber reconstruction will promote a better understanding of gray and white matter abnormalities in individuals with bipolar and unipolar disorders.

---

**Structural Imaging of White Matter:**

· Rarely compared unipolar and bipolar disorders directly

· Suggests that depression in bipolar and unipolar disorder may be distinguished by FA in right uncinate fasciculus

· Supports a hypothesis that unipolar depression demonstrates left- but not right-sided abnormalities in amygdala-orbitomedial prefrontal cortical structural connectivity

· Further suggests that differential patterns of abnormal right and left orbitomedial prefrontal cortical-limbic structural connectivity may predispose women to in both bipolar and unipolar disorders

---

## FUNCTIONAL NEUROIMAGING STUDIES IN BIPOLAR AND UNIPOLAR DISORDER

A large number of studies highlight the amygdala as a key neural region in the processing of emotionally-salient stimuli (McDonald, 2003; Sah et al., 2003; Swanson, 2003). Neuroimaging studies have therefore begun to focus on examination of amygdala activity in bipolar and unipolar depression (Siegle et al., 2007; Phillips, Ladouceur et al.,

2008; Frangou, 2009; Almeida et al., 2010). There are several questions that remain unanswered regarding amygdala dysfunction in bipolar and unipolar depression, however. First, it is unclear whether abnormal amygdala activity in response to emotional facial expressions is a persistent marker of bipolar disorder during both remission and depression, or whether abnormal amygdala activity to these stimuli is a state marker of depression, common to, or differentiating, bipolar and unipolar depression. Earlier studies suggested elevated amygdala activity to happy and fearful facial expressions in remitted, depressed and hypomanic adults with bipolar disorder (Blumberg et al., 2005). Later studies did not, however, demonstrate abnormal amygdala activity to either negative (fearful, disgust, sad) or positive (happy) emotional facial expressions in remitted or stabilized adults with bipolar disorder (Malhi et al., 2007; Hassel et al., 2008; Jogia et al., 2008; Robinson et al., 2008). Similarly, recent studies reported no abnormality in amygdala activity to fearful, angry or sad facial expressions in depressed adults with bipolar disorder (Chen et al., 2006; Altshuler et al., 2008). In depressed adults with unipolar disorder, studies reported abnormally elevated amygdala activity to masked, covertly-presented fear, happy and neutral facial expressions (Sheline et al., 2001; Abler et al., 2007; Dannlowski et al., 2007); increased amygdala blood flow at rest (Drevets et al., 1992); and pre-treatment abnormalities in capacity of amygdala activity, the response elicited by the difference between baseline and all facial trials taken together, to sad and neutral emotional expressions (Fu et al., 2004). Other studies, however, reported no increases in amygdala activity to either happy, sad or fearful facial expressions, even in a subliminal condition, in depressed adults with recurrent episodes of unipolar disorder (Lawrence et al., 2004; Surguladze et al., 2005; Fu et al., 2007; Dannlowski et al., 2008). These discrepant findings in amygdala activity in response to facial expressions in remitted and depressed adults with bipolar disorder and in depressed adults with unipolar disorder likely result from different paradigms and different neuroimaging measures across these studies.

In addition, it is unclear whether abnormally elevated amygdala activity occurs predominantly in response to negative or to positive emotional facial expressions in bipolar disorder and recurrent episodes of unipolar disorder. While previous studies reported abnormally elevated amygdala activity to both positive and negative emotional facial expressions in remitted adults with bipolar disorder (Lawrence et al., 2004) and in remitted, depressed and hypomanic adults with bipolar disorder (Blumberg et al., 2005), studies in depressed adults with recurrent episodes of unipolar disorder reported abnormally elevated amygdala activity mainly in response to negative emotional facial expressions (Sheline et al., 2001; Fu et al., 2004; Dannlowski et al., 2007). Some findings suggest abnormally elevated amygdala activity to positive emotional facial expressions in depressed adults with unipolar disorder, however (Sheline et al., 2001).

In a recent study, we first examined the extent to which abnormally elevated amygdala activity to emotional facial expressions was one of the following three possibilities: 1) a persistent marker of bipolar disorder during remission and depression, 2) a state marker of depression in both bipolar disorder and recurrent episodes of unipolar disorder, or 3) a specific marker of depression in either bipolar disorder or recurrent episodes of unipolar disorder. We then examined whether abnormally elevated amygdala activity occurred mainly to negative or to positive emotional facial expressions in each disorder. Our third aim was to examine the extent that abnormally elevated amygdala activity would be elicited by emotional facial expressions other than those displaying prototypical emotion: namely, mild, intense, and neutral facial expressions. We recruited remitted and depressed adults with bipolar disorder, depressed adults with unipolar disorder, and a group of age- and sex ratio-matched healthy adults. We employed a well-validated facial expression processing paradigm involving displays of negative (fear, sad) and positive (happy) facial expressions as important signals of socially-relevant emotions of social approval (happy), external threat (fear) and internal distress (sad) of both prototypical (intense) and mild intensities of each emotion, together with neutral expressions.

We found abnormally elevated left amygdala activity that was specific to depressed adults with bipolar disorder, and elicited by all facial expressions in the sad experiment, in particular by mild sad and neutral facial expressions (Figure 6.2). Remitted adults with bipolar disorder and depressed adults with unipolar disorder did not statistically differ from healthy adults.

Our finding of a bipolar depression-specific pattern of abnormally elevated amygdala activity is interesting given the inconsistent findings in the literature regarding amygdala activity in remitted and depressed adults with bipolar disorder, and depressed adults with unipolar disorder (Sheline et al., 2001; Fu et al., 2004; Lawrence et al., 2004; Malhi et al., 2004; Blumberg et al., 2005; Surguladze et al., 2005; Dannlowski et al., 2007; Malhi et al., 2007; Altshuler et al., 2008; Jogia et al., 2008). There are several points to highlight in these previous studies, however. First, no previous study directly compared amygdala activity to different emotional facial expressions in remitted and depressed adults with bipolar disorder and unipolar disorder. Second, the discrepancy of these findings may relate to using different paradigms and different neuroimaging measures across the studies. Third, while previous studies of depressed individuals with unipolar disorder reported elevated amygdala activity mainly to negative emotional facial expressions (Blumberg, Donegan et al., 2005), there are points to consider about these studies. In two of these studies (Sheline et al., 2001; Fu et al., 2004; Dannlowski et al., 2007), facial expressions were presented covertly in a backward masking paradigm; furthermore, elevated left amygdala activity was observed to happy, fearful and neutral masked facial expressions in one (Sheline et al., 2001; Dannlowski et al., 2007). The backward masking procedure may have made these emotional facial expressions appear more ambiguous and potentially threatening, that may in turn have contributed to the elevated amygdala activity observed in depressed adults with unipolar disorder relative to healthy subjects in this study. In another study, greater capacity of amygdala activity to sad facial expressions was demonstrated in depressed adults with unipolar disorder (Sheline et al., 2001), but the extent to which this relates to greater magnitude of amygdala activity to negative emotional expressions remains unclear. Additional studies reported relationships between pre-treatment amygdala activity to emotional facial expressions and symptom improvement after treatment (Fu et al., 2004) and with depression symptom severity (Canli et al., 2005), but did not show abnormally elevated amygdala activity to these facial expressions in depressed adults with unipolar disorder relative to healthy adults. Furthermore, we previously showed elevated ventral striatal, but not elevated amygdala, activity in response to sad facial expressions in depressed adults with unipolar disorder (Surguladze et al., 2005). These previous findings, together with the present findings of abnormally elevated amygdala activity in depressed adults with bipolar disorder (but not remitted adults with bipolar disorder or depressed adults with unipolar disorder), therefore, suggest that abnormally elevated amygdala activity may represent a pathophysiological process specific to depression in bipolar disorder.

Using an overt emotion labeling task may have contributed to our findings of abnormally elevated amygdala activity only in depressed adults with bipolar disorder, and not in depressed adults with unipolar disorder or remitted adults with bipolar disorder. Previous reports indicate that, unlike implicit emotion processing such as gender labeling, explicit emotion labeling of facial expressions is not consistently associated with robust amygdala activity in healthy adults, as it may be dependent on explicit appraisal and

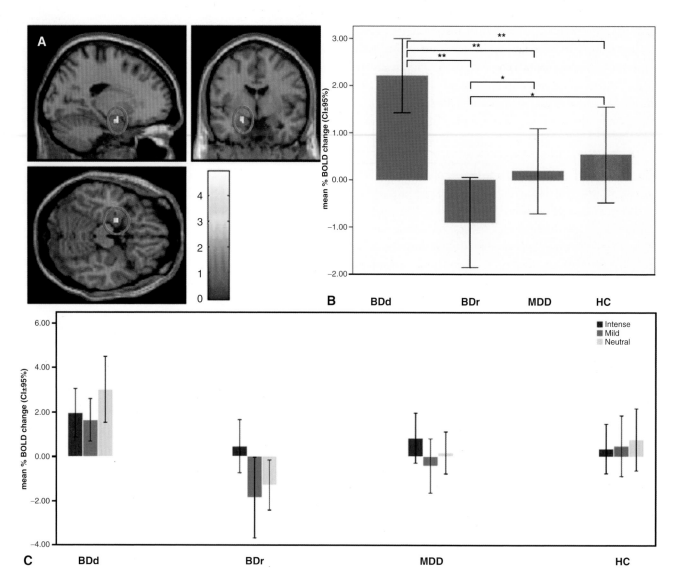

*Figure 6.2* Increased Amygdala Activity in Depressed Adults with Bipolar Disorder Panel A. Anatomical location of left amygdala activity where the main effect of group was statistically different during the sad experiment. Foci of significance were overlaid on sagittal, coronal and axial brain slices spatially normalized into the Montreal Neurologic Institute coordinates system (x = -18, y = -3, z = -18; cluster size = 11 voxels; F = 4.96; p = 0.003, corrected for multiple comparisons). Panel B. Mean left amygdala activity to faces in the sad experiment in each group (* trend toward significance; ** significant comparison after controlling for multiple comparisons). Panel C. Activity in the left amygdala in response to intense and mild sad and neutral faces in each group (Almeida, Versace et al. 2010).

re-appraisal processes supported by lateral prefrontal cortex rather than amygdala (Surguladze et al., 2005). Our finding of elevated amygdala activity in depressed adults with bipolar disorder in the present study may therefore reflect aberrant amygdala-lateral prefrontal cortical functional coupling during appraisal of emotion in depressed adults with bipolar, but not in depressed adults with unipolar disorder or in remitted adults with bipolar disorder, that could be examined in future studies using functional connectivity analyses. It is also possible that with larger numbers of participants, we would have been able to demonstrate significant increases in amygdala activity in depressed adults with unipolar

disorder and in remitted adults with bipolar disorder relative to healthy adults during the sad—or other emotion–experiments. The effect sizes in the significant *post hoc* pairwise between-group comparisons for the sad experiment (Cohen's d' = 1.02- d = 1.97) are similar to the effect sizes in previous between-group comparisons of amygdala activity (e.g., Lawrence et al., 2004), suggesting that our study was powered to detect meaningful between-group differences in amygdala activity during each emotion experiment consistent with previous findings.

Regarding our second aim, we found a negative-emotion specific pattern of abnormally elevated amygdala activity in depressed adults with bipolar disorder to all faces in the sad experiment relative to other groups. This finding is consistent with previous cognitive theories of depression proposing a negative emotion attentional bias in depression in general and in particular to self-relevant negative emotional material (Lange et al., 2003), such as mood-congruent, sad facial expressions in the present study. Our findings suggest, however, that the negative emotional attentional bias in bipolar disorder and recurrent depression in unipolar disorder may be associated with different pathophysiological processes in the two disorders.

We also previously demonstrated an attentional bias away from labeling "mild happy" facial expressions, but instead found a bias toward labeling "sad" facial expressions in depressed adults with unipolar disorder (Beck, 1967). These, together with the present, findings therefore suggest that recurrent depression in unipolar disorder may be characterized more by an inhibitory response to positive emotional facial expressions that may lead to an attentional bias away from these stimuli, rather than by attentional bias toward negative emotional facial expressions.

Regarding our third aim, depressed adults with bipolar disorder showed elevated amygdala activity to neutral and mild, rather than intense, sad facial expressions relative to remitted adults with bipolar disorder and depressed adults with unipolar disorder. Mild emotional and neutral facial expressions are often perceived as more ambiguous and potentially threatening than intense facial expressions (Surguladze et al., 2004), and may elicit amygdala activity because of the proposed role of this structure in processing ambiguity and potential threat (Calder et al., 2001; Surguladze et al., 2004). While depressed adults with bipolar disorder accurately labeled facial expressions in the sad and fear experiments, abnormally elevated amygdala activity to mild sad and neutral facial expressions may therefore suggest abnormal perception of potential threat in these faces, consistent with previous observations of abnormally elevated amygdala activity to neutral facial expressions appraised as hostile in youth with bipolar disorder (Davis & Whalen, 2001). Employment of subjective ratings of threat and hostility during facial expression emotion labeling in future studies in bipolar disorder could help clarify this.

The laterality of our amygdala findings in depressed adults with bipolar disorder is interesting. Previous studies report sustained response of the left rather than right amygdala during fearful facial expression processing in healthy adults (Rich et al., 2006), while studies that manipulated displays of facial expressions to prevent subjective awareness of these stimuli, most frequently through a backward masking procedure, reported right-sided lateralization

of amygdala activity (Phillips et al., 2001; Wright et al., 2001). In our analyses, we fitted a hemodynamic response function to the presentation of each facial stimulus, that models sustained rather than initial transient activity to all stimuli of a given emotion intensity in each experiment. Our finding of a between-group difference in left- rather than right-sided amygdala activity during facial emotion labeling therefore supports a more sustained and evaluative response of the left than right amygdala during emotion processing.

While there was no significant effect of group on emotion labeling in the sad experiment, all participants exhibited between 54 and 91 percent accuracy rather than nearer to 100 percent accuracy on labeling emotional faces. This was likely due to the known difficulty in accurately labeling mild emotional facial expressions from the facial expression series employed in our study (Morris et al., 1998). Previous studies in depressed adults indicated facial emotional expression labeling impairments in adults with bipolar and unipolar disorder (Calder et al., 1997). The more difficult facial expression labeling task that we used may have masked any between-group difference on task performance as all individuals had some difficulty with emotion face labeling.

Our exploratory analyses indicated few significant relationships between left amygdala activity to facial expressions in the sad experiment and clinical variables. Depressed adults with bipolar disorder with longer illness duration and higher medication load had lower amygdala activity to intense sad, but not mild sad or neutral, facial expressions. Previous findings in unipolar disorder indicate a reduction in amygdala capacity and activity after antidepressant treatment (Bozikas et al., 2006; Csukly et al., 2009; Rocca et al., 2009), which parallel our findings in medicated depressed adults with bipolar disorder in the present study. It is therefore possible that the combined effects of psychotropic medication and longer illness duration may have contributed to normalization of elevated left amygdala activity, at least to intense sad facial expressions, in depressed adults with bipolar disorder. The possible perception of the more ambiguous mild sad and neutral facial expressions as potentially threatening by depressed adults with bipolar disorder may have accounted for the absence of effects of illness duration and medication upon left amygdala activity to these stimuli. Greater left amygdala activity in remitted adults with bipolar disorder was associated with more accurate emotion labeling of all facial expressions, especially the more ambiguous mild sad facial expressions. Remitted adults with bipolar disorder taking antidepressant medication also showed greater left amygdala activity to the more ambiguous mild sad and neutral facial expressions, although did not differ from healthy adults on magnitude of left amygdala activity to these expressions. Together, these findings suggest that in remitted adults with bipolar disorder taking antidepressant medication, who are potentially more vulnerable to depression than remitted adults not taking antidepressant medication (since they require medication), greater left amygdala activity during emotion labeling of mild sad and neutral facial expressions may represent a persistent attentional bias to sad faces. A persistent attentional bias associated with more accurate sad emotion labeling may represent a vulnerability marker to depression in remitted adults with bipolar disorder. Depressed adults with unipolar disorder showed a positive correlation between left amygdala activity and age at scan and with age of unipolar illness onset, suggesting that older individuals with later age of illness onset had a pattern of left amygdala activity more similar to depressed adults with bipolar disorder.

**Functional imaging Studies:**

- Rarely compared unipolar and bipolar disorders directly

- Suggest abnormally elevated amygdala activity may represent a pathophysiological process specific to depression in bipolar disorder in response to emotional faces

- Suggest amygdala in bipolar disorder may be excessively responsive to mild emotional expressions

- Suggest increased left amygdala activation to emotional faces may represent a risk-marker for depression in bipolar disorder

## FUNCTIONAL AND EFFECTIVE CONNECTIVITY STUDIES OF BIPOLAR AND UNIPOLAR DISORDER

Few studies have examined the extent to which abnormal functional integration between amygdala and orbitomedial prefrontal cortex characterizes bipolar disorder. Functional connectivity refers to a correlation over time between activities in different neural regions. In contrast, effective connectivity refers to the impact that activity in one region exerts over that in another, and it can be used to estimate forward (bottom-up) versus back (top-down) connectivity between regions. Effective connectivity can be examined using dynamic causal modeling, a technique for estimating, and making inferences about, the negative or positive influence that one region exerts over another, and how this is

affected by experimental context (Fu et al., 2004; Canli et al., 2005). Only one study has examined functional connectivity in bipolar disorder. In this study reduced functional connectivity between ventrolateral prefrontal cortex and amygdala was reported in manic adults with bipolar disorder relative to healthy adults during an emotion-labeling task (Friston et al., 2003). Only two studies investigated effective connectivity using dynamic causal modeling in bipolar disorder (Foland et al., 2008). The first study compared remitted adults with bipolar disorder with healthy adults while performing an event-related functional magnetic resonance imaging paradigm, viewing mild and intense happy and neutral faces. Here, remitted adults with bipolar disorder had greater effective connectivity from the right parahippocampal gyrus to the subgenual cingulate cortex when compared to healthy adults, reflecting more rapid, and forward signaling.

Only one study directly compared effective connectivity in depressed adults with bipolar disorder vs. depressed adults with unipolar disorder (Almeida, Mechelli et al., 2009a; Almeida, Versace et al., 2009). In this study, we showed different patterns of abnormal left-sided top-down orbitomedial prefrontal cortex-amygdala during happy emotion labeling in depressed adults with bipolar and unipolar disorder relative to healthy adults. Additionally, depressed adults with bipolar disorder differed from depressed adults with unipolar disorder and from healthy adults on right-sided bottom-up amygdala-orbitomedial prefrontal cortex effective connectivity (Figure 6.3). Depressed adults with unipolar disorder showed significantly greater negative left-sided top-down orbitomedial prefrontal cortex-amygdala effective connectivity than healthy adults, while depressed adults with bipolar disorder showed significantly reduced positive left-sided top-down orbitomedial prefrontal cortex-amygdala effective connectivity and greater negative right-sided bottom-up amygdala-orbitomedial prefrontal cortex effective connectivity than healthy adults.

The reduced left-sided top-down effective connectivity in the happy experiment in depressed adults with bipolar disorder versus healthy adults may reflect reduced regulation of left amygdala by orbitomedial prefrontal cortex—that is, a disconnection—during positive emotion processing. This parallels previous functional neuroimaging studies in bipolar disorder reporting abnormally increased left-sided amygdala and striatal activity to happy faces (Almeida, Versace et al., 2009b), and abnormally decreased left-sided orbitomedial prefrontal cortex activity during emotion regulation (Lawrence et al., 2004; Blumberg et al., 2005; Hassel et al., 2008), that we previously highlighted

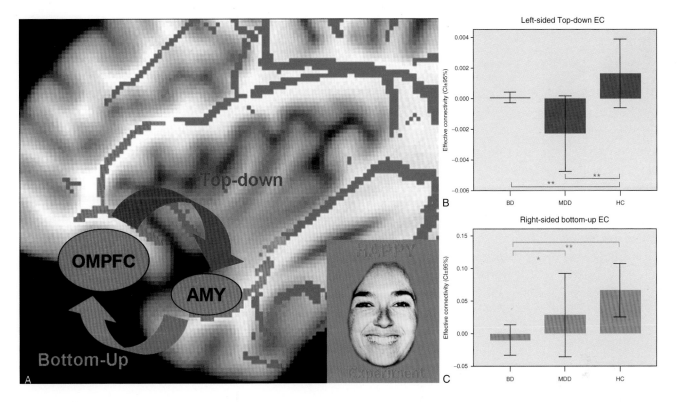

Figure 6.3 Effective Connectivity between Orbitomedial Prefrontal Cortex and Amygdala Panel A. Representation of the bottom-up (red arrow) and top-down (blue arrow) endogenous connection between left amygdala and left orbitomedial prefrontal cortex. Panel B. Left-sided top-down orbitomedial prefrontal cortex -amygdala effective connectivity in the happy experiment. Happy experiment: negative effective connectivity in depressed adults with unipolar disorder relative to healthy adults (**U = 52, p = 0.004; d = 0.95) A close to zero effective connectivity in depressed adults with bipolar disorder when relative to HC (**U = 52, p = 0.007; d = 0.65). There were no difference between the two depressed groups on this effective connectivity measure (*U = 83; p = 0.14; d = 0.67). Panel C. Right-sided bottom-up amygdala- orbitomedial prefrontal cortex effective connectivity in the happy experiment. Happy experiment: reduced effective connectivity in depressed adults with unipolar disorder relative to healthy adults (**U = 110, p = 0.5; d = 0.37). A close to zero effective connectivity in depressed adults with bipolar disorder relative to healthy adults (**U = 42, p = 0.002; d = 1.2). There was a trend difference between the two depressed groups on this effective connectivity measure (*U = 64; p = 0.027; d = 0.42)(Almeida et al. 2009).

(Blumberg et al., 2005). This left-sided reduction in top-down orbitomedial prefrontal cortex-amygdala effective connectivity, possibly reflecting reduced regulation of amygdala by orbitomedial prefrontal cortex during positive emotion processing, may represent a predisposition to elevated mood and mania in bipolar disorder. Conversely, depressed adults with unipolar disorder showed left-sided top-down negative orbitomedial prefrontal cortex-amygdala effective connectivity in the happy experiment. This finding may reflect increased inhibition of the left amygdala by left orbitomedial prefrontal cortex to positive emotional stimuli that parallels previous functional neuroimaging findings in depressed adults with unipolar disorder of abnormally reduced left striatal activity to positive emotional stimuli (Elliott et al., 2004). The increased negative orbitomedial prefrontal cortex-amygdala effective connectivity to happy faces may therefore represent an "over-regulation" by orbitomedial prefrontal cortex of the amygdala to these stimuli and a potential neural basis for

the increased negative and reduced positive emotional attentional bias that is frequently observed in major depression (Phillips, Ladouceur et al., 2008). Together, these findings suggest that different patterns of abnormal left-sided top-down orbitomedial prefrontal cortex-amygdala effective connectivity during positive emotion processing may reflect different neural mechanisms in bipolar and unipolar depression, and also support a role of the left hemisphere in positive emotion processing (Surguladze et al., 2005; Epstein et al., 2006).

Only depressed adults with bipolar disorder differed from healthy adults on right-sided bottom-up amygdala-orbitomedial prefrontal cortex effective connectivity during the happy experiment: This observation was positive in healthy and unipolar depressed adults, but negative in bipolar depressed adults, suggesting an inverse functional relationship between right amygdala and orbitomedial prefrontal cortex during happy emotion processing in depressed adults with bipolar disorder—that is, less amygdala activity associated with greater orbitomedial prefrontal cortex activity. This pattern of abnormal right amygdala-orbitomedial prefrontal cortex effective connectivity during the happy experiment is difficult to explain in the context of the hemispheric specialization of emotion theory previously discussed, but does suggest aberrant forward connectivity between right amygdala and right orbitomedial prefrontal cortex during emotion processing in bipolar more than unipolar depression. This finding also suggests that bipolar depression may be associated with functional abnormalities in neural systems supporting emotion regulation in both hemispheres, while unipolar depression may be associated with a functional abnormality predominantly within the left hemisphere, as previously observed in human lesion studies (Beck 1967). This interpretation is supported by the loss of normal left-right asymmetry in resting frontal activity in electroencephalogram studies of depression (Davidson and Irwin 1999). The involvement of functional abnormalities in both hemispheres in bipolar depression parallels our previous observation of abnormalities in left and right amygdala-orbitomedial prefrontal cortex white matter structure in bipolar disorder (Versace et al., 2008). (Table 6.3).

Therefore, taken together, these findings suggest that depressed adults with unipolar disorder may be better characterized by an inhibitory response to positive emotional facial expressions that may lead to an attentional bias away from these stimuli, rather than by attentional bias toward negative emotional facial expressions. By contrast, depressed adults with bipolar disorder may be characterized by an attentional bias to negative, mood-congruent expressions rather than an attentional bias away from happy faces.

**Functional & Effective Connectivity Studies Demonstrate That:**

- Bipolar & unipolar depression with abnormal left-sided top-down medial prefrontal—amygdala connectivity

- Bipolar depressed differ from unipolar depressed and healthy adults on right-sided bottom-up amygdala-medial prefrontal effective connectivity

- Unipolar depressed adults demonstrate attentional bias away from positive emotional stimuli, rather than toward negative emotional facial expressions

- Depressed bipolar disorder demonstrates attentional bias to negative, mood-congruent expressions rather than away from happy faces

## LIMITATIONS OF NEUROIMAGING STUDIES IN BIPOLAR DISORDER AND UNIPOLAR DISORDER

*Medication*: One potential limitation of neuroimaging studies of individuals with both bipolar and unipolar depression is the potential impact of psychotropic medication upon neuroimaging measures. Findings indicate, however, normalizing rather than confounding effects of psychotropic medication upon the majority of neuroimaging findings in individuals with bipolar and unipolar disorder (Robinson et al., 1984; Fedoroff et al., 1992; Jorge et al., 1993; Henriques & Davidson 1990; Allen et al., 1993; Haznedar et al., 2005; Blackhart et al., 2006; Versace et al., 2008; Versace, Almeida et al., 2010).

TABLE 6.3 FUNCTIONAL NEUROIMAGING STUDIES DIRECTLY COMPARING BD AND UD

| Study | Group (M/F) Age (yy) | Main findings |
|---|---|---|
| Lawrence et al. 2004 | 12 BD remission (7/5)<br>9 UD (5/4)<br>11 HI (7/4) | Elevated left amygdala activity to both positive and negative emotional facial expressions in remitted adults with BD compared to HI and adults with UD |
| Almeida, Versace et al. 2009 | 15 BD depression (1/14)<br>16 UD (3/13)<br>16 HC (4/12) | Left-sided, top-down orbitomedial prefrontal cortex -amygdala distinguished depressed adults with BD and UD from HI; and right-sided, bottom-up, amygdala-orbitomedial prefrontal cortex effective connectivity distinguished depressed adults with BD from depressed adults with UD during positive stimuli |
| Almeida et al. 2010 | 15 BD depression (1/14)<br>15 BD remission (5/10)<br>15 UD (2/13)<br>15 HI (3/12) | Elevated left amygdala activity to negative emotional facial expression in depressed adults with BD compared to remitted adults with BD, depressed adults with UD and HI |

BD: bipolar disorder; UD: unipolar disorder; HI: healthy individuals

*Sex Differences*: The sex ratio in studies of unipolar disorder, and to some extent studies of bipolar disorder, usually favor women, given the higher prevalence of mood disorders in women (Almeida et al., 2009b; Almeida et al., 2010). The extent to which pathophysiological processes in bipolar and unipolar disorder differ between men and women therefore remains little studied and should be a focus of future research.

## SUMMARY AND FUTURE DIRECTIONS

Together, converging findings from structural, diffusion tensor and, and functional neuroimaging studies indicate gray matter, structural and functional abnormalities in prefrontal cortical-amygdala neural circuitry supporting mood regulation in individuals with bipolar disorder and those with unipolar disorder. Only a small number of neuroimaging studies have directly compared depressed adults with bipolar disorder and those with unipolar disorder, but emerging findings suggest differential patterns of gray and white matter abnormalities, together with differential patterns of activity and effective connectivity, within this circuitry. In particular, these findings suggest that structural and functional effective connectivity abnormalities in prefrontal cortical-amygdala circuitry may be evident to a greater extent in depressed adults with bipolar disorder relative to depressed adults with unipolar disorder, and that abnormally elevated left amygdala activity to negative emotional stimuli may be a marker of depression in bipolar disorder more than unipolar disorder. Future studies can build on these findings to determine the extent to which these neuroimaging measures can yield biomarkers to help differentiate bipolar from unipolar disorder, especially in individuals presenting in depressed episode.

A new approach in psychiatric neuroimaging is to employ pattern recognition techniques to help classify individuals on a case-by-case basis into diagnostic groupings. Support vector machine learning is one example of a pattern recognition approach that identifies a decision boundary to discriminate groups based on a training dataset (e.g., structural, diffusion tensor, or functional neuroimaging data form whole brain or regions of interest) to then enable classification of new test data into different groupings based on the previously-identified decision function (Goodwin & Jamison, 2007). The classification procedure consists of two phases: training and testing. During the training phase, the support vector machine finds the decision boundaries that separate the highly correlated data (e.g., a region in the brain) according to their group (e.g., unipolar depression or bipolar depression). Once the boundaries are decided, it can be used to predict the group of new group of test individuals. These approaches therefore have potential to be used to identify neuroimaging measures that provide classifiers for individual subject classification (i.e., if a specific subject belongs to one group—unipolar depression; or to another—bipolar depression).

Another more recent approach has been to employ neuroimaging to examine abnormalities in neural circuitry supporting mood regulation that may predispose to future bipolar or unipolar disorder in individuals at risk for these illnesses in the future (Fu et al., 2008). Longitudinal neuroimaging studies are clearly needed to elucidate abnormal developmental trajectories of mood regulation circuitry in these individuals to help identify developmental trajectories predisposing to bipolar versus unipolar disorder that in turn can help provide biological targets for early interventions.

Finally, emerging findings from neuroimaging studies of depressed adults with unipolar disorder indicate that specific neuroimaging measures, in particular, magnitude of activity in rostral anterior cingulate cortex (Vapnik 1995; Mourao-Miranda, et al., 2005), may predict subsequent response to antidepressant treatment. There are almost no longitudinal neuroimaging studies of bipolar disorder, however, and no neuroimaging studies that have examined the extent to which neuroimaging measures may be used to help predict future treatment response.

In summary, promising findings from a variety of different structural neuroimaging, DTI and functional neuroimaging studies in adults with bipolar and unipolar disorder indicate that neuroimaging measures can help increase understanding of pathophysiological processes that may differentiate bipolar from unipolar disorder, particularly in the context of depression. New approaches can be used to help identify further neuroimaging measures that may differentiate the two illnesses; help identify neuroimaging measures that may help identify individuals most of risk of developing these illness; and help provide biological targets for treatment response prediction in bipolar and unipolar disorder.

## REFERENCES

Abler, B., Erk, S., Herwig, U., & Walter, H. 2007. Anticipation of aversive stimuli activates extended amygdala in unipolar depression. *Journal of Psychiatric Research,* 41(6), 511–522. doi: S0022-3956(06)00171-3 [pii] 10.1016/j.jpsychires.2006.07.020

Adler, C. M., Adams, J., DelBello, M. P., Holland, S. K., Schmithorst, V., Levine, A.... K., Strakowski, S.M. 2006. Evidence of white matter pathology in bipolar disorder adolescents experiencing their first episode of mania: a diffusion tensor imaging study. *American Journal of Psychiatry*, 163(2), 322–324. doi: 163/2/322 [pii] 10.1176/appi. ajp.163.2.322

Alexander, A. L., Lee, J. E., Lazar, M., & Field, A. S. 2007. Diffusion tensor imaging of the brain. *Neurotherapeutics,* 4(3), 316–329. doi: S1933-7213(07)00095-5 [pii] 10.1016/j.nurt.2007.05.011

Alexopoulos, G. S., Kiosses, D. N., Choi, S. J., Murphy, C. F., & Lim, K. O. 2002. Frontal white matter microstructure and treatment response of late-life depression: A preliminary study. *American Journal of Psychiatry*, 159(11), 1929–1932.

Allen, J. J., Iacono, W. G., Depue, R. A., & Arbisi, P. 1993. Regional electroencephalographic asymmetries in bipolar seasonal affective disorder before and after exposure to bright light. *Biological psychiatry*, 33(8-9), 642–646.

Almeida, J. R. C., Mechelli, A., Hassel, S., Versace, A., Kupfer, D. J., & Phillips, M. L. 2009. Abnormally increased effective connectivity between parahippocampal gyrus and ventromedial prefrontal regions during emotion labeling in bipolar disorder. *Psychiatry Research - Neuroimaging*, 174(3), 195–201.

Almeida, J. R., A. Versace, et al. (2009). Abnormal amygdala-prefrontal effective connectivity to happy faces differentiates bipolar from major depression. *Biological Psychiatry* 66(5): 451–459.

Almeida, J. R. C., Versace, A., Hassel, S., Kupfer, D. J., & Phillips, M. L. 2010. Elevated Amygdala Activity to Sad Facial Expressions: A State Marker of Bipolar but Not Unipolar Depression. [doi: DOI: 10.1016/j.biopsych.2009.09.027]. *Biological Psychiatry*, 67(5), 414–421.

Almeida, J. R. C., Versace, A., Mechelli, A., Hassell, S., Quevedo, K., Kupfer, D. J.... Phillips, M.L. 2009. Orbitomedial Prefrontal Cortical-Amygdala Effective Connectivity during Positive Emotion Processing Discriminates Bipolar from Major Depression. *Biological Psychiatry*, 65(8), 14.

Altshuler, L., Bookheimer, S., Townsend, J., Proenza, M. A., Sabb, F., Mintz, J.... Cohen, M.S. 2008. Regional brain changes in bipolar I depression: a functional magnetic resonance imaging study. *Bipolar Disord,* 10(6), 708–717. doi: BDI617 [pii] 10.1111/j.1399-5618. 2008.00617.x

Altshuler, L. L., Bartzokis, G., Grieder, T., Curran, J., & Mintz, J. 1998. Amygdala enlargement in bipolar disorder and hippocampal reduction in schizophrenia: An MRI study demonstrating neuroanatomic specificity. [Letter]. *Archives of General Psychiatry,* 55(7), 663–664.

Bae, J. N., MacFall, J. R., Krishnan, K. R. R., Payne, M. E., Steffens, D. C., & Taylor, W. D. 2006. Dorsolateral prefrontal cortex and anterior cingulate cortex white matter alterations in late-life depression. *Biological Psychiatry*, 60(12), 1356–1363.

Ballmaier, M., Toga, A. W., Blanton, R. E., Sowell, E. R., Lavretsky, H., Peterson, J. Kumar, A. 2004. Anterior cingulate, gyrus rectus, and orbitofrontal abnormalities in elderly depressed patients: An MRI-based parcellation of the prefrontal cortex. [Article]. *American Journal of Psychiatry*, 161(1), 99–108.

Barnea-Goraly, N., Chang, K. D., Karchemskiy, A., Howe, M. E., & Reiss, A. L. 2009. Limbic and corpus callosum aberrations in adolescents with bipolar disorder: a tract-based spatial statistics analysis. *Biological Psychiatry,* 66(3), 238–244. doi: S0006-3223(09)00292-3 [pii] 10.1016/j.biopsych.2009.02.025

Basser, P. J., Pajevic, S., Pierpaoli, C., Duda, J., & Aldroubi, A. 2000. In vivo fiber tractography using DT-MRI data. *Magnetic Resonance in Medicine,* 44(4), 625–632. doi: 10.1002/1522-2594(200010) 44:4<625::AID-MRM17>3.0.CO;2-O [pii]

Beck, A. T. 1967. *Depression: Causes and treatments.* Philadelphia: University of Pennsylvania Press.

Beyer, J. L., Taylor, W. D., MacFall, J. R., Kuchibhatla, M., Payne, M. E., Provenzale, J. M. Krishnan, K.R.R. 2005. Cortical white matter microstructural abnormalities in bipolar disorder. *Neuropsychopharmacology*, 30(12), 2225–2229.

Blackhart, G. C., Minnix, J. A., & Kline, J. P. 2006. Can EEG asymmetry patterns predict future development of anxiety and depression? A preliminary study. *Biological Psychology,* 72(1), 46–50.

Blumberg, H. P., Donegan, N. H., Sanislow, C. A., Collins, S., Lacadie, C., Skudlarski, P.... Krystal, J.H. 2005. Preliminary evidence for medication effects on functional abnormalities in the amygdala and anterior cingulate in bipolar disorder. *Psychopharmacology*, 183(3), 308–313. doi: 10.1007/s00213-005-0156-7

Blumberg, H. P., Fredericks, C., Wang, F., Kalmar, J. H., Spencer, L., Papademetris, X.... Krystal, J.H. 2005. Preliminary evidence for persistent abnormalities in amygdala volumes in adolescents and young adults with bipolar disorder. *Bipolar Disorders*, 7(6), 570–576.

Bozikas, V. P., Tonia, T., Fokas, K., Karavatos, A., & Kosmidis, M. H. 2006. Impaired emotion processing in remitted patients with bipolar disorder. *Journal of Affective Disorders,* 91(1), 53–56. doi: S0165-0327(05)00349-6 [pii] 10.1016/j.jad.2005.11.013

Brambilla, P., Harenski, K., Nicoletti, M., Sassi, R. B., Mallinger, A. G., Frank, E.... Soares, J.C. 2003. MRI investigation of temporal lobe structures in bipolar patients. [Proceedings Paper]. *Journal of Psychiatric Research*, 37(4), 287–295. doi: 10.1016/s0022-3956(03)00024-4

Brambilla, P., Nicoletti, M. A., Harenski, K., Sassi, R. B., Mallinger, A. G., Frank, E. Soares, J.C. 2002. Anatomical MRI study of subgenual prefrontal cortex in bipolar and unipolar subjects. [Article]. *Neuropsychopharmacology*, 27(5), 792–799.

Bremner, J. D., Narayan, M., Anderson, E. R., Staib, L. H., Miller, H. L., & Charney, D. S. 2000. Hippocampal volume reduction in major depression. [Article]. *American Journal of Psychiatry*, 157(1), 115–117.

Bremner, J. D., Vythilingam, M., Vermetten, E., Nazeer, A., Adil, J., Khan, S.... Charney, D.S. 2002. Reduced volume of orbitofrontal cortex in major depression. [Article]. *Biological Psychiatry,* 51(4), 273–279.

Bruno, S., Cercignani, M., & Ron, M. A. 2008. White matter abnormalities in bipolar disorder: a voxel-based diffusion tensor study. *Bipolar Disorders,* 10(4), 460–468.

Caetano, S. C., Kaur, S., Brambilla, P., Nicoletti, M., Hatch, J. P., Sassi, R. B.... Soares, J.C. 2006. Smaller cingulate volumes in unipolar depressed patients. [Proceedings Paper]. *Biological Psychiatry*, 59(8), 702–706. doi: 10.1016/j.biopsych.2005.10.011

Calder, A. J., Burton, A. M., Miller, P., Young, A. W., & Akamatsu, S. 2001. A principal component analysis of facial expressions. *Vision Research*, 41(9), 1179–1208. doi: S0042-6989(01)00002-5 [pii]

Calder, A. J., Young, A. W., Rowland, D., & Perrett, D. I. 1997. Computer-enhanced emotion in facial expressions. *Proceedings. Biological Sciences,* 264(1383), 919–925. doi: 10.1098/rspb. 1997.0127

Canli, T., Cooney, R. E., Goldin, P., Shah, M., Sivers, H., Thomason, M. E. Gotlib, I.H. 2005. Amygdala reactivity to emotional faces predicts improvement in major depression. *Neuroreport*, 16(12), 1267–1270. doi: 00001756-200508220-00003 [pii]

Chaddock, C. A., Barker, G. J., Marshall, N., Schulze, K., Hall, M. H., Fern, A.... McDonald, C. 2009. White matter microstructural impairments and genetic liability to familial bipolar I disorder. *British Journal of Psychiatry*, 194(6), 527–534. doi: 194/6/527 [pii] 10.1192/bjp.bp.107.047498

Chang, K., Karchemskiy, A., Barnea-Goraly, N., Garrett, A., Simeonova, D. I., & Reiss, A. 2005. Reduced amygdalar gray matter volume in familial pediatric bipolar disorder. [Proceedings Paper]. *Journal of the American Academy of Child and Adolescent Psychiatry*, 44(6), 565–573. doi: 10.1097/01.chi.0000159948.75136.0d

Chen, C. H., Lennox, B., Jacob, R., Calder, A., Lupson, V., Bisbrown-Chippendale, R.... Bullmore, E. 2006. Explicit and implicit facial affect recognition in manic and depressed States of bipolar disorder: a functional magnetic resonance imaging study. *Biological Psychiatry*, 59(1), 31–39. doi: S0006-3223(05)00714-6 [pii] 10.1016/ j.biopsych.2005.06.008

Conturo, T. E., Lori, N. F., Cull, T. S., Akbudak, E., Snyder, A. Z., Shimony, J. S.... Raichle, M.E. 1999. Tracking neuronal fiber pathways in the living human brain. *Proceedings of the National Academy of Sciences of the United States of America*, 96(18), 10422–10427.

Cotter, D. R., Mackay, D., Beasley, C. L., Everall, I. P., & Landau, S. 2002. The density, size and spatial pattern distribution of neurons and glia in area 9 prefrontal cortex in schizophrenia, bipolar disorder and major depression. *Schizophrenia Research*, 53(3), 107–108.

Csukly, G., Czobor, P., Szily, E., Takacs, B., & Simon, L. 2009. Facial expression recognition in depressed subjects: the impact of intensity level and arousal dimension. *Journal of Nervous and Mental Disease*, 197(2), 98–103. doi: 10.1097/NMD.0b013e3181923f82 00005053-200902000-00004 [pii]

Dannlowski, U., Ohrmann, P., Bauer, J., Deckert, J., Hohoff, C., Kugel, H.... Suslow, T. 2008. 5-HTTLPR biases amygdala activity in response to masked facial expressions in major depression. *Neuropsychopharmacology*, 33(2), 418–424. doi: 1301411 [pii] 10.1038/sj.npp.1301411

Dannlowski, U., Ohrmann, P., Bauer, J., Kugel, H., Arolt, V., Heindel, W.... Suslow, T. 2007. Amygdala reactivity to masked negative faces is associated with automatic judgmental bias in major depression: a 3 T fMRI study. *Journal of Psychiatry & Neuroscience*, 32(6), 423–429.

Davidson, R. J., & Irwin, W. 1999. The functional neuroanatomy of emotion and affective style. *Trends in Cognitive Sciences*, 3(1), 11–21.

Davis, M., & Whalen, P. J. 2001. The amygdala: vigilance and emotion. *Molecular Psychiatry*, 6(1), 13–34.

DelBello, M. P., Zimmerman, M. E., Mills, N. P., Getz, G. E., & Strakowski, S. M. 2004. Magnetic resonance imaging analysis of amygdala and other subcortical brain regions in adolescents with bipolar disorder. [Article]. *Bipolar Disorders*, 6(1), 43–52.

Dickstein, D. P., Milham, M. P., Nugent, A. C., Drevets, W. C., Charney, D. S., Pine, D. S.... Leibenluft, E. 2005. Frontotemporal alterations in pediatric bipolar disorder - Results of a voxel-based morphometry study. [Article]. *Archives of General Psychiatry*, 62(7), 734–741.

Drevets, W. C., Price, J. L., Simpson, J. R., Todd, R. D., Reich, T., Vannier, M.... M., Raichle, M.E. 1997. Subgenual prefrontal cortex abnormalities in mood disorders. [Article]. *Nature*, 386(6627), 824–827.

Drevets, W. C., Videen, T. O., Price, J. L., Preskorn, S. H., Carmichael, S. T., & Raichle, M. E. 1992. A functional anatomical study of unipolar depression. *Journal of Neuroscience*, 12(9), 3628–3641.

Elliott, R., Ogilvie, A., Rubinsztein, J. S., Calderon, G., Dolan, R. J., & Sahakian, B. J. 2004. Abnormal ventral frontal response during performance of an affective go/no go task in patients with mania. *Biological Psychiatry*, 55(12), 1163–1170.

Epstein, J., Pan, H., Kocsis, J. H., Yang, Y., Butler, T., Chusid, J.... Silbersweig, D.A. 2006. Lack of ventral striatal response to positive stimuli in depressed versus normal subjects. *American Journal of Psychiatry*, 163(10), 1784–1790.

Fedoroff, J. P., Starkstein, S. E., Forrester, A. W., Geisler, F. H., Jorge, R. E., Arndt, S. V.... Robinson, R.G. 1992. Depression in patients with acute traumatic brain injury. *American Journal of Psychiatry*, 149(7), 918–923.

Foland, L. C., Altshuler, L. L., Bookheimer, S. Y., Eisenberger, N., Townsend, J., & Thompson, P. M. 2008. Evidence for deficient modulation of amygdala response by prefrontal cortex in bipolar mania. *Psychiatry Research: Neuroimaging*, 162(1), 27.

Frangou, S. 2009. Functional neuroimaging in mood disorders. *Psychiatry*, 8(3), 102–104.

Frazier, J. A., Ahn, M. S., DeJong, S., Bent, E. K., Breeze, J. L., & Giuliano, A. J. 2005. Magnetic Resonance Imaging Studies in Early-Onset Bipolar Disorder: A Critical Review. *Harvard Review of Psychiatry*, 13(3), 125–140. doi: 10.1080/10673220591003597

Frazier, J. A., Breeze, J. L., Papadimitriou, G., Kennedy, D. N., Hodge, S. M., Moore, C. M.... Giuliano, A.J. 2007. White matter abnormalities in children with and at risk for bipolar disorder. *Bipolar Disorders*,

9(8), 799-809. doi: BDI482 [pii] 10.1111/j.1399-5618.2007.00482.x

Friston, K. J., Harrison, L., & Penny, W. 2003. Dynamic causal modelling. *NeuroImage*, 19(4), 1273–1302.

Frodl, T., Meisenzahl, E., Zetzsche, T., Bottlender, R., Born, C., Groll, C.... Moller, H.J. 2002. Enlargement of the amygdala in patients with a first episode of major depression. [Article]. *Biological Psychiatry*, 51(9), 708–714.

Fu, C. H., Mourao-Miranda, J., Costafreda, S. G., Khanna, A., Marquand, A. F., Williams, S. C.... Brammer, M.J. 2008. Pattern classification of sad facial processing: toward the development of neurobiological markers in depression. *Biological Psychiatry*, 63(7), 656–662. doi: S0006-3223(07)00877-3 [pii] 10.1016/j.biopsych.2007.08.020

Fu, C. H., Williams, S. C., Brammer, M. J., Suckling, J., Kim, J., Cleare, A. J.... Bullmore, E.T. 2007. Neural responses to happy facial expressions in major depression following antidepressant treatment. *American Journal of Psychiatry*, 164(4), 599–607. doi: 164/4/599 [pii] 10.1176/appi.ajp.164.4.599

Fu, C. H., Williams, S. C., Cleare, A. J., Brammer, M. J., Walsh, N. D., Kim, J. Bullmore, E.T. 2004. Attenuation of the neural response to sad faces in major depression by antidepressant treatment: a prospective, event-related functional magnetic resonance imaging study. *Archives of General Psychiatry*, 61(9), 877–889. doi: 10.1001/archpsyc.61.9.877 61/9/877 [pii]

Goodwin, F. K., & Jamison, K. R. 2007. *Manic-depressive illness : bipolar disorders and recurrent depression* (2 ed.). New York, N.Y.: Oxford University Press.

Harrison, P. J. 2002. The neuropathology of primary mood disorder. *Brain*, 125, 1428–1449.

Hasan, K. M., & Narayana, P. A. 2006. Retrospective measurement of the diffusion tensor eigenvalues from diffusion anisotropy and mean diffusivity in DTI. *Magnetic Resonance in Medicine*, 56(1), 130–137.

Hassel, S., Almeida, J. R. C., Kerr, N., Nau, S., Ladouceur, C. D., Fissell, K.... Phillips, M.L. 2008. Elevated striatal and decreased dorsolateral prefrontal cortical activity in response to emotional stimuli in euthymic bipolar disorder: no associations with psychotropic medication load. *Bipolar Disorders*, 10(8), 916–927.

Hastings, R. S., Parsey, R. V., Oquendo, M. A., Arango, V., & Mann, J. J. 2004. Volumetric analysis of the prefrontal cortex, amygdala, and hippocampus in major depression. [Article]. *Neuropsychopharmacology*, 29(5), 952–959. doi: 10.1038/sj.npp.1300371

Haznedar, M. M., Roversi, F., Pallanti, S., Baldini-Rossi, N., Schnur, D. B., LiCalzi, E. M.... Buchsbaum, M.S. 2005. Fronto-thalamo-striatal gray and white matter volumes and anisotropy of their connections in bipolar spectrum illnesses. *Biological Psychiatry*, 57(7), 733–742.

Heng, S., Song, A. W., & Sim, K. 2010. White matter abnormalities in bipolar disorder: insights from diffusion tensor imaging studies. *Journal of Neural Transmission*, 117(5), 639–654. doi: DOI 10.1007/s00702-010-0368-9

Henriques, J. B., & Davidson, R. J. 1990. Regional brain electrical asymmetries discriminate between previously depressed and healthy control subjects. *Journal of Abnormal Psychology*, 99(1), 22–31.

Hirschfeld, R. M., Lewis, L., & Vornik, L. A. 2003. Perceptions and impact of bipolar disorder: how far have we really come? Results of the national depressive and manic-depressive association 2000 survey of individuals with bipolar disorder. *Journal of Clinical Psychiatry*, 64(2), 161–174.

Hoptman, M.J., Gunning-Dixon, F.M., Murphy, C.F., Ardekani, B.A., Hrabe, J., Lim, K.O., ... Alexopoulos, G.S. 2009. Blood pressure and white matter integrity in geriatric depression. *Journal of Affective Disorders*, 115, 171–176.

Houenou, J., Wessa, M., Douaud, G., Leboyer, M., Chanraud, S., Perrin, M.... Paillere-Martinot, M.L. 2007. Increased white matter connectivity in euthymic bipolar patients: diffusion tensor tractography between the subgenual cingulate and the amygdalo-hippocampal complex. *Molecular Psychiatry, 12*(11), 1001–1010. doi: 4002010 [pii] 10.1038/sj.mp.4002010

Jogia, J., Haldane, M., Cobb, A., Kumari, V., & Frangou, S. 2008. Pilot investigation of the changes in cortical activation during facial affect recognition with lamotrigine monotherapy in bipolar disorder. *British Journal of Psychiatry, 192*(3), 197–201. doi: 192/3/197 [pii] 10.1192/bjp.bp.107.037960

Jones, D. K., & Cercignani, M. 2010. Twenty-five pitfalls in the analysis of diffusion MRI data. *NMR in Biomedicine, 23*(7), 803–820. doi: 10.1002/nbm.1543

Jones, D. K., Symms, M. R., Cercignani, M., & Howard, R. J. 2005. The effect of filter size on VBM analyses of DT-MRI data. *Neuroimage, 26*(2), 546–554. doi: S1053-8119(05)00095-9 [pii] 10.1016/j.neuroimage.2005.02.013

Jorge, R. E., Robinson, R. G., Arndt, S. V., Starkstein, S. E., Forrester, A. W., & Geisler, F. 1993. Depression following traumatic brain injury: a 1 year longitudinal study. *Journal of affective disorders, 27*(4), 233–243.

Kafantaris, V., Kingsley, P., Ardekant, B., Saito, E., Lencz, T., Lim, K.... Szeszko, P. 2009. Lower Orbital Frontal White Matter Integrity in Adolescents With Bipolar I Disorder. *Journal of the American Academy of Child and Adolescent Psychiatry, 48*(1), 79–86.

Kaur, S., Sassi, R. B., Axelson, D., Nicoletti, M., Brambilla, P., Monkul, E. S.... Soares, J.C. 2005. Cingulate cortex anatomical abnormalities in children and adolescents with bipolar disorder. [Proceedings Paper]. *American Journal of Psychiatry, 162*(9), 1637–1643.

Kleinman, L., Lowin, A., Flood, E., Gandhi, G., Edgell, E., & Revicki, D. 2003. Costs of bipolar disorder. *Pharmacoeconomics, 21*(9), 601–622.

Konarski, J. Z., McIntyre, R. S., Kennedy, S. H., Rafi-Tari, S., Soczynska, J. K., & Ketter, T. A. 2008. Volumetric neuroimaging investigations in mood disorders: bipolar disorder versus major depressive disorder. [Review]. *Bipolar Disorders, 10*(1), 1–37.

Lacerda, A. L. T., Keshavan, M. S., Hardan, A. Y., Yorbik, O., Brambilla, P., Sassi, R. B.... Soares, J.C. 2004. Anatomic evaluation of the orbitofrontal cortex in major depressive disorder. [Article]. *Biological Psychiatry, 55*(4), 353–358. doi: 10.1016/j.biopsych.2003.08.021

Lange, K., Williams, L. M., Young, A. W., Bullmore, E. T., Brammer, M. J., Williams, S. C.... Phillips, M.L. 2003. Task instructions modulate neural responses to fearful facial expressions. *Biological Psychiatry, 53*(3), 226–232. doi: S0006322302014555 [pii]

Lawrence, N. S., Williams, A. M., Surguladze, S., Giampietro, V., Brammer, M. J., Andrew, C.... Phillips, M.L. 2004. Subcortical and ventral prefrontal cortical neural responses to facial expressions distinguish patients with bipolar disorder and major depression. *Biological Psychiatry, 55*(6), 578–587. doi: 10.1016/j.biopsych. 2003.11.017 S0006322303012186 [pii]

Li, L. J., Ma, N., Li, Z. X., Tan, L. W., Liu, J., Gong, G. L.... Xu, L. 2007. Prefrontal white matter abnormalities in young adult with major depressive disorder: A diffusion tensor imaging study. *Brain Research, 1168*, 124–128.

Lin, F., Weng, S., Xie, B., Wu, G., & Lei, H. 2011. Abnormal frontal cortex white matter connections in bipolar disorder: A DTI tractography study. *Journal of Affective Disorders, In Press, Corrected Proof.* doi: DOI 10.1016/j.jad.2010.12.018

Lopez-Larson, M. P., DelBello, M. P., Zimmerman, M. E., Schwiers, M. L., & Strakowski, S. M. 2002. Regional prefrontal gray and white matter abnormalities in bipolar disorder. [Article]. *Biological Psychiatry, 52*(2), 93–100.

Lyoo, I. K., Kim, M. J., Stoll, A. L., Demopulos, C. M., Parow, A. M., Dager, S. R.... Renshaw, P.F. 2004. Frontal lobe gray matter density decreases in bipolar I disorder. [Article]. *Biological Psychiatry, 55*(6), 648–651. doi: 10.1016/j.biopsych.2003.10.017

Ma, N., Li, L. J., Shu, N., Liu, J., Gong, G. L., He, Z.... Jiang, T.Z. 2007. White 'Matter abnormalities in first-episode, treatment-naive young adults with major depressive disorder. *American Journal of Psychiatry, 164*(5), 823–826.

MacMillan, S., Szeszko, P. R., Moore, G. J., Madden, R., Lorch, E., Ivey, J.... Rosenberg, D.R. 2003. Increased amygdala: Hippocampal volume ratios associated with severity of anxiety in pediatric major depression. [Article]. *Journal of Child and Adolescent Psychopharmacology, 13*(1), 65–73.

Macritchie, K. A. N., Lloyd, A. J., Bastin, M. E., Vasudev, K., Gallagher, P., Eyre, R.... Young, A.H. 2010. White matter microstructural abnormalities in euthymic bipolar disorder. *British Journal of Psychiatry, 196*(1), 52–58. doi: DOI 10.1192/bjp.bp.108.058586

Mahon, K., Burdick, K. E., & Szeszko, P. R. 2010. A role for white matter abnormalities in the pathophysiology of bipolar disorder. *Neuroscience and Biobehavioral Reviews, 34*(4), 533–554. doi: DOI 10.1016/j.neubiorev.2009.10.012

Mahon, K., Wu, J., Malhotra, A. K., Burdick, K. E., Derosse, P., Ardekani, B. A.... Szeszko, P.R. 2009. A Voxel-Based Diffusion Tensor Imaging Study of White Matter in Bipolar Disorder. *Neuropsychopharmacology.*

Malhi, G. S., Lagopoulos, J., Sachdev, P. S., Ivanovski, B., Shnier, R., & Ketter, T. 2007. Is a lack of disgust something to fear? A functional magnetic resonance imaging facial emotion recognition study in euthymic bipolar disorder patients. *Bipolar Disorders, 9*(4), 345–357. doi: BDI485 [pii] 10.1111/j.1399-5618.2007.00485.x

Malhi, G. S., Lagopoulos, J., Ward, P. B., Kumari, V., Mitchell, P. B., Parker, G. B.... Sachdev, P. 2004. Cognitive generation of affect in bipolar depression: an fMRI study. *European Journal of Neuroscience, 19*(3), 741–754. doi: 3159 [pii]

McDonald, A. J. 2003. Is there an amygdala and how far does it extend? An anatomical perspective. *Annals of the New York Academy of Sciences, 985*, 1–21.

McIntosh, A. M., Maniega, S. M., Lymer, G. K. S., McKirdy, J., Hall, J., Sussmann, J. E. D.... Lawrie, S.M. 2008. White Matter Tractography in Bipolar Disorder and Schizophrenia. *Biological Psychiatry, 64*(12), 1088–1092.

Mori, S., Matsui, T., Kuze, B., Asanome, M., Nakajima, K., & Matsuyama, K. 1999. Stimulation of a restricted region in the midline cerebellar white matter evokes coordinated quadrupedal locomotion in the decerebrate cat. *Journal of Neurophysiology, 82*(1), 290–300.

Morris, J. S., Ohman, A., & Dolan, R. J. 1998. Conscious and unconscious emotional learning in the human amygdala. *Nature, 393*(6684), 467–470. doi: 10.1038/30976

Mourao-Miranda, J., Bokde, A. L., Born, C., Hampel, H., & Stetter, M. 2005. Classifying brain states and determining the discriminating activation patterns: Support Vector Machine on functional MRI data. *Neuroimage, 28*(4), 980–995. doi: S1053-8119(05)00478-7 [pii] 10.1016/j.neuroimage.2005.06.070

Murphy, C. F., Gunning-Dixon, F. M., Hoptman, M. J., Lim, K. O., Ardekani, B., Shields, J. K.... Alexopoulos, G.S. 2007. White-matter integrity predicts stroop performance in patients with geriatric depression. *Biological Psychiatry, 61*(8), 1007–1010. doi: DOI 10.1016/j.biopsych.2006.07.028

Nobuhara, K., Okugawa, G., Minami, T., Takase, K., Yoshida, T., Yagyu, T., Tajika, A., . . . Kinoshita, T. 2004. Effects of electroconvulsive therapy on frontal white matter in late-life depression: a diffusion tensor imaging study. *Neuropsychobiology 50*, 48–53.

Nobuhara, K., Okugawa, G., Sugimoto, T., Minami, T., Tamagaki, C., Takase, K.... Kinoshita, T. 2006. Frontal white matter anisotropy and symptom severity of late-life depression: a magnetic resonance diffusion tensor imaging study. *Journal of Neurology Neurosurgery and Psychiatry, 77*(1), 120–122.

Pavuluri, M. N., Yang, S., Kamineni, K., Passarotti, A. M., Srinivasan, G., Harral, E. M... Zhou, X.J. 2009. Diffusion Tensor Imaging Study of White Matter Fiber Tracts in Pediatric Bipolar Disorder and Attention-Deficit/Hyperactivity Disorder. *Biological Psychiatry, 65*(7), 586–593. doi: DOI 10.1016/j.biopsych.2008.10.015

Phillips, M., Ladouceur, C., & Drevets, W. 2008. A neural model of voluntary and automatic emotion regulation: implications for understanding the pathophysiology and neurodevelopment of bipolar disorder. *Molecular Psychiatry, 13*(9), 833–857.

Phillips, M. L., Medford, N., Young, A. W., Williams, L., Williams, S. C., Bullmore, E. T.... Brammer, M.J. 2001. Time courses of left and right amygdalar responses to fearful facial expressions. *Human Brain Mapping*, 12(4), 193–202. doi: 10.1002/1097-0193(200104)12:4<193::AID-HBM1015>3.0.CO;2-A [pii]

Phillips, M. L., Travis, M. J., Fagiolini, A., & Kupfer, D. J. 2008. Medication effects in neuroimaging studies of bipolar disorder. *American Journal of Psychiatry*, 165(3), 313–320. doi: appi. ajp.2007.07071066 [pii] 10.1176/appi.ajp.2007.07071066

Rajkowska, G. 2002. Cell pathology in bipolar disorder. [Review]. *Bipolar Disorders*, 4(2), 105–116.

Rajkowska, G., Miguel-Hidalgo, J. J., Wei, J. R., Dilley, G., Pittman, S. D., Meltzer, H. Y.... Stockmeier, C.A. 1999. Morphometric evidence for neuronal and glial prefrontal cell pathology in major depression. *Biological Psychiatry*, 45(9), 1085–1098.

Rich, B. A., Vinton, D. T., Roberson-Nay, R., Hommer, R. E., Berghorst, L. H., McClure, E. B.... Leibenluft, E. 2006. Limbic hyperactivation during processing of neutral facial expressions in children with bipolar disorder. *Proceedings of the National Academy of Sciences of the United States of America*, 103(23), 8900–8905. doi: 0603246103 [pii] 10.1073/pnas.0603246103

Robinson, J. L., Monkul, E. S., Tordesillas-Gutierrez, D., Franklin, C., Bearden, C. E., Fox, P. T.... Glahn, D.C. 2008. Fronto-limbic circuitry in euthymic bipolar disorder: evidence for prefrontal hyperactivation. *Psychiatry Research*, 164(2), 106–113. doi: S0925-4927(07)00250-8 [pii] 10.1016/j.pscychresns.2007.12.004

Robinson, R. G., Kubos, K. L., Starr, L. B., Rao, K., & Price, T. R. 1984. Mood disorders in stroke patients. Importance of location of lesion. *Brain : a journal of neurology*, 107 (Pt 1)(Pt 1), 81–93.

Rocca, C. C., Heuvel, E., Caetano, S. C., & Lafer, B. 2009. Facial emotion recognition in bipolar disorder: a critical review. *Rev Bras Psiquiatr*, 31(2), 171–180. doi: S1516-44462009000200015 [pii]

Sah, P., Faber, E. S., Lopez De Armentia, M., & Power, J. 2003. The amygdaloid complex: anatomy and physiology. *Revista Brasileira de Psiquiatria*, 83(3), 803–834. doi: 10.1152/physrev.00002.2003 83/3/803 [pii]

Sassi, R. B., Brambilla, P., Hatch, J. P., Nicoletti, M. A., Mallinger, A. G., Frank, E.... Soares, J.C. 2004. Reduced left anterior cingulate volumes in untreated bipolar patients. [Proceedings Paper]. *Biological Psychiatry*, 56(7), 467–475. doi: 10.1016/j.biopsych.2004.07.005

Sheline, Y. I., Barch, D. M., Donnelly, J. M., Ollinger, J. M., Snyder, A. Z., & Mintun, M. A. 2001. Increased amygdala response to masked emotional faces in depressed subjects resolves with antidepressant treatment: an fMRI study. *Biological Psychiatry*, 50(9), 651–658. doi: S000632230101263X [pii]

Sheline, Y. I., Gado, M. H., & Price, J. L. 1998. Amygdala core nuclei volumes are decreased in recurrent major depression. [Article]. *Neuroreport*, 9(9), 2023–2028.

Siegle, G. J., Thompson, W., Carter, C. S., Steinhauer, S. R., & Thase, M. E. 2007. Increased amygdala and decreased dorsolateral prefrontal BOLD responses in unipolar depression: related and independent features. *Biological Psychiatry*, 61(2), 198–209. doi: S0006-3223(06)00793-1 [pii] 10.1016/j.biopsych.2006.05.048

Smith, S. M., Jenkinson, M., Johansen-Berg, H., Rueckert, D., Nichols, T. E., Mackay, C. E.... Behrens, T.E.J. 2006. Tract-based spatial statistics: Voxelwise analysis of multi-subject diffusion data. *Neuroimage*, 31(4), 1487–1505.

Song, S. K., Sun, S. W., Ramsbottom, M. J., Chang, C., Russell, J., & Cross, A. H. 2002. Dysmyelination revealed through MRI as increased radial (but unchanged axial) diffusion of water. *Neuroimage*, 17(3), 1429–1436.

Steele, J.D., Bastin, M.E., Wardlaw, J.M., Ebmeier, K.P. 2005. Possible structural abnormality of the brainstem in unipolar depressive illness: a transcranial ultrasound and diffusion tensor magnetic resonance imaging study. *Journal of Neurology, Neurosurgery and Psychiatry*, 76, 1510–1515.

Strakowski, S. M., DelBello, M. P., Sax, K. W., Zimmerman, M. E., Shear, P. K., Hawkins, J. M.... Larson, E.R. 1999. Brain magnetic resonance imaging of structural abnormalities in bipolar disorder. [Proceedings Paper]. *Archives of General Psychiatry*, 56(3), 254–260.

Surguladze, S., Brammer, M. J., Keedwell, P., Giampietro, V., Young, A. W., Travis, M. J.... Phillips, M.L. 2005. A differential pattern of neural response toward sad versus happy facial expressions in major depressive disorder. *Biological Psychiatry*, 57(3), 201.

Surguladze, S. A., Young, A. W., Senior, C., Brebion, G., Travis, M. J., & Phillips, M. L. 2004. Recognition accuracy and response bias to happy and sad facial expressions in patients with major depression. *Neuropsychology*, 18(2), 212–218. doi: 10.1037/0894-4105.18.2.212 2004-12990-002 [pii]

Sussmann, J. E., Lymer, G. K. S., McKirdy, J., Moorhead, T. W. J., Maniega, S. M., Job, D.... McIntosh, A.M. 2009. White matter abnormalities in bipolar disorder and schizophrenia detected using diffusion tensor magnetic resonance imaging. *Bipolar Disorders*, 11(1), 11–18.

Swanson, L. W. 2003. The amygdala and its place in the cerebral hemisphere. *Annals of the New York Academy of Sciences*, 985, 174–184.

Taylor, W.D., Payne, M.E., Krishnan, K.R.R., Wagner, H.R., Provenzale, J.M., Steffens, D.C. & MacFall, J.R. 2001. Evidence of white matter tract disruption in MRI hyperintensities. *Biological Psychiatry* 50, 179–183.

Taylor, W. D., MacFall, J. R., Payne, M. E., McQuoid, D. R., Provenzale, J. M., Steffens, D. C.... Krishnan, K.R.R. 2004. Late-life depression and microstructural abnormalities in dorsolateral prefrontal cortex white matter. *American Journal of Psychiatry*, 161(7), 1293–1296.

Vapnik, V. 1995. *The Nature of Statistical Learning Theory*. New York: Springer-Verlag.

Versace, A., Almeida, J. R. C., Hassel, S., Walsh, N. D., Novelli, M., Klein, C. R.... Phillips, M.L. 2008. Elevated left and reduced right orbitomedial prefrontal fractional anisotropy in adults with bipolar disorder revealed by tract-based spatial statistics. *Archives of General Psychiatry*, 65(9), 1041–1052.

Versace, A., Almeida, J. R. C., Quevedo, K., Thompson, W. K., Terwilliger, R. A., Hassel, S.... Phillips, M.L. 2010. Right Orbitofrontal Corticolimbic and Left Corticocortical White Matter Connectivity Differentiate Bipolar and Unipolar Depression. *Biological Psychiatry*, 68(6), 560–567. doi: DOI: 10.1016/j.biopsych.2010.04.036

Versace, A., Ladouceur, C. D., Romero, S., Birmaher, B., Axelson, D. A., Kupfer, D. J.... Phillips, M.L. 2010. Altered Development of White Matter in Youth at High Familial Risk for Bipolar Disorder: A Diffusion Tensor Imaging Study. *Journal of the American Academy of Child and Adolescent Psychiatry*, 49(12), 1249–1259.e1241. doi: DOI: 10.1016/j.jaac.2010.09.007

Wang, F., Kalmar, J. H., He, Y., Jackowski, M., Chepenik, L. G., Edmiston, E. E.... Blumberg, H.P. 2009. Functional and Structural Connectivity Between the Perigenual Anterior Cingulate and Amygdala in Bipolar Disorder. *Biological Psychiatry*, 66(5), 516–521.

Wessa, M., Houenou, J., Leboyer, M., Chanraud, S., Poupon, C., Martinot, J. L.... Paillere-Martinot, M.L. 2009. Microstructural white matter changes in euthymic bipolar patients: a whole-brain diffusion tensor imaging study. *Bipolar Disorders*, 11(5), 504–514.

Wright, C. I., Fischer, H., Whalen, P. J., McInerney, S. C., Shin, L. M., & Rauch, S. L. 2001. Differential prefrontal cortex and amygdala habituation to repeatedly presented emotional stimuli. *Neuroreport*, 12(2), 379–383.

Xia, J., Lei, Y., Xu, H. J., Feng, W., Wu, X. L., & Liu, X. L. 2007. [Preliminary study of diffusion tensor imaging in treatment response assessment of major depression]. *Nan Fang Yi Ke Da Xue Xue Bao*, 27(12), 1905–1907.

Yang, Q., Huang, X. B., Hong, N., & Yu, X. 2007. White matter microstructural abnormalities in late-life depression. *International Psychogeriatrics*, 19(4), 757–766.

Yuan, Y. G., Zhang, Z. J., Bai, F., Yu, H., Shi, Y. M., Qian, Y.... You, J.Y. 2007. White matter integrity of the whole brain is disrupted in first-episode remitted geriatric depression. *Neuroreport*, 18(17), 1845–1849.

Yurgelun-Todd, D. A., Silveri, M. M., Gruber, S. A., Rohan, M. L., & Pimentel, P. J. 2007. White matter abnormalities observed in bipolar disorder: a diffusion tensor imaging study. *Bipolar Disorders*, 9(5), 504–512.

Zanetti, M. V., Jackowski, M. P., Versace, A., Almeida, J. R., Hassel, S., Duran, F. L.... Phillips, M.L. 2009. State-dependent microstructural white matter changes in bipolar I depression. *European Archives of Psychiatry and Clinical Neuroscience*, 259(6), 316–328. doi: 10.1007/s00406-009-0002-8

Zou, K., Huang, X. Q., Li, T., Gong, Q. Y., Li, Z., Luo, O. Y.... Sun, X.L. 2008. Alterations of white matter integrity in adults with major depressive disorder: a magnetic resonance imaging study. *Journal of Psychiatry & Neuroscience*, 33(6), 525–530.

# 7.

# NEUROIMAGING IN BIPOLAR DISORDER AND SCHIZOPHRENIA

## Heather C. Whalley, Jessika E. Sussmann, and Andrew M. McIntosh

## INTRODUCTION

Bipolar disorder and schizophrenia are common, disabling psychiatric disorders. There is considerable symptom heterogeneity among people with the same diagnosis, and no symptom is uniquely associated with either condition (Bora et al., 2008; Keck et al., 2003; Kempf et al., 2005; Murray et al., 2004; Siris, 2000). Furthermore, many of the associated risk factors, neurocognitive deficits (Bora et al., 2008; Krabbendam et al., 2005), and effective treatments (other than lithium) show little evidence of diagnostic specificity.

Structural and functional imaging studies have helped to clarify the neural basis of bipolar disorder and schizophrenia. Changes in structure and function have been found in the risk state and in people with established illness compared, even at the first episode of illness, with healthy subjects. However, debate continues as to whether these disorders are separate disease entities or whether they are points on a continuum of illness with many shared features and disease mechanisms. These issues can be addressed using in vivo brain imaging, and this chapter will review the literature of published studies directly comparing individuals with bipolar disorder and schizophrenia.

## STRUCTURAL IMAGING OF GREY MATTER IN SCHIZOPHRENIA VS. BIPOLAR DISORDER

Most grey matter imaging studies to date have used $T_1$-weighted images obtained from magnetic resonance imaging (MRI) using sequences optimized for grey-white contrast. The methods used to analyze these images can be divided into (i) region of interest methods, which seek to measure differences in brain structural volumes based on hypothesized regions (usually hand-traced), and (ii) voxel-based methods, which usually compare grey matter density at every voxel in the brain simultaneously.

## GREY MATTER: REGION OF INTEREST APPROACH

There are now many published MRI region of interest studies (e.g. see Figure 7.1) comparing individuals with bipolar disorder and healthy subjects, which have been summarized in meta-analyses (Arnone et al., 2009; McDonald et al., 2004b). One recent meta-analysis found evidence of whole brain and prefrontal volume reductions in bipolar disorder along with increased volume of the globus pallidus and lateral ventricles (Arnone et al., 2009). Many of these findings have also been made in schizophrenia (Wright et al., 2000); for example, ventricular and basal ganglia volume increases have also been reported in schizophrenia, although there is some evidence that the latter effect may be secondary to the effects of antipsychotic medication. While these findings suggest a degree of commonality between the disorders, inferences based on studies directly comparing bipolar disorder and schizophrenia within the same experiment may be more informative than comparing global or meta-analytic findings.

Two meta-analyses directly compared region of interest studies of people with bipolar disorder and schizophrenia studied within the same analysis paradigm. The first review (Kempton et al., 2008) demonstrated greater ventricular enlargement in schizophrenia than in bipolar disorder and larger hippocampal volumes in bipolar disorder compared to schizophrenia. These findings suggest that reductions of medial temporal lobe volume may be specific to the latter condition (Arnone et al., 2009). However, studies of hippocampal volume tended to show fewer small negative studies than expected, suggesting the possibility of publication bias. The meta-analysis also included studies using computed tomography, although it is not clear whether doing so added further heterogeneity to the analyses or alternatively, if it actually improved power. The second meta-analysis (Arnone et al., 2009) found overlapping findings, in which the finding of greater ventricular enlargement in schizophrenia was replicated. Individuals with bipolar

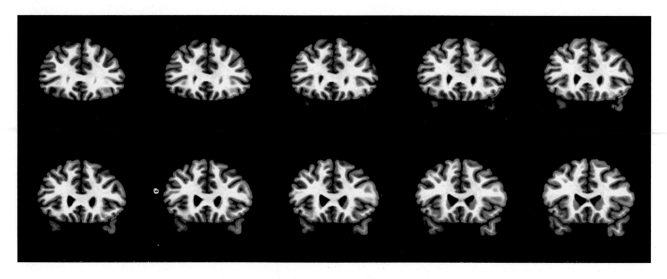

*Figure 7.1* Extracted prefrontal region(s) from a T$_1$-weighted image. (Source: McIntosh AM, Owens DC, Moorhead TWJ, Whalley HC, Stanfield AS, Hall J, Johnstone EC, and Lawrie SM. Longitudinal volume reductions in people at high genetic risk of schizophrenia as they develop psychosis. *Biological Psychiatry* 2011;69:953–958.)

disorder showed an increased volume of the right amygdala compared to individuals with schizophrenia, and no significant differences in the volume of the hippocampus. Although the volume of the amygdala and hippocampus are reduced in schizophrenia, the meta-analysis showed no significant differences in the volume of these structures in bipolar disorder compared to healthy subjects. In a subsequent analysis of between-study heterogeneity, amygdala volume was shown to be significantly influenced by the number of euthymic subjects in the bipolar disorder group, and hippocampal volumes were shown to be significantly influenced by the ages of the subjects.

The findings from these meta-analyses suggest that there may be quantitative structural differences between bipolar disorder and schizophrenia, with bipolar disorder being intermediate between the schizophrenia group and healthy subjects. Qualitative differences in the medial temporal lobe are probably more likely, although inconsistency within the bipolar disorder versus healthy subject literature about the direction of volumetric abnormalities in the hippocampus and (especially) the amygdala continue to make interpretation difficult. There is also emerging evidence in both conditions that these effects may vary as a function of age and medication status (Arnone et al., 2009; Hallahan et al., 2010). Since medication received by individuals with schizophrenia and bipolar disorder may differ considerably in its mode of action, the degree to which these effects confound any between-group differences is not known with any certainty.

In summary, 18 MRI studies included in the meta-analysis by Arnone et al. compared individuals with schizophrenia and bipolar disorder within the same experiment—and for some anatomical comparisons more than 400 people contributed data to the analyses. Findings from this analysis suggested that if there are as yet undiscovered structural differences between bipolar disorder and schizophrenia, their effect sizes are probably relatively small, and, therefore, there is likely to be significant overlap in neuroanatomic measures between the disorders.

**Gray Matter Structural Imaging—ROI: Schizophrenia Vs. Bipolar Disorder**

- Relatively few differences between schizophrenia and bipolar disorder have been reported

- Bipolar disorder associated with larger amygdala & hippocampus compared to schizophrenia

- Schizophrenia is associated with greater ventriculomegaly compared to bipolar disorder

## GREY MATTER: VOXEL-BASED STUDIES

Automated whole brain voxel-based analysis in bipolar disorder has grown considerably in recent years (see Table 7.1), and most studies now use this method instead of conventional region of interest analyses. This choice is driven partly by the economic advantages of voxel-based methods (the manpower demands are much lower), improvements in computing power, and by the fact that the region of interest technique is highly labor intensive and time-consuming. Voxel based methods are highly reliable and repeatable. Although these studies have given similar findings to region of interest studies in many respects, biological interpretation

**TABLE 7.1** SUMMARY OF VOXEL-BASED GREY-MATTER IMAGING STUDIES COMPARING SCHIZOPHRENIA (SCZ) AND BIPOLAR DISORDER (BD)

| Study | Sample | Results | |
|---|---|---|---|
| McIntosh (2004) | SCZ 20<br>BD 45<br>CTR 49<br>Relatives | SCZ vs. CTR | SCZ show reduced grey matter in left middle frontal gyrus, left inferior frontal gyrus and thalamus |
| | | BD vs. CTR | BD show reduced grey matter in left thalamus and caudate (family history BD only). Right inferior frontal gyrus and right insula (family history SCZ and BD) |
| | | BD vs. SCZ | No significant differences when directly compared |
| McDonald (2004, 2005) | SCZ 25<br>BD 37<br>Relatives | SCZ vs. CTR | SCZ associated with reduced grey matter in cerebellum, temporal cortex, medial temporal lobe, thalamus, prefrontal cortex, cingulate, insula, parietal lobe, precuneus, pre and post-central gyrii |
| | | BD vs. CTR | No significant differences |
| | | SCZ vs. BD | SCZ showed reduced grey matter in frontotemporal cortex, medial temporal lobe, lentiform, caudate, thalamus insula, precuneus, pre and post central gyrii compared to BD |
| Farrow (2005)<br>First episode study | SCZ 25<br>BD 8<br>CTR 22 | SCZ vs. CTR | Grey matter reduced in SCZ in right prefrontal cortex, anterior cingulate, pre-central gyrus, temporal cortex, parietal cortex and cerebellum |
| | | BD vs. CTR | Reduced grey matter in BD in right prefrontal cortex, bilateral temporal cortex, left insula and left posterior cingulate cortex |
| | | BD vs. SCZ | Reduced grey matter in the temporal cortex in BD, and reduced grey matter in the Frontal cortex and anterior cingulate cortex |
| Janssen (2008)<br>Fist episode adolescents—diagnosis made retrospectively | SCZ 25<br>BD 20<br>CTR 51 | SCZ vs. CTR | Reduced grey matter in left middle and medial prefrontal gyrus compared to CTR |
| | | BD vs. CTR | Reduced grey matter in left medial prefrontal gyrus |
| | | BD vs. SCZ | No significant differences reported |
| Cui (2011) | SCZ 23<br>BD 24<br>CTR 36 | SCZ vs. CTR | SCZ associated with reduced grey matter in right parietal lobule and right superior temporal gyrus and increased grey matter in the left putamen. |
| | | BD vs. CTR | BD associated with reduced grey matter in right middle frontal gyrus, left parietal lobule, right superior temporal gyrus, left middle temporal gyrus, bilateral caudate nuclei and right occipital cortex. |
| | | BD vs. SCZ | No significant differences |

of the findings is not entirely straightforward, and interpretation of many findings is still unclear. In part this is due to the many complex processing steps required for each image.

Voxel-based studies examine a particular tissue class between subjects, usually grey matter, once brain images have been warped to a common three-dimensional template. Once this warping (or transformation) has been conducted, the density at each specific voxel is then compared using methods based on t-tests or other parametric statistical techniques. A refinement to this technique involves adjusting for the amount of warping necessary to bring the brain into the same space as the standard template. In situations in which the subject's image has effectively been increased in volume to match the template image, each grey matter voxel's density is adjusted downwards in order that its value approximates the local grey matter tissue volume in the subject's native brain image (and vice versa for individuals with larger brains than the template).

The first study directly comparing bipolar disorder and schizophrenia in the same experiment (McDonald et al., 2005; McDonald et al., 2004a) reported no significant differences between bipolar disorder and healthy subjects, but a widespread pattern of frontotemporal and subcortical volume reductions in schizophrenia. Many of these findings were significant when the schizophrenia group was compared to the bipolar disorder group, implying that the bipolar disorder group was relatively similar to healthy subjects. In a follow-up publication on an extended study sample, widespread grey matter differences were found in association with a genetic liability measure for schizophrenia in bilateral fronto-striatal-thalamic and left lateral temporal regions, whereas the same measure in bipolar disorder was associated with only anterior cingulate grey matter volume reductions. However, no cingulate volumes were reported in the original patient study in bipolar disorder. In a similarly designed study, McIntosh et al. (2009, 2004) reported prefrontal and thalamic grey matter density reductions in schizophrenia and bipolar disorder in which medial temporal lobe reductions were specific to schizophrenia and striatal volume reductions were specific to bipolar disorder. However, the study relied on comparison of patient-healthy subject differences for their inferences, and when schizophrenia and bipolar disorder patients were compared directly, these differences were not significant. A further longitudinal first-episode study by Farrow et al. (2005) examined a group of eight patients with bipolar disorder and 25 with schizophrenia studied over a two-year period. The study also provided a direct comparison of bipolar disorder and schizophrenia at the baseline assessment showing significant reductions in prefrontal and temporal cortex in both disorders compared to healthy subjects. When the patient groups were compared to one another, there was evidence of greater grey matter deficit in bipolar disorder compared to schizophrenia in these regions and greater frontal an anterior cingulate grey matter loss in schizophrenia. A very recent study by Cui et al. (2011) in contrast found enlargement of the putamen in both schizophrenia (N = 23) and bipolar disorder (N = 24 with psychotic mania) and reduced volume of the superior temporal gyrus and parietal cortex. No differences were found between patients with schizophrenia and those with bipolar disorder. Although the effects in the striatum went in the opposite direction of preceding studies, the finding of an enlarged putamen in bipolar disorder is supported by a recent individual patient data meta-analysis (Hallahan et al., 2010). Although there were common reductions in both schizophrenia and bipolar disorder, the disorders could not be separated from each other on direct comparison.

Janssen at al. (2008) took an alternative approach of using imaging assessments in a group of people with first-episode psychosis, who were then retrospectively diagnosed after a one-year follow up. This study reported largely overlapping grey matter deficits in prefrontal areas common to both schizophrenia and bipolar disorder, but also reported no significant differences when the groups were compared directly (Janssen et al., 2008).

In summary, direct voxel-based comparisons between schizophrenia and bipolar disorder have been infrequent, and there remains considerable doubt about whether there are distinct anatomical differences. Two recent meta-analyses combined case control studies of each disorder using an anatomical likelihood based technique in order to make comparisons between the disorders. The results of these studies differed significantly, with one finding (Yu et al., 2010) common reductions in frontal lobe, thalamus, middle temporal gyrus, cingulate, and head of the caudate. The same study also found relatively specific amygdala and insula reductions in schizophrenia, and a relative excess of grey matter in the tail of the caudate. Excess grey matter in the putamen was common to both schizophrenia and bipolar disorder. In contrast, the review by Ellison-Wright and Bullmore (2010) found overlapping reductions in both

schizophrenia and bipolar disorder, with only anterior cingulate grey matter reductions showing a specific reduction in bipolar disorder. These studies illustrate the difficulties of comparing the disorders when the patient groups were not present within the same experiment and when original patient or study-level whole brain data are unavailable.

A further difficulty yet to be fully addressed in the literature is the relationship between grey matter deficits and psychotic symptoms. While most studies include patients with bipolar disorder with psychosis, it is not clear whether the common findings in schizophrenia relate to the presence of these symptoms, or whether the presence of psychosis in bipolar disorder is largely explained by illness severity. These subgroup analyses can only be facilitated by much larger studies than have been conducted to date and this would have the likely effect of improving the consistency of findings in general.

---

**Gray Matter Structural Imaging—Voxelwise: Schizophrenia Vs. Bipolar Disorder**

- The number and size of studies directly comparing schizophrenia and bipolar disorder are too few to make any clear conclusions

- Fronto-temporal grey matter reductions are of greater magnitude in schizophrenia in some studies

- Overall, the literature using voxel-based gray matter imaging studies suggests significant overlap in the anatomy of both conditions

---

## WHITE MATTER IMAGING IN SCHIZOPHRENIA AND BIPOLAR DISORDER

White matter consists of many myelinated and un-myelinated axons, as well as other non-neuronal cell types, and it is assumed to be the anatomical substrate of functional interaction between different brain regions. Regional disconnectivity in both schizophrenia and bipolar disorder directly implicates white matter (Friston & Frith, 1995) which in turn has led to increasing interest in this tissue class in both conditions.

A number of methods have been used to study white matter pathology in schizophrenia and bipolar disorder. These include the analysis of qualitative white matter abnormalities using $T_2$-weighted structural imaging, volumetric analysis of white matter segments from $T_1$-weighted imaging, and diffusion tensor imaging. The results of these studies will be reviewed, although unfortunately very few studies have directly compared white matter disruption in the two disorders within the same imaging protocol.

## WHITE MATTER HYPERINTENSITIES

White matter hyperintensities (WMHs) are identified as regions of high-signal on $T_2$-weighted MR images, usually occurring in deep brain white matter around subcortical structures and the ventricles. In the past, these abnormalities have been though to reflect ischemic damage, focal demyelination, axonal loss, lacunar infarctions or necrosis (Beyer et al., 2009). The presence of $T_2$-weighted hyperintensities in bipolar disorder and schizophrenia may relate to the as yet unidentified etiology of the conditions, although an increased prevalence of cardiovascular risk factors in these disorders may explain some of the positive findings reported. The way in which the presence of WMHs is recorded also differs among studies that simply record their number, to others which distinguish periventricular from other WMHs, and studies in which the volume of white matter occupied by WMHs is the main unit of analysis.

To the best of our knowledge seven studies directly compared white matter hyperintensities between schizophrenia and bipolar disorder. Although bipolar disorder has been associated with increased rates of white matter hyperintensities for a number of years, compared with healthy subjects (Lyoo et al., 2002; Pillai et al., 2002; Strakowski et al., 1993), individuals with bipolar disorder also seem to have higher rates of hyperintensities than individuals with schizophrenia (Lyoo et al., 2002; Pillai et al., 2002). Krabbendam et al. (2000) found a greater number of WMH in bipolar disorder, but this result was not significant. Three studies, however, reported negative findings (Breeze et al., 2003; Lewine et al., 1995; Persaud et al., 1997), although some studies (e.g., Breeze et al., 2003)) compared many other diagnostic groups simultaneously, and many individual studies to date may lack sufficient power to confidently identify differences between disorder.

The finding of increased WMHs in bipolar disorder compared to schizophrenia is consistent with the literature in schizophrenia in which results from meta-analysis do not support a statistically significant association (Beyer et al., 2009). A few studies suggest that WMHs are larger (Persaud et al., 1997; Pillai et al., 2002) and more severe (Pillai et al., 2002) in schizophrenia, even though there were fewer of them. Other factors that might impact rates or types of white matter hyperintensities include cardiovascular disease, greater than three hospital admissions, and lithium use in men (Breeze et al., 2003). Although age is implicated in increasing WMH, it is not clear that this is the case in

bipolar disorder (McDonald et al., 1999), as a study of adolescents did demonstrate significant differences between patient groups (Pillai et al., 2002). In summary, WMHs appear to be more frequent in bipolar disorder than in schizophrenia and may therefore reflect disorder-specific pathophysiology. Although an increased rate of cardiovascular risk factors has been suggested as a potential cause of these findings, WMHs may yet provide important clues to our understanding of the non-shared etiology of bipolar disorder. Studies examining the neuropathological basis of WMHs are problematic and therefore addressing the cellular basis of these findings is not straightforward.

---

**White Matter Hyperintensities: Schizophrenia Vs. Bipolar Disorder**

- White matter hyperintensities are increased in number and volume in bipolar disorder

- White matter hyperintensities may not be increased in schizophrenia

- White matter hyperintensities are related to cardiovascular risk factors although this does not explain their association with bipolar disorder

---

## WHITE MATTER DENSITY AND VOLUME

A number of voxel-based (VBM) studies extracted the white matter tissue segments from $T_1$-weighted images and measures of tissue concentration or volume between bipolar disorder and schizophrenia. Decreases in fronto-thalamic white matter density have been reported using VBM in both schizophrenia and bipolar disorder (McDonald et al., 2005; McIntosh et al., 2005) and in unaffected relatives of people with these disorders (McIntosh et al., 2009; McIntosh et al., 2005; McIntosh et al., 2006). A recent meta-analysis demonstrated that whole brain white matter volume did not differ between the disorders when compared directly, although the number of people available for this comparison was relatively small (Arnone et al., 2009). A study of individuals at the time of their first-episodes found significant whole brain white matter loss when comparing a combined sample of psychotic patients (eight with bipolar disorder and 25 with schizophrenia) with 22 healthy subjects, but no differences between the disorders. Bilateral frontotemporal and parietal white matter deficits were also reported in another sample (37 with bipolar disorder, 25 with schizophrenia) of both disorders compared to healthy subjects, but no findings remained significant when the clinical groups were compared directly (McDonald et al.,

2005). The anatomical localization of these deficits has shown some inconsistency, with abnormalities in longitudinal and inter-hemispheric tracts in one study (McDonald et al., 2005), while another study reported deficits in the anterior limb of the internal capsule (Sussmann et al., 2009a). These apparently discrepant findings may reveal a more generalized white matter density/volume reduction, differences in subject characteristics, or study methodology. In one study individuals with schizophrenia showed deficits in the right superior frontal gyrus that were not present in the bipolar group (McIntosh et al., 2005). This finding may reveal disorder-specific white matter abnormalities in a

specific region and may have important implications for our understanding of schizophrenia and bipolar disorder. Unfortunately, since these studies were conducted, few investigators have subsequently examined white matter density or volume, preferring instead to use diffusion tensor imaging (DTI) as their technique of choice. While findings within each disorder have been individually replicated using $T_1$-weighetd analyses, no direct comparisons have since been conducted—although these interesting initial findings may have important implications for our understanding of these conditions.

## DIFFUSION TENSOR IMAGING

Diffusion tensor imaging measures the diffusivity of water molecules within organized tissues *in vivo*. The movement of water molecules is highly constrained within a white matter tract, with increased diffusion along the length of the axon compared to the water motion occurring across the tract. This unequal, or anisotropic, water motion in organized brain tissue enables the reconstruction of white matter tracts and a measure of their integrity. Fractional anisotropy (FA , see Figure 7.2) is the most common measure of constrained diffusion and takes values between 0 (unconstrained motion, as would be the case in a glass of water) and 1 (constrained entirely along a single axis). Within the brain, FA has the highest values in white matter and the lowest in cerebrospinal fluid. FA can then be

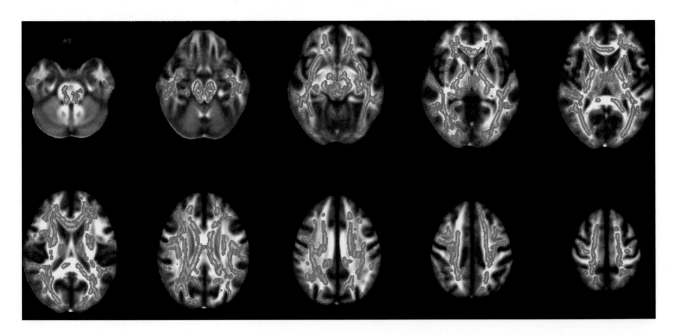

*Figure 7.2* Image showing diffusion tensor imaging finding of reduced white matter integrity in relatives of people with bipolar disorder. Significant findings are overlaid on a $T_1$-weighted image. (Source: Sprooten E, Sussmann JE, Clugston A, Peel A, McKirdy J, Moorhead TWJ, Anderson S, Shand AJ, Giles S, Bastin ME, Hall J, Johnstone EC, Lawrie SM and McIntosh AM. White matter integrity in individuals at high genetic risk of bipolar disorder. *Biological Psychiatry* 2011;70:350–356.)

compared between individuals on a voxel-by-voxel basis, such as in the TBSS (tract based spatial statistics) analysis package, or can incorporate directional information to enable the white matter connections to be reconstructed. Tractography uses this directional information to assess connectivity over specific fibre tracts.

Very few DTI studies have been published directly comparing these disorders. Using DTI (Sussmann et al., 2009b) and tractography (McIntosh et al., 2008b), reduced FA was found in the anterior thalamic radiation (McIntosh et al., 2008b; Sussmann et al., 2009b), left anterior limb of internal capsule (Sussmann et al., 2009b), the uncinate fasciculus (McIntosh et al., 2008b; Sussmann et al., 2009b) and the superior thalamic radiation (Sussmann et al., 2009b) in both schizophrenia and bipolar disorder compared with healthy subjects. Patient groups did not differ from each other implying that these findings showed no evidence of diagnostic specificity. A further study recruited patients (12 with bipolar disorder and three with major depressive disorder) into an affective psychosis group and compared them to individuals with schizophrenia and healthy subjects. All patients were within four years of diagnosis. Patients with schizophrenia had reduced FA in the uncinate fasciculus compared to healthy subjects (Kawashima et al., 2009). Comparisons with the affective psychosis group were however negative—consistent with the hypothesis that white matter abnormalities are common to both conditions and fail to show diagnostic specificity. Further studies are clearly needed to order to replicate and extend these studies—and much larger sample sizes will be required if evidence of anatomical specificity is to be obtained.

In summary, the literature on white matter imaging directly comparing bipolar disorder and schizophrenia is very small; as a result conclusions about the pathophysiological similarities and differences must be tentative. To date, studies implicate white matter abnormalities especially between frontotemporal and frontothalamic regions.

These abnormalities appear to be shared by both disorders, and there is evidence of similar abnormalities in unaffected relatives (Maniega et al., 2007) that implies that these findings are not merely secondary to medication or illness related factors.

## FUNCTIONAL IMAGING IN BIPOLAR DISORDER AND SCHIZOPHRENIA

Although the causes of bipolar disorder and schizophrenia are as yet unknown, genetic factors are unequivocally important to their etiology (Cannon et al., 1998; Cardno et al., 1999; Kendler et al., 1994; McGuffin et al., 2003) and, to date, many genetic risk factors have shown overlapping influences on both disorders (Craddock et al., 2005, 2006; Huang et al., 2010; Lichtenstein et al., 2009; Moskvina et al., 2009; Purcell et al., 2009). These findings, together with evidence of overlapping symptoms, treatment response and outcome infers overlapping pathological mechanisms (Craddock & Owen, 2010). This concept is far from new, with researchers questioning the traditional dichotomy between the disorders for several decades (Bramon & Sham, 2001; Cardno et al., 2002; Kerr & McClelland, 1991; Laursen et al., 2009). Although the evidence suggests that bipolar disorder and schizophrenia are not entirely separate disease entities, the fact that there are also non-shared risk factors (Craddock & Owen, 2005; Grozeva et al., 2010; Lichtenstein et al., 2009), indicates that they are also unlikely to be due to a single common mechanism. Various explanations have been proposed to account for these findings, including that they are two distinct illnesses with minimal overlap, to a large singular dimension of illness spectrum with affective components at one and psychotic features at the other.

There is therefore considerable interest in using functional imaging (Figure 7.3) in particular to explore the underlying neurobiological processes in order to determine whether there are diagnosis-specific or symptom-specific features of the disorders or whether they share abnormalities of functional neural architecture. Such studies may aid in the development of biologically plausible illness models that may be informative for diagnosis and treatment. In the following section we present a review of functional imaging studies that have directly compared then two disorders. Specifically, a review of the literature was carried out to identify studies that directly compared both disorders using fMRI. Studies were categorized into those describing (i) emotion, reward and memory tasks (i.e., with presumed primary involvement of limbic, sub-cortical, ventral prefrontal and medial temporal lobe regions), and (ii) those describing executive

> **Diffusion Tensor Imaging: Schizophrenia Vs. Bipolar Disorder**
>
> - Reduced integrity in fronto-temporal and fronto-thalamic tracts is found in both bipolar disorder and schizophrenia
>
> - The relatively small literature to date does not suggest any diagnostic specificity
>
> - Studies of unaffected relatives suggest a possible genetic basis to the observed findings

**TABLE 7.2** SUMMARY OF WHITE-MATTER IMAGING STUDIES COMPARING SCHIZOPHRENIA (SCZ) AND BIPOLAR DISORDER (BD)

| Study | Sample | Comparisons | Results | Comparisons | Results |
|---|---|---|---|---|---|
| **WHITE MATTER HYPERINTENSITIES** | | | | | |
| Lyoo 2002 (mean age 12.9) | SCZ 42 BD 56 HC 83 | BD>SCZ>HC | Both paediatric patient groups had more WMH than controls and more BD patients had WMH than SCZ | | |
| Pillai 2002 | BD 15 SCZ 19 HC 16 | | BD adolescents had more WMH than controls and SCZ | | |
| Strakowski 1993 | BD 18 SCZ 54 HC 15 | BD>HC | BD had more WMH than controls and SCZ | BD>SCZ | |
| Krabbendam 2000 | BD 22 SCZ 22 HC 22 | | no significant differences between groups | | |
| Lewine 1995 | BD 20 SCZ 108 HC 150 | | no significant differences between groups | | |
| Persaud 1997 | BD 26 SCZ 48 HC 34 | SCZ>HC | SCZ had significantly greater area of brain occupied by focal signal hyperintensities than BD or HC | SCZ>BD | |
| **VOXEL BASED MORPHOMETRY** | | | | | |
| McDonald 2005 | BD 37 SCZ 25 HC 52 | BD<HC SCZ<HC | Bilateral temporoparietal cortex, bilateral medial frontal lobes Brainstem Bilateral frontal lobe, right temporoparietal area | SCZ vs BD | No differences |
| McIntosh 2005 | BD 26 SCZ 26 HC 49 | SCZ<HC BD<HC | Bilateral subgyral frontal WM Genu of corpus callosum/left cingulum Left anterior internal capsule Left anterior internal capsule | | No direct comparison between patient groups |
| **DIFFUSION TENSOR IMAGING** | | | | | |
| Sussmann 2009 | BD 42 SCZ 28 HC 38 | BD<HC (whole brain) BD<HC (frontal SVC) SCZ<HC (frontal SVC) | Superior thalamic radiation Anterior thalamic radiation Uncinate fasciculus UF/anterior thalamic radiation/inf. fronto-occipital fasc. | SCZ vs. BD | No differences |
| McIntosh 2008 | BD 40 SCZ 25 HC 49 | BD<HC SCZ<HC | Uncinate fasciculus Anterior thalamic radiation Uncinate fasciculus Anterior thalamic radiation | SCZ vs. BD | No differences |
| Kawashima 2009 | Affective psychosis 15 SCZ 15 HC 15 | SCZ<HC | Uncinate fasciculus | SCZ vs. BD | No differences |

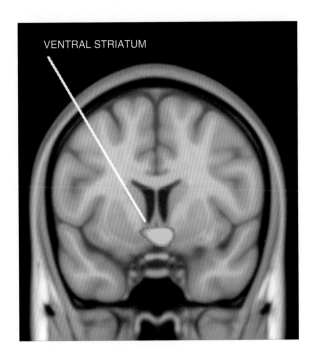

VENTRAL STRIATUM

*Figure 7.3* Image showing positive association between depression scores and activation in ventral striatum using fMRI, overlaid on a T$_1$ weighted image. (Image adapted from: Whalley HC, Sussmann JE, Chakirova G, Mukerjee P, Peel A, McKirdy J, Hall J, Johnstone EC, Lawrie SM, McIntosh AM. The Neural Basis of Familial Risk and Temperamental Variation in Individuals at High Risk of Bipolar Disorder *Biological Psychiatry*, 2011;70(4):343-349.)

function and language tasks (with presumed primary involvement of lateral prefrontal regions). Those not fitting into these categories are described separately. Studies examining associations with symptom measures are also described. In total 14 fMRI studies were identified by the review. Methodological and demographic details of these studies are summarized in Table 7.3, and Table 7.4 contains the primary findings listing all areas of difference reported in the papers, although the following review will focus on limbic areas and prefrontal regions. Specifically the focus was to explore evidence for differences in activation between the diagnoses.

## STUDIES OF EMOTION, REWARD AND EXECUTIVE TASKS

Four studies employed tasks involving emotion, reward, or memory to compare bipolar disorder and schizophrenia (Abler et al., 2008; Hall et al., 2009; Malhi et al., 2004; Whalley et al., 2009), and seven studies employed language tasks (Costafreda et al., 2009; Costafreda et al.,; Curtis et al., 2001; McIntosh et al., 2008a; Mechelli et al., 2008; Sommer et al., 2007), and working memory (Hamilton et al., 2009). Although there were methodological differences in the tasks employed, three of the four studies using emotion-type tasks reported relative over-activation of

medial temporal lobe structures or limbic/meso-limbic regions in bipolar disorder versus schizophrenia, see Table 7.2 (Hall et al., 2009; Malhi et al., 2004; Whalley et al., 2009). Regions implicated in these studies included the amygdala, hippocampus, parahippocampal gyrus and mid-cingulate cortex. For the reverse contrast (schizophrenia versus bipolar disorder), one study reported relative over-activation of the mid-cingulate cortex (Malhi et al., 2004), although this was a more anterior region to that described above.

In contrast to studies examining emotional, reward and memory tasks, none of the executive function/language studies reported over-activation of medial temporal lobe or meso-limbic regions in bipolar disorder versus schizophrenia. One study however reported over-activation in schizophrenia patients versus bipolar disorder in the wider network including the medial prefrontal cortex during a working memory task (Hamilton et al., 2009), and one study reported over-activation of the insula cortex during a sentence completion task (McIntosh et al., 2008a).

This pattern is generally consistent with the wider literature comparing the separate disorders with healthy subjects, in which there is a reported under-activation of medial temporal lobe structures in schizophrenia, and an over-activation of these structures in bipolar disorder. This pattern also fits with neurobiological models implicating the importance of these regions in the disorders (Phillips et al., 2003; Strakowski et al., 2005). In schizophrenia there are a number of reports of reduced responses of medial temporal regions to emotional versus neutral stimuli versus healthy subjects (Gur et al., 2002; Phillips et al., 1999; Schneider et al., 1998; Williams et al., 2004). These differences have more recently been proposed to derive from an increased response to the comparator neutral stimuli (Hall et al., 2008; Holt et al., 2006; Schwartz et al., 2003; Surguladze et al., 2006). Together with behavioral studies typically showing deficits in emotion recognition, especially for negative emotions, it appears that in schizophrenia there is an over-activation to, and misinterpretation of, ambiguous stimuli as being emotionally salient. This abnormality in turn may contribute to such clinical symptoms such as delusions, in which emotionally neutral stimuli may be perceived as threatening (Phillips et al., 2003). In contrast, increased activation of medial temporal lobe structures has been one of the most consistently reported findings in bipolar disorder (Cerullo et al., 2009; Phillips et al., 2008a). This increased activation to emotional stimuli has been proposed to represent an oversensitive, but dysfunctional system for determining emotional significance of stimuli, and hence may contribute to the production of abnormal affective states (Phillips et al., 2003). The differences in medial temporal

**TABLE 7.3** FUNCTIONAL MRI STUDIES COMPARING BIPOLAR DISORDER AND SCHIZOPHRENIA

| | General details | | Main findings |
|---|---|---|---|
| | | | Controls v BD |
| Study | Task | Task contrast | Direction |
| **EMOTION, REWARD AND MEMORY TASKS** | | | |
| Mitchell 2004 (40) | Emotional prosody | Pure emotional prosody (a) | C>BD |
| | | | C>BD |
| | | | C>BD |
| | | | C>BD |
| | | | C>BD |
| | | | C>BD |
| | | Unfiltered emotional prosody (b) | C>BD |
| | | | C>BD |
| | | | BD>C |
| Abler 2008 (41) | Reward task | Outcome: win v omission (a) | C > BD(m) |
| Hall 2009 (42) | Associative memory task | Early encoding (b) | - |
| | | Early retrieval | - |
| | | Late encoding | - |
| | | Late retrieval | - |
| Whalley 2009 (43) | Emotional memory | Emotion v neutral scenes (a) | BD >C |
| | | | BD >C |
| | | | BD >C |
| | | | BD >C |
| | | Emotional scenes v baseline (b) | - |
| | | Neutral scenes v baseline (c) | C>BD |
| | | | C>BD |
| **EXECUTIVE FUNCTION AND LANGUAGE TASKS** | | | |
| Curtis 2001 (44) | Verbal fluency | Verbal fluency (a) | BD>C |
| | | | BD>C |
| | | | BD>C |
| | | | BD>C |

Main findings

| | Controls v SCZ | | BD v SCZ | |
|---|---|---|---|---|
| Region | Direction | Region | Direction | Region |
| L + R superior temporal gyrus | SCZ>C | L inferior parietal lobule | SCZ>BD | R middle temporal gyrus |
| R amygdala | SCZ>C | R precentral gyrus | SCZ>BD | **R cingulate gyrus** |
| L uncus | | | SCZ>BD | L supramarginal gyrus |
| R inferior frontal gyrus | | | BD>SCZ | R middle temporal gyrus |
| R precentral gyrus | | | | |
| L postcentral gyrus | | | | |
| R hippocampus | C>SCZ | L superior temporal gyrus | SCZ>BD | L + R superior temporal gyrus |
| R supramarginal gyrus | C>SCZ | R precuneus | SCZ>BD | L middle temporal gyrus |
| L uncus | SCZ>C | L middle temporal gyrus | BD>SCZ | L superior temporal gyrus |
| | SCZ>C | L parahippocampal gyrus | BD>SCZ | **R parahippocampal gyrus** |
| | SCZ>C | R precentral gyrus | BD>SCZ | **L middle frontal gyrus (DPFC), BA6** |
| | | | BD>SCZ | R precentral gyrus |
| L nucleus accumbens | - | n/s | - | n/s |
| n/s | C>SCZ | Midline cerebellum | SCZ>BD | **L DPFC, BA8** |
| n/s | SCZ>C | L DLPFC | BD>SCZ | **R hippocampus** |
| | | | SCZ>BD | **L DMedPFC** |
| n/s | C>SCZ | L superior temporal cortex | - | n/s |
| | SCZ>C | L lingual gyrus | | |
| n/s | - | n/s | SCZ>BD | **L DMedPFC** |
| L hippocampus | | | BD> SCZ | **L hippocampus** |
| R posterior cingulate | | | BD> SCZ | L superior temporal sulcus |
| L superior temporal gyrus | | | BD> SCZ | R inferior parietal lobule |
| L precentral gyrus | | | BD> SCZ | **Left cingulate gyrus** |
| n/s | C>SCZ | L + R amygdala | - | n/s |
| L superior temporal sulcus | - | n/s | - | n/s |
| R calcarine suclus | | | | |
| R lingual gyrus | C>SCZ* | L inferior frontal gyrus | BD> SCZ | R medial parietal cortex |
| L inferior frontal gyrus | C>SCZ* | L middle frontal gyrus | BD> SCZ | L cerebellar vermis |
| R cerebellum | C>SCZ* | R medial parietal cortex | BD> SCZ | L + R fusiform |
| R medial parietal cortex | C>SCZ* | R inferior frontal gyrus | BD> SCZ | L middle temporal gyrus |

(Continued)

| | General details | | Main findings |
|---|---|---|---|
| Study | Task | Task contrast | Controls v BD |
| | | | BD>C |
| | | | BD>C |
| | | Semantic decision (b) | C>BD |
| | | | C>BD |
| | | | BD>C |
| Sommer 2007 (45) | Verb generation and semantic decision | | BD(m)>C |
| McIntosh 2008 (46) | Sentence completion | Sentence completion versus baseline (a) | C>BD |
| | | Parametric contrast (b) | BD>C |
| | | | BD>C |
| | | | BD>C |
| Mechelli 2008 (47) | Verbal fluency (effects of NRG1)* | | BD>C |
| Costafreda 2009 (48) | Verbal fluency | Verbal fluency | - |
| Hamilton 2009 (49) | Working memory | Working memory | C>BD |
| | | | C>BD |
| | | | C>BD |
| Costafreda et al., 2011 | Verbal fluency | Verbal fluency | BD>C |

| | Main findings | | | |
|---|---|---|---|---|
| | Controls v SCZ | | BD v SCZ | |
| Midline medial frontal lobe | SCZ>C* | R medial parietal cortex | | |
| L cerebellar vermis | | | | |
| R fusiform | C>SCZ** | L + R lingual gyrus | SCZ>BD | L lingual gyrus |
| L + R lingual gyrus | C>SCZ** | L + R middle occipital gyrus | BD>SCZ | R fusiform gyrus |
| R fusiform | C>SCZ** | R cuneus | | |
| | C>SCZ** | L fusiform | | |
| | C>SCZ** | L inferior temporal gyrus | | |
| | SCZ>C** | R fusiform | | |
| | SCZ>C** | R Supplementary motor area | | |
| | SCZ>C** | L middle frontal gyrus | | |
| Greater right sided language-related activation | SCZ>C | Greater right sided language-related activation | Not described | |
| L insula | C>SCZ | L insula | SCZ>BD | **R insula** |
| | C>SCZ | L middle temporal gyrus | BD>SCZ | **L DPFC, BA9** |
| | C>SCZ | R caudate | | |
| R ventral prefrontal cortex | n/s | - | n/s | - |
| R ventral striatum | | | | |
| L caudal middle temporal gyrus | | | | |
| L angular gyrus (trend) | SCZ>C | L angular gyrus | n/s | - |
| n/s | SCZ>C | L + R inferior frontal cortex, (VPFC), BA44 + 45 | SCZ>BD | **L + R inferior frontal cortex (VPFC), BA44 + 45** |
| L + R cuneus | C>SCZ | L inferior frontal gyrus | SCZ>BD | L postcentral gyrus |
| R lingual gyrus | C>SCZ | L insula | SCZ>BD | **L + R medial frontal gyrus (DPFC), BA6** |
| R inferior occipital gyrus | C>SCZ | L superior temporal gyrus | SCZ>BD | L precentral gyrus |
| | C>SCZ | L middle frontal gyrus | | |
| R + L precuneus | SCZ>C | L anterior cingulate | SCZ>BD | **R inferior frontal gyurs** |
| R angular gyrus | SCZ>C | L + R middle frontal gyrus | SCZ>BD | **R middle frontal gyrus** |
| R + L posterior cingulate | SCZ>C | R putamen | SCZ>BD | **R superior frontal gyrus** |
| | SCZ>C | R superior frontal gyrus | | |
| | SCZ>C | R inferior frontal gyrus | | |
| | SCZ>C | R +L precuneus | | |
| | SCZ>C | R angular gyrus | | |
| | SCZ>C | R + L posterior cingulate | | |

*(Continued)*

| | General details | | Main findings |
|---|---|---|---|
| Study | Task | Task contrast | Controls v BD |
| **OTHER:** | | | |
| Loeber 1999 (68) | Dynamic susceptibility constrast fMRI: | | Not described |
| Calhoun 2008 (69) | Auditory oddball task | Temporal lobe components (a) | C>BD<br>BD>C |
| | | Default mode components# (b) | C>BD |
| Ongur 2010 | Resting fMRI | | C>BD |
| | | | C>BD |
| | | | C>BD |
| | | | BD>C |
| | | | BD>C |
| | | | BD>C |
| | | | BD>C |
| | | | BD>C |

Regions in bold indicate primary regions of interest for the direct comparison of the two disorders

*—C V schizophrenia comparisons not explicitly detailed, published in previous paper Curtis et al., 1998, ** published in Curtis et al., 1999. # default mode components therefore could be interpreted as decreased activity during rest or positive task related activity, results presented having larger component voxel values between groups following ICA analysis.

functioning between the disorders appeared to be more specific to tasks involving emotion or memory, although caution should be taken as these suggestions may be in part attributable to the "region of interest" type analysis, which focused on these regions for emotional tasks, and conversely on prefrontal regions for executive tasks. There have been reports for example of abnormal over-activation of the amygdala to cognitive tasks in remitted bipolar disorder versus healthy subjects (Strakowski et al., 2004; Gruber et al., 2010) suggesting it could represent trait-related pathology.

Differences between the diagnoses were also reported in lateral prefrontal regions, although with less consistency than with the regions previously discussed. One study reported relative over-activation of the dorsal prefrontal cortex (BA6) in bipolar disorder versus schizophrenia during an emotional prosody task (Malhi et al., 2004), and

one study reported the reverse (schizophrenia versus bipolar disorder) for a task of associative memory in BA8 (Hall et al., 2009). For the executive type tasks, one study reported increased activation in bipolar disorder versus schizophrenia in dorsal regions (McIntosh et al., 2008a) and another studies reported increased activation in schizophrenia versus bipolar disorder in ventral (Costafreda et al., 2009; Costafreda et al.) and dorsal regions (Hamilton et al., 2009).

Along with medial temporal and limbic structures, neurophysiological models of these disorders also stress the importance of prefrontal regions in terms of their modulatory role. These considerations suggest that there was some evidence of general under-activation in dorsal prefrontal regions in schizophrenia versus bipolar disorder (Malhi et al., 2004; McIntosh et al., 2008a), although other studies reported over-activation (Costafreda et al., 2009; Hall et al.,

| Main findings | | | | |
|---|---|---|---|---|
| | Controls v SCZ | | BD v SCZ | |
| | | | | |
| | Not described | | SCZ>BD | L + R tonsil |
| Anterior temporal lobe<br>Posterior temporal lobe | C>SCZ | Anterior temporal lobe | BD>SCZ | Posterior temporal lobe |
| Lateral frontal regions | SCZ>C<br>SCZ>C | Posterior cingulate<br>Parietal cortex | SCZ>BD | **Lateral frontal regions** |
| R + L Medial PFC | C>SCZ | R + L anterior cingulate | BD>SCZ | L lateral parietal cortex |
| L fusiform | SCZ>C | L frontal polar cortex | BD>SCZ | L parietal operculum |
| L hippocampus | SCZ>C | L DLPFC | BD>SCZ | L fusiform gyrus |
| L lateral parietal cortex | SCZ>C | R basal ganglia | BD>SCZ | L primary visual cortex |
| L frontal polar cortex | | | BD>SCZ | L + R visual association cortex |
| R visual association cortex | | | SCZ>BD | L frontal polar cortex |
| L fusiform gyrus | | | SCZ>BD | R superior frontal gyrus |
| R auditory association cortex | | | SCZ>BD | R fusiform gyrus |
| | | | SCZ>BD | L middle temporal gyrus |

2009; Hamilton et al., 2009) which may relate to task type and difficulty, as will be discussed subsequently. There was also an indication of under-activation in ventral prefrontal regions in bipolar disorder versus schizophrenia (Costafreda et al., 2009). In comparisons with healthy subjects, there was a suggestion of differences in both dorsal as well as ventral regions in schizophrenia patients manifesting as both hyper- and hypofrontality, primarily for the executive type tasks (Costafreda et al., 2009; Curtis et al., 2001; Hamilton et al., 2009). Abnormal functioning of dorsal prefrontal regions has been widely reported in patients with schizophrenia. Whether this translates as hypo- or hyperfrontality is assumed to be dependent on task difficulty and performance (Manoach, 2003; Weinberger & Berman, 1996). The majority of studies described here did not report performance differences between the patient groups, but it could be the case that residual perceived task demand could

be influencing the direction of differences, particularly given the range of task types. For bipolar disorder versus healthy subjects, there were no differences reported in any of the studies in dorsal prefrontal regions; however three studies reported both hypo- and hyperfrontality in ventral regions (Curtis et al., 2001; Malhi et al., 2004; McIntosh et al., 2008a). The ventral prefrontal cortex is generally considered to be involved in affect regulation; hence it may contribute to the loss of affective homeostasis seen in bipolar disorder. Activation in these regions has been consistently reported to be abnormal in bipolar mania (Blumberg et al., 2003; Blumberg et al., 1999; Elliott et al., 2004), depression (Blumberg et al., 2003; Chen et al., 2006; Lawrence et al., 2004), and in euthymia (Blumberg et al., 2003; Strakowski et al., 2004; Kronhaus et al., 2006; Kruger et al., 2006). Taken together these studies indicate that there are patterns of activation differences in lateral

TABLE 7.4 SUMMARY OF MAIN fMRI FINDINGS BY REGION

| Region | BD>SCZ | SCZ>BD | C>BD | BD>C | C>SCZ | SCZ>C |
|---|---|---|---|---|---|---|
| Medial temporal lobe | (Hall et al., 2009) (Whalley et al., 2009) | | (Mitchell et al., 2004) | (Whalley et al., 2009) | (Whalley et al., 2009) | |
| Meso-limbic/ sub-cortical structures | (Mitchell et al., 2004) (Whalley et al., 2009) | (Mitchell et al., 2004) (Hamilton et al., 2009) (McIntosh et al., 2008) | (Mitchell et al., 2004) (Abler et al., 2008) | (Mitchell et al., 2004) (Whalley et al., 2009) (Curtis et al., 2001) (McIntosh et al., 2008) | (Hamilton et al., 2009) (McIntosh et al., 2008) | (Mitchell et al., 2004) |
| Dorsal prefrontal cortex (Middle frontal gyrus) | (Mitchell et al., 2004) (McIntosh et al., 2008) | (Hall et al., 2009) | | | (Curtis et al., 2001) (Hamilton et al., 2009) | (Hall et al., 2009) (Curtis et al., 2001) |
| Ventral prefrontal cortex (Inferior frontal gyrus) | | (Costafreda et al., 2009) | (Mitchell et al., 2004) | (Curtis et al., 2001) (McIntosh et al., 2008) | (Curtis et al., 2001) (Hamilton et al., 2009) | (Costafreda et al., 2009) |

prefrontal regions that may be important for distinguishing the two diagnoses. Indeed, in terms of the discriminant ability of fMRI, the two studies using such an approach implicated the importance of the dorsolateral prefrontal cortical activation as distinguishing the disorders (Hall et al., 2009; McIntosh et al., 2008a).

## SYMPTOMS

Two studies examined patients with mania versus schizophrenia and healthy subjects (Abler et al., 2008; Sommer et al., 2007), and three studies examined correlations with symptom measures (Hall et al., 2009; McIntosh et al., 2008a; Whalley et al., 2009). In a study of reward processing, Abler et al. (2008) reported that manic patients did not present the same pattern of responding to that seen in the healthy or schizophrenia subjects during receipt or omission of expected reward. Here the differential response for receipt versus omission of reward was significantly lower in the nucleus accumbens in bipolar mania compared to healthy subjects (Abler et al., 2008). This observation was interpreted as evidence for dysfunctional reward pathways in acute mania, specifically alterations in the coding of prediction error signals in the ventral striatum. This abnormality was proposed to underlie deficits seen in learning and decision-making in acutely manic patients.

Sommer et al. (2007) examined patients with psychotic mania and unipolar psychotic depression compared to an earlier sample of healthy subjects and patients with schizophrenia. The main findings were that there was decreased language lateralization in all patient groups versus healthy

subjects—that is, higher language related activation in the right hemisphere in all patient groups—and was not found to be related to the severity of psychosis.

Relationships between clinical measures and symptom scales were explored in three studies (Hall et al., 2009; McIntosh et al., 2008a; Whalley et al., 2009). In the first of these, the only significant relationship found was between activation in the orbitofrontal cortex and positive and negative symptoms scale (PANSS) positive scores in bipolar disorder subjects (McIntosh et al., 2008a). In the study by Hall and colleagues examining associative memory, a positive correlation was found between scores of mania from the young mania rating scale (YMRS) and activation in the hippocampus during early encoding, and a negative correlation was found in the schizophrenia patients (Hall et al., 2009). Finally, in a study of emotional memory, significant correlations were reported between scores for mania from the YMRS and activation in the anterior cingulate across both patient groups, and a negative correlation between activation in the dorsolateral prefrontal cortex with depression scores from the Hamilton depression rating scale (HDRS) (Whalley et al., 2009). For the correlation with mania ratings, the correlation values did not differ between groups, indicating a possible symptom specific rather than disease specific abnormality. In contrast for the correlation with depression there was a significant difference between the groups with the bipolar group having a significant negative correlation. Due to the small number of studies it is not possible to formulate a cohesive overview of these studies, but there appears to be some association between the presence or severity of mania and activation in limbic structures (Abler et al., 2008; Hall et al., 2009; Whalley et al., 2009)

## NON-TASK DRIVEN fMRI STUDIES

Of the three other studies that did not fit either of the above categories, one examined cerebellar blood volume in both disorders using dynamic susceptibility contrast (Loeber et al., 1999). In this study patients with schizophrenia were found to have the highest mean cerebellar blood volume and bipolar disorder patients had the lowest volume, although differences did not reach statistical significance. For sub-regions the only significant finding was in a similar direction for the right and left cerebellar tonsils.

The remaining studies used a computational approach (independent components analysis) to examine temporally synchronous fluctuations in fMRI activity to discriminate between the two patient groups (Calhoun et al., 2008; Ongur et al., 2010). The default mode network is considered to be a characteristic network of regions which display spontaneous fluctuation in fMRI activity at rest, or conversely regions whose activity decreases on performance of a task; abnormalities in this network have been implicated in both disorders (Raichle et al., 2001). The first study specifically examined temporal lobe regions of this network that had previously been shown in schizophrenia to fail to follow healthy deactivation (Fletcher et al., 1998). Here the three-way classification algorithm resulted in discrimination with an average sensitivity of 90% and specificity of 95%. The second study compared the wider default mode network between groups and reported differences between the diagnoses in frontal polar regions and superior frontal gyrus, along with posterior brain regions (schizophrenia>bipolar disorder). As in the previous section, the limited number of studies making direct comparisons between the disorders using such techniques means it is premature to summarize findings at the present time.

## COMMENTS ON FUNCTIONAL IMAGING IN BIPOLAR DISORDER AND SCHIZOPHRENIA

This section was intended as an early narrative summary of the current fMRI literature directly comparing bipolar disorder and schizophrenia. A more structured meta-analysis was not warranted at this time given the small number of studies in the various sub-categories and consequent heterogeneity in co-ordinates. It should be noted that we did not examine effects of medication, since not all studies examined such effects directly. Those that did generally reported that there were no effects of medication, typically examined as chlorpromazine equivalents, on the main findings of interest (Hall et al., 2009; Malhi et al., 2004; McIntosh et al., 2008a; Whalley et al., 2009). It should be cautioned however that a recent review of the wider literature of both anti-psychotic and lithium treatment were found to have some potential effects on regional brain activity (Phillips et al., 2008b)

Another limitation was that the prime focus of the studies reviewed was on identification of diagnostically specific features, rather than on similarities between disorders. This approach is complicated by the fact that deficits seen in bipolar disorder, particularly in euthymic phases, are generally less severe than those seen in schizophrenia. Consequently it may be the case, as in one study in this review (Hamilton et al., 2009), that differences are only significant in the schizophrenic versus healthy subject comparisons. More direct testing for similarities, perhaps with the application of conjunction analyses by the individual studies themselves, may therefore be appropriate to reveal regions of shared abnormal functional architecture.

In summary, the literature comparing schizophrenia and bipolar disorder indicates that there is evidence for functional differences in the neurobiological substrates of each disorder in medial temporal lobe structures, associated limbic regions, and in the lateral prefrontal cortex. From the studies described here it appears that these differences generally manifest as increased activation of limbic and associated regions in bipolar patients, with an increased involvement of dorsal rather than ventral prefrontal abnormalities in schizophrenia. Larger studies and the prospect of imaging across symptom dimensions in combination with investigating the influence of candidate risk genes in common between the disorders (Mechelli et al., 2008) may further the understanding of the underlying aetiological mechanisms behind these conditions.

---

**Functional Imaging: Schizophrenia Vs. Bipolar Disorder**

- Relatively few studies within task categories

- In those examining emotion, reward and memory, bipolar disorder associated with over-activation in limbic regions compared to schizophrenia

- Some evidence for greater involvement of dorsolateral prefrontal abnormalities in schizophrenia compared to bipolar disorder

## CONCLUSIONS AND SUMMARY

Schizophrenia and bipolar disorder are symptomatically overlapping syndromes for which there is considerable nosological uncertainty. Imaging has been applied to schizophrenia and bipolar disorder in an attempt to identify whether these two disorders are truly separate or are points on a continuum of illness.

The many imaging studies of bipolar disorder and schizophrenia conducted to date have revealed a rather complicated picture. Some findings from structural imaging (particularly of the medial temporal lobe) reveal that particular deficits may be present only in subjects with schizophrenia. Functional imaging also reveals qualitative differences between the disorders that are of sufficient magnitude to be of clinical utility, if the findings are subsequently replicated in larger cohorts with first illness episodes. On the other hand, many regions closely linked to the etiology of bipolar disorder and schizophrenia have been shown to be abnormal in both conditions.

A major issue with the current literature is the considerable amount of between-study heterogeneity and the relatively small sample sizes. In the systematic review by Kempton and colleagues (2008), most studies of patents with bipolar disorder compared to healthy subjects were grossly underpowered to address the differences they were designed to find. If this is the case for studies using healthy controls, this issue may be even greater in magnitude for studies comparing two overlapping clinical conditions.

## REFERENCES

Abler, B., Greenhouse, I., Ongur, D., Walter, H., & Heckers, S., 2008. Abnormal reward system activation in mania. *Neuropsychopharmacology*, 33: 2217–2227.

Arnone, D., Cavanagh, J., Gerber, D., Lawrie, S. M., Ebmeier, K. P., & McIntosh, A. M., 2009. Magnetic resonance imaging studies in bipolar disorder and schizophrenia: meta-analysis. *The British Journal of Psychiatry*, 195: 194–201.

Beyer, J. L., Young, R., Kuchibhatla, M., & Krishnan, K. R., 2009. Hyperintense MRI lesions in bipolar disorder: A meta-analysis and review. *International Review of Psychiatry*, 21: 394–409.

Blumberg, H. P., Leung, H. C., Skudlarski, P., Lacadie, C. M., Fredericks, C. A., Harris, B. C., . . . Peterson, B. S., 2003. A functional magnetic resonance imaging study of bipolar disorder: state- and trait-related dysfunction in ventral prefrontal cortices. *Archives of General Psychiatry*, 60: 601–609.

Blumberg, H. P., Stern, E., Ricketts, S., Martinez, D., de Asis, J., White, T., . . . Silbersweig, D. A., 1999. Rostral and orbital prefrontal cortex dysfunction in the manic state of bipolar disorder. *American Journal of Psychiatry*, 156: 1986–1988.

Bora, E., Yucel, M., Fornito, A., Berk, M., & Pantelis, C., 2008. Major psychoses with mixed psychotic and mood symptoms: are mixed psychoses associated with different neurobiological markers? *Acta Psychiatrica Scandinavica*, 118: 172–187.

Bramon, E., & Sham, P. C., 2001. The common genetic liability between schizophrenia and bipolar disorder: a review. *Current Psychiatry Reports*, 3: 332–337.

Breeze, J. L., Hesdorffer, D. C., Hong, X., Frazier, J. A., & Renshaw, P. F., 2003. Clinical significance of brain white matter hyperintensities in young adults with psychiatric illness. *Harvard Review of Psychiatry*, 11: 269–283.

Calhoun, V. D., Maciejewski, P. K., Pearlson, G. D., & Kiehl, K. A., 2008. Temporal lobe and "default" hemodynamic brain modes discriminate between schizophrenia and bipolar disorder. *Human Brain Mapping*, 29: 1265–1275.

Cannon, T. D., Kaprio, J., Lonnqvist, J., Huttunen, M., & Koskenvuo, M., 1998. The genetic epidemiology of schizophrenia in a Finnish twin cohort. A population-based modeling study. *Archives of General Psychiatry*, 55: 67–74.

Cardno, A. G., Marshall, E. J., Coid, B., Macdonald, A. M., Ribchester, T. R., Davies, N. J., . . . Murray, R. M., 1999. Heritability estimates for psychotic disorders: the Maudsley twin psychosis series. *Archives of General Psychiatry*, 56: 162–168.

Cardno, A. G., Rijsdijk, F. V., Sham, P. C., Murray, R. M., & McGuffin, P., 2002. A twin study of genetic relationships between psychotic symptoms. *American Journal of Psychiatry*, 159: 539–545.

Cerullo, M. A., Adler, C. M., DelBello, M. P., & Strakowski, S. M., 2009. The functional neuroanatomy of bipolar disorder. *International Review of Psychiatry*, 21: 314–322.

Chen, C. H., Lennox, B., Jacob, R., Calder, A., Lupson, V., Bisbrown-Chippendale, R., . . . Bullmore, E., 2006. Explicit and implicit facial affect recognition in manic and depressed States of bipolar disorder: a functional magnetic resonance imaging study. *Biological Psychiatry*, 59: 31–39.

Costafreda, S. G., Fu, C. H., Picchioni, M., Kane, F., McDonald, C., Prata, D. P., . . . McGuire, P. K., 2009. Increased inferior frontal activation during word generation: a marker of genetic risk for schizophrenia but not bipolar disorder? *Human Brain Mapping*, 30: 3287–3298.

Costafreda, S. G., Fu, C. H., Picchioni, M., Touloupoulou, T., McDonald, C., Walshe, M., . . . McGuire, P. K., Pattern of neural responses to verbal fluency shows diagnostic specificity for schizophrenia and bipolar disorder. *BMC Psychiatry*, 11: 18.

Craddock, N., O'Donovan, M. C., & Owen, M. J., 2005. The genetics of schizophrenia and bipolar disorder: dissecting psychosis. *Journal of Medical Genetics*, 42: 193–204.

Craddock, N., O'Donovan, M. C., & Owen, M. J., 2006. Genes for schizophrenia and bipolar disorder? Implications for psychiatric nosology. *Schizophrenia Bulletin*, 32: 9–16.

Craddock, N., & Owen, M. J., 2005. The beginning of the end for the Kraepelinian dichotomy. British *Journal of Psychiatry* 186: 364–366.

Craddock, N., & Owen, M. J., 2010. The Kraepelinian dichotomy—going, going. . . but still not gone. *British Journal of Psychiatry*, 196: 92–95.

Cui, L., Li, M., Deng, W., Guo, W., Ma, X., Huang, C., Jiang, L., Wang, Y., Collier, DA., Gong, Q., Li, T. 2011. Overlapping clusters of gray matter deficits in paranoid schizophrenia and psychotic bipolar mania with family history. *Neuroscience Letters*, 489(2): 94–98.

Curtis, V. A., Dixon, T. A., Morris, R. G., Bullmore, E. T., Brammer, M. J., Williams, S. C., . . . McGuire, P. K., 2001. Differential frontal activation in schizophrenia and bipolar illness during verbal fluency. *Journal of Affective Disorders*, 66: 111–121.

Elliott, R., Ogilvie, A., Rubinsztein, J. S., Calderon, G., Dolan, R. J., & Sahakian, B. J., 2004. Abnormal ventral frontal response during performance of an affective go/no go task in patients with mania. *Biol Psychiatry*, 55: 1163–1170.

Ellison-Wright, I., & Bullmore, E. 2010. Anatomy of bipolar disorder and schizophrenia: a meta-analysis. *Schizophrenia Research*, 117(1): 1–12.

Farrow, T.F.D., Whitford, T. J., Williams, L. M., Gomes, L., & Harris, A.W.F., 2005. Diagnosis-Related Regional Gray Matter Loss Over Two Years in First Episode Schizophrenia and Bipolar Disorder. *Biol Psychiatry*, 58: 713–723.

Fletcher, P. C., McKenna, P. J., Frith, C. D., Grasby, P. M., Friston, K. J., & Dolan, R. J., 1998. Brain activations in schizophrenia during a graded memory task studied with functional neuroimaging. *Archives of General Psychiatry*, 55: 1001–1008.

Friston, K. J., & Frith, C. D., 1995. Schizophrenia: a disconnection syndrome? *Clinical Neuroscience*, 3: 89–97.

Grozeva, D., Kirov, G., Ivanov, D., Jones, I. R., Jones, L., Green, E. K., . . . Craddock, N., 2010. Rare copy number variants: a point of rarity in genetic risk for bipolar disorder and schizophrenia. *Archives of General Psychiatry*, 67: 318–327.

Gruber, O., Tost, H., Henseler, I., Schmael, C., Scherk, H., Ende, G., . . . Rietschel, M., 2010. Pathological amygdala activation during working memory performance: Evidence for a pathophysiological trait marker in bipolar affective disorder. *Human Brain Mapping*, 31: 115–125.

Gur, R. E., McGrath, C., Chan, R. M., Schroeder, L., Turner, T., Turetsky, B. I., . . . Gur, R. C., 2002. An fMRI study of facial emotion processing in patients with schizophrenia. *American Journal of Psychiatry*, 159: 1992–1999.

Hall, J., Whalley, H. C., Marwick, K., McKirdy, J., Sussmann, J., Romaniuk, L., . . . Lawrie, S. M., 2009. Hippocampal function in schizophrenia and bipolar disorder. *Psychological Medicine*, 40(5): 761–770

Hall, J., Whalley, H. C., McKirdy, J. W., Romaniuk, L., McGonigle, D. J., McIntosh, A. M., . . . Young, A. W., 2008. Overactivation of fear systems to neutral faces in schizophrenia. *Biological Psychiatry*, 64: 70–73.

Hallahan, B., Newell, J., Soares, J. C., Brambilla, P., Strakowski, S. M., Fleck, D. E., . . . McDonald, C., 2010. Structural MRI in Bipolar Disorder: An international collaborative mega-analysis of individual adult patient data. *Biological Psychiatry*, 7(8): 764–785.

Hamilton, L. S., Altshuler, L. L., Townsend, J., Bookheimer, S. Y., Phillips, O. R., Fischer, J., . . . Narr, K. L., 2009. Alterations in functional activation in euthymic bipolar disorder and schizophrenia during a working memory task. *Human Brain Mapping*, 30: 3958–3969.

Holt, D. J., Kunkel, L., Weiss, A. P., Goff, D. C., Wright, C. I., Shin, L. M., . . . Heckers, S., 2006. Increased medial temporal lobe activation during the passive viewing of emotional and neutral facial expressions in schizophrenia. *Schizophrenia Research*, 82: 153–162.

Huang, J., Perlis, R. H., Lee, P. H., Rush, A. J., Fava, M., Sachs, G. S., . . . Smoller, J. W., 2010. Cross-Disorder Genomewide Analysis of Schizophrenia, Bipolar Disorder, and Depression. *American Journal of Psychiatry*, 167: 1254–1263.

Janssen, J., Reig, S., Parellada, M., Moreno, D., Graell, M., Fraguas, D., . . . Arango, C., 2008. Regional gray matter volume deficits in adolescents with first-episode psychosis. *J Am Acad Child Adolesc Psychiatry*, 47: 1311–1320.

Kawashima, T., Nakamura, M., Bouix, S., Kubicki, M., Salisbury, D. F., Westin, C. F., . . . Shenton, M. E., 2009. Uncinate fasciculus abnormalities in recent onset schizophrenia and affective psychosis: a diffusion tensor imaging study. *Schizophrenia Research*, 110: 119–126.

Keck, P. E., Jr., McElroy, S. L., Havens, J. R., Altshuler, L. L., Nolen, W. A., Frye, M. A., . . . Post, R. M., 2003. Psychosis in bipolar disorder: phenomenology and impact on morbidity and course of illness. *Comprehensive Psychiatry*, 44: 263–269.

Kempf, L., Hussain, N., & Potash, J. B., 2005. Mood disorder with psychotic features, schizoaffective disorder, and schizophrenia with mood features: trouble at the borders. *International Review of Psychiatry*, 17: 9–19.

Kempton, M. J., Geddes, J. R., Ettinger, U., Williams, S. C., & Grasby, P. M., 2008. Meta-analysis, database, and meta-regression of 98 structural imaging studies in bipolar disorder. *Archives of General Psychiatry*, 65: 1017–1032.

Kendler, K. S., Gruenberg, A. M., & Kinney, D. K., 1994. Independent diagnoses of adoptees and relatives as defined by DSM-III in the provincial and national samples of the Danish Adoption Study of Schizophrenia. *Archives of General Psychiatry*, 51: 456–468.

Kerr, A., & McClelland, H., 1991. *Concepts of Mental Disorder: A Continuing Debate*. London: Gaskell.

Krabbendam, L., Arts, B., van Os, J., & Aleman, A., 2005. Cognitive functioning in patients with schizophrenia and bipolar disorder: a quantitative review. *Schizophrenia Research*, 80: 137–149.

Krabbendam, L., Honig, A., Wiersma, J., Vuurman, E. F., Hofman, P. A., Derix, M. M., . . . Jolles, J., 2000. Cognitive dysfunctions and white matter lesions in patients with bipolar disorder in remission. *Acta Psychiatrica Scandinavica*, 101: 274–280.

Kronhaus, D. M., Lawrence, N. S., Williams, A. M., Frangou, S., Brammer, M. J., Williams, S. C., . . . Phillips, M. L., 2006. Stroop performance in bipolar disorder: further evidence for abnormalities in the ventral prefrontal cortex. *Bipolar Disorders*, 8: 28–39.

Kruger, S., Alda, M., Young, L. T., Goldapple, K., Parikh, S., & Mayberg, H.S., 2006. Risk and resilience markers in bipolar disorder: brain responses to emotional challenge in bipolar patients and their healthy siblings. *American Journal of Psychiatry*, 163: 257–264.

Laursen, T. M., Agerbo, E., & Pedersen, C. B., 2009. Bipolar disorder, schizoaffective disorder, and schizophrenia overlap: a new comorbidity index. *Journal of Clinical Psychiatry*, 70: 1432–1438.

Lawrence, N. S., Williams, A. M., Surguladze, S., Giampietro, V., Brammer, M. J., Andrew, C., . . . Phillips, M. L., 2004. Subcortical and ventral prefrontal cortical neural responses to facial expressions distinguish patients with bipolar disorder and major depression. *Biological Psychiatry*, 55: 578–587.

Lewine, R. R., Hudgins, P., Brown, F., Caudle, J., & Risch, S. C., 1995. Differences in qualitative brain morphology findings in schizophrenia, major depression, bipolar disorder, and normal volunteers. *Schizophrenia Research*, 15: 253–259.

Lichtenstein, P., Yip, B. H., Bjork, C., Pawitan, Y., Cannon, T. D., Sullivan, P. F., & Hultman, C.M., 2009. Common genetic determinants of schizophrenia and bipolar disorder in Swedish families: a population-based study. *Lancet*, 373: 234–239.

Loeber, R. T., Sherwood, A. R., Renshaw, P. F., Cohen, B. M., & Yurgelun-Todd, D. A., 1999. Differences in cerebellar blood volume in schizophrenia and bipolar disorder. *Schizophrenia Research*, 37: 81–89.

Lyoo, I. K., Lee, H. K., Jung, J. H., Noam, G. G., & Renshaw, P. F., 2002. White matter hyperintensities on magnetic resonance imaging of the brain in children with psychiatric disorders. *Comprehensive Psychiatry*, 43: 361–368.

Malhi, G. S., Lagopoulos, J., Sachdev, P., Mitchell, P. B., Ivanovski, B., & Parker, G. B., 2004. Cognitive generation of affect in hypomania: an fMRI study. *Bipolar Disorders*, 6: 271–285.

Maniega, S. M., Lymer, G. K., Bastin, M. E., Marjoram, D., Job, D. E., Owens, D. G., . . . Lawrie, S. M., 2007. Diffusion tensor MRI in subjects at high risk of schizophrenia. *Schizophrenia Bulletin*, 33: 348–348.

Manoach, D. S., 2003. Prefrontal cortex dysfunction during working memory performance in schizophrenia: reconciling discrepant findings. *Schizophrenia Research*, 60: 285–298.

McDonald, C., Bullmore, E., Sham, P., Chitnis, X., Suckling, J., MacCabe, J., . . . Murray, R. M., 2005. Regional volume deviations of brain structure in schizophrenia and psychotic bipolar disorder: computational morphometry study. *British Journal of Psychiatry*, 186: 369–377.

McDonald, C., Bullmore, E. T., Sham, P. C., Chitnis, X., Wickham, H., Bramon, E., & Murray, R.M., 2004a. Association of genetic risks for schizophrenia and bipolar disorder with specific and generic brain structural endophenotypes. *Archives of General Psychiatry*, 61: 974–984.

McDonald, C., Zanelli, J., Rabe-Hesketh, S., Ellison-Wright, I., Sham, P., Kalidindi, S., . . . Kennedy, N., 2004b. Meta-analysis of magnetic resonance imaging brain morphometry studies in bipolar disorder. *Biological Psychiatry*, 56: 144–417.

McDonald, W. M., Tupler, L. A., Marsteller, F. A., Figiel, G. S., DiSouza, S., Nemeroff, C. B., & Krishnan, K.R., 1999. Hyperintense lesions on magnetic resonance images in bipolar disorder. *Biological Psychiatry*, 45: 965–971.

McGuffin, P., Rijsdijk, F., Andrew, M., Sham, P., Katz, R., & Cardno, A., 2003. The heritability of bipolar affective disorder and the genetic relationship to unipolar depression. *Archives of General Psychiatry*, 60: 497–502.

McIntosh, A. M., Hall, J., Lymer, G.K.S., Sussmann, J.E.D., & Lawrie, S. M., 2009. Genetic risk for white matter abnormalities in bipolar disorder. *Int ernationalReviews of Psychiatry*, 21: 387–393.

McIntosh, A. M., Job, D. E., Moorhead, T. W., Harrison, L. K., Lawrie, S. M., & Johnstone, E. C., 2005. White matter density in patients with schizophrenia, bipolar disorder and their unaffected relatives. *Biological Psychiatry*, 58: 254–257.

McIntosh, A. M., Job, D. E., Moorhead, W. J., Harrison, L. K., Whalley, H. C., Johnstone, E. C., & Lawrie, S. M., 2006. Genetic liability to schizophrenia or bipolar disorder and its relationship to brain structure. *American Journal pf Medical Genetics B,* 141: 76–83.

McIntosh, A. M., Job, D., Moorhead, T. W. J., Harrison, L. K., Forrester, K., Lawrie, S. M., & Johnstone, E. C., 2004. Voxel-Based morphometry of patients with schizophrenia or bipolar disorder and their unaffected relatives. *Biological Psychiatry*, 56: 544–552.

McIntosh, A. M., Whalley, H. C., McKirdy, J., Hall, J., Sussmann, J. E., Shankar, P., . . . Lawrie, S. M., 2008a. Prefrontal function and activation in bipolar disorder and schizophrenia. *American Journal of Psychiatry*, 165, 378–384.

McIntosh, A. M., Whalley, H. C., McKirdy, J., Hall, J., Sussmann, J. E., Shankar, P., . . . Lawrie, S. M., 2008b. Prefrontal function and activation in bipolar disorder and schizophrenia. *American Journal of Psychiatry*, 165: 378–384.

Mechelli, A., Prata, D. P., Fu, C. H., Picchioni, M., Kane, F., Kalidindi, S., . . . McGuire, P. K., 2008. The effects of neuregulin1 on brain function in controls and patients with schizophrenia and bipolar disorder. *Neuroimage*, 42: 817–826.

Moskvina, V., Craddock, N., Holmans, P., Nikolov, I., Pahwa, J. S., Green, E., . . . O'Donovan, M. C., 2009. Gene-wide analyses of genome-wide association data sets: evidence for multiple common risk alleles for schizophrenia and bipolar disorder and for overlap in genetic risk. *Molecular Psychiatry*, 14: 252–260.

Murray, R. M., Sham, P., van Os, J., Zanelli, J., Cannon, M., & McDonald, C., 2004. A developmental model for similarities and dissimilarities between schizophrenia and bipolar disorder. *Schizophrenia Research*, 71: 405–416.

Ongur, D., Lundy, M., Greenhouse, I., Shinn, A. K., Menon, V., Cohen, B. M., & Renshaw, P. F., 2010. Default mode network abnormalities in bipolar disorder and schizophrenia. *Psychiatry Research*, 183: 59–68.

Persaud, R., Russow, H., Harvey, I., Lewis, S. W., Ron, M., Murray, R. M., & du Boulay, G., 1997. Focal signal hyperintensities in schizophrenia. *Schizophrenia Research*, 27: 55–64.

Phillips, M. L., Drevets, W. C., Rauch, S. L., & Lane, R., 2003. Neurobiology of emotion perception II: Implications for major psychiatric disorders. *Biological Psychiatry*, 54: 515–528.

Phillips, M. L., Ladouceur, C. D., & Drevets, W. C., 2008a. A neural model of voluntary and automatic emotion regulation: implications for understanding the pathophysiology and neurodevelopment of bipolar disorder. *Molecular Psychiatry*, 13: 829.

Phillips, M. L., Travis, M. J., Fagiolini, A., & Kupfer, D. J., 2008b. Medication effects in neuroimaging studies of bipolar disorder. *American Journal of Psychiatry*, 165: 313–320.

Phillips, M. L., Williams, L., Senior, C., Bullmore, E. T., Brammer, M. J., Andrew, C., . . . David, A. S., 1999. A differential neural response to threatening and non-threatening negative facial expressions in paranoid and non-paranoid schizophrenics. *Psychiatry Research*, 92: 11–31.

Pillai, J. J., Friedman, L., Stuve, T. A., Trinidad, S., Jesberger, J. A., Lewin, J. S., . . . Schulz, S. C., 2002. Increased presence of white matter hyperintensities in adolescent patients with bipolar disorder. *Psychiatry Research*, 114: 51–56.

Purcell, S. M., Wray, N. R., Stone, J. L., Visscher, P. M., O'Donovan, M. C., Sullivan, P. F., & Sklar, P., 2009. Common polygenic variation contributes to risk of schizophrenia and bipolar disorder. *Nature*, 460: 748–752.

Raichle, M. E., MacLeod, A. M., Snyder, A. Z., Powers, W. J., Gusnard, D. A., & Shulman, G. L., 2001. A default mode of brain function. *Proceedings of the National Academy of Sciences of the United States of America*, 98: 676–682.

Schneider, F., Weiss, U., Kessler, C., Salloum, J. B., Posse, S., Grodd, W., & Muller-Gartner, H. W., 1998. Differential amygdala activation in schizophrenia during sadness. *Schizophrenia Research*, 34: 133–142.

Schwartz, C. E., Wright, C. I., Shin, L. M., Kagan, J., Whalen, P. J., McMullin, K. G., & Rauch, S. L., 2003. Differential amygdalar response to novel versus newly familiar neutral faces: a functional MRI probe developed for studying inhibited temperament. *Biological Psychiatry*, 53: 854–862.

Siris, S.G., 2000. Depression in schizophrenia: perspective in the era of "Atypical" antipsychotic agents. *American Journal of Psychiatry*, 157: 1379–1389.

Sommer, I. E., Vd Veer, A. J., Wijkstra, J., Boks, M. P., & Kahn, R.S., 2007. Comparing language lateralization in psychotic mania and psychotic depression to schizophrenia; a functional MRI study. *Schizophrenia Research*, 89: 364–365.

Strakowski, S. M., Adler, C. M., Holland, S. K., Mills, N., & DelBello, M. P., 2004. A preliminary FMRI study of sustained attention in euthymic, unmedicated bipolar disorder. *Neuropsychopharmacology*, 29: 1734–1740.

Strakowski, S. M., DelBello, M. P., & Adler, C. M., 2005. The functional neuroanatomy of bipolar disorder: a review of neuroimaging findings. *Molecular Psychiatry*, 10: 105–116.

Strakowski, S. M., Woods, B. T., Tohen, M., Wilson, D. R., Douglass, A. W., & Stoll, A. L., 1993. MRI subcortical signal hyperintensities in mania at first hospitalization. *Biological Psychiatry*, 33: 204–206.

Surguladze, S., Russell, T., Kucharska-Pietura, K., Travis, M.J., Giampietro, V., David, A.S., & Phillips, M.L., 2006. A reversal of the normal pattern of parahippocampal response to neutral and fearful faces is associated with reality distortion in schizophrenia. *Biological Psychiatr,y* 60: 423–431.

Sussmann, J. E., Lymer, G. K., McKirdy, J., Moorhead, T. W., Maniega, S. M., Job, D., . . . McIntosh, A. M., 2009a. White matter abnormalities in bipolar disorder and schizophrenia detected using diffusion tensor magnetic resonance imaging. *Bipolar Disorders*, 11: 11–18.

Sussmann, J. E., Lymer, G. K., McKirdy, J., Moorhead, T. W., Munoz Maniega, S., Job, D., . . . McIntosh, A. M., 2009b. White matter abnormalities in bipolar disorder and schizophrenia detected using diffusion tensor magnetic resonance imaging. *Bipolar Disorders*, 11: 11–18.

Weinberger, D. R., & Berman, K. F., 1996. Prefrontal function in schizophrenia: confounds and controversies. *Philosophical Transactions of the Royal Society of London—Series B: Biological Sciences*, 351: 1495–1503.

Whalley, H. C., McKirdy, J., Romaniuk, L., Sussmann, J., Johnstone, E. C., Wan, H., . . . Hall, J., 2009. Functional imaging of emotional memory in bipolar disorder and schizophrenia. *Bipolar Disorders*, 11(80): 840–856.

Williams, L. M., Das, P., Harris, A. W., Liddell, B. B., Brammer, M. J., Olivieri, G., . . . Gordon, E., 2004. Dysregulation of arousal and amygdala-prefrontal systems in paranoid schizophrenia. *American Journal of Psychiatry*, 161: 480–489.

Wright, I. C., Rabe-Hesketh, S., Woodruff, P. W., David, A. S., Murray, R. M., & Bullmore, E. T., 2000. Meta-analysis of regional brain volumes in schizophrenia. *American Journal of Psychiatry*, 157: 16–25.

Yu K, Cheung C, Leung M, Li Q, Chua S, & McAlonan G. 2010. Are Bipolar Disorder and Schizophrenia Neuroanatomically Distinct? An anatomical likelihood meta-analysis. *Frontiers in Human Neurosciences*, 4 (Oct 26): 189.

# PART II

## HOW GENETIC RESEARCH INFORMS MODELS OF BIPOLAR DISORDER

# 8.

# GENETIC TECHNIQUES AND THEIR APPLICATION TO BIPOLAR DISORDER

## Aaron C. Vederman and Melvin G. McInnis

### BEGINNING AND CHALLENGES

With the turn of the twenty-first century it was widely anticipated and assumed that with the combination of research advances in knowledge and technology, the field of neuroscience and psychiatry would appreciate a revolutionary advance in the nosology, phenomenology, and treatment of psychiatric conditions. These advances were expected to radically transition mental health care to a more biologically mechanistic paradigm. At the very least, such methodologies brought into clinical practice would herald the transition of treatment practices from a clinically subjective approach to a research-based objectively anchored neuroscience approach to psychiatric disorders. While treatments in overlapping medical and psychiatric conditions have been heavily influenced by the field of pharmacogenetics (exemplified by the need to monitor CYP2D6 status in the management of depression in breast cancer patients when tamoxifen is used), the daily practice of psychiatry has not been influenced as many had expected.

The primary reason for the current minimal influence of genetics and technological advances from the laboratory on advancing psychiatry is that findings so far are modest; there are statistically significant, but clinically negligible, risks of illness that are associated with genetic variants. In the current understanding of psychiatric disorders there is little value that the knowledge of genetic variants adds to the understanding of the etiology of psychiatric disorders. A major contributor to this lack of clarity is related to the clinical heterogeneity of the illnesses, which confound classification of psychiatric cases and, consequently, genetics study. This explanation has been invoked generously whenever challenges are encountered, however, without identifying potential solutions to the problem. The recent results from genome wide association (GWAS) and linkage analyses have certainly emphasized this reality. In many regards,

results from GWAS, epigenetics, and pharmacogenetics have impressed upon researchers the truly unchartered nature of the nosology and etiology of psychiatric illness. One prominent feature of the unchartered terrain is the protean nature of the expression and function of the genome. Integrating biology, psychology, physiology, and environmental effects will remain a challenge for the coming generation of investigators. Behavior and environmental factors impact genetic expression and biology in dramatic ways. An example from the biology of aging is the profound effect that dietary or caloric restriction produces by reducing morbidity and mortality and increasing maximal lifespan across species; this effect has been studied extensively for over 70 years (McCay, 1934). However, recently research at the genetic and cellular levels has shed light on how an environmental stressor, such as caloric restriction, may act upon specific pathways of gene expression (Medvedik et al., 2007; Kenyon, 2010). A review of this topic in detail is well beyond the scope of this chapter, however, broadly it is possible to comment that caloric restriction may act upon gene expression and cell signaling which in our evolutionary path ensured survival by shifting growth and reproduction of the organism to protection and maintenance of the biological system. This line of research has continued through many investigations of both environmental manipulations that extend lifespan as well as direct manipulation of the genome in animal models to influence lifespan. For a more extensive reading, see Kenyon's (2010) comprehensive review. Such research is changing our understanding of aging from a simplistic model of biological inevitability, to one based upon specific cellular pathways with genetic foundations (Kenyon, 2010; Selman & Withers, 2011).

So too within the sphere of psychiatric illness, a movement away from classic clinical phenotypic observation and categorical characterization and toward a more sophisticated model that incorporates dimensional measures of the research domain criteria (RDoC) (Insel et al., 2010) and biological parameters is emphasized. Like genetic pathways in aging, environmental factors will moderate and therefore obfuscate the phenotypic expression of high-risk genes, in ways that are dynamic and yet to be determined. A manifold approach is necessary and will include simple organisms as well as research with human subjects. Modeling aging or metabolism is straightforward in simple biological organisms in which experimental manipulations may be implemented and their outcomes recorded. The approach to studying psychiatric illness is more challenging because modeling major depression, schizophrenia, or bipolar disorder in animal models is difficult. Nevertheless, productive research in animal models has been conducted and is reviewed in the following chapter. Finally, the disjunctive categorical nature of psychiatric diagnosis is highly likely to be contributing to diagnostic heterogeneity; there are many combinations of DSM-IV symptoms that can bring the patient into a category.

Exploring the genetic basis of bipolar disorder has its root in the nineteenth-century work of Emil Kraepelin (Kraepelin, 1921; Goodwin & Ghaemi, 1998). The familial basis of the disorder is clearly evident in family (Gershon et al., 1982), twins (Bertelsen, 1978), and adoption (Mendlewicz, 1977) studies. Several studies have estimated the heritability of bipolar disorder to be around 80% (McGuffin et al., 2003) (Kieseppa et al., 2004). Given the high heritability, the paucity of identified genetic markers remains somewhat of an enigma. The heritability of other psychiatric disorders more generally presents a similar confound. Burmeister et al. (2008) suggest that heritability estimates for psychiatric illness may be distorted due to high genetic heterogeneity in the form of *de novo* mutations and epigenetic changes. They also conclude that after more than a decade of intensive research that major risk variants for most psychiatric diseases may contribute only marginal increases in risk (odds ratios in the 1.2 to 1.3 range). Investigations into the genetics of bipolar disorder are complicated by several factors beyond locus heterogeneity, lack of specificity in defining traits of interest, and incomplete penetrance that include unmeasured moderating nongenetic variables from the environment, internal and external. This inherent complexity is further compounded by diagnostic overlap among conditions; while clinical (and biological) phenomena may be more often associated with one specific category, it may be present in others. Psychotic symptoms (delusions or hallucinations) may be present in a number of psychiatric diagnoses including depression, bipolar disorder, or any of the heterogeneous presentations of schizophrenia. Typically, studies will attempt to correct for this by adopting very rigid classification systems when applying psychiatric diagnoses, and the use of a consensus for final diagnosis processes is common in genetics studies. The problems of heterogeneity will remain until biological parameters can unequivocally define membership in specific disease states; these definitions may ultimately be somewhat different than what is now current.

Despite the challenges faced in the study of complex human diseases, there is a palpable energy in the field that is driven by the emerging technology that has provided opportunities for data generation that have surpassed expectations. An integrated research paradigm that adapts biology with clinical measures will redefine psychiatry and neuroscience.

---

**Beginning and Challenges**

· Greater sophistication has been gained in understanding the scope of genetics in psychiatric illness with appreciation for environmental influences on the malleable nature of the gene

· Single genes as comprehensive risks for a bipolar disorder phenotype have been supplanted by a broader model which may account for additive effect of multiple small risk associated variants

· Challenges inherent in the study of psychiatric genetics were discussed including etiological heterogeneity and comorbidities in the observed clinical phenotype

---

## MAIN APPROACHES TO SEQUENCING

### LINKAGE

Genetic linkage analysis remains very useful for identifying single gene disorders in families in which disorders appear to segregate in a Mendelian manner. Linkage refers to the coinheritance of two genetic loci that are physically close to each and tend to stay together during meiosis; one of the markers being a measurable genetic marker and the other the putative disease locus. There was initial optimism for the discovery of single genes contributing significantly to bipolar disorder and other psychiatric illness that was fueled by linkage studies for bipolar, which mapped a locus onto chromosomes X (Baron et al., 1987) and 11p (Egeland et al., 1987). These early findings generated by linkage studies in psychiatric illness were not replicated (Hodgkinson et al., 1987; Kelsoe et al., 1989; Gershon 1991). The linkage era (1980–2005) for bipolar studies identified two loci, 8q and 6q (McQueen et al., 2005) likely to harbor susceptibility loci; however further fine mapping on 8q has not yielded evidence for a specific gene (Zhang, Xiang et al., 2010). Overall the linkage analyses have failed to identify any individual locus that could be replicated across multiple independent samples (Burmeister et al., 2008; Cichon et al., 2009).

While linkage studies are powerful for the discovery of single gene mutations in diseases of a Mendelian nature, they have not been successful for multifactorial disorders of complex inheritance; that is, those that clearly have a genetic basis but do not show a Mendelian inheritance pattern (Cichon et al., 2009). This observation has been true despite the accrual of large numbers of pedigrees and combining data sets for integrated analyses (Segurado et al., 2003; McQueen et al., 2005); regions of interest remain, but no clear candidates have emerged from linkage. While disagreement as to ideal methodology continues, it is agreed that linkage studies are of low power when risk variants have small individual effect sizes or if there is heterogeneity between samples of pedigrees; both highly probable in psychiatric research.

Linkage disequilibrium refers to the non-random association of specific alleles at two loci (generally one being the presumed disease state), and is a character of the reproducing population of study. That is, linkage disequilibrium also refers to a combination of alleles with greater or lesser frequency than is expected based on their naturally occurring frequencies in the population. While better powered to detect polymorphisms with a low individual risk, linkage disequilibrium studies have also generated findings that supported previous linkage findings (Glaser et al., 2005), but in general have not been replicated. A 2008 meta-analysis of linkage disequilibrium studies generated several candidate gene associations for psychiatric illness, although these may fall short of genome-wide level of statistical significance (Allen et al., 2008).

Applying the principles of linkage disequilibrium to the entire genome was proposed by Risch and Merikangas (1996) in order to detect small risk contributions from multiple SNPs. Single nucleotide polymorphisms (SNPs) are single point mutations in the genome that differ between chromosomes within an individual. A SNP that falls within a coding sequence of DNA does not necessarily result in functional disruptions to the resulting protein. A given SNP frequency also may vary within different geographical populations and thus definitive statements on frequency may sometimes need to be qualified. Although the feasibility of linkage disequilibrium methods to study the entire genome was limited at the time of Risch and Merikangas's

writing in the mid 1990s, this study design became a reality with the development of high-throughput genotyping chips (a microchip containing probes which recognize DNA samples) as well as the ability of investigators to reference the large number of identified SNPs generated from the HapMap Project (www.hapmap.org; Frazer, et al., 2007). With the steady fall in costs associated with genome-wide assay of large SNP sets, the genome wide association study (GWAS) became the standard methodology for the study of complex diseases. GWAS methods are described later in this chapter. In GWAS, samples were combined for meta-analyses, highlighted by type II diabetes research in which several investigators (Zeggini et al., 2008) combined over 60,000 individuals (cases and controls) to study prior findings that had not reached genome-wide significance. However, with increased sample size, six SNPs emerged with p values $<5 \times 10^{-8}$ with odds ratios from 1.09 to 1.15. A more recent meta-analysis of type II diabetes with a combined case and control sample of 141,454 individuals further identified. It is estimated that loci with odds ratios between 1.1 and 1.2 require from 10,000 to over 20,000 individuals to achieve 80% power to detect a locus of significant effect (Cichon et al., 2009). Thus, GWAS research in other human diseases brought into focus the scope of effort that would be required in psychiatric research.

---

**Linkage Studies**

- Linkage analyses have been a powerful approach for single gene mutations seen in Mendelian diseases. However, they have proven less useful for diseases with a multifactorial etiology.

- Linkage analyses generally have low power when genetic risk variants have small individual effect sizes or when there is heterogeneity in samples of pedigrees. Thus their suitability for investigation of psychiatric illness is constrained.

---

## GWAS IN PSYCHIATRIC DISORDERS

The essence of GWAS is the statistical comparison of the observed frequency of alleles (i.e., different variants of the same gene) in the risk (affected) population with the expected frequency found in the control (unaffected) population derived from the same breeding group. Association studies are advantageous over linkage studies when individual genetic variants have a small effect on risk estimates; this advantage persists even after controlling for multiple comparisons. Originally association studies focused on candidate genes selected on the basis of known or suspected biological function or chromosomal position. Often, selection of candidate genes in psychiatric illness has been based on mechanisms of action of psychiatric medications affecting monoamine neurotransmission, knowledge that dates back to the 1960s. Primarily these have included functional polymorphisms in dopaminergic and serotonergic pathways. However, thus far none of these candidate genes have been reliably shown to associate (with independent replication) with risk of psychiatric illness to a generally acceptable level of significance (Cichon et al., 2009).

There are three genes with variants that have been associated with bipolar disorder and replicated. They include CACNA1C and ANK3 (Baum et al., 2008; Ferreira et al., 2008; Sklar et al., 2008) and Syne1 (Belmonte Mahon et al., 2011). Several additional variants have been identified and remain to be replicated (Ferreira et al., 2008; Baum et al., 2008; Sklar et al., 2008). However, even when replication is reported, variants were not replicated by the study's initial samples (Sklar et al., 2008; Ferreira et al., 2008). Further, it has been reported that two separate SNPs within the ANK3 gene appear to carry independent risk for bipolar disorder with some replication of these findings across separate samples (Schulze et al., 2009). Mutations in the ANK3 gene have been an exciting area of investigation and further studies will need to explore the relationship these polymorphisms have with biological and neuroimaging pathways seen in the phenotype of bipolar disorder.

Continuous advances in genomics are underway such as the 1,000 Genomes Project that will generate sequence on a large number of people providing a base resource for human genetic variation. The goal of the 1,000 Genomes Project endeavors to identify variants with at least 1% frequency in the human population (www.1000genomes.org). This project may allow for identification of most, but not all, genetic variants. The challenge then becomes the interpretation of the results. GWAS will be subject to false positives (type 1 error), in particular for reasons of ethnic stratification, lack of correction for multiple testing, and publication bias in favor of positive findings. Finally, when considering the results of GWAS standards for declaring significance and replication (Chanock et al., 2007; Sullivan 2007), there are no established and universally accepted criteria.

Efforts are underway to increase sample sizes approaching the targets seen in other diseases such as diabetes with >38,000 samples obtained. By using this large approach more robust findings in bipolar disorder may emerge. The pattern observed in bipolar disorder mirrors trends in non-psychiatric diseases such that combining smaller samples with modestly significant p-values produced significant findings as more samples became available (Cichon et al., 2009). Furthermore it has been suggested that the future of GWAS will include increasingly large analyses of common SNP and copy number variants as well as individual resequencing to target rare variants (Cichon et al., 2009). Ultimately whole genome sequencing will provide a comprehensive study of variation.

While optimism for the future of GWAS with increasing sample sizes is permissible, it should be noted that even with increasing sample size, thus far the clarity of the findings remains opaque and the Odds Ratios for the identified alleles are low (1.2—1.4) (McInnis, 2009). Clearly a larger sample confers greater power to the analyses, and statistical significance will emerge, but may be compromised with concomitant increases in heterogeneity, a potential major pitfall for GWAS that is difficult to fully accommodate in the analyses. For instance, large samples of bipolar individuals combined from across multiple collaborative sites may contain sources of error, including ascertainment biases and variation in diagnostic schemes. Testing a smaller number with specific clinical subtypes may be preferable if they are well defined, measureable, heritable, and uncommon (Burmeister et al., 2008).

The phenotype selected for study is critical to the approach. Phenotypes have commonly been defined in terms of binary diagnostic categories. Such an approach presents a substantial problem as diagnostic categories in psychiatry are disjunctive and therefore heterogeneous at the clinical observational level. The current approach to distill clinical characteristics into meaningful entities for correlation is to use quantitative measurements of traits that could be physiological, psychological, or biological. This philosophy is captured in the research domain criteria (Insel et al., 2010) wherein it is appreciated that while it is not yet possible to define what it is that should be measured as a phenotype, a dimensional measure of the phenotype should be integral to the assessment. The phenotype can be directly observed; Langenecker et al. (2010) found that clusters of neuropsychological measures grouped into factor scores offered potential markers for intermediate cognitive phenotypes in bipolar disorder. Specifically, they found that processing speed and interference resolution, fine motor processing, and visual memory factors significantly differentiated bipolar disorder from healthy individuals. Prior studies also identified dysfunction in executive functions, attention, memory, and fine motor skills (McIntosh et al., 2005; Nehra et al., 2006; Thompson et al., 2005; Zubieta et al., 2001). Phenotypes may not be direct complements to the clinical phenomenon; endophenotypes are measurable clinical phenomena that are generally not considered a part of the clinical syndrome (Gottesman & Gould, 2003), aberrant eye tracking movements in schizophrenia being a classic example (Thaker et al., 2004). Regardless of whether disjunctive categories of clinical disorders or endophenotypes are identified, a measure along a dimension of intensity or severity is likely to be helpful for assessing the degree of correlation between clinical, physiological, and biological parameters.

---

### Genome Wide Association Studies (GWAS)

- GWAS applied the methodology of simpler association studies to the entire genome. The feasibility of GWAS for large samples increases with the falling cost of sequencing the genome.

- Original association studies focused on selection of candidate genes with hypothesized relationship to disease outcome. GWAS tests for associations across the entire genome and thus are generally absent of a priori hypotheses.

- Given the large number of statistical tests, appropriate corrections for multiple testing are critical to reduce the chances of reporting type 1 errors.

---

## GENOME SEQUENCING

In order to capture the detail of genetic variability and appreciate the relationship between genes and regulatory elements at the individual level it is necessary to know the complete genetic sequence of that individual. It is now over 10 years since the initial report of sequencing of the human genome (Lander et al., 2001) and as noted in the previous section, efforts are underway to provide a reference sequence from 1,000 individuals (www.1000genomes.org). It is anticipated that whole genome sequencing will become sufficiently inexpensive to be the method of choice for interrogation of genome, in place of the use of SNPs or other polymorphisms. There remain several challenges and include the observation that there remain some gaps, approximately 1% of the genome is considered inaccessible using current technology. The depth of coverage dictates the cost and the level of detail of assembly to provide a high likelihood of accuracy. While screening the genome at perhaps four-fold average coverage is the most cost-effective

approach, it may also result in too high an error rate acceptable for research. A fifty-fold coverage of the entire genome is likely to capture the variability accurately, although it is still too high in price for practical application, especially given the ever increasing sample sizes needed for non-Mendelian psychiatric illnesses.

One proposed compromise is to sequence the genome at a four-fold coverage and to separately sequence the DNA coding regions (exomes) at a higher level of fifty-fold. Since there are about 180,000 exons comprising only about 1% of the human genome, this approach may provide a cost-benefit ratio acceptable to current investigators. Nevertheless, the face of this debate will necessarily change with the pace of emerging technologies as well as projected falling cost of whole genome sequencing. While no institutions have currently met the arbitrarily marked $1,000 genome, costs have dramatically fallen and will continue to do so.

The technology behind sequencing is an evolving science of biological engineering. A challenge has been issued by the X Prize Foundation to the first team of researchers that can build a device used to sequence 100 human genomes within 10 days or less. A further benchmark of progress is defined as an accuracy of no more than one error in every 100,000 bases sequenced, with sequences accurately covering at least 98% of the genome. Finally, the X Prize Foundation stipulates that the recurring cost should be no more than $10,000 (US) per genome. A complete review of sequencing technologies is beyond the scope of this chapter; reviews of the technologies are emerging frequently (Zhang, et al., 2011).

The emerging future technologies include the use of microscopy-based and microfluidic technologies (Kan et al., 2004; Edwards et al., 2005) that use nanotechnologies in order to achieve the high throughput at lower costs using more advanced technology. Continued research is ongoing and will meet the challenges.

---

### Genome Sequencing

- Genome sequencing can be performed with fewer iterations that incurs lower cost, but a larger risk of errors. One goal is to sequence the genome at no more than one error per every 100,000 base pairs.

- A proposed compromise between the difficulties of shallow and deep sequencing may be to sequence the genome at four-fold coverage and conduct separate fifty-fold separate sequence of the exomes which comprise only 1% of the human genome.

---

## ENVIRONMENTAL FACTORS IN PSYCHIATRIC ILLNESS

As noted previously, heritability for psychiatric illness in general is quite high although much of the remaining risk may be associated with unique environmental factors including measurement error (McGue & Bouchard, 1998). Interest in accounting for the variance in psychiatric phenotypes is not a new concern, but one that extends to the work and concepts of psychobiology of the prominent academic psychiatrist Adolf Meyer (1866–1950) (McInnis, 2009). Meyer suggested that the clinical presentation of the individual and their illness was an integration of biology and life experiences in an environment that shaped the manifestation of the disorder (see figure 8.1). This concept became the basis for the biopsychosocial model of Engel (1980) and the perspectives of psychiatry, both of which represent a pluralistic base that integrates with a systems biology approach to the understanding of psychiatric disorders.

Detailed studies of environmental factors on the development of psychiatric illness remain relatively limited, and most genetic studies do not consider environmental factors. Stressful life events and parental maltreatment have been implicated in the onset and course of depression (Caspi et al., 2003). These same studies provided evidence for an interaction between genetic (5HTTLPR promoter allelic variation) and environmental factors leading to development of depression.

Psychosocial stressors affect the onset and course of illness in bipolar disorder, (Glassner & Haldipur, 1983; Bidzinska 1984; Miklowitz et al., 1988). Swendsen and colleagues (1995) found that stress and personality variables such as introversion and obsessionality were the strongest predictors of mood episode relapse in bipolar disorder. According to their findings, stress and personality characteristics were stronger predictors than markers of illness burden such as age of onset, number of lifetime mood episodes, and family history which did not distinguish between relapse and nonrelapse in their participants. A contrary view holds that stress and negative life events play a diminishing role as bipolar illness progresses over time. Such a "kindling" model predicts that as bipolar disorder progresses, mood episodes will reoccur even in the absence of any precipitating stressor. Some evidence for this model is supported by the observation that severe childhood abuse is found in approximately half of individuals with bipolar disorder, and that multiple forms of abuse predict greater morbidity (Garno et al., 2005).

Stressful life events have a significant role throughout the course of bipolar disorder (Swendsen et al., 1995; Hlastala et al., 2000; Post & Leverich, 2006). While social rejection has been rarely studied in bipolar disorder, the factor of social support is thought to be associated with morbidity in bipolar disorder such that those with more supportive relationships had fewer mood episodes and fewer hospitalizations (Cohen et al., 2004). These researchers also found that stress (measured with a scale of negative

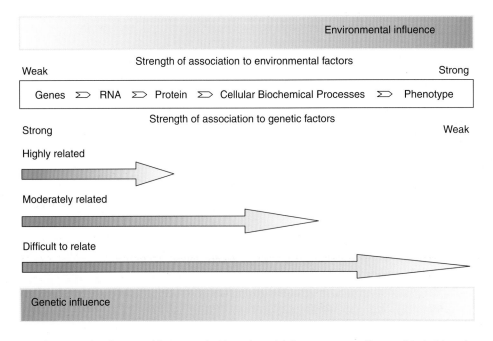

*Figure 8.1* The associations of genes and environmental factors on the biopsychosocial disease process. (Source: Adapted from Arranz & Kapur, 2008.)

life events) independently predicted recurrence of mood episode in a one year follow-up period. While it is not surprising that lower levels of perceived social support are risk factors for episode recurrence in bipolar disorder (Johnson et al., 1999; O'Connell et al., 1985), explanatory mechanisms of hormonal and neurobiological variables are not yet well established.

## EPIGENETICS

Epigenetics is the study of heritable changes in phenotype and gene expression caused by mechanisms other than changes in the underlying DNA sequence. Examples of histone acetylation and methylation in gene expression caused by environmental stressors or drugs in animal models may have implications for psychiatric illness and are described later. These changes in gene expression may remain through cell divisions for the remainder of the life of the organism and may impact behavior across multiple generations. However, there is no change in the underlying DNA sequence of the organism; instead, non-genetic factors cause the organism's genes to behave (or express themselves) differently. The complexities of genetic influence on phenotype including epigenetic mechanisms is presaged in Conrad Waddington's classic "developmental landscape" (Waddington, 1957) (figure 8.2) which is still a useful visual analogy to genetic and epigenetic expression.

A vast and largely unsurveyed territory of exploration in psychiatric disorders is represented by the study of epigenetic mechanisms of mental illness. While this area of research is still in its infancy, insights into the inter-individual and inter-generational formation and transmission of psychiatric behavioral disturbances have begun to emerge. Already there is evidence that epigenetic mechanisms are involved in neurogenesis, neuronal plasticity, learning, memory, cognitive dysfunction and in psychiatric disorders such as depression, addiction, and schizophrenia. Much attention has been directed at histone modification, DNA methylation, and chromatin remodeling in animal models of epigenetics. A detailed explanation of the complex processes involved in gene expression is beyond the scope of this chapter. However, it should be understood that the process of translating DNA into proteins early in the chain involves the structure of histone and histone tails around which DNA is wrapped in the cell nucleus. Portions of histone may become methylated and thus repressing transcription, or subject to acetylation which is associated with transcription availability. For instance, following chronic cocaine administration, acetylation of histone and binding of a transcription factor is seen in the striatum that is noted to be a brain region important for the behavioral effects of that drug (Kumar et al., 2005; Tsankova, et al., 2007).

Although the epigenetics of bipolar disorder is a new area of research, some review of the findings of epigenetics in major depressive disorder may prove translatable. Previous work in a rat model examined changes in histone modifications after chronic electroconvulsive seizures (ECS) in the hippocampus (Tsankova, et al., 2004). They found that levels of histone H4 acetylation correlated with increased levels of gene expression including c-*fos*, *BDNF*, and *CREB* mRNA levels after acute and chronic ECS. Further, the up-regulated expression of BDNF and Creb has been shown to mediate antidepressant activity in animal models (Duman, 2004; Tsankova, et al., 2007; Monteggia et al., 2004; Monteggia et al., 2007). Further, like real-world environmental factors that may alter gene expression, differences in chromatin remodeling were seen in chronic ECS versus acute ECS. Studies examining epigenetics of chronic stress in depression have produced some interesting initial findings. Chronic social stress in a rat model resulted in altered chromatin regulation in BDNF in the hippocampus. The behavioral changes associated with exposure to such stress such as social avoidance were reportedly reversed by chronic administration of antidepressant agents (Berton et al., 2006; Tsankova, et al., 2006). These investigations also suggest that there were other changes in histone modification that persisted for several weeks after cessation of stressor and were resistant to pharmacological treatment.

The role of epigenetics in transgenerational transmission of vulnerability to psychiatric illness using rat models

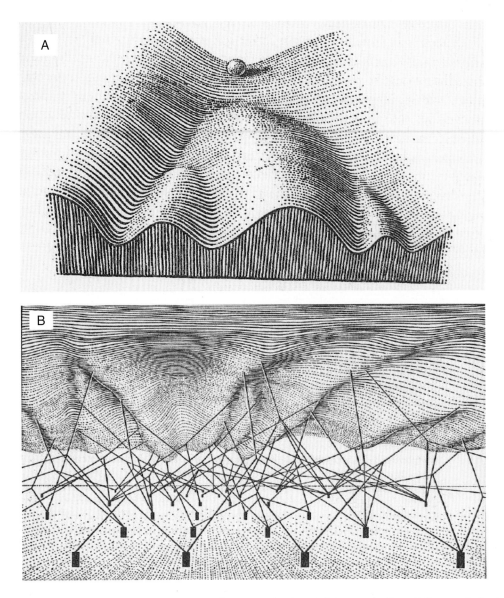

Figure 8.2 Conrad Waddington's "developmental landscape" *Figure A*: Represents the phenotypic topography *Figure B*: Represents the genetic parameters (black pegs) that pull on the surface to determine its features These figures nicely capture the complexity of gene-by-gene interactions known as epistatic effects, represented by the links between strings originating from the genetic loci. These figures illustrate by analogy the phenotypic developmental trajectory of an organism by the course of the ball over the surface. The diagram illustrates the fact that the effect of any one genetic loci is often affected by the expression of all other loci in the system. Another important concept that these figures introduce is that of the relative importance a gene loci has on the developmental phenotype. That is, a gene with an affect on a surface peak will have little or no impact on the course of the ball across the terrain, where as a loci or locus affecting the configuration of a valley may exert a huge affect on the course of the ball. The influence of environment and epigenetics on both figure A and B can easily be included, though the original visual model proposed by Waddington remains essentially current. (Source: Reprinted from Waddington, 1957.)

provided evidence that may be applied to human models of psychiatric illness. In rats some mothers display a high degree of nurturing behaviors to their offspring in the form of licking, grooming, and nursing, whereas other mothers are naturally lower in these behaviors. Compared to offspring of low nurturing mother, pups of high-nurturing mothers have been found to have increased expression of glucocorticoid receptor mRNA and protein in the hippocampus and lower corticosterone response to stress. Further, increased methylation at other gene regions was found to emerge early; it occurred in the first week of life and persisted throughout their lives. Another study comparing differences in high and low nurturing in rats on offspring further elaborated this mechanism by reporting that in low-nurtured pups their methylated glucocorticoid receptor promoter prevented binding of a transcriptional enhancer (NGFI-A), which in turn disrupted the normal regulation of the glucocorticoid receptor gene (Weaver et al., 2004).

The investigation of epigenetic mechanisms of psychiatric illness is a critical component in forming a clearer understanding of how environmental factors influence the expression of psychiatric illness. This approach is particularly true for other brain regions outside of the hippocampus and involving other genes besides BDNF and glucocorticoid receptor genes. It will also be important to increase our understanding of epigenetics in neurodevelopment. That is, are organisms truly sensitive to epigenetic influence only early during early imprinting and canalization periods or is epigenetic plasticity a factor in adulthood as well?

---

### Epigenetics

- Epigenetics is the study of changes in gene expression not caused by changes to the underlying DNA sequence. Environmental stressors, exposure to drugs, and differential patterns of mother-offpring rearing are examples of exogenous factors that may alter gene expression.

- Research on the epigenetics of depression may prove translatable in some instances to bipolar disorder, although the epigenetics unique to this condition has yet to be addressed.

---

## FUNCTIONAL GENETICS

While traditional sequencing techniques provide information on what proteins an organism's cell could potentially produce, gene expression studies provide information on what any given differentiated cell is actually doing. That is, in any given cell only some of the genes are active in the production of mRNA, while others are silenced. For instance, skin, nerve, and liver cells, though all containing a complete copy of the genome, are each differentiated in the genes that they express.

Gene expression studies directly measure the relative amount of mRNA expressed under experimental conditions. Examining the activity of cells in brain regions thought to be involved in affect regulation may be particularly promising in understanding the etiology of bipolar disorder, as well as developing targeted therapies. In psychiatric disorders such studies have presently been limited to brain autopsy samples. One difficulty with this method is that such samples may also be affected by long-term

exposure to medications, substance abuse, and smoking, which may confound conclusions (Sawa & Cascella, 2009). Expression studies in schizophrenia have uncovered abnormalities in smell perception and the olfactory epithelium (Arnold et al., 2001; Sawa & Cascella, 2009). Moreover, first-degree relatives of schizophrenia patients also demonstrated a relative decrease on a test of smell identification compared to the general population, suggesting that abnormalities in this ability may represent a genetic predisposition to the disorder (Kopala et al., 2001; Roalf et al., 2006). At this juncture the basic biological science suggests that a disruption in the intracellular signaling molecule cyclic adenosine monophosphate (cAMP) may be one link between hyposmia and signal transduction in schizophrenia (Turetsky & Moberg, 2009).

A review of the broad literature of functional genetics is outside the scope of this introductory chapter. For a more comprehensive overview see Einat and Manji's review (2006). Signaling pathways may be of significance: Phosphoinositide has been implicated in mood disorders secondary to findings that inositol levels have been detected to be affected in individual's blood plasma (Barkai et al., 1978). The inositol depletion hypothesis of bipolar disorder also found support from studies on the effect of lithium on this signaling pathway as well as from imaging studies showing reduced levels of inositol in lithium treated individuals (Berridge, 1989; Davanzo et al., 2001; Moore et al., 1999). Other genetic pathways of interest include glycogen synthase kinase-3 (Gould & Manji, 2005) and protein kinase C (Young et al., 1999). Very well known and investigated is the role of brain derived neurotrophic factor (BDNF) in stress and mood dysregulation (see the review by Einat & Manji 2006 for a more comprehensive treatment of the subject). It appears that BDNF is modulated by environmental factors such that it is down regulated by chronic stress in animal models and appears to further be targeted by anti-depressant medications (Nibuya et al., 1995). The multiple influences on neuroplasticity and resilience in mood disorder is highlighted in figure 8.3. This adapted figure (Manji, et al. 2001) illustrates how stress and depression may downregulate levels of BDNF, upregulate glutamate and cortisol, and reduce the cells energy capacity. See Manji et al. (2001) for a more detailed explanation of the functional genetic model of mood disorders. In animal models, BDNF has been up-regulated by antidepressants as well as non-pharmacological interventions including dietary or calorie restriction as well as exercise (Stranahan et al., 2009; Lutter et al., 2008). It remains to be seen whether dietary regulation interventions in humans could confer similar benefits of decreased morbidity and

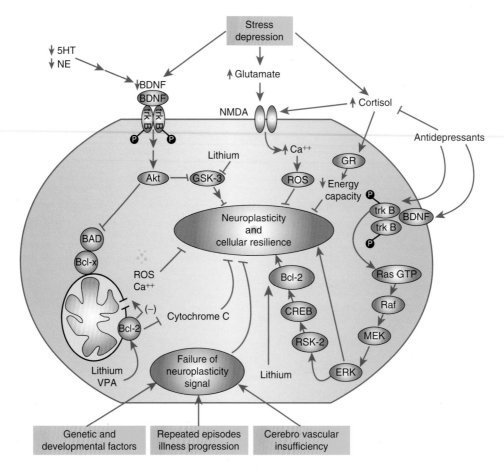

*Figure 8.3* Neuroplasticity and celluclar resilience in mood disorders. (Source: Reprinted from Manji et al., 2001 with permission from the publisher.)

mortality seen in animal models, as well as possible mood regulation.

Functional genetic studies will be facilitated by the emergence of technologies to create inducible pluripotent stem (iPS) cells. These cells are created from somatic cells (usually fibroblasts) and "induced" to grow into selected cell types such as neurons (Kim, 2010; Chiang et al., 2011). Additional cell types will include lymphoblastoid cell lines and olfactory cells (Sawa & Cascella, 2009). Functional studies will involve cell biology and assessment of biological functions (including gene expression patterns) of the cell under experimental conditions.

## PHARMACOGENETICS

Pharmacogenentics is the study of variations in genes and their effect on clinical response to pharmacological agents. This is especially salient to the treatment of mental illnesses, in which tailoring psychotropic treatments may involve a prolonged period of trial-and-error experimentation

### Functional Genetics

- Functional genetics involves the investigation of the behavior of differentiated cells in which only some of the genes are active. Although each cell contains the entire genome, only a fraction of genes are active which differentiate the cell as a nerve, skin, or kidney cell.

- By creating pluripotent stem cells, the genetic expression of a neuron (for instance) in a given bipolar individual may be studied in vitro. This will expand upon the current investigations that have been limited to autopsy samples.

- Functional genetics allows the field to progress from genetic studies alone and toward investigations of cell behavior and response to experimental manipulation.

with several agents in combination or in isolation. Evidence that genetic factors may play a role in response to psychotropic agents comes from early studies in antidepressant response between first-degree family members, which

THE BIPOLAR BRAIN

found significantly concordant clinical responses among these individuals (Pare et al., 1962; Pare & Mack, 1971; Franchini et al., 1998). Fewer studies have been conducted for other psychiatric medication classes and research specific to bipolar disorder will require further developments in the field.

Studies thus far have primarily focused on mechanisms of action in dopamine and serotonin since a number of psychotropic medications have a high affinity for these systems. In particular most studies have focused on the variations in the DRD2, DRD4, and CYP2D6 genotypes (Malhotra et al., 2004). There is evidence that homozygous genotypes in the DRD2 Taq1A polymorphism confer a decreased response to haloperidol (Schafer et al., 2001). Considerable research has also been focused on the over 70 variants of CYP2d6 which codes for an enzyme which metabolizes many tricylic and SSRI antidepressants. Much has been published to date on the change in metabolism associated with various alleles of this gene (Johansson et al., 1993; Raimundo et al., 2000; Sachse et al., 1997; Marez et al., 1997), although negative findings of no association between polymorphism and clinical outcome have also been reported (Murphy et al., 2003). For a more comprehensive review on serotonin and dopamine gene polymorphisms affecting medication response see (Malhotra et al., 2004). Identifying and stratifying metabolic rate for various drugs is crucial since sub-therapeutic plasma concentrations or overall therapeutic failure may result when conventional dosages are administered to some patients. Conversely slow metabolizers are at greater risk for concentration dependent adverse effects. Given the fact that as many as 25% of all drugs are metabolized in part by CYP2D6, assessing enzyme activity for this, as well as CYP2C19, quickly through breath-test technology is looming on the horizon (Ingelman-Sundberg, 2004; Modak, 2009).

## Pharmacogenetics

- Pharmacogenetics is the study of how genes impact upon response to medication either through difference in metabolism or somatic response to that drug.

- Early investigations have linked polymorphisms in the DRD2 gene with decreased response to haloperidol. Other studies have focused on variation in gene-coded enzymes which metabolize tricylic and SSRI antidepressants. It is unclear how genetic differences between patient groups may impact upon treatment with mood stabilizing agents and the pharmacogenetics of bipolar disorder is a promising area of research.

## SYSTEMS BIOLOGY

According to Leroy Hood's comprehensive review (2002), systems biology is "the study of all elements in a biological system (all genes, mRNAs, proteins, etc.) and their relationships one to another in response to perturbations – a contrast to the one gene or one protein at-a-time studies so successful in biology over the preceding 30 years or so." Such an integrated approach to the study of biology, and by extension the genetics of complex diseases, is gaining importance in empirical investigations. Such a paradigm naturally requires cross-disciplinary collaboration, often between the fields of biology, chemistry, and engineering. Hood goes on to illustrate that in contrast to other scientific disciplines, the core of biology is digital (the genome). Further, the genome contains two major types of digital information: the individual genes and regulatory networks that control the behavior of the genes. When considering systems biology, it is important to keep both of these in mind, as well as the fact that biological information is essentially hierarchical. That is, information moves sequentially from the DNA, RNA, protein, protein interactions, and biomodules (in which a constellation of proteins converge to perform a phenotypic operation). Hood (2002) states that for the purposes of a systems biology approach, data should be gathered from as many of these hierarchical levels as is feasible.

The scope of data collection and interpretation in the study of psychiatrically complex diseases is challenging at first view. That is, in studying non-Mendelian type diseases, the sequencing of the genome must be broad and attempt to account for the interaction between many genetic variants with individually low to moderate risks. But even after accomplishing this sequencing, it may be that establishing a meaningful etiology of psychiatric illness will need to include epigenetic mechanisms, as well as other data gathered from within a systems biology approach.

While still searching for the most parsimonious understanding of mental illness, the investigator will need to become comfortable with complexity that is orders of magnitude above more basic reductionist biological models of disease. Such complexity will likely encompass a landscape greater than any one individual in any single discipline can tread alone. This brings into focus the increasing importance not only of interdepartmental collaboration, but also collaborations among disciplines. This greater emphasis on mutually interdependent sub-systems is the focus of a systems biology approach. Despite the challenges evident in the undertaking itself, researchers in the field of psychiatric genetics need not be crestfallen, as exponential development of technologies will continue to make this research possible.

## CONCLUSIONS

The perhaps unavoidable message for researchers in the field of psychiatric genetics to keep in mind is the magnitude and scope of the task at hand of understanding psychopathology and human mental disease. Furthermore, collaboration will be crucial to generate the sample sizes needed to identify allelic, biological, and physiological signatures of shared and unique features of psychiatric illness. Moreover, investing the time and resources to follow through on preliminary findings is much needed in the field. All too often suggested candidate genes or biological mechanisms are added to the published corpus, but then left for others to investigate the basic biology at a later time. The findings linger in the literature. Although it is only within the scope of any single lab or any single project to carve out a limited area of research, one difficulty with progress in the field thus far is the apparent piecemeal nature of the work without a clear network of organization by which we may fashion a useable garment. Although the task of such tailoring is indeed beyond the scope of any micro- or mesosystem, greater integration and collaboration between genetic, biological, and phenomenological researchers will best serve to tell a more complete story behind the etiologies of various mental illnesses.

One of the tasks at hand is to distill parsimony from the complexity of the human bio-psycho-social system. It has been suggested that the human brain contains

characteristics of a probabilistic recursive fractal (Kitzbichler et al., 2009) such that a relatively simple coding design generates tremendous variability in observed presentation. By analogy, the Mandelbrot set is a mathematical equation containing only six characters (Devaney, 2011), yet due to the iterative application of this data, tremendous complexity is permitted in its expressed "phenotype". Similarly, the molecular language of the genome (and therefore biology) is relatively simple and for humans potentially constrained to roughly 25,000 protein coding genes with over 2,000 of those *specific* for the brain. In some regards GWA studies appear to be akin to looking for a recognizable pattern in a visual fractal array (similar to the Mandelbrot set) based upon variation in underlying coding design. While such an approach is not without merit, more in-depth study of other noncoding factors influencing phenotypic expression such as early environmental condition, life stressors, and nutrition is needed. Much like attempting to predict patterns of growth in trees by examining only the underlying genome (of course there will be an estimation of height), coding data must be considered along with soil constitution, light patterns, exposure to toxins, and the larger physical environment. Without detailed examination of these variables the most likely conclusion will be that single or combined variations in genetic coding each result in widely varying phenotypic expression. Such a conclusion offers little in the way of predictive medicine or individualized treatment such that additional information is crucial to the interpretation of the genetic and biological data.

With these thoughts in mind, two factors will be important to move the field forward. The first is to consider a broad view of the contributing factors to the phenotype of bipolar disorder. Despite any particular researcher's narrow focus, collaboration between disciplines is not only important, but fundamental to the science of human health and disease. Second, advances in technology, including rapid and inexpensive whole genome sequencing as well as advancement in computing that permit reverse engineered computer models of the human nervous system, will propel our field forward in the decades to come.

## REFERENCES

1000 Genomes: A deep Catalog of Human Genetic variation. 2011. Available from http://www.1000genomes.org/, accessed April 24, 2011.

Allen, N. C., Bagade, S., McQueen, M. B., Ioannidis, J. P. A., Kavvoura, F. K. Khoury, M. J., . . . Bertram, L. 2008. Systematic meta-analyses and field synopsis of genetic association studies in schizophrenia: the SzGene database. *Nature Genetics*, 40(7): 827–834.

Arnold, S. E., Han, L. Y., Moberg, P. J., Turetsky, B. I., Gur, R. E., Trojanowski, J. Q., . . . Hahn, C. G. 2001. Dysregulation of olfactory receptor neuron lineage in schizophrenia. *Archives of General Psychiatry*, 58(9): 829–835.

Barkai, A. I., Dunner, D. L., Gross, H. A., Mayo, P., & Fieve, R. R. 1978. Reduced myo-inositol levels in cerebrospinal fluid from patients with affective disorder. *Biological Psychiatry*, 13(1): 65–72.

Baron, M., Risch, N. J., Hamburger, R., Mandel, B., Kushner, S., Newman, M., Drumer, D., & Belmaker, R. H. 1987. Genetic linkage between X-chromosome markers and bipolar affective illness. *Nature*, 326(6110): 289–292.

Baum, A. E., Akula, N., Cabanero, M., Cardona, I., Corona, W., Klemens, B., . . . McMahon, F. J. 2008. A genome-wide association study implicates diacylglycerol kinase eta (DGKH) and several other genes in the etiology of bipolar disorder. *Molecular Psychiatry*, 13(2): 197–207.

Belmonte Mahon, P., Pirooznia, M., Goes, F. S., Seifuddin, F., Steele, J., Lee, P. H., . . . Zandi, P. P. 2011. Genome-wide association analysis of age at onset and psychotic symptoms in bipolar disorder. *American Journal of Medical Genetics Part B: Neuropsychiatric Genetics*, 156(3): 370–378.

Berridge, M. J. 1989. Inositol 1,4,5-trisphosphate-induced calcium mobilization is localized in Xenopus oocytes. *Proceedings of the Royal Society London B: Biological Sciences*. 238(1292): 235–243.

Bertelsen, A., Harvald, B., & Hauge, M. 1977. A Danish twin study of manic-depressive disorders. *The British Journal of Psychiatry* 130: 330–351.

Berton, O., McClung, C. A., DiLeone, R. J., Krishnan, V., Renthal, W., Russo, S. J., . . . Nestler, E. J. 2006. Essential role of BDNF in the mesolimbic dopamine pathway in social defeat stress. *Science*, 311(5762): 864–868.

Bidzinska, E. J. 1984. Stress factors in affective diseases. *British Journal of Psychiatry*, 144: 161–166.

Burmeister, M., McInnis, M. G., & Zollner, S. 2008. Psychiatric genetics: progress amid controversy. *Nature Reviews Genetics*, 9(7): 527–540.

Caspi, A., Sugden, K., Moffitt, T. E., Taylor, A., Craig, I. W., Harrington, H., . . . Poulton, R. 2003. Influence of life stress on depression: moderation by a polymorphism in the 5-HTT gene. *Science*, 301(5631): 386–389.

Chanock, S. J., Manolio, T., Boehnke, M., Boerwinkle, E., Hunter, D. J., Thomas, G., . . . Collins, F. S. 2007. Replicating genotype-phenotype associations. *Nature*, 447(7145): 655–660.

Chiang, C. H., Su, Y., Wen, Z., Yoritomo, N., Ross, C. A., Margolis, R. L., . . . Ming, G. I. 2011. Integration-free induced pluripotent stem cells derived from schizophrenia patients with a DISC1 mutation. *Molecular Psychiatry*, 16(4): 358–360.

Cichon, S., Craddock, N., Daly, M., Faraone, S. V., Gejman, P. V., Kelsoe, J., . . . Sullivan, P. F. 2009. Genomewide association studies: history, rationale, and prospects for psychiatric disorders. *American Journal of Psychiatry*, 166(5): 540–556.

Cohen, A. N., Hammen, C., Henry, R. M., & Daley, S. E. 2004. Effects of stress and social support on recurrence in bipolar disorder. *Journal of Affective Disorders*, 82(1): 143–147.

Davanzo, P., Thomas, M. A., Yue, K., Oshiro, T., Belin, T., Strober, M., & McCracken, J. 2001. Decreased anterior cingulate myo-inositol/creatine spectroscopy resonance with lithium treatment in children with bipolar disorder. *Neuropsychopharmacology*, 24(4): 359–369.

Devaney, R.L. 2011. Available from http://math.bu.edu/DYSYS/FRACGEOM/FRACGEOM.html

Duman, R. S. 2004. Role of neurotrophic factors in the etiology and treatment of mood disorders. *Neuromolecular Medicine*, 5(1): 11–25.

Edwards, J. R., Ruparel, H., & Jingyue, J. 2005. Mass-spectrometry DNA sequencing. *Mutation Research*, 573(1–2): 3–12.

Egeland, J. A., Gerhard, D. S., Pauls, D. L., Sussex, J. N., Kidd, K. K., Alien, C. R., . . . Housman, D. E. 1987. Bipolar affective disorders linked to DNA markers on chromosome 11. *Nature*, 325(6107): 783–787.

Einat, H. & Manji, H. K. 2006. Cellular plasticity cascades: genes-to-behavior pathways in animal models of bipolar disorder. *Biological Psychiatry*, 59(12): 1160–1171.

Engel, G. L. 1980. The clinical application of the biopsychosocial model. *American Journal of Psychiatry*, 137(5): 535–544.

Ferreira, M. A., O'Donovan, M. C., Meng, Y. A., Jones, I. R., Ruderfer, D. M., Jones, L., . . . Craddock, N. 2008. Collaborative genome-wide association analysis supports a role for ANK3 and CACNA1C in bipolar disorder. *Nature Genetics*, 40(9): 1056–1058.

Franchini, L., Serretti, V., Gasperini, M., & Smeraldi, E. 1998. Familial concordance of fluvoxamine response as a tool for differentiating mood disorder pedigrees. *Journal of Psychiatric Research*, 32(5): 255–259.

Frazer, K. A., Ballinger, D. G., Cox, D. R., Hinds, D. A., Stuve, L. L., Gibbs, R. A., . . . Stewart, J. 2007. A second generation human haplotype map of over 3.1 million SNPs. *Nature*, 449(7164): 851–861.

Garno, J. L., Goldberg, J. F., Ramirez, P. M., & Ritzler, B. A. 2005. Impact of childhood abuse on the clinical course of bipolar disorder. *The British Journal of Psychiatry*, 186: 121–125.

Gershon, E. S. 1991. Marker genotyping errors in old data on X-linkage in bipolar illness. *Biological Psychiatry*, 29(7): 721–729.

Gershon, E. S., Hamovit, J., Guroff, J. J., Dibble, E., Leckman, J. F., Sceery, W., . . . Bunney, W. E. Jr., 1982. A family study of schizoaffective, bipolar I, bipolar II, unipolar, and normal control probands. *Archives of General Psychiatry*, 39(10): 1157–1167.

Glaser, B., Kirov, G., Green, E., Craddock, N., & Owen, M. J. 2005. Linkage disequilibrium mapping of bipolar affective disorder at 12q23-q24 provides evidence for association at CUX2 and FLJ32356. *American Journal of Medical Genettics B Neuropsychiatric Genetics*, 132B(1): 38–45.

Glassner, B., & Haldipur, C. V. 1983. Life events and early and late onset of bipolar disorder. *American Journal of Psychiatry*, 140(2): 215–217.

Goodwin, F. K., & Ghaemi, S. N. 1998. Understanding manic-depressive illness. *Archives of General Psychiatry*, 55(1): 23–25.

Gottesman, I. I., & Gould, T. D. 2003. The endophenotype concept in psychiatry: etymology and strategic intentions. *American Journal of Psychiatry*, 160(4): 636–645.

Gould, T. D., & Manji, H. K. 2005. Glycogen synthase kinase-3: a putative molecular target for lithium mimetic drugs. *Neuropsychopharmacology*, 30(7): 1223–1237.

Hlastala, S. A., Frank, E., Kowalski, J., Sherrill, J. T., Tu, X. M., Anderson, B., & Kupfer, D. J. 2000. Stressful life events, bipolar disorder, and the "kindling model." *Journal of Abnormal Psychology*, 109(4): 777–786.

Hodgkinson, S., Sherrington, R., Gurling, H., Matchbanks, R., Reeders, S., Mallet, J., . . . Brynjolfsson, J. 1987. Molecular genetic evidence for heterogeneity in manic depression. *Nature*, 325(6107): 805–806.

Hood, L. 2002. A personal view of molecular technology and how it has changed biology. *Journal of Proteome Research*, 1(5): 399–409.

Ingelman-Sundberg, M. 2004. Pharmacogenetics of cytochrome P450 and its applications in drug therapy: the past, present and future. *Trends in Pharmacological Science*, 25(4): 193–200.

Insel, T., Cuthbert, B., Garvey, M., Heinssen, R., Pine, D. S., Quinn, K., . . . Wang, P. 2010. Research domain criteria (RDoC): toward a new classification framework for research on mental disorders. *American Journal of Psychiatry*, 167(7): 748–751.

Johansson, I., Lundqvist, E., Bertilsson, L., Dahl, M. L., Sjoqvist, F., & Ingelman-Sundberg, M. 1993. Inherited amplification of an active gene in the cytochrome P450 CYP2D locus as a cause of ultrarapid metabolism of debrisoquine. *Proceedings of the National Academy of Science of the United States of America*, 90(24): 11825–11829.

Johnson, S. L., Winett, C. A., Meyer, B., Greenhouse, W. J., & Miller, I. 1999. Social support and the course of bipolar disorder. *Journal of Abnormal Psychology*, 108(4): 558–566.

Kan, C. W., Fredlake, C. P., Doherty, E. A., & Barron, A. E. 2004. DNA sequencing and genotyping in miniaturized electrophoresis systems. *Electrophoresis*, 25(21–22): 3564–3588.

Kelsoe, J. R., Ginns, E. I., Egeland, J. A., Gerhard, D. S, Goldstein, A. M., Bale, S. J., . . . Paul, S. M. 1989. Re-evaluation of the linkage relationship between chromosome 11p loci and the gene for bipolar affective disorder in the Old Order Amish. *Nature*, 342(6247): 238–243.

Kenyon, C. J. 2010. The genetics of ageing. *Nature*, 464(7288): 504–512.

Kieseppa, T., Partonen, T., Haukka, J., Kaprio, J., & Lonngvist, J. 2004. High concordance of bipolar I disorder in a nationwide sample of twins. *American Journal of Psychiatry*, 161(10): 1814–1821.

Kim, K. S. 2010. Induced pluripotent stem (iPS) cells and their future in psychiatry. *Neuropsychopharmacology*, 35(1): 346–348.

Kitzbichler, M. G., Smith, M. L., Christensen, S. R., & Bullmore, E. 2009. Broadband criticality of human brain network synchronization. *PLoS Computational Biology*, 5(3): e1000314.

Kopala, L. C., Good, K. P., Morrison, K., Bassett, A. S., Alda, M., & Honer, W. G. 2001. Impaired olfactory identification in relatives of patients with familial schizophrenia. *American Journal of Psychiatry*, 158(8): 1286–1290.

Kraepelin, E. 1921. *Manic-depressive Insanity and Paranoia*. Edinburgh: Livingstone.

Kumar, A., Choi, K. H., Renthal, W., Tsankova, N. M., Theobald, D. E., Truong, H. T., . . . Nestler, E. J. 2005. Chromatin remodeling is a key mechanism underlying cocaine-induced plasticity in striatum. *Neuron*, 48(2): 303–314.

Lander, E. S., Linton, L. M., Birren, B., Nusbaum, C., Zody, M. C., Baldwin, J., . . . Morgan, M. J. 2001. Initial sequencing and analysis of the human genome. *Nature,* 409(6822): 860–921.

Langenecker, S. A., Saunders, E. F., Kade, A. M., Ransom, M. T., & McInnis, M. G. 2010. Intermediate: cognitive phenotypes in bipolar disorder. *Journal of Affective Disorders*, 122(3): 285–293.

Lutter, M., Krishnan, V., Russo, S. J., Jung, S., McClung, C. A., & Nestler, E. J. 2008. Orexin signaling mediates the antidepressant-like effect of calorie restriction. *The Journal of Neuroscience*, 28(12): 3071–3075.

Malhotra, A. K., Murphy, G. M., & Kennedy, J. L. 2004. Pharmacogenetics of psychotropic drug response. *American Journal of Psychiatry*, 161(5): 780–796.

Manji, H. K., W. C. Drevets, et al. (2001). "The cellular neurobiology of depression." *Nature Medicine*, 7(5): 541–547.

Marez, D., Legrand, M., Sabbagh, N., Lo Guidice, J. M., Spire, C., Lafitte, J. J., Meyer, U. A., & Broly, F. 1997. Polymorphism of the cytochrome P450 CYP2D6 gene in a European population: characterization of 48 mutations and 53 alleles, their frequencies and evolution. *Pharmacogenetics*, 7(3): 193–202.

McCay, C. C., & Crowell, M. F. 1934. Prolonging the Life Span. *The Scientific Monthly*, 39(5): 405–414.

McGue, M., &Bouchard, T. J. 1998. Genetic and environmental influences on human behavioral differences. *Annual Review of Neuroscience*, 21: 1–24.

McGuffin, P., Rijsdijk, F., Andrew, M., Sham, P., Katz, R., & Cardno, A. 2003. The heritability of bipolar affective disorder and the genetic relationship to unipolar depression. *Archives of General Psychiatry*, 60(5): 497–502.

McInnis, M. G. 2009. "Paradigms lost: rethinking psychiatry in the post-genome era." *Depression and Anxiety* 26(4): 303–306.

McIntosh, A. M., Harrison, L. K., Forrester, K., Lawrie, S. M., & Johnstone, E. C. 2005. Neuropsychological impairments in people with schizophrenia or bipolar disorder and their unaffected relatives. *British Journal of Psychiatry*, 186: 378–385.

McQueen, M. B., Devlin, B., Faraone, S. V., Nimgaonkar, V. L., Sklar, P., Smoller, J. W., . . . Laird, N. M. 2005. Combined analysis from eleven linkage studies of bipolar disorder provides strong evidence of susceptibility loci on chromosomes 6q and 8q. *The American Journal of Human Genetics*, 77(4): 582–595.

Medvedik, O., Lamming, D. W., Kim, K. D., & Sinclair, D. A. 2007. MSN2 and MSN4 link calorie restriction and TOR to sirtuin-mediated lifespan extension in Saccharomyces cerevisiae. *PLoS Biology*, 5(10): e261.

Mendlewicz, J., & Rainer, J. D. 1977. Adoption study supporting genetic transmission in manic-depressive illness. *Nature*, 268(5618): 327–332.

Miklowitz, D. J., Goldstein, M. J., Nuechterlein, K. H., Snyder, K. S., & Mintz, J. 1988. Family factors and the course of bipolar affective disorder. *Archives of General Psychiatry*, 45(3): 225–231.

Monteggia, L. M., Barrot, M., Powell, C. M., Berton, O., Galanis, V., Gemelli, T., . . . Nestler, E. J. 2004. Essential role of brain-derived neurotrophic factor in adult hippocampal function. *Proceedings from the National Academy of Science U S A*, 101(29): 10827–10832.

Modak, A. S. 2009. Single time point diagnostic breath tests: a review. *Journal of Breath Research*, 4(1): 017002.

Monteggia, L. M., Luikart, B., Barrot, M., Theobold, D., Malkovska, I., Nef, S., Parada, L. F., & Nestler, E. J. 2007. Brain-derived neurotrophic factor conditional knockouts show gender differences in depression-related behaviors. *Biological Psychiatry*, 61(2): 187–197.

Moore, G. J., Bebchuk, J. M., Parrish, J. K., Faulk, M. W., Arfken, C. L., Strahl-Bevacqua, J., & Manji, H. K. 1999. Temporal dissociation between lithium-induced changes in frontal lobe myo-inositol and clinical response in manic-depressive illness. *American Journal of Psychiatry*, 156(12): 1902–1908.

Murphy, G. M., Kremer, C., Rodrigues, H. E., & Schatzberg, A. F. 2003. Pharmacogenetics of antidepressant medication intolerance. *American Journal of Psychiatry*, 160(10): 1830–1835.

Nehra, R., Chakrabarti, S., Pradhan, B. K., & Khehra, N. 2006. Comparison of cognitive functions between first- and multi-episode bipolar affective disorders. *Journal of Affective Disorders*, 93(1–3): 185–192.

Nibuya, M., Morinobu, S., & Duman, R. S. 1995. Regulation of BDNF and trkB mRNA in rat brain by chronic electroconvulsive seizure and antidepressant drug treatments. *The Journal of Neuroscience*, 15(11): 7539–7547.

Pare, C. M., & Mack, J. W. 1971. Differentiation of two genetically specific types of depression by the response to antidepressant drugs. *Journal of Medical Genetics*, 8(3): 306–309.

O'Connell, R. A., Mayo, J. A., Eng, L. K., Jones, J. S., & Gabel, R. H. 1985. Social support and long-term lithium outcome. *British Journal of Psychiatry*, 147: 272–275.

Pare, C. M., Rees, L., & Sainsbury, M. J. 1962. Differentiation of two genetically specific types of depression by the response to anti-depressants. *Lancet*, 2(7270): 1340–1343.

Post, R. M., & Leverich, G. S. 2006. The role of psychosocial stress in the onset and progression of bipolar disorder and its comorbidities: the need for earlier and alternative modes of therapeutic intervention. *Development and Psychopathology*, 18(4): 1181–1211.

Raimundo, S., Fischer, J., Eichelbaum, M., Griese, E. U., Schwab, M., & Zanger, U. M. 2000. Elucidation of the genetic basis of the common 'intermediate metabolizer' phenotype for drug oxidation by CYP2D6. *Pharmacogenetics*, 10(7): 577–581.

Risch, N., & Merikangas, K. 1996. The future of genetic studies of complex human diseases. *Science*, 273(5281): 1516–1517.

Roalf, D. R., Turetsky, B. I., Owzar, K., Balderston, C. C., Johnson, S. C., Brensinger, C. M., . . . Moberg, P. J. 2006. Unirhinal olfactory function in schizophrenia patients and first-degree relatives. *The Journal of Neuropsychiatry & Clinical Neuroscience*, 18(3): 389–396.

Sachse, C., Brockmoller, J., Bauer, S., & Roots, I. 1997. Cytochrome P450 2D6 variants in a Caucasian population: allele frequencies and phenotypic consequences. *The American Journal of Human Genetics*, 60(2): 284–295.

Sawa, A., & Cascella, N. G. 2009. Peripheral olfactory system for clinical and basic psychiatry: a promising entry point to the mystery of brain mechanism and biomarker identification in schizophrenia. *American Journal of Psychiatry*, 166(2): 137–139.

Schafer, M., Rujescu, D., Giegling, I., Guntermann, A., Erfurth, A., Bondy, B., & Moller, H. J. 2001. Association of short-term response to haloperidol treatment with a polymorphism in the dopamine D(2) receptor gene. *American Journal of Psychiatry*, 158(5): 802–804.

Schulze, T. G., Detera-Wadleigh, S. D., Akula, N., Gupta, A., Kassem, L., Steele, J., . . . McMahon, F. J. 2009. Two variants in Ankyrin 3 (ANK3) are independent genetic risk factors for bipolar disorder. *Molecular Psychiatry*, 14(5): 487–491.

Segurado, R., Detera-Wadleigh, S. D., Levinson, D. F., Lewis, C. M., Gill, M., Nurnberger, J. I., . . . Akarsu, N. 2003. Genome scan meta-analysis of schizophrenia and bipolar disorder, part III: Bipolar disorder. *The American Journal of Human Genetics*, 73(1): 49–62.

Selman, C., & Withers, D. J. 2011. Mammalian models of extended healthy lifespan. *Philosophical Transactions of the Royal Society of London B Biological Sciences*, 366(1561): 99–107.

Sklar, P., Smoller, J. W., Fan, J., Ferriera, M. A., Perlis, R. H., Chambert, K., . . . Purcell, S. M. 2008. Whole-genome association study of bipolar disorder. *Molecular Psychiatry*, 13(6): 558–569.

Stranahan, A. M., Lee, K., Martin, B., Maudsley, S., Golden, E., Cutler, R. G., & Mattson, M. P. 2009. Voluntary exercise and caloric restriction enhance hippocampal dendritic spine density and BDNF levels in diabetic mice. *Hippocampus*, 19(10): 951–961.

Sullivan, P. F. 2007. Spurious genetic associations. *Biological Psychiatry*, 61(10): 1121–1126.

Swendsen, J., Hammen, C., Heller, T., & Gitlin, M. 1995. Correlates of stress reactivity in patients with bipolar disorder. *American Journal of Psychiatry*, 152(5): 795–797.

Thaker, G. K., Wonodi, I., Avila, M. T., Hong, L. E., & Stine, O. C. 2004. Catechol O-methyltransferase polymorphism and eye tracking in schizophrenia: a preliminary report. *American Journal of Psychiatry*, 161(12): 2320–2322.

Tsankova, N. M., Berton, O., Renthal, W., Kumar, A., Neve, R. L., & Nestler, E. J. 2006. Sustained hippocampal chromatin regulation in a mouse model of depression and antidepressant action. *Nature Neuroscience*, 9(4): 519–525.

Tsankova, N., Renthal, W., Kumar, A., & Nestler, E. J. 2007. Epigenetic regulation in psychiatric disorders. *Nature Reviews Neuroscience*, 8(5): 355–367.

Thompson, J. M., Gallagher, P., Hughes, J. H., Watson, S., Gray, J. M., Ferrier, I. N., & Young, A.H. 2005. Neurocognitive impairment in euthymic patients with bipolar affective disorder. *British Journal of Psychiatry*, 186: 32–40.

Tsankova, N. M., Kumar, A., & Nestler, E. J. 2004. Histone modifications at gene promoter regions in rat hippocampus after acute and chronic electroconvulsive seizures. *The Journal of Neuroscience*, 24(24): 5603–5610.

Turetsky, B. I., & Moberg, P. J. 2009. An odor-specific threshold deficit implicates abnormal intracellular cyclic AMP signaling in schizophrenia. *The American Journal of Psychiatry*, 166(2): 226–233.

Waddington, C. H. (1957). The Strategy Of The Genes. London, George Allen & Unwin.

Weaver, I. C., Cervoni, N., Champagne, F. A., D'Alessio, A. C., Sharma, S., Seckl, J. R., Dymov, S., Szyf, M., & Meaney, M. J. 2004. Epigenetic programming by maternal behavior. *Nature Neuroscience*, 7(8): 847–854.

Young, L. T., Wang, J. F., Woods, C. M., & Robb, J. C. 1999. Platelet protein kinase C alpha levels in drug-free and lithium-treated subjects with bipolar disorder. *Neuropsychobiology*, 40(2): 63–66.

Zeggini, E., Scott, L. J., Saxena, R., Voight, B. F., Marchini, J. L., Hu, T., . . . Altshuler, D. 2008. Meta-analysis of genome-wide association data and large-scale replication identifies additional susceptibility loci for type 2 diabetes. *Nature Genetics*, 40(5): 638–645.

Zhang, J., Chiodini, R., Badr, A., & Zhang, G. 2011. The impact of next-generation sequencing on genomics. *Journal of Genetics & Genomics*, 38(3): 95–109.

Zhang, P., Xiang, N., Chen, Y., Sliwerska, E., McInnis, M. G., Burmeister, M., & Zollner, S. 2010. Family-based association analysis to finemap bipolar linkage peak on chromosome 8q24 using 2,500 genotyped SNPs and 15,000 imputed SNPs. *Bipolar Disorders*, 12(8): 786–792.

Zubieta, J. K., Huguelet, P., O'Neil, R. L., & Giordani, B. J. 2001. Cognitive function in euthymic bipolar I disorder. *Psychiatry Research*, 102(1): 9–20.

# 9.

# GENERAL GENETICS OF BIPOLAR DISORDER

## John I. Nurnberger, Jr.

Research into the genetics of major medical disorders is important because it provides a direct window into the biology of illness. The actions of specific single genes are revealed in the developmental expression of specific proteins in the brain and other organs; the expression and control of the expression of these proteins provides a substrate for the development of disease. In recent years, it has become clear that psychiatric disorders, like other common medical conditions, result from complex genetic factors and interactions. That is, for the major disorders that we study such as depression, drug and alcohol dependence, schizophrenia, and bipolar disorder, multiple genes are involved. This conclusion has dramatically affected the methods that we use in psychiatric genetics.

At the same time, a scientific revolution has occurred in the field of genetics with the advent of molecular biological techniques. It is now possible to study DNA variants directly, and to study these variants within the context of examining the entire genome rather than single genes. Using these techniques, genes influencing risk for many neuropsychiatric diseases have been identified. Initially, Mendelian single-gene conditions, such as Huntington's disease, were studied and resolved; in the last few years, research into conditions with complex genetic pathophysiology, such as alcohol dependence and schizophrenia, has informed multigene models underlying illness expression. Some of this work has been facilitated by the study of endophenotypes or biologic vulnerability markers. Technological gains now permit investigation of genetic effects in complex behavioral disorders such as bipolar disorder that involve complex, multi-gene interactions with environmental risk factors to lead to these conditions. In this chapter, we review various findings within these and other genetic investigations that inform the potential molecular substrate of bipolar disorder.

## CLINICAL EPIDEMIOLOGY: TWIN, FAMILY, AND ADOPTION STUDIES

Clinical epidemiology permits determination of how a condition distributes within a population and, consequently, whether it clusters in families. These techniques provide starting points to decide whether a condition might have a genetic basis. Three types of population genetic studies are typically conducted to ascertain whether a particular human phenomenon is substantially genetically influenced:

### FAMILY STUDIES

Family studies can answer three critical questions concerning the inheritance of a disorder:

1. Are relatives of an affected subject at increased risk for the disorder compared to relatives of comparison (unaffected) subjects?

2. What other disorders may share a common genetic vulnerability with the phenomenon in question?

3. Can a specific mode of inheritance be discerned?

A family study typically begins with a proband (i.e., an index patient or case), whose relatives are then studied. Family studies in mood disorder have continually demonstrated aggregation of illness in relatives (Tsuang & Faraone, 1990). For example, in a study at the National Institute of Mental Health (NIMH) Intramural Research Program, 25% of relatives of bipolar probands were found to have bipolar or unipolar illness (we use the latter term interchangeably with major depression in this chapter), compared with 20% of relatives of unipolar probands and 7% of

TABLE 9.1 **LIFETIME RISK FOR MAJOR AFFECTIVE DISORDER IN DIFFERENT GROUPS**

| General Population | Relatives of probands with depression | Relatives of probands with bipolar illness | Relatives of probands with acute schizoaffective Disorder | Children of two ill parents | Identical twin ill |
|---|---|---|---|---|---|
| 7% | 20% | 25% | 40% | 50% + | 65% |

**TABLE 9.2** **LIFETIME RISK FOR BIPOLAR DISORDER IN DIFFERENT GROUPS**

| Controls | Relatives of probands with depression | Relatives of probands with bipolar disorder | Relatives of probands with acute schizoaffective disorder | Identical twin with bipolar disorder |
|---|---|---|---|---|
| 0.5—1% | 3% | 8% | 17% | 80% |

relatives of healthy subjects (Gershon et al., 1982). In the same study 40% of the relatives of schizoaffective probands demonstrated mood disorder at some point in their lives (Table 9.1, Table 9.2, Figure 9.1). These data demonstrate increased risk for mood disorders in relatives of patients with mood disorders. These studies also suggested that the various forms of mood disorder appear to be related in a hierarchical way; namely, relatives of schizoaffective probands more often have schizoaffective illness than probands of other mood disorders. However relatives of schizoaffective disorder are more likely to have bipolar or unipolar illness than schizoaffective disorder, so transmission of symptom complexes (i.e., syndromes) is not necessarily pure. Similarly, relatives of bipolar probands are more likely to express bipolar disorder than relatives of other probands, yet they exhibit major depression more often than bipolar illness. Some of these relationships are illustrated graphically in Figure 9.1.

The familial nature of mood disorders has been recognized for centuries, but recent evidence suggests that the rates of these mood disorders in the population may be changing. Specifically, a birth cohort effect has been observed in recent family studies: There is an increasing prevalence of mood disorder among persons born in more recent decades (especially since 1970) in comparison to those born earlier. . The cohort effect appears to be true for schizoaffective and bipolar disorders as well as major depression (Gershon et al., 1989). The cohort effect appears among relatives at risk to a greater degree than in the general population, an observation that may be ascribed to a gene-by-environment interaction. The critical environmental variable(s) have not yet been identified.

In order to clarify these obviously complex relationships among the various mood disorders, investigators have tried to identify clinical characteristics that might define more homogeneous subgroups, presumably identifying a more circumscribed genetic risk. For example, age at onset may be useful for this purpose because early onset probands have increased morbid risk of illness in relatives in comparison to probands with later onset illness in most data sets (Faraone et al., 2004). Other *subphenotypes,* such as affective cycling frequency and the presence of comorbid anxiety or substance use disorders, have also been studied, as we will discuss later in this chapter. In terms of the questions that may be answered by family studies, bipolar disorder is clearly a familial condition. Other diagnoses that may aggregate in relatives of bipolar I disorder probands include bipolar II disorder, major (unipolar) depression, and schizoaffective disorder, bipolar type; this question of familial aggregation is treated in more detail later in this chapter ("The Mood Disorders Spectrum"). In terms of mode of inheritance, segregation analyses of family data (a comparison of the actual distribution of illness within families to the distribution that would be predicted under specific genetic models) has

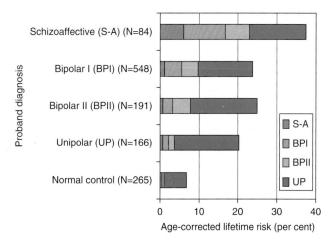

*Figure 9.1* Risk of mood disorders among relatives of probands with different specific mood-disorder diagnoses and relatives of healthy subjects (data from Gershon et al, 1982).

generally favored multi-factorial inheritance (Nurnberger & Berrettini, 1998), which implies a mixture of multiple genetic and environmental factors acting together to cause illness, rather than the impact of a single gene, as occurs in Huntington's disease.

## TWIN STUDIES

Twin studies are based on the fact that monozygotic (MZ) or identical twins represent a natural experiment in which two individuals have exactly the same genes. This relationship is in contrast to dizygotic (DZ) or fraternal twins who share 50% of their genes and are no more genetically similar than any pair of siblings Consequently, characteristics which are under genetic control should be more concordant (similar) in monozygotic than dizygotic twins.

Twin studies for major mood disorders show consistent evidence for heritability. A commonly used formula to calculate heritability (often designated $H^{2)}$ is the Holzinger Index:

$$H^2 = (\% \text{ MZ concordance} - \% \text{ DZ concordance})/ (100 - \% \text{ DZ concordance}).$$

On average, in mood disorders, monozygotic twin pairs show diagnostic concordance 65% of the time and dizygotic twin pairs demonstrate diagnostic agreement 14% of the time (Nurnberger & Berrettini, 2000). When divided by polarity, twin probands with bipolar illness show about 80% concordance (Bertelsen et al., 1977; 1979). Bienvenu et al. (2010) summarize three recent twin studies of bipolar disorder and calculated a heritability of 85%. This implies that about 85% of the variance in whether a person in the population will experience bipolar disorder is explained by genetic factors. This rate of heritability in bipolar disorder is higher than other psychiatric illnesses and most complex medical conditions.

## ADOPTION STUDIES

Adoption studies provide a natural experiment to separate the effects of environment from those of genes. These types of studies are particularly relevant for complex disorders that are likely to involve multiple genes interacting with the environment, such as bipolar disorder. In adoption studies the risk for the disorder may be evaluated among four combinations of adoptees and adoptive and biological relatives: the adoptive and biological relatives of affected adoptees (probands) and the adoptive and biological relatives of comparison (unaffected) adoptees. If the disorder is heritable, one should find an increased risk among the biological relatives of affected probands, compared to the other three groups of relatives. One can also compare risk for illness in adopted-away children of ill parents versus adopted-away children of well parents. Several adoption studies have been performed examining these relationships in mood disorders generally and bipolar disorder specifically: The results have been consistent with hypotheses that genetic effects significantly explain illness variance in cases and families (Nurnberger & Berrettini, 1998). Namely, bipolar probands growing up in an adoptive family will have more biological relatives with mood disorder than control probands growing up in an adoptive family. One of the more striking examples of adoption studies in mood disorders was the excess of suicide found in the biological relatives of adoptees with depression compared to control adoptees, with no excess of suicide in adoptive relatives of either group (Wender et al., 1986). This finding suggests that even relatively specific behavioral symptoms may be significantly influenced by genetic effects.

In summary, genetic epidemiologic studies of bipolar illness provide strong evidence not only for familiality, but also for a predominance of genetic effects in the etiology of the disorder. These genetic effects, though, are complex, and one should not expect to identify single genes that explain a major portion of the variance. Moreover, since monozygotic twins do not show a 100% concordance rate of bipolar disorder, environmental factors clearly also contribute to the risk of developing bipolar illness (Table 9.2).

### Clinical Epidemiology Key Points:

- Mood disorders run in families and bipolar disorder is strongly heritable

- Twin and adoption studies suggest that the phenomenology of bipolar disorder is under strong genetic control, but environmental factors are also relevant

- Mood disorder inheritance is hierarchical, meaning that more severe disorders (e.g. Bipolar I and Schizoaffective Disorder Bipolar Type) tend to confer more risk in relatives although in all groups of relatives major depression is the most common expression of illness

- Population rates of mood disorders seem to be increasing, particularly in relatives of persons with mood disorders

A spectrum of disorders generally refers to a set of disorders related by family studies or that share a number of overlapping symptoms. As noted in the previous discussion in this chapter, if you examine relatives of bipolar I probands, you will find an excess of not only bipolar I disorder, but also bipolar II, major (unipolar) depression, and schizoaffective disorder—bipolar type. In this section, we examine these disorders that appear to be genetically related to bipolar I disorder in more detail.

*Bipolar I Disorder*: Bipolar I disorder is so-called classic manic-depressive illness and is defined by the occurrence of mania, but in most cases also includes episodes of major depression that are typically more frequent than manic episodes.

*Bipolar II disorder*: Bipolar II disorder is defined by the occurrence of hypomania plus at least one episode of major depression. Hypomania shares the same symptoms as mania, but is distinguished from it by not being as severe in terms of functional impairment. Bipolar II disorder appears to be genetically related to both Bipolar I disorder and unipolar disorder on the basis of family studies. There is also some evidence in such studies for an excess of bipolar II disorder in relatives of bipolar II probands (Heun & Meier, 1993), suggesting that there may be some genetic specificity for this condition. Consistent with that notion, bipolar II disorder tends to be a stable lifetime diagnosis; that is, patients with bipolar II do not frequently convert to bipolar I disorder, at least among adults (Coryell et al., 1995).

*Major Depression*: Major depression is also known as unipolar disorder, as noted previously. This condition is highly familial, especially in early onset cases, and it is also related to bipolar I disorder. The classic twin studies that we reviewed typically included both unipolar and bipolar cases. Unipolar depression is the most common psychiatric illness among the relatives of probands with bipolar disorder (Tsuang & Faraone, 1990), although it is also quite common in the general population.

*Rapid Cycling*: Rapid-cycling represents a clinical course subtype of both bipolar I and II disorders. It has been the subject of great theoretical and clinical interest, as it can be very difficult to treat. Typically, rapid cycling is defined as four or more episodes in a year. Rapid cycling tends to be temporally limited, and may be related to environmental factors; for example, a link with thyroid pathology has been proposed. Rapid cycling may arise from heritable factors which might produce aggregation within families (Saunders et al., 2008, but see Nurnberger et al., 1988).

Rapid switching of mood, which is related to rapid cycling, also appears to be familial (MacKinnon et al., 2003).

*Unipolar mania*: By definition, patients who experience unipolar mania (i.e., never develop major depression) meet criteria for bipolar I disorder, but their course of illness is atypical. Nonetheless, this relatively uncommon group is not distinguishable from other bipolar I patients on the basis of family pattern of illness (Nurnberger et al., 1979).

*Cyclothymia*: This is a condition of repetitive high and low mood swings that do not meet criteria for full manic or depressive episodes. Cyclothymia often does not require clinical intervention, but may be genetically related to bipolar disorder (Akiskal & Pinto, 1999). Cyclothymia has been considered a personality disorder, rather than an Axis I condition by some investigators.

*Schizoaffective Disorder*: Schizoaffective disorder is differentiated from psychotic mood disorders by the persistence of psychosis for at least two weeks in the absence of prominent mood symptoms, and from schizophrenia by the occurrence of significant mood symptoms throughout a substantial portion of the course of illness. It is further subdivided into bipolar and depressive subtypes based on whether mood symptoms include mania or only depression, respectively. This group of patients has an increase in mood disorder and an increase in schizophrenia in relatives, which suggests a genetic relationship to both conditions. This group may have the highest genetic load (total risk for mood disorder or schizophrenic illness in relatives) of any diagnostic category (Gershon et al., 1988). More specifically, those patients with schizoaffective disorder, bipolar type may carry genes related to both bipolar illness and schizophrenia. Patients with schizoaffective disorder, depressed type also confer risk for both chronic psychosis and mood disorder to relatives but have less overall genetic load than those with schizoaffective disorder, bipolar type.

*Schizophrenia*: In recent years, an overlap in chromosomal linkage areas and vulnerability genes between bipolar I disorder and schizophrenia has been identified (International Schizophrenia Consortium, 2009), especially in genes related to glutamate neurotransmission. These findings will be discussed in more detail later in this chapter.

*Eating disorders*: Family studies of anorexia and bulimia have generally found an excess of mood disorder in relatives. Relatives of anorexics may have a similar risk for mood disorders to that of relatives of bipolar probands (Nurnberger & Berrettini, 2000).

*Attention-deficit hyperactivity disorder (ADHD)*: Children with ADHD appear to have increased depression in their relatives. Some studies, but not others, report increased risk of ADHD in the offspring of probands with bipolar disorder, which has led to hypotheses that ADHD may be a premorbid expression of bipolar illness (see summary in Nurnberger et al., 2011). The co-occurrence of bipolar disorder and attention deficit disorder has been proposed to be a potentially distinct familial illness (Faraone et al., 1997; Faraone & Wilens, 2003).

*Alcohol Dependence*: There may be overlapping vulnerability traits between alcohol dependence and mood disorders. Alcohol dependence is commonly *comorbid* with unipolar depression and especially, bipolar disorders; likewise persons with primary alcohol problems have an increased risk for *comorbid* mood disorders. There is some evidence that alcoholism with mood disorder may itself aggregate within families (Nurnberger et al., 2007).

Since family and genetic studies are particularly sensitive to the correct identification of affected individuals (i.e., cases), identifying appropriate diagnostic boundaries is a critical component of identifying genetic associations. Unfortunately, behavioral symptoms across different diagnostic conditions are often continuous, rather than distinct, making case identification a challenge at times. The use of spectrums may help to alleviate some of this problem by suggesting a variable phenotype within specific genetic models that can be used to identify gene effects. However, more research in the validity of this proposed mood spectrum is needed to maximize benefit from this approach.

## ENDOPHENOTYPES

An endophenotype is a biological characteristic that may substitute for a diagnosis in a genetic analysis. The advantage is that an endophenotype may be closer to the underlying pathophysiology of the illness, and therefore may be more easily demonstrated to be linked or associated with specific genetic markers. Sometimes an endophenotype is also easier to define using objective criteria. Endophenotypes may be important clues to the underlying biological mechanisms of illness. The term endophenotype was first used in this context by Gottesman (see Hasler et al., 2006). Criteria for an endophenotype have been derived from those proposed by Gershon and Goldin (1986):

1. The endophenotype must be associated with illness in the general population.

2. The endophenotype should be a stable, state-independent characteristic; that is, it should be observable even when the patient is in partial or complete remission.

3. The endophenotype should be heritable.

4. The endophenotype should segregate with illness within families.

Gottesman has also called attention to the following criterion:

5. Among family members of a proband with the endophenotype, the endophenotype should occur at a higher rate than it does in the general population.

Comments on selected endophenotypes for bipolar disorder are included in Table 9.3. A limitation of many of the endophenotypes studied so far is that they are difficult to measure and unlikely to be applied to large samples (see Scalability). However, they are certainly suitable for candidate gene studies. Some of the brain imaging phenotypes, such as amygdala activation in fMRI studies, may now be appropriate for larger-scale testing. The reader is directed to the review by Hasler et al. (2006) for a more extended discussion.

### EPIGENETIC STUDIES/GENE EXPRESSION STUDIES

Epigenetics is the study of biological modifiers of DNA transcription. The most common mechanisms studied thus far are DNA methylation and chromatin remodeling. Methylation of DNA generally prevents transcription of a particular gene. Chromatin (the protein framework supporting DNA in the nucleus) may exist in an active state (allowing transcription) or an inactive state (preventing

---

**The Mood Disorders Spectrum:**

- Mood disorders may exist in a spectrum of genetic liability and phenotypic expression

- Primary conditions within this spectrum include:

  Bipolar I Disorder

  Bipolar II Disorder

  Major (Unipolar) Depression

  Schizoaffective Disorder, Bipolar Type

- Other conditions mentioned above, such as schizophrenia and alcohol dependence, may also have some genetic overlap with the mood disorders.

| Marker and Primary Reference | Current Status | Scalability | Comments |
|---|---|---|---|
| REM sleep induction by cholinergic drugs (Sitaram et al., 1980) | likely confirmed | poor | Index of muscarinic cholinergic sensitivity |
| White matter hyperintensities on MRI (Altshuler et al., 1995) | Heritability not clear | good | Well replicated |
| Amygdala activation on fMRI (Strakowski et al., 2005) | Needs confirmation in euthymic subjects; heritability is unclear | possible | Anatomically specific |
| Hippocampal size (Hallahan et al., 2011) | Inconsistent results | good | Anatomically specific |
| Response to tryptophan depletion (Delgado et al., 1991) | True for unipolar patients; not clear if relevant for bipolar disorder | moderate | Index of serotonergic sensitivity |
| Response to sleep deprivation (Wehr et al., 1987) | Heritability is not clear; Neurobiology not clear | poor | Index of circadian rhythms disturbance |
| Melatonin suppression by light (Lewy et al., 1985) | Needs replication in euthymic subjects | poor | Index of circadian rhythms disturbance |

transcription). Various stimuli, including environmental events, may be responsible for epigenetic changes that turn genes on or off. Of course, substantial additional gene regulation occurs at the RNA level, much of which may be captured by gene expression studies that measure RNA directly.

Epigenetic mechanisms have not been demonstrated to be critical in clinical studies of traditional psychiatric disorders to date. Differential methylation does appear to be important however in Prader-Willi syndrome, which includes mental retardation and sometimes mood disorders as part of the clinical picture. This condition is related to *imprinting* on 15q; the DNA segment that is transcribed for this chromosomal region is generally the segment from the father. The mother's DNA from that region tends to be methylated and not transcribed. In Prader-Willi there is deletion of the father's DNA in that region, so neither segment is functional.

Two animal models are of some interest. One has been described by Eric Nestler and includes differential methylation (and perhaps chromatin remodeling) in social defeat, with susceptible mice demonstrating decreased BDNF and cyclic AMP response element binding protein (CREB), and consequently presumably decreased neuronal growth. This effect is preventable with chronic antidepressant treatment (Benton et al., 2006). The other model (studied by Frances Champagne at Columbia) involves maternal licking/grooming in rodents. Low licking/grooming is associated with increased methylation of the estrogen receptor promoter in the offspring, decreased production of that receptor, and many behavioral changes suggesting greater responsivity to stress (but also increased sexual interest and more offspring). The most interesting aspect of this model is that differential methylation appears to be transmitted from the offspring to their offspring (i.e. the F2 generation) as well. This finding is an unusual instance of apparent inheritance of acquired characteristics, or an example that would seem to suggest a variation on the discredited theories of Lamarck and Lysenko (Champagne, 2008).

Ogden et al. (2004) have summarized gene expression data related to bipolar disorder. They used a convergent approach that integrated human brain gene expression data with results from a pharmacologic mouse model. This approach identified several candidate genes including DARPP-32 (dopamine- and cAMP-regulated phosphoprotein of 32 kDa) located at 17q12, PENK (preproenkephalin) located at 8q12.1, and TAC1 (tachykinin 1, substance P) located at 7q21.3. These findings suggest that genes associated with the experiences of pleasure and pain in animals may play a role in emotional expression in humans. Le-Niculescu et al. (2009) expanded this work by including data from genome-wide association studies as well as postmortem gene expression studies and expression studies in lymphocytes (and other lines of evidence including animal models). The candidate genes determined to be most likely involved in bipolar disorder pathogenesis were ARNTL, BDNF, ALDH1A1, and KLF12.

## HIGH-RISK STUDIES

High-risk studies are of great use for testing endophenotypes and for observing the predictive utility of risk gene variants. High-risk studies in bipolar disorder typically involve evaluating children, who may or may not be ill, of bipolar parents and comparing them to children of healthy parents. When performed longitudinally, these studies are also useful for observing developmental changes of expression in the phenotype of bipolar disorder. More offspring of bipolar patients than healthy subjects have a diagnosed Axis I disorder. Offspring of bipolar parents may be more prone to respond to dysphoric feeling states and by disinhibitory behavior than children of healthy parents (Nurnberger et al., 1988). Recent studies of offspring at risk for bipolar disorder have identified children with anxiety disorders or externalizing disorders as being at increased risk for development of adolescent mood disorder (Duffy et al., 2009; Nurnberger et al., 2011). The reader is referred to chapter 5 of this textbook for a more detailed discussion of findings that have been reported from high-risk studies.

## LINKAGE STUDIES

At any given genetic locus, each individual carries two copies (*alleles*) of the DNA sequence that defines that locus. One of these alleles is inherited from the mother and the other is from the father. If two genetic loci are close to each other on a chromosome, their alleles tend to be inherited together (not independently) and they are known as linked loci. During meiosis, crossing over (also known as *recombination*) can occur between homologous chromosomes, thus accounting for the observation that alleles of linked loci are not always inherited together.

The rate at which crossing over occurs between two linked loci is directly proportional to the distance separating them on the chromosome. In fact, the genetic distance between two linked loci is defined in terms of the percentage of recombination between the two loci (this value is known as *theta*). Loci that are far apart on a chromosome will have a 50% chance of being inherited together and consequently are not linked. Therefore, the maximum value for theta is 0.5, which represents random association, whereas the minimum value is 0, implying that two loci are so close that they are virtually always linked. Linkage analysis is a method for estimating theta for two or more loci. The probability that two loci are linked is the probability that theta < 0.5, while the probability that the two loci are not linked is the probability that theta = 0.5. This relationship is typically represented by a LOD (logarithm of the odds ratio) score for a family or set of families, which is defined by the following formula:

**LOD score = ($\log_{10}$ probability of theta < 0.5)/ (probability of theta = 0.5)**

Although it is possible to perform such calculations by hand, LOD scores are usually calculated using computer programs such as GENEHUNTER or Merlin. Since a LOD score is a log value, scores from different families can be summed. For complex conditions collections of affected sibling pairs may be studied rather than large families. A LOD score of 1.0 indicates that linkage is 10 times more likely than non-linkage. For simple genetic conditions, a LOD score of 3 or greater is evidence for linkage, while a score of -2 or less is sufficient to exclude linkage for the sample studied. For disorders with more complex forms of inheritance (including most psychiatric disorders), a higher positive LOD score is required (3.6 for definite linkage and 2.2 for suggestive linkage) to protect against chance associations being interpreted as meaningful findings. See Lander and Kruglyak (1995) for further discussion on this topic.

Linkage for bipolar disorder (LOD scores of > 3.6 in single studies or equivalent evidence) has been demonstrated on (chromosome and arm) 4p, 6q, 8q, 13q, 18p, 18q, and 22q. Other areas are "close" to significant, including 12q, 21q, and Xq (Hayden & Nurnberger, 2006). Meta-analyses have supported linkage on 6q and 8q (McQueen et al., 2005), and 13q and 22q (Badner & Gershon, 2002). A large single sample analysis implicated 16p using a dominant model (Ross et al., 2008). It is clear that multiple chromosomal regions are linked to bipolar disorder; presumably

**Linkage studies:**

· Identify whether a gene marker occurs more often with illness within families than would be expected by chance, suggesting that the chromosomal region includes one or more risk-related genes

· A LOD score is one measure of linkage typically used in research reports; other measures include the NPL or non-parametric linkage score

· Linkages for bipolar disorder have been identified at chromosomes 4p, 6q, 8q, 13q, 16p, 18p, 18q, & 22q

**TABLE 9.5 CANDIDATE GENES RELATED TO BIPOLAR DISORDER IN MULTIPLE STUDIES**

| Gene | Location | References |
|---|---|---|
| G72/G30 (DAOA) | 13q33 | Hattori et al., 2003; Chen et al., 2004; Bass et al., 2009 |
| BDNF | 11p15 | Sklar et al., 2002; Neves-Perreira et al., 2002; Liu et al., 2008 |
| FKBP5 | 6p21.31 | Binder et al., 2009; Willour et al., 2009 |
| DISC1 | 1q42 | Millar et al., 2005; Thomason et al. 2005 |
| 5HTT (SLC6A4) | 17q11.2 | Cho et al. 2005 (meta-analysis) |
| MAOA | Xp11.3 | Preisig et al., 2000; Fan et al., 2010 (meta-analysis) |
| TPH1 | 11p15.3-p14 | Chen et al., 2011 (meta-analysis) |
| TPH2 | 12q21.1 | Lopez et al., 2007; Harvey et al., 2007; Cichon et al., 2008 |

all of these contain a specific gene or (more likely) a number of genes that influence vulnerability to the disorder

## ASSOCIATION/CANDIDATE GENE STUDIES

Studies of numerous candidate gene studies have been reported in the literature for bipolar disorder. Several genes have emerged with replicated findings or positive meta-analyses from multiple studies (Tables 9.4 and 9.5). In this section, we will review some of the more promising findings. References in text and table are not exhaustive, but feature the largest studies and meta-analyses.

**Candidates identified in genome-wide association studies:**

*Ankyrin 3 (ANK3)*: The first gene identified in a major psychiatric disorder using GWAS methods was ankyrin 3 (Ferreira et al., 2008; Schulze et al., 2008; Smith et al., 2009) This gene codes for a structural membrane protein related to sodium channels. Sodium transport has been reported to be abnormal in studies of bipolar disorder and major depression since the 1960s (El-Mallakh & Huff, 2001).

The calcium channel gene *CACNA1C* reached genome-wide significance in the report of Ferreira et al. (2008). Recent data show *CACNA1C* with the most significant

**TABLE 9.4 SINGLE GENES RELATED TO BIPOLAR DISORDER IN GENOME-WIDE ASSOCIATION STUDIES (GWAS)**

| Gene | Location | Reference |
|---|---|---|
| ANK3 | 10 | Ferreira et al., 2008; Schulze et al., 2008; Smith et al., 2009 |
| CACNA1C | 12 | Ferreira et al., 2008 |
| NCAN | 19 | Cichon et al., 2011 |

association results for any gene in a 16,000 subject consortium analysis of bipolar GWAS data (Psychiatric GWAS Consortium Bipolar Disorder Working Group, submitted for publication).

*NCAN* was recently identified by a large international consortium studying bipolar illness and using GWAS methods (Cichon et al., (2011). it codes for an extracellular matrix glycoprotein. In the mouse, this is localized in cortical and hippocampal brain areas.

**Candidates identified in multiple individual studies:**

*G72 or D-Amino Acid Oxidase Activator (DAOA)*: This gene (together with G30) is one of two implicated together in association studies on chromosome 13q. The gene G30 is a DNA sequence which is reverse transcribed within G72. The association with bipolar disorder was first identified by Hattori et al. (2003) after work by Chumakov and colleagues (2002) in schizophrenia. It has been supported by several other independent groups (Chen et al., 2004, Williams et al., 2006), but the implicated variants have not always been the same (see meta-analyses by Detera-Wadleigh and McMahon, 2006, Shi et al., 2008, and Muller et al., 2011). The function of DAOA is to oxidize serine, which is a potent activator of glutamate transmission via a modulatory site on the NMDA (n-methyl-d-aspartate) receptor. Inadequate DAOA function might be hypothesized to lead to problems in modulating the glutamate signal in areas of the brain such as the prefrontal cortex, which are likely to be involved in the expression of bipolar disorder (please see chapter 2 for detailed discussions of bipolar neuroanatomy). Existing evidence from animal studies suggests that glutamate antagonists may have antidepressant effects, and that depression may be associated with inadequate modulation of glutamate neurotransmission. A subsequent report, however, emphasized the role of G72 in dendritic arborization rather than serine oxidation (Kvajo et al., 2008). Dendritic arborization could be relevant for underlying findings of prefrontal and other regional brain abnormalities observed in bipolar disorder.

*Brain-derived Neurotrophic Factor (BDNF)*: This gene is a candidate based both on position (11p14, near reported linkage peaks in several family series) and function (as a neuronal growth factor, it is implicated in several recent hypotheses of depression and bipolar mood disorder—see Verhagen et al., 2010). Polymorphisms in BDNF have shown significant association in three independent reports in family-based data, but not in several case-control series. Two reports suggested association in child/adolescent onset bipolar disorder, and two additional series show association in rapid-cycling subgroups of bipolar patients. A meta-analysis was positive (Fan & Sklar, 2008). However a population study (Petryshen et al., 2010) has shown significant ethnic variation in the most widely studied variant (the val-66met promoter polymorphism), and this effect must be carefully considered in case/control studies. Several studies have shown that antidepressant administration is associated with increased central BDNF levels in experimental animals, and administration of BDNF itself has been associated with antidepressant-like activity. Depression has been postulated to be associated with decreased neurogenesis in the hippocampus, which is dependent on neurotrophic factors, including BDNF. Mood stabilizing medications used in bipolar disorder are thought to have neuroprotective effects that may be mediated through BDNF expression. The val/met polymorphism appears to be directly functional in the brain, as variation is associated with hippocampal activity and memory function (Hariri et al., 2003). It is also associated with HPA reactivity (Goodyer et al., 2010; Dougherty et al., 2010; Vinberg et al., 2009; Alexander et al., 2010; Shalev et al., 2009)

*FKBP5*: Binder (2009) reviewed evidence suggesting a role for *FKBP5* in glucocorticoid receptor sensitivity, and also evidence for alleles at this locus being involved with bipolar and unipolar mood disorders. Our collaborative group (Willour et al., 2009) has participated in a positive family-based association study of SNPs in this gene and bipolar disorder as well.

*Disrupted in Schizophrenia 1 (DISC1)*: This gene, located on chromosome 1q, was identified in a Scottish family with a genetic translocation and with multiple cases of psychiatric disorders, primarily schizophrenia. However DISC1 variants were associated with mood disorders in family members as well. Later studies in an independent series of bipolar patients in Scotland were positive for association (Thomson et al., 2005). A study in Wales of schizo-affective patients showed a linkage peak in the same chromosomal location. This gene is expressed in multiple brain regions, including the hippocampus, where it is differentially expressed in neurons. It is associated with microtubules that may contribute to cortical structural development; in mice, disruption of DISC1 leads to abnormal neuronal migration in the developing cerebral cortex. DISC1 appears to interact with phosphodiesterase 4B, which may play a role in mood regulation (Millar et al., 2005).

*5HTT (SLC6A4), MAOA, COMT*: These three genes have been shown in meta-analyses to be associated with bipolar disorder, even though no strong effects were shown in any one study. The effect size for each appears to be in the range of 10%–20% increase in risk. Each of these genes has been shown to be associated with other behavioral phenotypes, and each has been reported to interact with environmental factors to increase risk for specific disorders (major depression, antisocial personality disorder, and schizophrenia respectively). Note that a second meta-analysis of COMT and bipolar disorder was not positive (Craddock et al., 2006).

*Tryptophan hydroxylase (TPH1 and 2)*: These two enzymes catalyze the first and rate-limiting, step of serotonin synthesis. TPH1 is peripherally expressed and TPH2 is brain-expressed. Both genes contain variants that have been associated with bipolar disorder in several, but not all, studies (Roche & McKeon 2009).

**Other candidate genes:**

*P2RX7 (aka P2X7, P2X7R)*: This gene on 12q24 was identified in a French-Canadian case-control series following linkage studies using large pedigrees from the same population (Barden et al., 2006). It codes for a calcium-stimulated ATPase. The association was also seen in a German series of patients with major depression (Lucae et al., 2006), but not in a large UK series (Green et al., 2009). Its relevance for bipolar disorder remains somewhat uncertain.

*GRK3*: GRK3 is the only candidate gene identified using animal model studies, specifically a mouse model employing methamphetamine. The original gene expression studies were followed by association studies in several samples as well as expression studies in human lymphoblasts (Barrett et al., 2003; 2007). Independent replication has not yet occurred. This gene participates in down-regulation of G protein coupled receptors.

As genetic techniques continue to improve, and as we better understand possible endophenotypes underlying the expression of bipolar disorder, it is likely that some of these genes will turn out to play a significant role in conferring risk for bipolar disorder, whereas others will be only peripherally involved, or will be false positives. However, the examples discussed in this section demonstrate the promise of this approach.

### Association/Candidate Gene Studies:

- Candidate gene studies have identified several genes that may be involved in the expression of bipolar disorder

- None of the currently identified candidate genes demonstrate large effect sizes, suggesting multiple genes combine to accumulate risk of bipolar disorder

- Candidate genes include: DAOA, BDNF, Ankyrin 3, DISC1, 5HTT, MAOA, TPH1 & 2, P2RX7,GRK3, NCAN, and CACNA1C

- These candidate genes are involved with neural development and structure, monoamine regulation, and sodium and calcium channel regulation

## THE DEVELOPMENT OF GENOME-WIDE ASSOCIATION STUDIES (GWAS)

Genome-wide association studies (GWAS) were introduced in 2006. They were made possible by chip technology in which up to 2.5 million SNPs may be tested within a single experiment. This methodology enables examination of virtually every gene in the genome with multiple SNPs, and, because of linkage disequilibrium (the fact that nearby variants tend to be transmitted together within a population), even detection of variation some distance from the actual SNP tested (GAIN Collaborative Research Group, 2007). The major limitation of GWAS studies is in interpreting the data, since the number of simultaneous tests is massive, and requires statistical corrections that are complex, since not all events are independent due to linkage disequilibrium in the population as noted above. The presently accepted standard is a p value of $< 5\times10e\text{-}8$ for a SNP association with illness in a GWAS study (Altshuler et al., 2008), based on empirical probability of a type I error.

Since the effect size of variants associated with psychiatric disorders is generally quite small (odds ratios of 1.1–1.2 are the norm), achieving p values that meet this threshold requires very large sample sizes. Complex traits such as height, and risk for type II diabetes have now been analyzed extensively with GWAS methods, but success required samples in the tens of thousands or even hundreds of thousands (Lango Allen et al., 2010). These samples are achievable now only by extensive collaboration involving multiple sites, usually from international sources. Each set of cases should be matched with controls from a similar ethnic background because of the extensive variation in SNP genotype frequencies on the basis of ancestry. This ethnic variability is generally assessed formally using multidimensional scaling (MDS) or a similar method.

GWAS methods have now proven to be useful in psychiatric disorders, with several loci meeting stringent criteria in both schizophrenia and bipolar disorder (Ripke et al, 2011; Psychiatric GWAS Consortium Bipolar Disorder Working Group, 2011). Several of the loci described previously are the product of GWAS investigations (e.g., ANK3, CACNA1C, NCAN).

GWAS datasets have also been used for additional studies that extend the reach of the association methodology: polygenic score analyses and pathway analyses. The polygenic score method was introduced in neuropsychiatric disorders by Shaun Purcell as part of the International Schizophrenia Consortium (**2009**) report on GWAS findings in an initial dataset. The idea is to assign a score to each risk allele (i.e. the variant of the gene that is more common in cases than in controls) that is even nominally associated with disease (using a weighting factor based on the ratio of allele frequency in cases to allele frequency in controls) and then add the scores for each individual based on the number of risk alleles that individual carries. The risk alleles from one population may be tested to see whether they predict illness in a second population. In the ISC paper, risk scores for a group with schizophrenia successfully predicted illness in a second population with schizophrenia, and also in a separate population with bipolar disorder, but not in groups with several other medical conditions. This suggested substantial genetic overlap between the schizophrenia and bipolar disorder samples.

Pathway analyses start with the premise that multiple genes (each one explaining a small portion of the overall genetic variance) are involved in the predisposition for complex neuropsychiatric disorders and that it will be more parsimonious and heuristic to explain their effects in terms of the biological pathways that they participate in rather than considering them individually. SNPs that show evidence for association (even though not meeting the stringent criteria discussed in the section Association/Candidate Gene Studies in this chapter) are considered markers for genes that they reside in or are very close to. The gene lists generated in this manner are compared with **canonical pathways** or gene lists designated in bioinformatic databases. Commonly used databases for this purpose include Gene Ontology (GO, www.geneontology.org) or KEGG (www.genome.jp/kegg/), or the proprietary database Ingenuity (www.ingenuity.com/). Statistical analysis may be conducted at the pathway level, usually correcting for gene size, which varies over several orders of magnitude. Schork has published a report on pathways in bipolar disorder (Torkamani et al., **2008**) and several other reports are in preparation. Using this approach, Torkamani et al. (**2008**) suggested that regulation of dopamine signaling represents a significant risk pathway for bipolar disorder.

> **Genome-wide Association Studies (GWAS):**
>
> - GWAS examines the entire human genome, looking for regions associated with a condition
>
> - GWAS studies are beginning to identify genes that are related to bipolar disorder, such as ANK3, CACNA1C and NCAN
>
> - Pathway analyses have been developed to help interpret large GWAS

## SEQUENCING STUDIES

Sequencing studies have been initiated in a number of major psychiatric disorders including bipolar disorder. Sequencing (also referred to as re-sequencing) now uses next-generation methods that are many times cheaper and more efficient than the common PCR-based methods in use several years ago. The two strategies generally employed are whole genome sequencing and exome sequencing, the former involving determination of every base pair in a subject's genome and the latter involving just the ~2% of the genome that is directly transcribed or in known regulatory regions. An important variable in sequencing endeavors is the "read frequency" or the number of times that an area is analyzed for sequence information. Up to 30x coverage may be necessary to identify some rare mutations precisely, but 8x may be sufficient to identify most variants. The major advantage of sequencing over GWAS is that sequencing is better for identifying rare variants (e.g., less than 1% frequency

in cases), some of which are anticipated to have large effects on illness vulnerability.

Analysis of sequence data presents currently unsolved computational problems, since there are $3 \times 10e9$ data points per person, including several hundred thousand rare variants per person (Ng et al., 2008); each of us appears to carry 250–300 loss-of-function variants in annotated genes and 50-100 variants previously implicated in inherited disorders (1000 Genomes Project Consortium, 2010). How does one identify the truly pathogenic variants within these huge datasets? Current studies have relied on lists of genes previously reported to be associated with the disorder in question, as well as strategies of collapsing different variants within single genes or even single regions. We expect that statistical methods will evolve quickly in this area to help answer these questions and strengthen the value of sequencing methods for defining the genetics of bipolar, and other, disorders.

## COPY NUMBER VARIATION (CNV)

Studies of copy number variation (CNVs) have been ongoing for several years in neuropsychiatric disorders. CNVs are cytogenetic abnormalities that are too small to resolve using microscopic examination of the chromosomes, but still large enough to involve hundreds or thousands of base pairs. They are, therefore, mini-duplications or deletions of genetic material. They have been found to be widespread in healthy individuals, but have also been reported to be concentrated in areas of possible significance for autism (Pinto et al., 2010), intellectual disability (Morrow, 2010), and schizophrenia (Walsh et al., 2008). They may either be *inherited* or *de novo,* and the *de novo* events have appeared to be of more importance, at least for the childhood onset disorders. *De novo* status is demonstrated by examination of the parents' genomes and confirmation of the absence of the event in them.

Rare CNVs were reported to be elevated in a study by Zhang et al. (2009) in subjects with bipolar disorder from the NIMH Genetics Initiative Database. A subsequent study showed increased CNVs in patients with bipolar disorder who had early onset (< 21), but not patients with later onset (Priebe et al., 2011). However other studies have not seen an elevation in CNVs (Grozeva et al., 2010). In order for these reports to be biologically meaningful, the identification and confirmation of specific loci, or genes, involved in the putative increased CNV burden in bipolar illness, will be necessary. One study has implicated 16p11.2 (McCarthy et al., 2009) and one study has reported increased CNVs in the *GSK3beta* gene (Lachman et al., 2007) in bipolar disorder. CNVs may now be detected using dedicated microchips, and thus these studies are expected to be more commonly performed in the future.

## PHARMACOGENETICS OF LITHIUM RESPONSE

Genetic evidence may be useful not only to identify pathophysiology and prediction of risk for illness, but also in identification of treatment mechanisms and prediction of treatment response. In a series of studies, Grof and his coworkers have described a method for strict classification of lithium responders and nonresponders among bipolar patients (Turecki et al., 2001). Their evidence suggests that lithium response is familial and probably genetic. Data from their group (Turecki et al., 2001) suggests linkage of lithium response to an area on chromosome 15q.

Specific genetic associations have not yet been identified and replicated for lithium response. Perlis et al. (2009) have published a genomewide association study of lithium response from the STEP-BD dataset but did not report

unambiguous signals. Additional GWAS in this area are awaited.

## GENETIC COUNSELING

The lifetime risk (also described as age-corrected morbid risk) for severe (incapacitating) mood disorder in the general population is about 7%. Risk is increased to about 20% in first-degree relatives of unipolar depressed probands, and 25% in first-degree relatives of bipolar probands. Risk is about 40% in relatives of schizoaffective patients. The risk to offspring of two affected parents is in excess of 50% (Figure 9.1 and Tables 1 & 2; data from the family study described in Gershon et al., 1982). Overall prevalence figures appear to be rising in recent years, but more so in relatives of patients than in the general population (keeping at about a 3:1 ratio).

First episodes of bipolar illness almost always occur before age 50. Fully 50% of subjects with bipolar disorder develop an initial episode (either depressive or manic) prior to age 20 (see Figure 9.2).; for unipolar depression, the

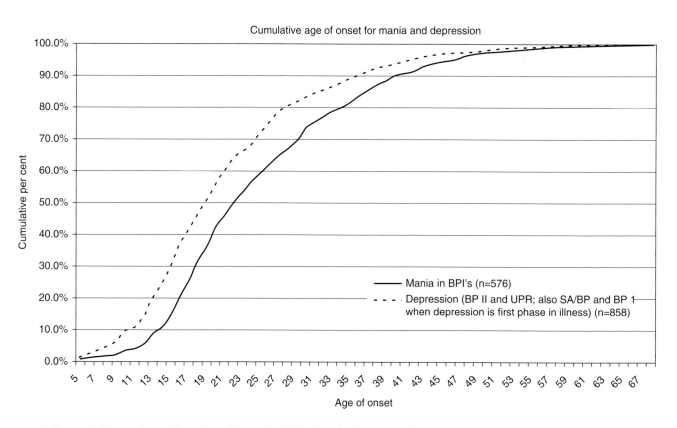

*Figure 9.2* The cumulative age of onset for mania and depression in bipolar and unipolar mood disorders (data from the NIMH Genetics Initiative Study as described in Dick et al, 2003).

THE BIPOLAR BRAIN

median onset age would be 25. This age distribution should be considered when assessing risk. For example, an unaffected 40-year-old son of a bipolar parent has already passed through most of the age at risk, and thus, his risk is substantially less than 25% to develop major mood disorder. An estimate of ~2% would be more accurate in this case.

The subject of genetic counseling is discussed in greater detail elsewhere (Nurnberger and Berrettini, 1998) Nurnberger and Beirut (2007; Smoller et al, 2008). It is anticipated that genotypic methods will be adapted for use in genetic counseling in the coming years. Such methods are not yet clinically applicable. Most experts feel that genotypic screening for persons with multifactorial disorders would still be premature; however some products are already on the market, and it seems likely that the predictive power of such methods will approach clinical utility within the next decade. As our understanding of the genetics of bipolar disorder evolves, it is likely that we will first be able to define specific subgroups within the larger bipolar population, then develop tests to make diagnoses and, ultimately, use the information from these genetic analyses to improve treatments. As we integrate genetic studies with neuroimaging, treatment trials and other research methods, our ability to impact the lives of our bipolar patients should substantially improve.

## ACKOWLEDGMENTS

Some sections of this chapter were modified from a chapter by Drs. Nurnberger, Wade Berrettini, and A. Niculescu in *The Medical Basis of Psychiatry*, H. Fatemi and P. Clayton, Saunders Publishers, 2008, and were used with permission.

## REFERENCES

1000 Genomes Project Consortium, 2010. A map of human genome variation from population-scale sequencing. *Nature*, 467:1061–1074.

Akiskal, H. S., & Pinto, O. 1999. The evolving bipolar spectrum. Prototypes I, II, III, and IV. *The Psychiatric Clinics of North America*, 22(3):517–534, vii.

Alexander, N., Osinsky, R., Schmitz, A., Mueller, E., Kuepper, Y., & Hennig J. 2010. The BDNF Val66Met polymorphism affects HPA-axis reactivity to acute stress. *Psychoneuroendocrinology*, i(6): 949–953.

Altshuler, D., Daly, M. J., & Lander, E. S. 2008. Genetic mapping in human disease. Science, 322 (5903): 881–889.

Altshuler, L. L., Curran, J. G., Hauser, P., Mintz, J., Denicoff, K., & Post, R. 1995. T2 hyperintensities in bipolar disorder: magnetic resonance imaging comparison and literature meta-analysis. *American Journal of Psychiatry*, 152(8):1139–1144.

Badner, J. A., & Gershon, E. S. 2002. Meta-analysis of whole-genome linkage scans of bipolar disorder and schizophrenia. *Molecular l Psychiatry*, 7(4):405–411.

Barden, N., Harvey, M., Gagné, B., Shink, E., Tremblay, M., Raymond, C., . . . Müller-Myhsok, B. 2006. Analysis of single nucleotide polymorphisms in genes in the chromosome 12Q24.31 region points to P2RX7 as a susceptibility gene to bipolar affective disorder. *Am J Med Genet B Neuropsychiatr Genet*, American Journal of Medical Genetics Part B (Neuropsychiatric Genetics) 141B(4): 374–382.

Bass, N. J., Datta, S. R., McQuillin, A., Puri, V., Choudhury, K., Thirumalai, S., . . . Gurling. H. M. 2009. Evidence for the association of the DAOA (G72) gene with schizophrenia and bipolar disorder but not for the association of the DAO gene with schizophrenia. *Behav Brain Funct*, 8(5): 28.

Barrett, T. B., Emberton, J. E., Nievergelt, C. M., Liang, S. G., Hauger, R. L., Eskin, E., . . . Kelsoe, J. R. 2007. Further evidence for association of GRK3 to bipolar disorder suggests a second disease mutation. *Psychiatric Genetics*, 17(6): 315–322.

Barrett, T. B., Hauger, R. L., Kennedy, J. L., Sadovnick, A. D., Remick, R. A., Keck, P. E., . . . Kelsoe, J. R. 2003. Evidence that a single nucleotide polymorphism in the promoter of the G protein receptor kinase 3 gene is associated with bipolar disorder. *Molecular Psychiatry*, 8(5): 546–557.

Berton, O., McClung, C. A., Dileone, R. J., Krishnan, V., Renthal, W., Russo, S. J., . . . Nestler, E. J. 2006. Essential role of BDNF in the mesolimbic dopamine pathway in social defeat stress. *Science*, 311(5762): 864–868.

Bertelsen, A. 1979. In *Origins, Prevention, and Treatment of Affective Disorders*, M. Schou and E. Stromgren eds., (pp 227–239). London: Academic Press.

Bertelsen, A., Harvald, B., & Hauge, B. 1977. A Danish twin study of major affective disorders. *British Journal of Psychiatry*, 130 (Apr): 330–351.

Bienvenu, O. J., Davydow, D. S., Kendler, K. S. 2011. Psychiatric "diseases" versus behavioral disorders and degree of genetic influence. *Psychological Medicine*, 41(1): 33–40.

Binder, E. B. 2009. The role of FKBP5, a co-chaperone of the glucocorticoid receptor in the pathogenesis and therapy of affective and anxiety disorders. *Psychoneuroendocrinology*, 34 (Suppl 1): S186–195.

Champagne, F. A. 2008. Epigenetic mechanisms and the transgenerational effects of maternal care. *Front Neuroendocrinol*, 29(3): 386–397.

Chen D, Liu F, Yang C, Liang X, Shang Q, He W, Wang Z. (2011) Association between the TPH1 A218C polymorphism and risk of mood disorders and alcohol dependence: Evidence from the current studies. *Journal 0f Affective Disorders*, May 19.

Chen, Y. S., Akula, N., Detera-Wadleigh, S. D., Schulze, T. G., Thomas, J., Potash, J. B., . . . McMahon, F. J. 2004. Findings in an independent sample support an association between bipolar affective disorder and the G72/G30 locus on chromosome 13q33. *Molecular Psychiatry*, 2004 Jan;9(1):87–92; image 5. Erratum in: *Molecular Psychiatry*, 9(8): 811.

Cho, H. J., Meira-Lima, I., Cordeiro, Q., Michelon, L., Sham, P., Vallada, H., & Collier, D.A. 2005. Population-based and family-based studies on the serotonin transporter gene polymorphisms and bipolar disorder: a systematic review and meta-analysis. *Molecular Psychiatry*, 10(8): 771–781.

Chumakov I, Blumenfeld M, Guerassimenko O, Cavarec L, Palicio M, Abderrahim H, et al. (2002) Genetic and physiological data implicating the new human gene G72 and the gene for D-amino acid oxidase in schizophrenia. *Proceedings of National Academy of Sciences U S A*. Oct 15;99(21):13675–13680. Epub 2002 Oct 3. Erratum in: *Proceedings of National Academy of Sciences U S A* 2002 Dec 24;99(26):17221.

Cichon, S., Mühleisen, T. W., Degenhardt, F. A., Mattheisen, M., Miró, X., Strohmaier, J., . . . Nöthen, M.M. 2011. Genome-wide association study identifies genetic variation in neurocan as a susceptibility factor for bipolar disorder. *American Journal of Human Genetics*, 88(3): 372–381.

Cichon, S., Winge, I., Mattheisen, M., Georgi, A., Karpushova, A., Freudenberg, J., . . . Nöthen, M.M. 2008. Brain-specific tryptophan hydroxylase 2 (TPH2): a functional Pro206Ser substitution and variation in the 5'-region are associated with bipolar affective disorder. *Human Molecular Genetics*, 17(1): 87–97.

Coryell, W., Endicott, J., Maser, J. D., Keller, M. B., Leon, A. C., & Akiskal, H. S. 1995. Long-term stability of polarity distinctions in the affective disorders. *American Journal of Psychiatry*, 152(3): 385–390.

Delgado, P. L., Price, L. H., Miller, H. L., Salomon, R. M., Licinio, J., Krystal, J. H., . . . Charney, D. S. 1991. Rapid serotonin depletion as a provocative challenge test for patients with major depression: relevance to antidepressant action and the neurobiology of depression. *Psychopharmacology Bulletin*, 27(3): 321–330.

Detera-Wadleigh, S. D., McMahon, F. J. 2006. G72/G30 in schizophrenia and bipolar disorder: review and meta-analysis. *Biological Psychiatry*, 60(2): 106–114.

Dick DM, Foroud T, Flury L, Bowman ES, Miller MJ, Rau NL . . .Nurnberger JI Jr. Genomewide linkage analyses of bipolar disorder: a new sample of 250 pedigrees from the National Institute of Mental Health Genetics Initiative. *American Journal of Human Genetics*. 2003 Jul;73(1):107–14. Epub 2003 May 27. Erratum in: American Journal of Human Genetics. 2003 Oct;73(4):979

Dougherty, L. R., Klein, D. N., Congdon, E., Canli, T., & Hayden, E. P. 2010. Interaction between 5-HTTLPR and BDNF Vall66Met polymorphisms on HPA axis reactivity in preschoolers. *Biological Psychology*, 83(2): 93–100

Duffy, A., Alda, M., Hajek, T., Sherry, S. B., & Grof, P. 2009. Early stages in the development of bipolar disorder. *Journal of Affective Disorders*, 121(1–2): 127–135.

El-Mallakh, R. S., & Huff, M. O. 2001. Mood stabilizers and ion regulation. *Harvard Review of Psychiatry*, 9(1): 23–32.

Fan, J., & Sklar, P. 2008. Genetics of bipolar disorder: focus on BDNF Val66Met polymorphism. *Novartis Foundation Symposium*, 289: 60–72; discussion 72–3, 87–93.

Fan, M., Liu, B., Jiang, T., Jiang, X., Zhao, H., & Zhang, J. 2010. Meta-analysis of the association between the monoamine oxidase-A gene and mood disorders. *Psychiatric Genetics*, 20(1): 1–7.

Faraone, S. V., Biederman, J., Mennin, D., Wozniak, J., & Spencer, T. 1997. Attention-deficit hyperactivity disorder with bipolar disorder: a familial subtype? *Journal of the American Academy of Child and Adolescent Psychiatry*, 36(10): 1378–1387.

Faraone, S. V., Glatt, S. J., Su, J., & Tsuang, M. T. 2004. Three potential susceptibility loci shown by a genome-wide scan for regions influencing the age at onset of mania. *American Journal of Psychiatry*, 161(4): 625–630.

Faraone, S. V., & Wilens, T. 2003. Does stimulant treatment lead to substance use disorders? *Journal of Clinical Psychiatry*, 64, (Suppl 11): 9–13.

Ferreira, M. A., O'Donovan, M. C., Meng, Y. A., Jones, I. R., Ruderfer, D. M., Jones, L., . . . Welcome Trust Case Control Consortium. 2008. Collaborative genome-wide association analysis supports a role for ANK3 and CACNA1C in bipolar disorder. *Nature Genetics*, 40(9): 1056–1058.

GAIN Collaborative Research Group, Collaborative Association Study of Psoriasis, International Multi-Center ADHD Genetics Project, Molecular Genetics of Schizophrenia Collaboration, Bipolar Genome Study, Major Depression Stage 1 Genomewide Association in Population-Based Samples Study, Genetics of Kidneys in Diabetes (GoKinD) Study. 2007. New models of collaboration in genome-wide association studies: the Genetic Association Information Network. *Nature Genetics*, 39(9): 1045–1051.

Gershon, E. S., DeLisi, L. E., & Hamovit, J., Nurnberger JI Jr, Maxwell ME, Schreiber J . . .Guroff JJ. 1988. A controlled family study of chronic psychoses. Schizophrenia and schizoaffective disorder. *Archives of General Psychiatry*, 45(4): 328–336.

Gershon, E. S., & Goldin, L. R. 1986. Clinical methods in psychiatric genetics. I. Robustness of genetic marker investigative strategies. *Acta Psychiatrica Scandinavica*, 74(2): 113–118.

Gershon, E. S., Hamovit, J., & Guroff, J. J., Dibble E, Leckman JF, Sceery W . . .Bunney WE Jr. 1982. A family study of schizoaffective, Bipolar I, Bipolar II, unipolar, and normal control probands. *Archives of General Psychiatry*, 39(10): 1157–1167.

Gershon, E. S., Martinez, M., Goldin, L., Gelernter, J., & Silver, J. 1989. Detection of marker associations with a dominant disease gene in genetically complex and heterogeneous diseases. *American Journal of Human Genetics*, 45(4): 578–585.

Goodyer, I. M., Croudace, T., Dudbridge, F., Ban, M., & Herbert, J. 2010. Polymorphisms in BDNF(Val66Met) and 5-HTTLPR, morning cortisol and subsequent depression in at-risk adolescents. *British Journal of Psychiatry*, 197: 365–371.

Green, E. K., Grozeva, D., Raybould, R., Elvidge, G., Macgregor, S., Craig, I., . . . Craddock, N. 2009. P2RX7: A bipolar and unipolar disorder candidate susceptibility gene? *American Journal of Medical GeneticsPart B: Neuropsychiatric Genetics*, 150B(8): 1063–1069.

Grozeva, D., Kirov, G., Ivanov, D., Jones, I. R., Jones, L., Green, E. K., . . . Wellcome Trust Case Control Consortium. 2010. Rare copy number variants: a point of rarity in genetic risk for bipolar disorder and schizophrenia. *Archives of General Psychiatry*, 67(4): 318–327.

Hallahan, B., Newell, J., Soares, J. C., Brambilla, P., Strakowski, S. M., Fleck, D. E., . . . McDonald, C. 2011. Structural magnetic resonance imaging in bipolar disorder: an international collaborative mega-analysis of individual adult patient data. *Biological Psychiatry*, 69(4): 326–335.

Hariri, A. R., Goldberg, T. E., Mattay, V. S., Kolachana, B. S., Callicott, J. H., Egan, M. F., & Weinberger, D. R. 2003. Brain-derived neurotrophic factor val66met polymorphism affects human memory-related hippocampal activity and predicts memory performance. *Journal of Neuroscience*, 23(17): 6690–6694.

Harvey, M., Gagné, B., Labbé, M., & Barden, N. 2007, Polymorphisms in the neuronal isoform of tryptophan hydroxylase 2 are associated with bipolar disorder in French Canadian pedigrees. *Psychiatr Genet*, 17(1): 17–22.

Hasler, G., Drevets, W. C., Gould, T. D., Gottesman, I. I., & Manji, H. K. 2006, Toward constructing an endophenotype strategy for bipolar disorders. *Biological Psychiatry*, 60(2): 93–105.

Hattori, E., Liu, C., Badner, J. A., Bonner TI, Christian SL, Maheshwari M . . .Gershon ES. 2003. Polymorphisms at the G72/G30 gene locus, on 13q33, are associated with bipolar disorder in two independent pedigree series. *American Journal of Human Genetics*, 72(5): 1131–1140.

Hayden, E. P., & Nurnberger, J. I., Jr. 2006. Molecular genetics of bipolar disorder. *Genes, Brain, and Behavior*, 5(1): 85–95.

Heun, R., & Maier, W. 1993. The distinction of Bipolar II disorder from Bipolar I and recurrent unipolar depression: results of a controlled family study. *Acta Psychiatrica Scandinavica*, 87(4): 279–284.

International Schizophrenia Consortium, Purcell, S. M., Wray, N. R., Stone, J. L., Visscher, P. M., O'Donovan, M. C., Sullivan, P. F., & Sklar, P. 2009. Common polygenic variation contributes to risk of schizophrenia and bipolar disorder. *Nature*, 460(7256): 748–752.

Kvajo, M., Dhilla, A., Swor, D. E., Karayiorgou, M., & Gogos, J. A. 2008. Evidence implicating the candidate schizophrenia/bipolar disorder susceptibility gene G72 in mitochondrial function. *Molecular Psychiatry*, 13(7): 685–696.

Lachman, H. M., Pedrosa, E., Petruolo, O. A., Cockerham, M., Papolos, A., Novak, T., . . . Stopkova, P. 2007. Increase in GSK3beta gene copy number variation in bipolar disorder. *Am J Med Genet B Neuropsychiatr Genet*, 144B(3): 259–265

Lander, E., & Kruglyak, L. 1995. Genetic dissection of complex traits: guidelines for interpreting and reporting linkage results. *Nature Genetics*, 11(3): 241–247.

Lango Allen, H., Estrada, K., Lettre, G., Berndt, S. I., Weedon, M. N., Rivadeneira, F., . . . Hirschhorn, J. N. 2010. Hundreds of variants clustered in genomic loci and biological pathways affect human height. *Nature*, 467(7317): 832–838.

Le-Niculescu, H., Patel, S. D., Bhat, M., Kuczenski, R., Faraone, S. V., Tsuang, M. T., . . . Niculescu, III A. B. 2009. Convergent functional genomics of genome- wide association data for bipolar disorder: Comprehensive identification of candidate genes, pathways and mechanisms. *American Journal of Medical Genetics Part B*, 150B(2): 155–181.

Lewy AJ, Nurnberger JI Jr, Wehr TA, Pack D, Becker LE, Powell RL, Newsome DA. Supersensitivity to light: possible trait marker for manic-depressive illness. *American Journal of Psychiatry*. 1985 Jun;142(6):725–7.

Liu, L., Foroud, T., Xuei, X., Berrettini, W., Byerley, W., Coryell, W., . . . Nurnberger, Jr. J. I. 2008. Evidence of association between brain-derived neurotrophic factor (BDNF) gene and bipolar disorder. *Psychiatric Genetics*, 18(6): 267–274.

Lopez, V. A., Detera-Wadleigh, S., Cardona, I., National Institute of Mental Health Genetics Initiative Bipolar Disorder Consortium, Kassem, L., & McMahon, F. J. 2007. Nested association between genetic variation in tryptophan hydroxylase II, bipolar affective disorder, and suicide attempts. *Biological Psychiatry*, 61(2): 181–186.

Lucae, S., Salyakina, D., Barden, N., Harvey, M., Gagné, B., Labbé, M., . . . Müller-Myhsok, B. 2006. P2RX7, a gene coding for a purinergic ligand-gated ion channel, is associated with major depressive disorder. *Human Molecular Genetics*, 15(16): 2438–2445.

MacKinnon, D. F., Zandi, P. P., Gershon, E., Nurnberger, J. I., Jr., Reich, T., & DePaulo, J. R. 2003. Rapid switching of mood in families with multiple cases of bipolar disorder. *Archives of General Psychiatry*, 60(9): 921–928.

McCarthy, S. E., Makarov, V., Kirov, G., Addington, A. M., McClellan, J., Yoon, S., . . . Sebat, J. 2009. Microduplications of 16p11.2 are associated with schizophrenia. *Nature Genetics*, 41(11): 1223–1227.

McQueen, M. B., Devlin, B., Faraone, S. V., Nimgaonkar, V. L., Sklar, P., Smoller, J. W., . . . Laird, N. M. 2005. Combined analysis from eleven studies of bipolar disorder provides strong evidence of susceptibility loci on chromosomes 6q and 8q. *American Journal of Human Genetics*, 77(4): 582–595.

Millar, J. K., Pickard, B. S., Mackie, S., James, R., Christie, S., Buchanan, S. R., . . . Porteous, D. J. 2005. DISC1 and PDE4B are interacting genetic factors in schizophrenia that regulate cAMP signaling. *Science*, 310(5751): 1187–1191.

Morrow, E. M. 2010. Genomic copy number variation in disorders of cognitive development. *J Am Acad Child Adolesc Psychiatry*, 49(11): 1091–1104.

Müller, D. J., Zai, C. C., Shinkai. T., Strauss, J., & Kennedy, J. L. 2011. Association between the DAOA/G72 gene and bipolar disorder and meta-analyses in bipolar disorder and schizophrenia. *Bipolar Disorders*, 13(2): 198–207.

Neves-Pereira, M., Mundo, E., Muglia, P., King, N., Macciardi, F., & Kennedy, J. L. 2002. The brain -derived neurotrophic factor gene confers susceptibility to bipolar disorder: evidence from a family-based association study. *American Journal Human Genetics*, 71(3): 651–655.

Ng, P. C., Levy, S., Huang, J., Stockwell, T. B., Walenz, B. P., Li, K., . . . Venter, J. C. 2008. Genetic variation in an individual human exome. *PLoS Genetics*, 4(8):

Nurnberger, J. I., & Bierut, L. J. 2007. Seeking the connections: alcoholism and our genes. *Scientific American*, 296(4): 46–53.

Nurnberger, Jr. J. I., Guroff, J. J., Hamovit, J., Berrettini, W., & Gershon, E. S. 1998. A family study of rapid–cycling bipolar illness. *Journal of Affective Disorders*, 15(1): 87–91.

Nurnberger, J. I., Hamovit, J., Hibbs, E., Pellegrini, D., Guroff, J., Maxwell, M. E., . . . Gershon, E. S. 1988. A high risk study of primary affective disorder: I. Selection of subjects, initial assessment, and 12 year follow-up. In D. L. Dunner, E. G., J. E. Barrett, ed. *Relatives at Risk for Mental Disorder,* (pp. 161–177). New York: Raven Press.

Nurnberger, J. I. Jr., & Berrettini, W. 2000. Psychiatric genetics. In Ebert, M., Loosen, P. T., & Nurcombe, B, eds. *Current Diagnosis & Treatment in Psychiatry,* (pp. 61–79). New York: Lange Medical Books/McGraw Hill.

Nurnberger, J. I., Jr., & Berrettini, W. H. 1998. *Psychiatric Genetics*. London: Chapman & Hall.

Nurnberger, J. I., Kuperman, S., Flury-Wetherill, L., Meyer ET, Lawson WB, and MacKinnon DF. 2007. Genetics of comorbid mood disorder and alcohol dependence. *Journal of Dual Diagnosis*, 3(2): 31–46.

Nurnberger, Jr. J. I. 2008. A simulated genetic structure for bipolar illness. *Am J Med Genet B Neuropsychiatric Genetics*, 147B(6): 952–956.

Nurnberger, J. I. Jr., McInnis, M., Reich, W., Kastelic, E., Wilcox, H. C., Glowinski, A., . . . Monahan, P. O. 2011. A high-risk study of bipolar disorder: Childhood clinical phenotypes as precursors of major mood disorders. *Archives of General Psychiatry*, 68(10): 1012–20.

Nurnberger, Jr. J. I., Roose, S. P., Dunner, D. L., & Fieve, R. R. 1979. Unipolar mania: A distinct clinical entity? *American Journal of Psychiatry*, 136(11): 1420–1423.

Ogden, C. A., Rich, M. E., Schork, N. J., Paulus MP, Geyer MA, Lohr JB . . . Niculescu AB.l. 2004. Candidate genes, pathways and mechanisms for bipolar (manic-depressive) and related disorders: an expanded convergent functional genomics approach. *Molecular Psychiatry*, 9(11): 1007–1029.

Perlis RH, Smoller JW, Ferreira MA, McQuillin A, Bass N, Lawrence J, Sachs GS, Nimgaonkar V, Scolnick EM, Gurling H, Sklar P, Purcell S. 2009**.** A genomewide association study of response to lithium for prevention of recurrence in bipolar disorder. *American Journal of Psychiatry*. Jun;166(6):718–25.

Petryshen, T. L., Sabeti, P. C., Aldinger, K. A., Fry, B., Fan, J. B., Schaffner, S. F., . . . Sklar, P. 2010. Population genetic study of the brain-derived neurotrophic factor (BDNF) gene. *Molecular Psychiatry*, 15(8): 810–815.

Pinto, D., Pagnamenta, A. T., Klei, L., Anney, R., Merico, D., Regan, R., . . . Betancur, C. 2010. Functional impact of global rare copy number variation in autism spectrum disorder. *Nature*, 466(7304): 368–372.

Preisig M, Bellivier F, Fenton BT, Baud P, Berney A, Courtet P, Hardy P, Golaz J, Leboyer M, Mallet J, Matthey ML, Mouthon D, Neidhart E, Nosten-Bertrand M, Stadelmann-Dubuis E, Guimon J, Ferrero F, Buresi C, Malafosse A. Association between bipolar disorder and monoamine oxidase A gene polymorphisms: results of a multicenter study. *American Journal of Psychiatry*. 2000 Jun;157(6):948–55.

Priebe, L., Degenhardt, F. A., Herms, S., Haenisch, B., Mattheisen, M., Nieratschker, V., . . . Mühleisen, T. W. 2011. Genome-wide survey implicates the influence of copy number variants (CNVs) in the development of early-onset bipolar disorder. *Molecular Psychiatry*.

Psychiatric GWAS Consortium Bipolar Disorder Working Group. Combined analysis of 11 genomewide association studies of bipolar disorder identifies strong evidence for multiple susceptibility loci. *Nature Genetics*. 2011 Sep 18; 43(10), 977–983.

Ripke S, Sanders AR, Kendler KS, Levinson DF, Sklar P, Holmans PA, et al. 2011. Genome-wide association study identifies five new schizophrenia loci. *Nature Genetics*. Sep 18;43(10):969–977.

Roche, S., & McKeon, P. 2009. Support for tryptophan hydroxylase-2 as a susceptibility gene for bipolar affective disorder. *Psychiatric Genetics*, 19(3): 142–146.

Ross, J., Berrettini, W., Coryell, W., Gershon, E. S., Badner, J. A., Kelsoe, J. R., . . . Byerley, W. 2008. Genome-wide parametric linkage analyses of 644 bipolar pedigrees suggest susceptibility loci at chromosomes 16 and 20. *Psychiatric Genetics*, 18(4): 191–198.

Saunders, E. H., Scott, L. J., McInnis, M. G., & Burmeister, M. 2008. Familiality and diagnostic patterns of subphenotypes in the National Institutes of Mental Health bipolar sample. *Am J Med Genet B Neuropsychiatric Genetics*, 147B(1): 18–26

Schulze, T. G., Detera-Wadleigh, S. D., Akula, N., Gupta, A., Kassem, L., Steele, J., . . . McMahon, F. J. 2009. Two variants in *Ankyrin 3 (ANK3)* are independent genetic risk factors for bipolar disorder. *Molecular Psychiatry*, 14(5):487–91.

Shalev, I., Lerer, E., Israel, S., Uzefovsky, F., Gritsenko, I., Mankuta, D., . . . Kaitz, M. 2009. BDNF Val66Met polymorphism is associated with HPA axis reactivity to psychological stress characterized by genotype and gender interactions. *Psychoneuroendocrinology*, 34(3): 382–388.

Shi, J., Badner, J. A., Gershon, E. S., & Liu, C. 2008. Allelic association of G72/G30 with schizophrenia and bipolar disorder: a comprehensive meta-analysis. *Schizophrenia Research*, (1–3): 89–97.

Sitaram N, Nurnberger JI Jr, Gershon ES, Gillin JC. (1980) Faster cholinergic REM sleep induction in euthymic patients with primary affective illness. *Science*. 208(4440):200–2.

Sklar, P., Gabriel, S. B., McInnis, M. G., Bennett, P., Lim, Y. M., Tsan, G., . . . Lander, E. S. 2002. Family-based association study of 76 candidate genes in bipolar disorder: BDNF is a potential risk locus. Brain-derived neutrophic factor. *Molecular Psychiatry*, 7(6): 579–593.

Smith, E. N., Bloss, C. S., Badner, J. A., Barrett, T., Belmonte, P. L., Berrettini, W., . . . Kelsoe, J. R. 2009. Genome-wide association study of Bipolar Disorder in European American and African American individuals. *Molecular Psychiatry*, 14(8): 755–763.

Smoller JW, Sheidley BR, and Tsuang MT. (2008) Psychiatric Genetics: Applications in clinical practice. Washington DC: American Psychiatric Publishing.

Thomson, P. A., Wray, N. R., Millar, J. K., Evans, K. L., Hellard, S. L., Condie, A., . . . Porteous, D. J. 2005. Association between the TRAX/DISC locus and both bipolar disorder and schizophrenia in the Scottish population. *Molecular Psychiatrics*, 10(7): 657–668.

Strakowski SM, Adler CM, Holland SK, Mills NP, DelBello MP, Eliassen JC. Abnormal FMRI brain activation in euthymic bipolar disorder patients during a counting Stroop interference task. *American Journal of Psychiatry*. 2005 Sep;162(9):1697–705.

Torkamani, A., Topol, E. J., & Schork, N. J. 2008. Pathway analysis of seven common diseases assessed by genome-wide association. *Genomics*, 92(5): 265–272.

Tsuang, M. T., & Faraone, S. V. 1990. *The Genetics of Mood Disorders*. Baltimore: Johns Hopkins University Press.

Turecki, G., Grof, P., Grof, E., D'Souza, V., Lebuis, L., Marineau, C., . . . Alda, M. 2001. Mapping susceptibility genes for bipolar disorder: a pharmacognetic approach based on excellent response to lithium. *Molecular Psychiatry*, 6(5): 570–578.

Verhagen, M., van der Meij, A., van Deurzen, P. A., Janzing, J. G., Arias-Vasquez, A., Buitelaar, J. K., & Franke, B. 2010. Meta-analysis of the BDNF Val66Met polymorphism in major depressive disorder: effects of gender and ethnicity. *Mol Psychiatry*, 15(3): 260–271.

Vinberg, M., Trajkovska, V., Bennike, B., Knorr, U., Knudsen, G. M., & Kessing, L. V. 2009. The BDNF Vall66Met polymorphism: relation to familiar risk of affective disorder, BDNF levels and salivary cortisol. *Psychoneuroendocrinology*, 34(9): 1380–1389

Walsh, T., McClellan, J. M., McCarthy, S. E., Addington, A. M., Pierce, S. B., Cooper, G. M., . . . Sebat, J. 2008. Rare structural variants disrupt multiple genes in neurodevelopmental pathways in schizophrenia. *Science*, 320(5875): 539–543.

Wehr, T. A., & Sack, D. A, 1987. Rosenthal NE.Sleep reduction as a final common pathway in the genesis of mania. *American Journal of Psychiatry*, 144(2): 201–204.

Wender, P. H., Kety, S. S., Rosenthal, D., Schulsinger, F., Ortmann, J., & Lunde, I. (1986). Psychiatric disorders in the biological and adoptive families of adopted individuals with affective disorders. *Arch Gen Psychiatry*, 43(10): 923–929.

Williams, N. M., Green, E. K., Macgregor, S.,Dwyer S, Norton N, Williams H ...Craddock N. (2006). Variation at the DAOA/G30 locus influences susceptibility to major mood episodes but not psychosis in schizophrenia and bipolar disorder. *Archives of General Psychiatry*, 63(4): 366–373.

Willour, V. L., Chen, H., Toolan, J., Belmonte, P., Cutler, D. J., Goes, F. S., . . . Potash, J. B. (2009). Family-based association of FKBP5 in bipolar disorder. *Molecular Psychiatry*, 14(3): 261–268.

Zhang, D., Cheng, L., Qian, Y., Alliey-Rodriguez, N., Kelsoe, J. R., Greenwood, T., . . . Gershon, E. S. (2009). Singleton deletions throughout the genome increase risk of bipolar disorder. *Molecular Psychiatry*, 14(4): 376–380.

# 10.

## GENETICS OF BIPOLAR DISORDER AND SCHIZOPHRENIA

Michael E. Talkowski, Kodavali V. Chowdari, Hader Mansour, Konasale M. Prasad, Joel Wood, and Vishwajit L. Nimgaonkar

## INTRODUCTION

There has been vigorous debate about the etiological and psychopathological relationship between schizophrenia and bipolar I disorder throughout the modern psychiatric era (Crow, 1990). The arguments for and against a continuum between schizophrenia and bipolar I disorder (with schizoaffective disorder as an intermediate phenotype) have not been resolved, perhaps reflecting the complexity of the problem (Brockington & Leff, 1979; Gershon et al., 1988; Kendler & Diehl, 1993; Valles et al., 2000). The question is not merely of academic interest. It impacts the nosological status of these disorders, and its resolution may have a larger impact on diagnosis and even treatment.

In this chapter, we review data and hypotheses related to the concept that there are shared genetic etiological factors for bipolar disorder and schizophrenia. We first provide a historical overview of the bipolar disorder/schizophrenia classification system. Next, we review empirical data concerning genetic sharing between disorders. We then provide perspectives from family-based studies, as well as gene-mapping studies. Finally, we end by synthesizing these data and proposing directions for future research.

## HISTORICAL OVERVIEW

The early Greeks observed that manic and melancholic states were related (Marneros & Angst, 2000). Almost seventeen centuries later, Falret and Baillarger rediscovered these concepts based on their observations in French mental asylums (Akiskal, 2002). Furthermore, a cyclical illness with a short recovery and a very poor outcome was also described, foreshadowing today's concept of rapid cycling and ultra-rapid cycling bipolar disorder. A firm distinction between affective and non-affective psychotic disorders based on empirical observations did not really develop until

Kraepelin's work, circa 1900 (Kraepelin, 1919). At that time, several disease entities were being carved out of global concepts such as insanity, dementia and delirium, heavily influenced by the postulates put forth by Robert Koch (Koch, 1882). Kraepelin's careful and astute clinical observations of chronically institutionalized patients lead to the concept of a pattern of illnesses based on the disease onset, natural history and outcome. Such clinical observations were necessary because there was no apparent cause or pathogenic model to anchor the classification of diseases. From these early efforts, two major patterns emerged: dementia praecox, an early-onset condition characterized by steadily deteriorating personality and psychological functions, and manic depressive illness, a cyclical illness of recurrent affective states with relatively good recovery between episodes. These disorders were later rechristened as schizophrenia and bipolar disorder, respectively. The refinement of these concepts awaited further progress in etiological and pathophysiological research during the nineteenth and the early part of the twentieth centuries. Though impressive advances have been made in both arenas, clear and comprehensive explanations for the symptoms of schizophrenia and bipolar disorder are still unavailable. Moreover, in the absence of etiological causes, the considerable overlap in cross-sectional symptomatology of these two conditions makes it difficult to identify a specific distinguishing characteristic; hence, the evolution of spectrum hypotheses that attempt to unify these disorders in an overarching etiological model. With this brief historical framework in mind, we will use Robins and Guze's formulation of classification based on familial aggregation as an anchor in the schizophrenia/bipolar disorder debate (Robins & Guze, 1970). This formulation is based on the earlier notion that a biologically based diagnostic entity should breed true within families if it is to be used as a yardstick for classification (Robins & Guze, 1970).

Bipolar disorder and schizophrenia share several features in terms of familial aggregation. Relatives of both sets of patients have elevated risk for these disorders. In both conditions, the sibling recurrence risk ratio, defined as the risk to sibling of a patient divided by the population prevalence is 8–10 (Risch, 1990). Additionally, twin and family studies have established relatively high heritability estimates for both disorders, in excess of 60% (Gottesman, 1991; Tsuang & Faraone, 2000). Segregation analyses have repeatedly favored a multi-factorial polygenic inheritance model (Gottesman, 1991; Tsuang & Faraone, 2000). This model posits a combined effect of several genetic factors acting against variable environmental backgrounds; individuals are affected when a hypothetical threshold of liability is exceeded. Family-based studies can also help inform genetic etiologic overlap for bipolar disorder and schizophrenia. If genetic factors underlying these disorders are non-overlapping, they would be expected to "breed true." Indeed, classical studies that ascertained family based samples using bipolar I disorder or schizophrenia probands suggested that the morbid risk for bipolar disorder was increased among relatives of bipolar disorder cases. For example, it was reported in a US bipolar disorder sample that the morbid risks were 6% for siblings and 4.1%–6.4% among parents (Rice et al., 1987). Likewise, the average risks for schizophrenia are estimated at 9% among siblings and 6% among parents of probands with schizophrenia (Weissman et al., 1984; Gottesman, 1991; Ivleva et al., 2008). However, a recent study that evaluated a much larger unselected national sample reported contrasting findings (Lichtenstein et al., 2009). By cross-linking national Swedish registers for hospital discharges with a multi-generation register, data on over nine million individuals from two million families were analyzed over a 31-year period. In contrast to earlier studies, it was found that first-degree relatives of schizophrenia probands had elevated risk for schizophrenia *or* bipolar disorder. Likewise, when relatives of bipolar disorder patients were evaluated, elevated risk for schizophrenia was observed for all degrees of family relationships. Further multivariate analyses of the data suggested that shared genetic factors common to both disorders appeared to explain the co-morbidity between these disorders. Indeed, the authors suggested that 63% of the co-morbidity could be attributed to additive genetic effects common to both disorders, suggesting a model of shared genetic factors between these distinct disorders.

Whether there is shared genetic etiologic overlap between bipolar and schizophrenic disorders could also be addressed by examining offspring of marriages between parents concordant or discordant for bipolar disorder or schizophrenia. A recent Danish national registry-based study suggested that unions between parents concordant for schizophrenia or bipolar disorder lead to elevated risk for schizophrenia or bipolar disorder in the offspring, respectively, but not for the other disorder (Gottesman et al., 2010). Notably, among offspring born to parents concordant for bipolar disorder, there was an elevated risk for schizophrenia, albeit lower than in offspring of dual schizophrenia marriages.

A final line of investigation involves studies of schizoaffective disorder, which has clinical features that overlap with both bipolar disorder and schizophrenia. There has been, and continues to be, considerable variation within the diagnostic criteria for schizophrenia and schizoaffective disorder, leading to variable results from family-based studies. A recent Danish case-registry based analysis suggested that schizoaffective disorder may be genetically linked to both schizophrenia and bipolar disorder (Laursen et al., 2005). The risk for schizoaffective disorder in this study was elevated if a person's first-degree relative had any history of a mental illness. The risks for schizoaffective disorder were similar if the first-degree relative had a history of schizophrenia, bipolar disorder, or schizoaffective disorder (relative risks: 2.57, 3.23, or 1.92 respectively). In other words, risk factors for schizoaffective disorder could be shared with bipolar disorder or schizophrenia. In contrast to the Lichtenstein study, it was reported that bipolar disorder in a relative was by far the strongest risk for bipolar disorder in the proband, and schizophrenia was the largest risk factor for schizophrenia patients. The status of schizoaffective disorder at an intermediate position between schizophrenia and bipolar disorder is also supported by recent twin studies. Older twin studies focused on index twins with schizophrenia or bipolar disorder and suggested that these

> **Findings from Family Based Studies of Schizophrenia and Bipolar Disorder**
>
> - Disorders were initially thought to "breed true"
>
> - However, a recent large Swedish national study suggests significant overlap in risk for schizophrenia and bipolar disorder
>
> - Schizoaffective disorder may share genetic risk factors with either condition
>
> - The question of shared genetic etiological factors for schizophrenia and bipolar disorder remains unresolved

disorders "bred true." In contrast, recent analyses based on syndromal classifications suggest shared genetic risk factors for schizophrenia, schizoaffective and manic syndromes (Cardno et al., 2002).

In summary, older studies conceptualized on the basis of schizophrenia/bipolar disorder dichotomy generally suggested that familial risks for these disorders are distinct. A recent large scale study from Sweden, as well as some studies of schizoaffective disorder contradict these results and suggest significant sharing of genetic risk factors.

## OVERLAP BETWEEN BIPOLAR DISORDER AND SCHIZOPHRENIA: GENE MAPPING STUDIES

Rapid advances in molecular genetics during the 1980s provided renewed hopes that specific genetic etiological factors for bipolar 1 disorder and schizophrenia would be found. It was believed that such searches would enable a better understanding of heterogeneity within and across the disorder, enabling biological dissection.

## LINKAGE ANALYSIS

Linkage studies seek shared chromosomal segments that are consistently inherited among affected family members in an effort to find genomic regions harboring causative mutations. Despite extensive efforts, there has been considerable difficulty identifying consistently replicated regions of linkage for bipolar 1 disorder or schizophrenia (Moldin, 1997). When meta-analyses were completed, evidence for linkage emerged at chromosome segments 2q, 5q, 3p, 11q, 6p, 1q, 22q, 8p, 20q and 14p for schizophrenia and at 9p,

10q and 14q for bipolar 1 disorder, but the highest-ranked linked regions do not overlap (Lewis et al., 2003; Segurado et al., 2003).

## ASSOCIATION STUDIES

In contrast to linkage studies, genetic association studies typically identify relatively small genomic regions that confer risk. Therefore, association studies are arguably better tools than traditional linkage studies to examine whether individual risk loci are shared between bipolar 1 disorder and schizophrenia.

*Candidate Gene Association Studies* Historically, association studies focused on relatively discrete candidate genes or regions, and these studies then generally evaluated a small proportion of the total genetic variation within a gene, usually by genotyping single nucleotide polymorphisms (SNPs). A SNP is a genetic variation in a DNA sequence that occurs when a single nucleotide in a genome is altered. Very few, if any, early candidate gene studies yielded statistically significant associations that were replicated in multiple independent samples. The recent association studies using larger panels of SNPs have increased in sophistication and size, leading to somewhat more consistent results. These studies suggested several possible shared risk loci, including dysbindin (*DTNBP1*), brain derived neurotrophic factor (*BDNF*), catechol-o-methyltransferase (*COMT*), disrupted in schizophrenia 1 (*DISC1*), the dopamine transporter (*SLC6A3*), neuregulin-1 (*NRG1*), and the MAM domain containing glycosylphosphatidylinositol (*MDGA1*) (Li et al., 2011; Craddock et al., 2005; Mick et al., 2008; Talkowski et al., 2010). For many of these genes, the risk conferred for either bipolar disorder or schizophrenia is modest (odds ratios, OR ⊠1.2), the alleles contributing to the association signals are uncertain, and the data need to be confirmed in additional replicate studies (Shirts & Nimgaonkar, 2004; Gill et al., 2010).

---

**Observations from Linkage Studies of Schizophrenia and Bipolar Disorder**

- Schizophrenia linkages were found at chromosome regions 2q, 5q, 3p, 11q, 6p, 1q, 22q, 8p, 20q and 14p

- Bipolar linkages were found at chromosome regions 9p, 10q and 14

- Traditional linkage studies suggest little overlap for schizophrenia and bipolar 1 disorder

- There has been limited consensus among linkage studies in either disorder

- Linkage studies paved the way for larger genome-wide association studies

---

**Findings from Candidate Gene Association Studies of Schizophrenia and Bipolar Disorder**

- There may be shared loci for schizophrenia and bipolar 1 disorder: DTNBP1, BDNF, COMT, DISC1, SLC6A3, NRG1, MDGA1

- Effect sizes have been small for individual variations

- A very limited proportion of the overall genetic variance has been explained by these studies

---

Recently, candidate gene studies have been supplanted by GWAS that included representative, relatively frequent SNPs. These studies are designed to agnostically evaluate associations at a significant proportion of the common genetic variants in the human genome simultaneously, unbiased by prior biological hypotheses, and rigorously corrected for population substructure and statistical significance at a genome-wide level. Several GWAS have yielded promising sets of risk variants that remain statistically significant despite correcting for all genome-wide hypotheses tested. They include alleles of calcium channel voltage-dependent L type alpha 1C subunit (*CACNA1C*), transcription factor 4 (*TCF4*), neurogranin (*NRGN*), and polybromo-1 (*PBRM1*) for bipolar 1 disorder (Green et al., 2010; Stefansson et al., 2009; McMahon et al., 2010). Risk variants for schizophrenia include SNPs at the locus encoding zinc finger binding protein 804A (*ZNF804A*) (Williams et al., 2010) and an extended region covering the major histocompatability (MHC) locus on chromosome 6 (Purcell et al., 2009; Stefansson et al., 2009; Shi et al., 2009). The GWAS for bipolar 1 disorder and schizophrenia utilized different sets of cases and controls, so it is necessary to combine the datasets thoughtfully and synthesize the results in order to address the question of genetic overlap. Several such studies are in progress, and their rationale is further discussed by Cichon et al. (2009). One such combined analysis suggests that the same variants at *ZNF804* may confer risk for both bipolar 1 disorder and schizophrenia (Williams et al., 2010). Gene-based analyses have suggested other chromosomal regions that may be involved in the expression of both schizophrenia and bipolar disorder (Moskvina et al., 2009). Another combined dataset analysis suggested associations for both disorders at rs11789399 (chromosome 9q33.1), as well as additional SNPs (Wang et al., 2010). In a novel approach, Francks and colleagues adapted GWAS datasets for linkage analyses and suggested shared risk factors at chromosome segment 19q13 (Francks et al., 2010).

Despite these encouraging results, some caveats are noteworthy. The effect sizes for the GWAS based associations are modest. In addition, recent simulations of GWAS data suggest that literally dozens, or even hundreds, of common risk polymorphisms with similar effect sizes may be present, supporting the long hypothesized model of complex polygenic inheritance for these disorders (Purcell et al., 2009; Gottesman & Shields, 1967).

GWAS data can also help identify relatively large, submicroscopic chromosomal aberrations, or copy number variations (CNVs) (Sebat et al., 2009; Cook & Scherer, 2008). A CNV is conventionally defined as a segment of DNA (1kb or larger in size) that is present at a variable number of copies compared to a reference genome. Several case-control studies have suggested substantial risk for schizophrenia from CNVs within chromosomal regions 22q12, 1q21.1, 15q11.2, 15q13.3 and 16p11.2 (Walsh et al., 2008; Xu et al., 2008; Consortium, 2008; Stefansson et al., 2009). In contrast to the common SNPs, effect sizes for associations are substantial, with odds ratios in the 8–13 range. Some of these CNVs may also confer risk for other disorders such as autism (McCarthy et al., 2009; Sebat et al., 2007; Cusco et al., 2009; Szatmari et al., 2007). Systematic studies of CNVs and bipolar disorder have been completed (Zollner et al., 2009; Alaerts & Del-Favero, 2009; Yang et al., 2009). Despite early leads, analyses of large bipolar disorder samples have not revealed associations of the same magnitude observed in schizophrenia, suggesting that CNVs conferring risk may not be shared between bipolar disorder and schizophrenia (Grozeva et al., 2010; Zhang et al., 2009; Lachman et al., 2007).

---

**Results form GWAS Studies of Schizophrenia and Bipolar Disorder**

- Rapid technological advances and conservative statistical evaluations have yielded significant results from GWAS

- For bipolar disorder findings include: CACNA1C, TCF4, NRGN, PBRM1

- For schizophrenia, findings include: ZNF804A and an extended region covering the major histocompatability gene locus on chromosome 6

- Similar variants at ZNF804 and within chromosome segment 19q13 may impart increased risk for both conditions

- Individual effect sizes for common variants remain modest

- Simulations using GWAS data sets continue to suggest a polygenic model including many risk variants of small effect for both disorders

## ASSOCIATION ANALYSIS OF GENE NETWORKS

Cellular functions are typically mediated by networks of proteins. Therefore, comprehensively examining variants that map to specific networks of functionally linked genes is appealing, particularly if risk conferred by sets of variants is greater than risk conferred by individual variants alone, that is, epistatic interactions (Prasad et al., 2009). Potentially informative associations that are shared between bipolar disorder and schizophrenia have been identified for pathways involved in neuronal cell adhesion and membrane scaffolding (O'Dushlaine et al., 2011). Our earlier investigations of biologically related circadian genes did not reveal substantial evidence for shared risk factors (Mansour et al., 2009).

Dopamine (DA) dysfunction has long been implicated in the pathophysiology of schizophrenia and to a lesser extent bipolar disorder (Talkowski et al., 2007). Hence, we

TABLE 10.1 LIST OF DOPAMINERGIC GENES ANALYZED

| Chr | Gene | Name | Tag SNPs | Gene-based test (Hotelling's T2) | |
| --- | --- | --- | --- | --- | --- |
| | | | | P value (SZ) | p value (BP1) |
| 22 | ADRBK2 | adrenergic, beta, receptor kinase 2 | 3 | 0.756 | 0.700 |
| 22 | CACNG2 | calcium channel, voltage-dependent, gamma subunit 2 | 6 | 0.247 | 0.374 |
| 21 | CLIC6 | chloride intracellular channel 6 | 6 | 0.881 | 0.734 |
| 22 | COMT | catechol-O-methyltransferase | 31 | 0.804 | 0.518 |
| 7 | COPG2 | Gamma COP | 6 | 0.801 | 0.615 |
| 17 | DARPP32 | protein phosphatase 1, regulatory (inhibitor) subunit 1B | 1 | 0.179 | 0.849 |
| 9 | DBH | dopamine beta-hydroxylase | 29 | 0.617 | 0.878 |
| 7 | DDC | dopa decarboxylase | 40 | 0.391 | 0.708 |
| 5 | DRD1 | dopamine receptor 1 | 5 | 0.400 | 0.988 |
| 10 | DRD1IP | dopamine receptor D1 interacting protein | 4 | 0.090 | 0.063 |
| 11 | DRD2 | dopamine receptor D2 | 22 | 0.433 | 0.813 |
| 3 | DRD3 | dopamine receptor D3 | 20 | 0.007 | 0.013 |
| 11 | DRD4 | dopamine receptor D4 | 2 | 0.745 | 0.095 |
| 4 | DRD5 | dopamine receptor D5 | 1 | 0.597 | 0.577 |
| 12 | DRIP78 | dopamine receptor interacting protein | 3 | 0.496 | 1.000 |
| 1 | EPB41 | erythrocyte membrane protein band 4.1 | 15 | 0.818 | 0.109 |
| X | FLNA | Filamin A | 2 | 0.060 | 0.208 |
| 9 | FREQ | frequenin homolog | 21 | 0.776 | 0.376 |
| 5 | GNB2L1 | Receptor for activated C kinase1 | 4 | 0.150 | 0.419 |

(Continued)

TABLE 10.1 (CONTINUED)

| Chr | Gene | Name | Tag SNPs | Gene-based test (Hotelling's T2) | |
|---|---|---|---|---|---|
| | | | | P value (SZ) | p value (BP1) |
| 17 | GRB2 | growth factor receptor-bound protein 2 | 8 | 0.373 | 0.715 |
| 11 | GRK2 | adrenergic, beta, receptor kinase 1 | 2 | 0.671 | 0.447 |
| 8 | Hey1 | Hesr1/Hey1 | 7 | 0.992 | 0.156 |
| 16 | HIC5 | Focal adhesion protein | 2 | 0.828 | 0.360 |
| X | MAOA | monoamine oxidase A | 8 | 0.336 | 0.481 |
| X | MAOB | monoamine oxidase B | 8 | 0.268 | 0.296 |
| 3 | NCK1 | NCK adaptor protein | 6 | 0.826 | 0.977 |
| 8 | NEF3 | Neurofilament M | 8 | 0.342 | 0.286 |
| 2 | NR4A2 | nuclear receptor subfamily 4, group A, member 2 | 2 | 0.682 | 0.643 |
| 22 | PICK1 | Protein interacting with C Kinase1 | 6 | 0.697 | 0.931 |
| 17 | PPP1R9B | Spinophilin | 5 | 0.396 | 0.095 |
| 5 | PPP2CA | Protein Phosphatase | 1 | 0.566 | 1.000 |
| 8 | SLC18A1 | solute carrier family 18 (vesicular monoamine), member 1 | 22 | 0.761 | 0.113 |
| 10 | SLC18A2 | solute carrier family 18 (vesicular monoamine), member 2 | 18 | 0.420 | 0.393 |
| 5 | SLC6A3 | Dopamine Transporter | 47 | 0.479 | 0.818 |
| 20 | SNAP25 | synaptosomal-associated protein | 34 | 0.334 | 0.375 |
| 4 | SNCA | Synuclein | 12 | 0.753 | 0.614 |
| 7 | Sp4 | Sp4 transcription factor | 3 | 0.105 | 0.963 |
| 7 | STX1A | Syntaxin1A | 2 | 0.572 | 0.956 |
| 16 | SYNGR3 | synaptogyrin 3 | 2 | 0.650 | 0.885 |
| 11 | TH | tyrosine hydroxylase | 7 | 0.247 | 0.252 |

*Abbreviations*: Chr: chromosome; SNP: single nucleotide polymorphism

conducted a focused search for disorder-specific risk loci and shared associations with bipolar disorder/schizophrenia in the genes encoding DA function-related proteins. The list included 18 genes that directly impact DA function, reported earlier (Talkowski et al., 2008), and 22 additional genes that interact with the DA pathway (Table 10.1). Representative tag SNPs were genotyped in 527 patients with schizophrenia/schizoaffective disorder (DSM IV criteria) from Pittsburgh (Mansour et al., 2009), 526 bipolar disorder cases from the Systematic Treatment Enhancement Program for Bipolar Disorder (STEP-BD) study (Sachs et al., 2003; Sklar et al., 2008), and 477 adult controls, using the hybridization based Illumina GoldenGate Assay (www.Illumina.com) (Steemers &

Gunderson, 2007). We tested for individual SNP associations and obtained a summary statistic for all SNPs within a gene, then corrected all test statistics for the effective number of independent tests among SNPs within each gene using published methods (40 genes, 165.4 effective independent SNP tests in each disorder) (Conneely & Boehnke, 2007; Roeder et al., 2005). We also tested for population substructure using a variation of the genomic control (GC) method (Devlin and Roeder, 1999; Bacanu et al., 2000; Devlin et al., 2004) and found no meaningful differences between groups (Mansour et al., 2009).

Thirty-seven of the 422 SNPs tested reached nominal significance for bipolar disorder (8.8%) and 25 SNPs were nominally associated with schizophrenia/schizoaffective disorder (6.2%, p < 0.05). Of these 25 nominal associations, 15 SNPs (60%) were also associated with bipolar disorder. The top ranked association signal was the same *DRD3* SNP/allele in both disorders, rs9868039 (uncorrected p = 0.0017 and 0.0032 in bipolar disorder and schizophrenia/ schizoaffective disorder, respectively). However, no results remained significant after correcting for multiple testing across all SNP tests (p > 3.0x10$^{-4}$ in each disorder) (Table 10.2). Gene-based tests supported the shared SNP results at *DRD3* (empirical p = 0.007 and 0.013 in schizophrenia and bipolar disorder, respectively). No other genes reached nominal significance following permutation and no results were significant after correction for the number of gene tests conducted (Table 10.2). Furthermore, no significant associations were detected from available GWAS studies (Consortium, 2007; Shi et al., 2009; Sklar et al., 2008). Under a dominant transmission model, the sample had 81% power to detect a nominally significant association (OR 1.5) for a risk allele with 15% minor allele frequency (MAF) in the population, using a type I error threshold of 5%. However, the sample had less than 20% power to detect an association at odds ratios of 1.1—1.2. Despite some consistent nominal associations between diagnostic groups at *DRD3*, none of our analyses were statistically significant following corrections for multiple comparisons, and power was relatively low to detect common alleles of small effects. Therefore, common genetic risk factors of large effect for schizophrenia or bipolar disorder etiology were not detected and appear unlikely given the coverage of common variants in our samples and those from GWAS. These analyses

**TABLE 10.2** DOPAMINERGIC GENES WITH NOMINALLY SIGNIFICANT SNP ASSOCIATIONS

| | | | | SNP Associations | | | | Gene-Based Test | |
|---|---|---|---|---|---|---|---|---|---|
| Associated Phenotype | Gene | Tag SNPs | Effective tests | # SNPs p<0.05 (SZ) | Best SZ p-value | # SNPs p<0.05 (BP1) | Best BP1 p-value | Best Model p-value (SZ) | Best Model p-value (BP1) |
| SZ/SZA and BP1 | *DRD3* | 20 | 6.7 | 10 | 0.003* | 8 | 0.002* | 0.028 | 0.005 |
| | *DDC* | 40 | 11.9 | 6 | 0.029 | 11 | 0.002* | 0.259 | 0.054 |
| | *MAOB* | 8 | 3.3 | 2 | 0.019 | 2 | 0.042 | 0.051 | 0.023 |
| | *DRD1IP* | 4 | 1.9 | 1 | 0.012* | 2 | 0.008* | 0.013 | 0.013 |
| SZ/SZA Only | *DRD2* | 22 | 8.3 | 3 | 0.037 | 0 | 0.261 | 0.231 | 0.331 |
| | *SLC6A3* | 47 | 16.9 | 1 | 0.045 | 0 | 0.118 | 0.668 | 0.756 |
| | *NEF3* | 8 | 3.5 | 1 | 0.044 | 0 | 0.075 | 0.058 | 0.370 |
| | *Sp4* | 3 | 1.1 | 1 | 0.016* | 0 | 0.687 | 0.058 | 0.572 |
| | *SLC18A2* | 18 | 7.7 | 2 | 0.041 | 0 | 0.095 | 0.275 | 0.202 |
| | *GRB2* | 8 | 3.4 | 1 | 0.037 | 0 | 0.208 | 0.106 | 0.511 |
| BP1 Only | *FREQ* | 21 | 8.1 | 0 | 0.056 | 5 | 0.011 | 0.501 | 0.061 |
| | *SLC18A1* | 22 | 8.7 | 0 | 0.233 | 2 | 0.005* | 0.883 | 0.067 |
| | *SNAP25* | 34 | 13.3 | 0 | 0.064 | 2 | 0.012 | 0.667 | 0.228 |
| | *COMT* | 31 | 10.6 | 0 | 0.217 | 1 | 0.050 | 0.084 | 0.177 |
| | *SNCA* | 12 | 4.9 | 0 | 0.128 | 1 | 0.038 | 0.148 | 0.052 |
| | *DBH* | 29 | 11.2 | 0 | 0.124 | 1 | 0.045 | 0.386 | 0.492 |
| | *PPP1R9B* | 5 | 1.9 | 0 | 0.068 | 1 | 0.019* | 0.277 | 0.078 |
| | *EPB41* | 15 | 4.9 | 0 | 0.138 | 1 | 0.022 | 0.556 | 0.207 |

* Significant after correction for effective number of SNP tests within the gene (gene-wide significance). No results were significant at an experiment-wide threshold.
*Abbreviations*: SZ: schizophrenia; SZA: schizoaffective disorder; BP1: bipolar I disorder. SNP p-values were uncorrected for multiple comparisons

demonstrate the potential pitfalls in candidate gene association studies, where many sound biological hypotheses have failed to yield substantial genetic risk, even in a relatively comprehensive design.

Recently, efforts have been made to weave different genetic approaches in order to obtain more consistent etiologic explanations. For example an approach called convergent functional genomics (CFG) combines gene expression and genetic data from human and animal model studies to explore GWAS datasets (Patel et al., 2010). Such approaches deserve to be explored, but the major limitation is likely to be the availability of appropriate datasets.

## DISCUSSION AND CONCLUSIONS

We reviewed different lines of inquiry brought to bear on the question of shared genetic etiological factors for bipolar 1 disorder and schizophrenia. The early familial aggregation studies on the whole did not support shared risk factors, but recent Swedish national database analyses have breathed new life into the debate (Lichtenstein et al., 2009). By their nature, such studies cannot definitively identify specific shared risk factors. Gene mapping studies can potentially be informative in this respect, but linkage and candidate gene association studies have been of limited value; linkage studies typically identify relatively large genomic regions, and candidate gene studies are biased in terms of the genes selected for investigation. GWAS provide an opportunity for unbiased estimates, but the few replicated risk variants discovered to date explain only a small fraction of the heritability for either schizophrenia or bipolar disorder. Among these variants, there is limited evidence for shared risk, the most convincing being variants within *ZNF804* (Williams et al., 2010). Since models based on a single causative genetic variant or set of genes that explains a major proportion of the etiologic variance are unlikely to be substantiated, it is clear that many more risk factors remain to be identified. Until very recently, gene mapping studies have remained somewhat limited in locus coverage or the statistical power to find subtle pathway effects. The anticipated availability of denser microarrays on the order of several million common, intermediate, and rare variations will enable much greater coverage in forthcoming GWAS. Indeed, whole genome sequencing will provide the ultimate refinement from this perspective (Cirulli & Goldstein, 2010). One should be mindful that genetic association studies at various degrees of sophistication can only reveal genetic variants that may be associated with a given trait or may be shared in association by two traits.

Establishing them as causal variants or contributing to the etiology need to be pursued using additional techniques such as gene expression studies, animal studies, cellular models, imaging and other behavioral studies. The anticipated small effect sizes detected with these studies should not deter the pursuit of their discovery as small effects may still meaningfully contribute to the risk or the etiology of the disease(s) in question and have a substantial impact in targeted therapeutics.

Another major hurdle to overcome for identifying shared risk factors continues to be the inability thus far to explain the major portion of the heritability for bipolar 1 disorder and schizophrenia. This inability, also called the missing heritability, has been a difficult problem to unravel across most genetic studies of complex disorders (Manolio et al., 2009; Collins, 2010). It is likely due to many factors, including genetic heterogeneity—that is, presence of different susceptibility variants in the same gene or different risk factors across many genes, lack of power to detect very small effects in all studies to date, or over-estimated heritability (Manolio et al., 2009). Other models have also been proposed, for example, the presence of uncommon or rare risk alleles that are present in relatively few families, but collectively may explain a substantial portion of the missing heritability (McClellan & King, 2010). Risk may also accrue from other sources that have not been investigated extensively, such as mitochondrial DNA, epistatic interactions such as gene-to-gene or SNP-to-SNP interactive effects, epigenetic factors like DNA methylation and histone modifications, and environmental risk modifiers such as infectious agents (Petronis, 2004; Dickerson et al., 2004; Bamne et al., 2008; Shirts et al., 2008; Prasad et al., 2009). Analyses of these models will require refinement in our current statistical methods.

As we proceed to test such models, we recommend a broader framework than the current simplistic view of bipolar 1 disorder and schizophrenia dichotomy (Craddock & Owen, 2010). Some suggestions are illustrated in Figure 10.1. They include the independent model: that is, bipolar 1 disorder, schizophrenia, and other disorders such as autism or major depressive disorders have independent causes (Figure 10.1A). The heuristic shared model for bipolar disorder and schizophrenia is illustrated in Figure 10.1B. We advocate extension of this model to include overlap with other disorders, such as between autism/developmental disorders and schizophrenia; or between major depressive disorder and bipolar disorder and schizophrenia, as shown in Figure 10.1B. Another intriguing model is one in which different environmental factors act against a largely shared genetic background lead to the distinctive

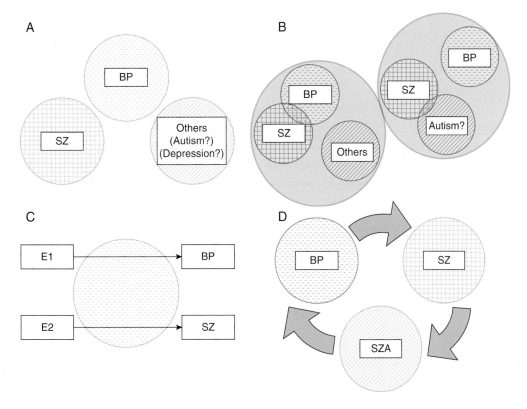

*Figure 10.1* Possible models of genetic associations among bipolar disorder (BP), schizophrenia (SZ) and other conditions (e.g., autism). Panel A represents the independent model, in which BP, SZ, and other disorders such as autism or major depressive disorders have independent genetic (and environmental) causes. The heuristic shared model for BP/SZ is illustrated in Panel B. This model may include overlap with other disorders, for example, between autism/developmental disorders and schizophrenia; or between major depressive disorder and bipolar disorder and schizophrenia. Another intriguing model is one in which different environmental factors act against a largely shared genetic background lead to the distinctive manifestations of bipolar disorder and schizophrenia (Panel C; E1 = first environmental factor; E2 = second, separate, environmental factor). This model can be extended to one in which clinical presentation can vary through an individual's life, the presentations across episodes being governed by unidentified factors (Panel D). Such a model is supported by published reports of affected identical triplets whose manifestations changed through their lifetimes. (Source: McGuffin et al., 1982.)

manifestations of bipolar disorder and schizophrenia (Figure 10.1C). This model can be extended to one in which clinical presentation can vary through an individual's life, the presentations across episodes being governed by unidentified factors (Figure 10.1D). Such a model is supported by published reports of affected identical triplets whose manifestations changed through their lifetimes (McGuffin et al., 1982). This model would advocate investigating endophenotypes that form the hypothetical substrate for both bipolar disorder and schizophrenia (Gould & Gottesman, 2006).

In conclusion, the question of shared genetic etiological factors for bipolar disorder and schizophrenia has been investigated extensively in recent years, but comprehensive or unambiguous conclusions remain elusive. There are several lines of evidence that suggest overlap in a small proportion of the etiologic space. Emerging genomic technologies promise more refined examination of this question. We propose that the search be extended from a simple bipolar

disorder/schizophrenia dichotomy to include additional related psychiatric disorders.

## REFERENCES

Akiskal, H. S. (2002). Classification, Diagnosis and Boundaries of Bipolar Disorders. In M. Maj, H. S. Akiskal, J. J. López-Ibor and N. Sartorius. *Bipolar Disorder*, (Vol. 5, pp. 1–52). Chichester, UK: John Wiley & Sons, Ltd.

Alaerts, M. & Del-Favero, J. 2009. Searching genetic risk factors for schizophrenia and bipolar disorder: learn from the past and back to the future. *Human Mutation*, 30: 1139–1152.

Bacanu, S. A., Devlin, B. & Roeder, K. 2000. The Power of Genomic Control. *American Journal of Human Genetics*, 66: 1933–1944.

Bamne, M. N., Talkowski, M. E., Moraes, C. T., Manuck, S. B., Ferrell, R. E., Chowdari, K. V. & Nimgaonkar, V. L. 2008. Systematic association studies of mitochondrial DNA variations in schizophrenia: focus on the ND5 gene. *Schizophrenia Bulletin*, 34: 458–465.

Brockington, I. F. & Leff, J. P. 1979. Schizo-affective psychosis: definitions and incidence. *Psychological Medicine*, 9: 91–99.

Cardno, A. G., Rijsdijk, F. V., Sham, P. C., Murray, R. M. & McGuffin, P. 2002. A twin study of genetic relationships between psychotic symptoms. *American Journal of Psychiatry*, 159: 539–545.

Cichon, S., Craddock, N., Daly, M., Faraone, S. V., Gejman, P. V., Kelsoe, J., . . . Sullivan, P. F. 2009. Genomewide association studies: history, rationale, and prospects for psychiatric disorders. *American Journal of Psychiatry,* 166: 540–556.

Cirulli, E. T. & Goldstein, D. B. 2010. Uncovering the roles of rare variants in common disease through whole-genome sequencing. *Nature Reviews Genetics,* 11: 415–425.

Collins, F. 2010. Has the revolution arrived? *Nature,* 464: 674–675.

Conneely, K. N. & Boehnke, M. 2007. So Many Correlated Tests, So Little Time! Rapid Adjustment of P Values for Multiple Correlated Tests. *American Journal of Human Genetics,* 81.

Consortium, T. I. S. 2008. Rare chromosomal deletions and duplications increase risk of schizophrenia. *Nature,* 455: 237–241.

Consortium, T. W. T. C. C. 2007. Genome-wide association study of 14,000 cases of seven common diseases and 3,000 shared controls. *Nature,* 447: 661–678.

Cook, E. H., JR. & Scherer, S. W. 2008. Copy-number variations associated with neuropsychiatric conditions. *Nature,* 455: 919–923.

Craddock, N. & Owen, M. J. 2010. The Kraepelinian dichotomy—going, going. . . but still not gone. *British Journal of Psychiatry,* 196: 92–95.

Craddock, N., O'Donovan, M. C. & Owen, M. J. 2005. The genetics of schizophrenia and bipolar disorder: dissecting psychosis. *Journal of Medical Genetics,* 42: 193–204.

Crow, T. J. 1990. The continuum of psychosis and its genetic origins. The sixty-fifth Maudsley lecture. *British Journal of Psychiatry,* 156: 788–797.

Cusco, I., Medrano, A., Gener, B., Vilardell, M., Gallastegui, F., Villa, O., . . . Perez-Jurado, L. A. 2009. Autism-specific copy number variants further implicate the phosphatidylinositol signaling pathway and the glutamatergic synapse in the etiology of the disorder. *Human Molecular Genetics,* 18:1795–1804.

Devlin, B. & Roeder, K. 1999. Genomic control for association studies. *Biometrics,* 55: 997–1004.

Devlin, B., Bacanu, S. A. & Roeder, K. 2004. Genomic Control to the extreme. *Nature Genetics,* 36: 1129–1130.

Dickerson, F. B., Boronow, J. J., Stallings, C., Origoni, A. E., Cole, S., Krivogorsky, B. & Yolken, R. H. 2004. Infection with herpes simplex virus type 1 is associated with cognitive deficits in bipolar disorder. *Biological Psychiatry,* 55: 588–593.

Francks, C., Tozzi, F., Farmer, A., Vincent, J. B., Rujescu, D., St Clair, D. & Muglia, P. 2010. Population-based linkage analysis of schizophrenia and bipolar case-control cohorts identifies a potential susceptibility locus on 19q13. *Molecular Psychiatry,* 15: 319–325.

Gershon, E. S., Delisi, L. E., Hamovit, J., Nurnberger, J. I., JR., Maxwell, M. E., Schreiber, J., . . . Guroff, J. J. 1988. A controlled family study of chronic psychoses. Schizophrenia and schizoaffective disorder. *Archives of General Psychiatry,* 45: 328–336.

Gill, M., Donohoe, G. & Corvin, A. 2010. What have the genomics ever done for the psychoses? *Psychological Medicine,* 40: 529–540.

Gottesman, I. 1991. *Schizophrenia Genesis: The Origins of Madness.* New York: WH Freeman.

Gottesman, I. I. & Shields, J. 1967. A polygenic theory of schizophrenia. *Proceedings of the National Academy of Sciences,* 58: 199–205.

Gottesman, II, Laursen, T. M., Bertelsen, A. & Mortensen, P. B. 2010. Severe mental disorders in offspring with 2 psychiatrically ill parents. *Archives of General Psychiatry,* 67: 252–257.

Gould, T. D. & Gottesman, II 2006. Psychiatric endophenotypes and the development of valid animal models. *Genes Brain and Behavior,* 5: 113–119.

Green, E. K., Grozeva, D., Jones, I., Jones, L., Kirov, G., Caesar, S., . . . Craddock, N. 2010. The bipolar disorder risk allele at CACNA1C also confers risk of recurrent major depression and of schizophrenia. *Molecular Psychiatry,* 15: 1016–1022.

Grozeva, D., Kirov, G., Ivanov, D., Jones, I. R., Jones, L., Green, E. K., . . . Craddock, N. 2010. Rare copy number variants: a point of rarity in genetic risk for bipolar disorder and schizophrenia. *Archives of General Psychiatry,* 67: 318–327.

Ivleva, E., Thaker, G. & Tamminga, C. A. 2008. Comparing genes and phenomenology in the major psychoses: schizophrenia and bipolar 1 disorder. *Schizophrenia Bulletin,* 34: 734–742.

Kendler, K. S. & Diehl, S. R. 1993. The genetics of schizophrenia: a current, genetic-epidemiologic perspective. [Review]. *Schizophrenia Bulletin,* 19: 261–285.

Koch, R. (ed.) 1882. *Die Aetiologie der Tuberculose.* New York: Dover Publications.

Kraepelin, E. 1919. *Dementia Praecox and Paraphrenia.* R. M. Barclay & G. M. Robertson, trans. Edinburgh: E&S Livingstone.

Lachman, H. M., Pedrosa, E., Petruolo, O. A., Cockerham, M., Papolos, A., Novak, T., . . . Stopkova, P. 2007. Increase in GSK3beta gene copy number variation in bipolar disorder. *American Journal of Medical Genetics Part B Neuropsychiatric Genetics,* 144B: 259–265.

Laursen, T. M., Labouriau, R., Licht, R. W., Bertelsen, A., Munk-Olsen, T. & Mortensen, P. B. 2005. Family history of psychiatric illness as a risk factor for schizoaffective disorder: a Danish register-based cohort study. *Archives of General Psychiatry,* 62: 841–848.

Lewis, C. M., Levinson, D. F., Wise, L. H., Delisi, L. E., Straub, R. E., Hovatta, I., . . . Helgason, T. 2003. Genome scan meta-analysis of schizophrenia and bipolar disorder, part II: Schizophrenia. *American Journal of Human Genetics,* 73: 34–48.

Li, J., Liu, J., Feng, G., Li, T., Zhao, Q., Li, Y., . . . Shi, Y. 2011. The MDGA1 gene confers risk to schizophrenia and bipolar disorder. *Schizophrenia Research,* 125: 194–200.

Lichtenstein, P., Yip, B. H., Bjork, C., Pawitan, Y., Cannon, t. D., Sullivan, P. F. & Hultman, C. M. 2009. Common genetic determinants of schizophRENIA AND bipolar disorder in Swedish families: a population-based study. *Lancet,* 373: 234–239.

Manolio, T. A., Collins, F. S., Cox, N. J., Goldstein, D. B., Hindorff, L. A., Hunter, . . . Visscher, P. M. 2009. Finding the missing heritability OF Complex diseases. *Nature,* 461: 747–753.

Mansour, H. A., Talkowski, M. E., Wood, J., Chowdari, K. V., McClain, L., Prasad, K., . . . Nimgaonkar, V. L. 2009. Association study of 21 circadian genes with bipolar I disorder, schizoaffective disorder, and schizophrenia. *Bipolar Disorders,* 11: 701–710.

Marneros, A. & Angst, J. 2000. *Bipolar Disorders: 100 Years After Manic Depressive Insanity.* Dordrecht; Kluwer.

McCarthy, S. E., Makarov, V., Kirov, G., Addington, A. M., McClellan, J., Yoon, S., . . . Sebat, J. 2009. Microduplications of 16p. 11.2 are associated with schizophrenia. *Nature Genetics,* 41: 1223–1227.

McClellan, J. & King, M. C. 2010. Genetic heterogeneity in human disease. *Cell,* 141: 210–217.

McGuffin, P., Reveley, A. & Holland, A. 1982. Identical triplets: non-identical psychosis? *British Journal of Psychiatry,* 140: 1–6.

McMahon, F. J., Akula, N., Schulze, T. G., Muglia, P., Tozzi, F., Detera-Wadleigh, S. D., . . . Rietschel, M. 2010. Meta-analysis of genome-wide association data identifies a risk locus for major mood disorders on 3p. 21.1. *Nature Genetics,* 42: 128–131.

Mick, E., Kim, J. W., Biederman, J., Wozniak, J., Wilens, T., Spencer, T., . . . Faraone, S. V. 2008. Family based association study of pediatric bipolar disorder and the dopamine transporter gene (SLC6A3). *American Journal of Medical Genetics Part B Neuropsychiatric Genetics,* 147B: 1182–1185.

Moldin, S. O. 1997. The maddening hunt for madness genes. *Nature Genetics,* 17: 127–129.

Moskvina, V., Craddock, N., Holmans, P., Nikolov, I., Pahwa, J. S., Green, E., . . . O'Donovan, M. C. 2009. Gene-wide analyses of genome-wide association data sets: evidence for multiple common risk alleles for schizophrenia and bipolar disorder and for overlap in genetic risk. *Molecular Psychiatry,* 14: 252–260.

O'Dushlaine, C., Kenny, E., Heron, E., Donohoe, G., Gill, M., Morris, D. & Corvin, A. 2011. Molecular pathways involved in neuronal cell adhesion and membrane scaffolding contribute to schizophrenia and bipolar disorder susceptibility. *Molecular Psychiatry,* 16: 286–292.

Patel, S. D., Le-Niculescu, H., Koller, D. L., Green, S. D., Lahiri, D. K., McMahon, F. J., . . . Niculescu, A. B., III 2010. Coming to grips with complex disorders: genetic risk prediction in bipolar disorder using panels of genes identified through convergent functional genomics. *American Journal of Medical Genetics Part B Neuropsychiatric Genetics,* 153B: 850–877.

Petronis, A. 2004. The origin of schizophrenia: genetic thesis, epigenetic antithesis, and resolving synthesis. *Biological Psychiatry,* 55: 965–970.

Prasad, K. M., Talkowski, M. E., Chowdari, K. V., McClain, L., Yolken, R. H. & Nimgaonkar, V. L. 2009. Candidate genes and their interactions with other genetic/environmental risk factors in the etiology of schizophrenia. *Brain Research Bulletin,* 83: 86–92.

Purcell, S. M., Wray, N. R., Stone, J. L., Visscher, P. M., O'Donovan, M. C., Sullivan, P. F. & Sklar, P. 2009. Common polygenic variation contributes to risk of schizophrenia and bipolar disorder. *Nature,* 460: 748–752.

Rice, J., Reich, T., Andreasen, N. C., Endicott, J., Van Eerdewegh, M., Fishman, R., . . . Klerman, G. L. 1987. The familial transmission of bipolar illness. *Archives of General Psychiatry,* 44: 441–447.

Risch, N. 1990. Linkage strategies for genetically complex traits. I. Multilocus models. *American Journal of Human Genetics,* 46: 222–228.

Robins, E. & Guze, S. B. 1970. Establishment of diagnostic validity in psychiatric illness: its application to schizophrenia. *American Journal of Psychiatry,* 126: 983–987.

Roeder, K., Bacanu, S. A., Sonpar, V., Zhang, X. & Devlin, B. 2005. Analysis of single-locus tests to detect gene/disease associations. *Genetic Epidemiology,* 28: 207–219.

Sachs, G. S., Thase, M. E., Otto, M. W., Bauer, M., Miklowitz, D., Wisniewski, S. R., . . . Rosenbaum, J. F. 2003. Rationale, design, and methods of the systematic treatment enhancement program for bipolar disorder (STEP-BD). *Biological Psychiatry,* 53: 1028–1042.

Sebat, J., Lakshmi, B., Malhotra, D., Troge, J., Lese-Martin, C., Walsh, T., . . . Wigler, M. 2007. Strong association of de novo copy number mutations with autism. *Science,* 316: 445–449.

Sebat, J., Levy, D. L. & McCarthy, S. E. 2009. Rare structural variants in schizophrenia: one disorder, multiple mutations; one mutation, multiple disorders. *Trends in Genetics,* 25: 528–535.

Segurado, R., Detera-Wadleigh, S. D., Levinson, D. F., Lewis, C. M., Gill, M., Nurnberger, J. I., JR., . . . Akarsu, N. 2003. Genome scan meta-analysis of schizophrenia and bipolar disorder, part III: Bipolar disorder. *American Journal of Human Genetics,* 73: 49–62.

Shi, J., Levinson, D. F., Duan, J., Sanders, A. R., Zheng, Y., Pe'er, I., . . . Gejman, P. V. 2009. Common variants on chromosome 6p. 22.1 are associated with schizophrenia. *Nature,* 460: 753–757.

Shirts, B. H. & Nimgaonkar, V. 2004. The genes for schizophrenia: finally a breakthrough? *Current Psychiatry Rep,* 6: 303–312.

Shirts, B. H., Prasad, K. M., Pogue-Geile, M. F., Dickerson, F., Yolken, R. H. & Nimgaonkar, V. L. 2008. Antibodies to cytomegalovirus and Herpes Simplex Virus 1 associated with cognitive function in schizophrenia. *Schizophrenia Research,* 106: 268–274.

Sklar, P., Smoller, J. W., Fan, J., Ferreira, M. A., Perlis, R. H., Chambert, K., . . . Purcell, S. M. 2008. Whole-genome association study of bipolar disorder. *Molecular Psychiatry,* 13: 558–569.

Steemers, F. J. & Gunderson, K. L. 2007. Whole genome genotyping technologies on the BeadArray platform. *Journal of Biotechnology,* 2: 41–49.

Stefansson, H., Ophoff, R. A., Steinberg, S., Andreassen, O. A., Cichon, S., Rujescu, D., . . . Collier, D. A. 2009. Common variants conferring risk of schizophrenia. *Nature,* 460: 744–747.

Szatmari, P., Paterson, A. D., Zwaigenbaum, L., Roberts, W., Brian, J., Liu, X. Q., . . . Langemeijer, M., et al. 2007. Mapping autism risk loci using genetic linkage and chromosomal rearrangements. *Nature Genetics,* 39: 319–328.

Talkowski, M. E., Bamne, M., Mansour, H. & Nimgaonkar, V. L. 2007. Dopamine genes and schizophrenia: case closed or evidence pending? *Schizophrenia Bulletin,* 33: 1071–1081.

Talkowski, M. E., Kirov, G., Bamne, M., Georgieva, L., Torres, G., Mansour, H., . . . Nimgaonkar, V. L. 2008. A network of dopaminergic gene variations implicated as risk factors for schizophrenia. *Human Molecular Genetics,* 17: 747–758.

Talkowski, M. E., McCann, K. L., Chen, M., McClain, L., Bamne, M., Wood, J., . . . Nimgaonkar, V. L. 2010. Fine-mapping reveals novel alternative splicing of the dopamine transporter. *American Journal of Medical Genetics Part B Neuropsychiatric Genetics,* 153B: 1434–1447.

Tsuang, M. T. & Faraone, S. V. 2000. The genetic epidemiology of bipolar disorder. *In:* Marneros, A. & Angst, J. eds. *Bipolar Disorders: 100 Years After Manic-Depressive Insanity.* Zurich: Kluwer Academic.

Valles, V., Van Os, J., Guillamat, R., Gutierrez, B., Campillo, M., Gento, P. & Fananas, L. 2000. Increased morbid risk for schizophrenia in families of in-patients with bipolar illness. *Schizophrenia Research,* 42: 83–90.

Walsh, T., McClellan, J. M., McCarthy, S. E., Addington, A. M., Pierce, S. B., Cooper, G. M., . . . Sebat, J. 2008. Rare structural variants disrupt multiple genes in neurodevelopmental pathways in schizophrenia. *Science,* 320: 539–543.

Wang, K. S., Liu, X. F. & Aragam, N. 2010. A genome-wide meta-analysis identifies novel loci associated with schizophrenia and bipolar disorder. *Schizophrenia Research,* 124: 192–199.

Weissman, M. M., Gershon, E. S., Kidd, K. K., Prusoff, B. A., Leckman, J. F., Dibble, E., . . . Guroff, J. J. 1984. Psychiatric disorders in the relatives of probands with affective disorders. The Yale University—National Institute of Mental Health Collaborative Study. *Archives of General Psychiatry,* 41: 13–21.

Williams, H. J., Norton, N., Dwyer, S., Moskvina, V., Nikolov, I., Carroll, L., . . . O'Donovan, M. C. 2010. Fine mapping of ZNF804A and genome-wide significant evidence for its involvement in schizophrenia and bipolar disorder. *Molecular Psychiatry,* in press.

Xu, B., Roos, J. L., Levy, S., Van Rensburg, E. J., Gogos, J. A. & Karayiorgou, M. 2008. Strong association of de novo copy number mutations with sporadic schizophrenia. *Nature Genetics,* 40: 880–885.

Yang, S., Wang, K., Gregory, B., Berrettini, W., Wang, L. S., Hakonarson, H. & Bucan, M. 2009. Genomic landscape of a three-generation pedigree segregating affective disorder. *PLoS One,* 4: e4474.

Zhang, D., Cheng, L., Qian, Y., Alliey-Rodriguez, N., Kelsoe, J. R., Greenwood, T., . . . Gershon, E. S. 2009. Singleton deletions throughout the genome increase risk of bipolar disorder. *Molecular Psychiatry,* 14: 376–380.

Zollner, S., Su, G., Stewart, W. C., Chen, Y., McInnis, M. G. & Burmeister, M. 2009. Bayesian EM algorithm for scoring polymorphic deletions from SNP data and application to a common CNV on 8q24. *Genetic Epidemiology,* 33: 357–368.

# 11.

# MITOCHONDRIAL GENETICS AND BIPOLAR DISORDER

## Hayley B. Clay, Satoshi Fuke, Tadafumi Kato, and Christine Konradi

## MITOCHONDRIAL ANATOMY

Mitochondria are intracellular organelles that perform a number of critical functions within the cytoplasm of nearly all eukaryotic cells, most prominently adenosine-5'-triphosphate (ATP) production through oxidative phosphorylation (Wallace & Fan, 2010). Mitochondria are distributed throughout the cell and allocated almost equally during cell division. They undergo dynamic changes in morphology due to movement along the cytoskeletal network, and through the processes of fusion and fission. Mitochondria contain a highly permeable outer membrane with many pores through which small molecules pass, and a largely impermeable inner membrane. This impermeability to most small molecules and ions is required to maintain an electrochemical gradient needed for production of ATP in the respiratory chain (Shao et al., 2008; Clay et al., 2010). Between the two mitochondrial membranes lies the intermembrane space (Smoly et al., 1970). The surface area of the inner membrane is larger than that of the outer membrane and folds into the matrix. The mitochondrial matrix contains the mitochondrial DNA (mtDNA) and the enzymes and metabolites required for the tricarboxylic acid cycle and ß-oxidation (Figure 11.1A, B). The five complexes of the mitochondrial respiratory chain that mediate oxidative phosphorylation are located in the inner mitochondrial membrane (Figure 11.1C). Because of the volatile nature of free electrons needed for oxidative phosphorylation, mitochondria are a source of reactive oxygen species, although they are also equipped with enzymes that scavenge these molecules (Wallace, 1999; Starkov, 2008). In addition to synthesizing ATP, mitochondria are vital for buffering intracellular calcium and for regulating apoptotic cell death (Orrenius et al., 2003).

## MITOCHONDRIA CONTAIN THEIR OWN LIMITED GENOME

Mitochondria likely originated from a symbiotic relationship between an anaerobic proto-eukaryotic cell and an aerobic proteobacterium (Esser et al., 2004), as indicated by certain bacterial characteristics of mitochondria, including the circular mtDNA and the ability to independently transcribe and translate genes (Fernandez-Silva et al., 2003; Wallace, 2005; Gilkerson, 2009). Unlike the Mendelian inheritance pattern of nuclear genes, mtDNA exhibits a maternal inheritance pattern (Youssoufian & Pyeritz, 2002; Wallace, 2005). This inheritance pattern is due to an excess of mtDNA in oocytes and the exclusion of sperm-derived mitochondria from the zygote (Danan et al., 1999; He et al., 2010). Although mtDNA appeared very early in eukaryotic evolution, the contents of mtDNA are relatively conserved across many species (Fernandez-Silva et al., 2003; Wallace, 2005; Clay Montier et al., 2009).

Human mtDNA is a 16.6 kb circular, double-stranded molecule that encodes two ribosomal RNAs, 22 transfer RNAs (tRNAs, denoted by stars in Figure 11.1B), and 13 mRNAs for the respiratory chain (Youssoufian & Pyeritz, 2002; Fernandez-Silva et al., 2003; Clay et al., 2010; Wallace & Fan, 2010), (Figure 11.1B). Respiratory chain complex assembly proteins encoded by mtDNA include seven complex I genes (ND1, ND2, ND3, ND4, ND4L, ND5, and ND6), three complex III genes (CO1, CO2, and CO3), one complex IV gene (Cyt $b$), and two complex V genes (ATP6 and ATP8). MtDNA contains a guanine-rich heavy strand, which encodes most mitochondrial genes, and a cytosine-rich light strand, which encodes ND6 and a small number of tRNAs (Fernandez-Silva et al., 2003; Clay Montier et al., 2009). In addition to the 37 transcripts, mtDNA contains a major non-coding region, which includes the heavy-strand promoter, the light-strand promoter, and a triple-stranded region, known as displacement-loop (D-loop) regulatory region (Kasamatsu et al., 1971; Crews et al., 1979). Although the D-loop has a high degree of variability, this region contains the origin of replication for the heavy strand ($O_H$), (Chang & Clayton, 1984). The origin of light strand replication ($O_L$) is located between the coding areas for CO1 and ND2, two-thirds down the mtDNA (Figure 11.1B), (Tapper & Clayton, 1981). Recently, alternative origins with bidirectional replication were reported in the noncoding region (discussed subsequently in this chapter), (Bowmaker et al., 2003; Yasukawa et al., 2005).

## THE MAJORITY OF MITOCHONDRIAL PROTEINS ARE ENCODED IN NUCLEAR DNA

MtDNA encodes only 13 of the approximately 1,500 protein-coding genes necessary for mitochondrial function (Wallace, 2005; Pagliarini et al., 2008). The remaining mitochondria-relevant proteins are encoded in the nuclear genome and translated in the cytoplasm (Wallace, 2005; DiMauro & Schon, 2008; Shao et al., 2008; Wallace & Fan, 2010). An N-terminal mitochondrial-targeting sequence on the protein is recognized for import into the mitochondria by translocases of the outer and inner mitochondrial membranes, (Wallace, 1999; Endo et al., 2003; Wallace, 2005; DiMauro & Schon, 2008; Clay Montier et al., 2009). Nuclear-encoded mitochondrial proteins are essential for many functions of mitochondria, including mtDNA maintenance and transcription, protein translation, and fusion, fission, biogenesis, and degradation of mitochondria. Because mtDNA still retains crucial genes for energy production, mtDNA and nuclear DNA are clearly highly interdependent.

## REPLICATION OF MTDNA

The mechanism underlying mtDNA replication is not fully elucidated. Three models of mtDNA replication have been described in mammals: an asynchronous strand displacement model, a strand-coupled bidirectional replication model, and ribonucleotide incorporation throughout the lagging strand (RITOLS) model (Figure 11.2), (reviewed in Krishnan et al., 2008).

In the asynchronous strand displacement model, DNA synthesis for each strand is initiated in an asymmetric fashion from two separate locations on mtDNA, the origin of heavy strand replication ($O_H$) and the origin of light strand replication ($O_L$) (Figure 11.2B), (Shadel & Clayton, 1997). Heavy-strand replication is initiated first with an RNA primer synthesized by DNA-directed RNA polymerase at the light strand promotor (Fernandez-Silva et al., 2003). Upon reaching $O_H$, DNA polymerase γ extends the RNA primer with deoxyribonucleotides and replicates the heavy-strand (Shadel & Clayton, 1997; Fernandez-Silva et al., 2003). When the replication fork reaches $O_L$, a stem-loop structure is formed which provides access for RNA primer synthesis of the light-strand by DNA-directed RNA polymerase, followed by light-strand replication by polymerase γ (Clay Montier et al., 2009; Fuste et al., 2010).

In the bidirectional replication model, mtDNA replication is initiated bidirectionally at multiple origins (Figure 11.2C), (Bowmaker et al., 2003). This model was suggested by an analysis of replication intermediates, which initially identified not only partially single-stranded replication intermediates, indicating asynchronous displacement, but also fully duplex replication intermediates, indicating bidirectional replication (Holt et al., 2000). Subsequent analyses suggested that partially single-stranded replication intermediates may be an experimental artifact caused by degradation of RNA in RNA/DNA hybrids that appear in mtDNA replication, and that nearly all replication intermediates are RNA/DNA or DNA/DNA duplexes (Yang et al., 2002). Furthermore, two mtDNA replication initiation clusters were identified: one at the previously identified $O_H$, and another a few hundred nucleotides upstream of $O_H$ (Yasukawa et al., 2005).

The recent ribonucleotide incorporation throughout the lagging strand (RITOLS) model proposes that the lagging strand is laid down initially as RNA (Figure 11.2D), (Yasukawa et al., 2006). This model has some similarities to the asynchronous strand displacement model. A key point of conversion of nascent RNA strands to DNA is in the vicinity of $O_L$, which could explain the data that created the asynchronous model. RITOLS was furthermore supported by findings that mitochondrial DNA replication intermediates are predominantly duplex with extensive RNA tracts on one strand (Pohjoismaki et al., 2010).

Although the replication models are still under debate, they likely involve the same proteins. The polymerase γ complex, a heterotrimer consisting in humans of one catalytic subunit (polymerase γ 1) and two accessory subunits (polymerase γ 2), plays a central role in mtDNA replication (Graziewicz et al., 2006). The catalytic subunit has a polymerase domain and a 3'-5' exonuclease domain for proofreading activity. The accessory subunit is required to enhance DNA-binding activity and to support high levels

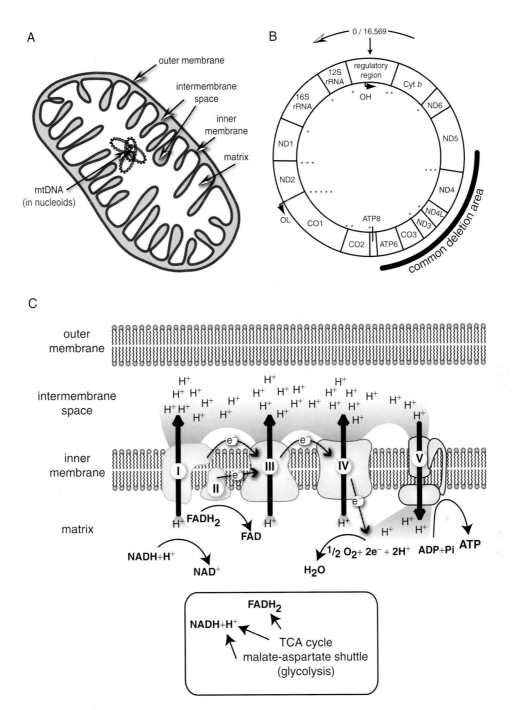

Figure 11.1 ANATOMY, GENETICS AND PHYSIOLOGY OF MITOCHONDRIA  *(A) Mitochondrial physiology:* Mitochondria share many similarities with α-proteobacteria, from which they are likely derived (Esser et al., 2004). They contain an outer and inner membrane, separated by the intermembrane space. The membranes of mitochondria are similar in lipid composition to the membranes of bacteria, while the intermembrane space is similar to the bacterial periplasm (Kutik et al., 2009). The inner membrane folds into cristae, which allow for greater space for the proteins of the mitochondrial respiratory chain, located within the inner membrane. The mitochondrial matrix contains the enzymes of the tricarboxylic acid cycle and varying numbers of mitochondrial DNA (mtDNA) are packed into nucleoids. *(B) Organization of the mtDNA plasmid*: The human mtDNA plasmid is 16,569 bp long and contains the coding sequences for 13 polypeptides of the electron transport chain, two ribosomal RNAs (rRNAs) and 22 transfer RNAs (tRNAs, denoted by stars), all contiguous and without introns (polycistronic). MtDNA has a guanine-rich heavy strand, which encodes most mitochondrial genes, and a cysteine-rich light strand, which encodes NADH dehydrogenase 6 (ND6) and a small number of tRNAs. The regulatory region contains the promoters for both strands, as well as the origin of replication for the heavy strand ($O_H$), (Tapper & Clayton, 1981). The light strand origin of replication ($O_L$) is located two-thirds of the way around the genome from $O_H$. Stars denote locations of tRNAs. The common deletion area is delineated with a black bar. *(C) The mitochondrial respiratory chain:* The five complexes of the mitochondrial respiratory chain are located in the inner mitochondrial membrane. During oxidative phosphorylation, electrons are captured from NADH in complex I, or $FADH_2$ in complex II, and shuttled through complexes III and IV. NADH and $FADH_2$ are provided by the tricarboxylic acid cycle in the mitochondrial matrix, and by the malate-aspartate shuttle, which uses NADH from cytosolic glycolysis (insert). The energy released during electron transport is used to pump protons into the intermembrane space. Four electrons are transferred to oxygen in complex IV and the protons are released through complex V, which uses the proton gradient to synthesize ATP from ADP and inorganic phosphate ($P_i$). Not shown are two molecules, ubiquinone between CI and CIII, and cytochrome c between CIII and CIV.

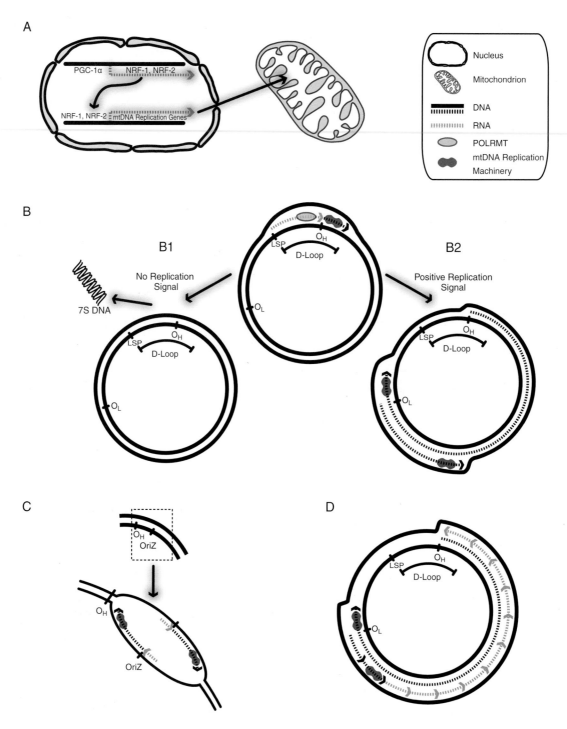

*Figure 11.2* MTDNA REPLICATION *(A)* In the nucleus, the transcription factor PGC-1α promotes the expression of nuclear respiratory factors 1 and 2, which, in turn, lead to the expression of several components of the mtDNA replication machinery, including mitochondrial transcription factor A. After protein synthesis in the cytoplasm, mtDNA replication factors encoded in the nucleus are imported into mitochondria. *(B) Asynchronous displacement*: Mitochondrial RNA polymerase (POLRMT) transcribes an RNA primer from the light strand promoter (LSP) to $O_H$, after which polymerase γ begins mtDNA replication to the end of the D-loop. *(B1)* If no signal to replicate the entire mtDNA is received, the initial DNA fragment encompassing the displacement loop (D-loop) is released as 7S DNA. *(B2)* When a signal to replicate the entire mtDNA is received, polymerase γ replicates the heavy strand until $O_L$ is reached, after which the light strand is replicated in the opposite direction. *(C) Bidirectional replication*: In this model, mitochondrial RNA polymerase transcribes an RNA primer and DNA replication begins from a zone of replication (OriZ) bidirectionally with coupled leading- and lagging-strand synthesis. *(D) Ribonucleotide incorporation throughout the lagging strand (RITOLS)*: Mitochondrial RNA polymerase transcribes an RNA primer and replication of the heavy strand begins around $O_H$. The light strand (lagging strand) is composed of RNA fragments. Once the light strand reaches $O_L$, conversion to DNA is initiated. However, conversion can also be initiated at other sites (Yasukawa et al., 2006; Krishnan et al., 2008).

of DNA synthesis. Together with mitochondrial single-strand DNA-binding protein and the mitochondrial DNA helicase Twinkle, polymerase γ forms the minimal replication machinery *in vitro* (Korhonen et al., 2004). In addition, DNA-directed RNA polymerase, which synthesizes RNA primers, and mitochondrial topoisomerase 1, which is required to unwind the supercoiled mtDNA, participate in mtDNA replication *in vivo* (Zhang et al., 2001; Fuste et al., 2010).

## TRANSCRIPTION OF MTDNA

Since mtDNA encodes crucial genes for energy production, mitochondrial transcription plays a critical role in cellular function. Polycistronic transcription, whereby one messenger RNA molecule carries the information of multiple genes and proteins, is observed in mammalian mitochondria. Transcription initiates at two heavy-strand promoters, heavy-strand promoter 1 and heavy-strand promoter 2 (also known as H1 and H2), and one light-strand promoter. Heavy-strand promoter 1 and the light-strand promoter lie in the non-coding region, and heavy-strand promoter 2 is found outside the non-coding region. When transcription is initiated at heavy-strand promoter 1, a relatively short RNA is produced, containing the two mitochondrial rRNAs (16S and 12S rRNA), and two tRNAs. In contrast, transcripts from heavy-strand promoter 2 and the light-strand promoter are long, polycistronic products. Transcription beginning at heavy-strand promoter 2 results in synthesis of the entire heavy strand mtRNA. Light-strand transcripts comprise eight tRNAs and ND6 which are synthesized by transcription starting at the light-strand promoter (Fernandez-Silva et al., 2003).

The core components required for mitochondrial transcription are known. RNA synthesis in mitochondria is mediated by DNA-directed RNA polymerase, which is a ~140 kDa single-subunit protein (Tiranti et al., 1997). The mitochondrial transcription factor A facilitates the initiation of mitochondrial transcription (Fisher et al., 1992; Parisi & Clayton, 1991), and it can wrap, unwind, and bend DNA (Thomas and Travers, 2001). The two mitochondrial transcription factors B1 and B2 are also needed to activate transcription through interaction with DNA-directed RNA polymerase and transcription factor A (Falkenberg et al., 2002; McCulloch & Shadel, 2003). It is thought that promoter-bound transcription factor A recruits DNA-directed RNA polymerase and transcription factor B1 or transcription factor B2 complexes, resulting in enhanced mitochondrial transcription.

The nuclear transcription co-activator PPARγ coactivator-1α (PGC-1α) promotes the expression of the transcription factors nuclear respiratory factors 1 and 2, which in turn promote the expression of mitochondrial oxidative phosphorylation genes and transcription and replication machinery, such as transcription factor A (Figure 11.2A), (Fernandez-Silva et al., 2003; Lee & Wei, 2005; Wallace, 2005; Clay Montier et al., 2009).

## MTDNA COPY NUMBER VARIES WITH PHYSIOLOGICAL STATE AND TISSUE TYPE

Unlike the static number of nuclear DNA copies in a cell, mtDNA copy number can vary with cell type or physical condition (Lee & Wei, 2005; Shao et al., 2008; Clay Montier et al., 2009; Clay et al., 2010). Altered physiological states, such as oxygen or nutrient deprivation or changes in pH, lead to an adjustment in mtDNA levels (Fernandez-Silva et al., 2003; Lee & Wei, 2005; Naydenov et al., 2007; Vawter et al., 2006; Shao et al., 2008). Since mtDNA replication is not restricted to a particular cell cycle stage, replication rates can be tuned to the cellular needs by balancing synthesis and degradation (Clay Montier et al., 2009).

Tissues that require large amounts of energy, including brain and muscle, contain more mitochondria and mtDNA than other cell types (Bai et al., 2004; Fattal et al., 2006; Shao et al., 2008). Within the brain, neurons require more energy than glia, and so have more mitochondria (Pysh & Khan, 1972; Galluzzi et al., 2009; Clay et al., 2010). Moreover, MtDNA levels vary among different brain regions. The cerebellum has fewer mitochondria and mtDNA copies (Pysh & Khan, 1972; Frahm et al., 2005; Clay et al., 2010), while the ventral tegmental area and substantia nigra, both of which contain dopaminergic neurons, show the highest levels of mtDNA copy number (Fuke et al., 2011).

The exact mechanism of mtDNA copy number regulation has not yet been elucidated, but it is known that transcription factor A levels correlate with mtDNA copy number, and transcription factor A knockdown causes mtDNA loss (Fernandez-Silva et al., 2003; Lee & Wei, 2005; Clay Montier et al., 2009; Gilkerson, 2009). Overexpression of transcription factor A increases mtDNA copy number and has detrimental effects *in vivo* (Ekstrand et al., 2004; Ylikallio et al., 2010). Knockdown of a transcriptional regulator of transcription factor A, PGC-1α, results in reduced mitochondrial metabolism (Kelly & Scarpulla, 2004; Wallace & Fan, 2010). Polymerase γ mutations can also result in mtDNA loss, but polymerase γ mRNA expression levels do not appear to correlate with mtDNA levels (Lee & Wei, 2005; Ashley et al., 2008; Gilkerson, 2009). During oxidative stress, mtDNA replication and degradation rates increase (Lee & Wei, 2005; Clay Montier et al., 2009). Elevated mtDNA replication during stress is accompanied by an up-regulation of nuclear respiratory factor-1 and transcription factor A (Lee & Wei, 2005), but the exact regulatory mechanisms are not fully understood. Given the complicated interaction between nuclear DNA and mtDNA, and the dynamic regulation of mtDNA copy number, a multitude of scenarios can be imagined by which mtDNA copy number and energy output can fall below optimal levels. Tissues with high energy demand, such as neurons, would be particularly sensitive and might not be able to fulfill their bioenergetic needs, particularly under metabolic stress.

## MtDNA IS NOT PROTECTED BY HISTONES, BUT IS PACKAGED INTO NUCLEOIDS

mtDNA lacks histones and is not packaged into chromatin like nuclear DNA (Kato, 2001; Clay et al., 2010). Within the mitochondrial network, mtDNA molecules are compacted into protein–DNA clusters called nucleoids (Iborra et al., 2004; Clay Montier et al., 2009; Gilkerson, 2009; Clay et al., 2010). Nucleoid organization is important for the maintenance, transcription, translation, inheritance, and segregation of mtDNA (Garrido et al., 2003; Bogenhagen et al., 2008). Similar to bacterial nucleoids, mitochondrial nucleoids attach to the inner mitochondrial membrane (Clay Montier et al., 2009). In human cell lines, each nucleoid has an average diameter of approximately 100 nm and frequently contains only a single copy of mtDNA together with many of the protein components required for mtDNA metabolism, transcription, and replication including transcription factor A, polymerase γ, Twinkle, and single-strand DNA-binding protein (Fernandez-Silva et al., 2003; Iborra et al., 2004; Legros et al., 2004; Lee & Wei, 2005; Clay Montier et al., 2009; Gilkerson, 2009; Clay et al., 2010; Kukat et al., 2011). Transcription factor A may serve a similar function as histones with nuclear DNA, covering and packaging the mtDNA molecule (Alam et al., 2003; Kaufman et al., 2007; Gilkerson, 2009).

MtDNA is particularly vulnerable to damage and mutation, with a mutation rate 10 times that of nuclear DNA (Kato & Kato, 2000; Youssoufian & Pyeritz, 2002; Fernandez-Silva et al., 2003; Wallace, 2005; Shao et al., 2008). The location of mtDNA next to the reactive oxygen species-producing complexes of the electron transport chain, and polymerase γ's limited repair abilities are contributing factors (Kato & Kato, 2000; Kato, 2001; Fernandez-Silva et al., 2003; Quiroz et al., 2008; Clay et al., 2010). The high mutation rate may be responsible for the relatively frequent rate of heteroplasmy, that is, multiple variants of mtDNA sequence within an organism (Youssoufian & Pyeritz, 2002; Wallace, 2005; He et al., 2010).

## A COMMON MtDNA DELETION ACCUMULATES IN THE BRAIN OVER TIME

In addition to inherited or acquired mtDNA point mutations, a 4,977 bp deletion, termed the "common deletion", often appears in cells with high reactive oxygen species levels or mutations in mtDNA replication factors, such as Twinkle or polymerase γ (Kato, 2005; DiMauro & Schon, 2008), (Figure 11.1B). High levels of the common deletion result in increased reactive oxygen species production at baseline and after exposure to stressors, increased rates of death after apoptotic stimuli, and decreased overall viability (Liu et al., 2004; Jou et al., 2005; Liu et al., 2007).

The common deletion is associated with a number of mitochondrial diseases and can produce myopathies and hearing and vision deficits, among other symptoms (Kato, 2005; Fattal et al., 2006). In the brain, the common deletion is reported to occur most frequently in the substantia nigra and the basal ganglia in Parkinson's disease (Bender et al., 2006; Kraytsberg et al., 2006; DiMauro & Schon, 2008; Gilkerson, 2009; McInerny et al., 2009; Naydenov et al., 2010). Accumulation of the common deletion shows age-dependency, regional variation, and sex differences in the human brain (Corral-Debrinski et al., 1992; Soong et al., 1992; Wallace, 1999; Bender et al., 2006; Kraytsberg et al., 2006; Fuke et al., 2008). Mice with increased mtDNA mutation rates have an accelerated rate of aging (Wallace & Fan, 2010). The common deletion is also found in some cancers (Wallace, 1999; Bai et al., 2004; Fattal et al., 2006; DiMauro & Schon, 2008; Mancuso et al., 2008; McInerny et al., 2009; Wang & Lu, 2009).

While researchers have examined the levels of mtDNA mutations and the common deletion in neurodegenerative diseases and brain areas associated with these disorders, it is conceivable that similar analyses in brain areas of higher function, such as cortex or hippocampus, might lead to similar findings in psychiatric disorders such as bipolar disorder.

## MITOCHONDRIA CAN BE HETEROPLASMIC AND CAUSE MOSAICISM

Mitochondrial heteroplasmy (more than one type of mtDNA in a cell) and mosaicism (cells with different variants of mtDNA) can restrict a genetic defect in mitochondria to some tissues while sparing others (Kato & Kato, 2000; Kato, 2005; Quiroz et al., 2008; Clay Montier et al., 2009; Gilkerson, 2009; He et al., 2010), (Figure 11.3A,B). Mammalian cells are polyploid for mtDNA, that is, they have multiple mtDNAs in each mitochondrion, and they have multiple mitochondria per cell (Kato & Kato, 2000; Fernandez-Silva et al., 2003; Kato, 2005; Lee & Wei, 2005; Clay Montier et al., 2009; Gilkerson, 2009). Given the presence of multiple mitochondria in each cell, mtDNA copy number can comprise 1%–10% of the cell's total DNA content (Wallace, 1999; Kato & Kato, 2000; Youssoufian & Pyeritz, 2002; Fernandez-Silva et al., 2003; Lee & Wei, 2005; Shao et al., 2008; McInerny et al., 2009; Wallace & Fan, 2010). Because mammalian cells are polyploid for mtDNA, the mitochondrial phenotype exhibited by a heteroplasmic cell depends on the gene expression pattern exhibited by the overall population of mtDNAs (Gilkerson, 2009).

During mitosis, mtDNAs randomly distribute to daughter cells (Wallace, 2005; DiMauro & Schon, 2008). If the parent cell is heteroplasmic, each daughter cell can receive an uneven share of mtDNA species (Youssoufian & Pyeritz, 2002; Wallace, 2005; DiMauro & Schon, 2008; Wallace & Fan, 2010), (Figure 11.3B). Interestingly, recent evidence shows that although some heteroplasmic variants can be inherited from the mother, many variants are due to somatic mutations that likely occur during early embryonic development (He et al., 2010). Consequently, environmental influences during development can have a significant impact on mitochondrial function of the developing embryo independent of the predicted maternal inheritance. Somatic mutations might have some impact on brain function and behavior, leading to psychiatric disorders but not to classical mitochondrial disorders.

## HETEROPLASMY AND MOSAICISM DETERMINE SYMPTOMS AND DEGREES OF PATHOLOGY IN INHERITED MITOCHONDRIAL DISEASES

In the case of heteroplasmy with disease-causing mutations, daughter cells may arise with large proportions of mutant mtDNA, resulting in cell-specific mitochondrial pathology. During embryogenesis, large sections of tissue can become enriched with mutant mtDNA, while other sections are spared, leading to mosaicism (Youssoufian & Pyeritz, 2002), (Figure 11.3C). In inherited mitochondrial disorders, offspring with the same mtDNA mutation may exhibit different mitochondrial disease symptoms due not only to differences in the tissues affected by the mutation, but also due to the varying proportion of mutated founder mtDNA in the oocyte or early cell division state (Figure 11.3), (Marchington et al., 1998; Wallace, 1999; He et al., 2010). Within a given range of mutation load, wild-type mtDNA can compensate for the deficient gene expression of mutant mtDNAs (DiMauro & Schon, 2008). In the case of the mitochondrial disorder MELAS (mitochondrial myopathy, encephalopathy, lactic acidosis, and stroke), normal levels of oxygen consumption in cells are maintained with only 10% of wild-type mtDNA. Once the mutation load exceeds the threshold by which the remaining wild-type mtDNA copies can compensate for mutant mtDNAs, the cell's mitochondrial function becomes deficient, and the cell becomes symptomatic for mitochondrial pathology (Wallace, 1999; Youssoufian & Pyeritz, 2002; Wallace, 2005; Gilkerson, 2009; Wallace & Fan, 2010). While a higher ratio of wild-type to mutated mtDNA might not lead to overt pathology, it could still affect cellular function and diminish the capacity to produce ATP. Neurons, with their high energy demand, might be unable to consistently maintain their membrane potential if ATP production is insufficient, resulting in abnormal neuronal function.

## MITOCHONDRIAL ENERGY PRODUCTION AND THE ELECTRON TRANSPORT CHAIN

The most prominent function of mitochondria is ATP production via the respiratory chain. The respiratory chain uses energy from oxidation of molecules derived from dietary substances to synthesize ATP, and it consists of five protein complexes located in the inner mitochondrial membrane (Figure 11.1C), (Shao et al., 2008). Each respiratory chain complex is an assembly of multiple protein subunits, most of which are encoded in nuclear DNA (Wallace & Fan, 2010). Complexes I, III, IV, and V also contain mtDNA-encoded subunits (Wallace & Fan, 2010). In the cytosol, dietary carbohydrates are metabolized to pyruvate through glycolysis. Pyruvate is transferred into mitochondria and converted to acetyl-CoA, a metabolite that enters the tricarboxylic acid cycle in the mitochondrial matrix. The tricarboxylic acid cycle produces the electron donors NADH and $FADH_2$. Electrons are removed

## A, heteroplasmy within mitochondria

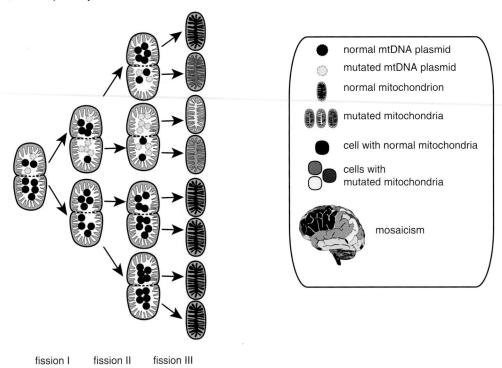

fission I  fission II  fission III

## B, heteroplasmy within cells

## C, mosaicism in the brain

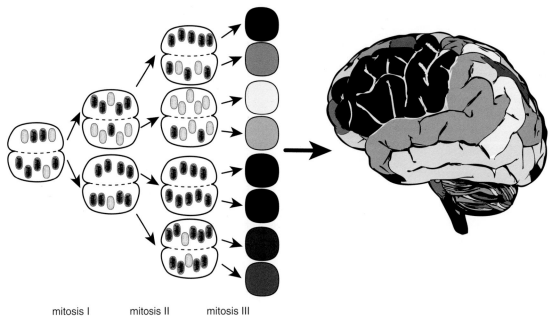

mitosis I  mitosis II  mitosis III

*Figure 11.3* HETEROPLASMY AND MOSAICISM  Because each mitochondrion contains typically 5 to 10 copies of mtDNA, and each cell can have hundreds of mitochondria (Legros et al., 2004), mtDNA variants with different polymorphisms can populate the same mitochondrion (A), the same cell (B), and the same organism. Recently developed high-throughput sequencing techniques have led to the realization that this heteroplasmy is more frequent than previously assumed, and often occurs *de novo* during early embryonic development (He et al., 2010). Uneven distribution of these mtDNA variants can lead to mosaicism (C), that is, the presence of genetically distinct cell lines in a single individual or organ. Though many mtDNA variants are not disease-causing, we chose an example of a disease-causing variant (mutation) creating mosaicism in the brain.

from NADH or FADH$_2$ and shuttled through the complexes of the electron transport chain until they combine with oxygen in complex IV (Figure 11.1C). The energy released by electron transport is used to generate a proton gradient across the mitochondrial inner membrane. Protons move down the gradient into the matrix through ATP synthase, releasing the energy needed to synthesize ATP from ADP and inorganic phosphate (P$_i$) (Figure 11.1C).

## MITOCHONDRIA PRODUCE AND SCAVENGE REACTIVE OXYGEN SPECIES

Electrons that are released prematurely from the electron transport chain combine with molecular oxygen to produce the superoxide anion (Wallace, 2005). The superoxide anion, along with hydrogen peroxide and the hydroxyl radical are the main reactive oxygen species, which damage lipids, proteins, and nucleic acids and increase mutation rates (Wallace, 1999; Ouyang & Giffard, 2004; Kato, 2005; Lee and Wei, 2005; Wallace, 2005; Quiroz et al., 2008; Shao et al., 2008; Wallace & Fan, 2010). In the normal state, 1%–5% of all oxygen consumed by mitochondria contributes to the formation of reactive oxygen species (Ouyang & Giffard, 2004; Lee & Wei, 2005). Electron transport chain inhibition or nutrient overload increases reactive oxygen species production rates, leading to premature release of electrons from the electron transport chain (Russell et al., 2002; Ouyang & Giffard, 2004; Lee & Wei, 2005; Wallace, 2005; Wallace & Fan, 2010). Conversely, nutrient deprivation can also lead to reactive oxygen species production (Isaev et al., 2008). Antioxidant enzymes such as manganese superoxide dismutase, copper/zinc superoxide dismutase, or glutathione peroxidase detoxify reactive oxygen species (Wallace, 1999; Lee & Wei, 2005; Wallace, 2005; Wallace & Fan, 2010). Knockout of these enzymes makes cells more susceptible to apoptotic cell death, while overexpression of antioxidant enzymes increases cellular resilience (Galluzzi et al., 2009). When the level of reactive oxygen species production exceeds the rate of detoxification, the cell experiences oxidative stress and a reduced capacity to generate ATP (Wallace, 1999; Ouyang & Giffard, 2004; Yuan, 2006; Quiroz et al., 2010; Wallace & Fan, 2010).

## MITOCHONDRIA BUFFER INTRACELLULAR CALCIUM LEVELS

Mitochondria, like the endoplasmic reticulum, are critical for maintaining calcium dynamics in the cell (Kato, 2008).

Mitochondrial calcium uptake is mediated by the mitochondrial calcium uniporter (Kato & Kato, 2000; Kato, 2005; Rizzuto & Pozzan, 2006; Wallace & Fan, 2010), which has a low affinity for calcium and only takes up calcium when levels are significantly elevated (Orrenius et al., 2003; Ouyang & Giffard, 2004; De Stefani et al, 2011; Baughman et al, 2011). Calcium is released through inositol trisphosphate receptors on the endoplasmic reticulum and high calcium concentrations are achieved in microdomains between endoplasmic reticulum and mitochondria. Through these microdomains, the mitochondrial calcium uniporter is exposed to locally high calcium concentrations and takes up calcium into the mitochondria (Orrenius et al., 2003; Quiroz et al., 2010).

Mitochondrial calcium uptake prevents cytosolic calcium concentrations from reaching toxic levels, but it can quickly have deleterious effects on the mitochondria (Clay et al., 2010). Calcium is pumped out of the mitochondria by the sodium-calcium exchanger, but when calcium levels overwhelm the exchanger, the mitochondrial permeability transition pore opens and the mitochondrial membrane potential is lost (Figure 11.4), (Kato & Kato, 2000; Kato, 2005; Shalbuyeva et al., 2007; Stelmashook et al., 2009; Quiroz et al., 2010). High mitochondrial calcium concentrations can also induce production of reactive oxygen species (Brown & Yamamoto, 2003). Loss of the mitochondrial membrane potential or excessive reactive oxygen species production leads to release of cytotoxic molecules from the mitochondria followed by apoptosis (Figure 11.4), (Orrenius et al., 2003; Ouyang & Giffard, 2004; Kato, 2005). Milder versions of calcium dysregulation and reactive oxygen species production might cause cell stress and reduced ATP production. In the brain, calcium is involved in synaptic plasticity and neurotransmitter release, and calcium dysregulation could have deleterious consequences for neuronal functions (Kato, 2008). Calcium can quickly overwhelm a neuron that is hyperactivated by excitatory neurotransmitters (Szydlowska & Tymianski, 2010). Consequently, calcium, excitotoxicity and deficient bioenergetic mechanisms combine to cause neuronal malfunction.

## MITOCHONDRIA ARE IMPORTANT MEDIATORS OF APOPTOSIS

Apoptosis, or programmed cell death (Wallace, 2005; Clay Montier et al., 2009), can be initiated either by the stimulation of cell-surface death receptors or by release of cytochrome c and other apoptosis-inducing proteins from the mitochondria (Yuan, 2006; Galluzzi et al., 2009; Hotchkiss et al., 2009). Mitochondria respond to pro-apoptosis

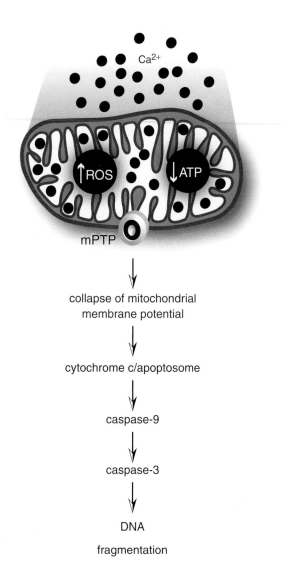

Ca²⁺

↑ROS   ↓ATP

mPTP

↓

collapse of mitochondrial
membrane potential

↓

cytochrome c/apoptosome

↓

caspase-9

↓

caspase-3

↓

DNA

fragmentation

*Figure 11.4* CALCIUM (CA²⁺), REACTIVE OXYGEN SPECIES (ROS) AND THE DIMINISHED CAPACITY TO GENERATE ATP CAN CAUSE APOPTOSIS Excessive calcium influx can induce reactive oxygen species production and reduce the cell's capacity to generate ATP. Each of these conditions can interchangeably trigger the others and lead to the opening of the mitochondrial permeability transition pore (mPTP) and disruption of the mitochondrial membrane potential. Mitochondrial swelling and bursting causes release of cytotoxic molecules from the mitochondria. In the cytosol, cytochrome c and apoptotic protease activating factor 1 combine with ATP to form the apoptosome, which proteolytically activates caspase-9. Caspase-9 activates caspase-3, which causes DNA fragmentation and degradation of the cytoskeleton.

signals such as nutrient deprivation, nutrient overload, reduced electron transport chain function, oxidative stress, or high mitochondrial calcium levels by opening the mito-chondrial permeability transition pore (Wallace, 1999; Russell et al., 2002; Orrenius et al., 2003; Ouyang and Giffard, 2004; Kato, 2005; Wallace, 2005; Galluzzi et al., 2009; Hotchkiss et al., 2009; Stelmashook et al., 2009; Wallace & Fan, 2010). The mitochondrial permeability

transition pore is a protein complex composed of cyclophi-lin D, the adenine nucleotide translocator and the voltage-dependent anion channel (porin), and is found at sites of close apposition of the inner and outer mitochondrial membranes (Orrenius et al., 2003; Kato, 2005; Wallace, 2005; Yuan, 2006; Galluzzi et al., 2009). Opening of the mitochondrial permeability transition pore abolishes the mitochondrial membrane potential and ATP production (Ouyang & Giffard, 2004; Wallace, 2005; Shalbuyeva et al., 2007; Quiroz et al., 2008; Galluzzi et al., 2009; Wallace & Fan, 2010). Opening of the mitochondrial permeability transition pore also causes mitochondria to swell and burst, and to release pro-apoptotic molecules such as cytochrome c, endonuclease G, apoptosis-inducing factor, and procas-pases (Figure 4), (Wallace, 1999; Ouyang and Giffard, 2004; Wallace, 2005; Quiroz et al., 2008; Clay Montier et al., 2009; Galluzzi et al., 2009; Wallace & Fan, 2010). In the cytosol, cytochrome c and apoptotic protease activating factor 1 (APAF1) combine with ATP to form the apopto-some, which proteolytically activates caspase-9 (Wallace, 2005; Yuan, 2006; Hotchkiss et al., 2009). Caspase-9 is an initiator caspase, which activates caspase-3, an executioner caspase (Galluzzi et al., 2009; Hotchkiss et al., 2009).

## Facts about Mitochondria with Implications for Bipolar Disorder

- Mitochondria meet cellular energy requirements and manage cellular stress.

- Mitochondria have their own DNA, which is liable to mutations and is close to a major source of reactive oxygen species.

- The majority of proteins needed for mitochondrial function are encoded in the nuclear genome, requiring highly regulated communication between the nuclear genome and mitochondria. This communication presents points for potential disruption.

- MtDNA mutations can be unevenly distributed during embryogenesis, causing selective accumulation in some cells while sparing others.

- If mtDNA mutations selectively accumulate in parts of the brain, it is difficult to trace in diagnostic tests.

- Because the brain is uniquely dependent on mitochondria for its energy requirements and cellular health, minor disruptions in mitochondrial function have the potential to lead to selective disturbances in affective networks.

Caspase-3 mediates the events that lead to apoptotic cell death, such as DNA fragmentation and degradation of the cytoskeleton (Orrenius et al., 2003; Yuan, 2006; Chipuk & Green, 2008; Galluzzi et al., 2009; Hotchkiss et al., 2009; Clay et al., 2010).

## SIMILARITIES BETWEEN MITOCHONDRIAL DISORDERS AND BIPOLAR DISORDER

Mutations in mitochondria-related genes, whether in the nuclear genome or mtDNA, can result in mitochondrial disease (Kato, 2001; Young, 2007; Shao et al., 2008; Wallace & Fan, 2010). Point mutations of mtDNA are maternally inherited, although it is known that mtDNA mutations can also appear *de novo* (Danan et al., 1999; Lebon et al., 2003; Pulkes et al., 2003; McFarland et al., 2004; He et al., 2010). Mitochondrial disorders caused by mutations in nuclear DNA are inherited in a Mendelian fashion (Kato & Kato, 2000; Campos et al., 2001; Kato, 2005; Fattal et al., 2006; DiMauro & Schon, 2008; Wallace & Fan, 2010). Mutations of nuclear genes can cause secondary mutations in mtDNA. Due to heteroplasmy and random segregation of mutant and wild-type mtDNAs to daughter cells, mitochondrial diseases can appear in a tissue-specific or mosaic pattern, and may affect only a few cells or cells types (Kato, 2001; Wallace, 2005; Ashley et al., 2008). Mitochondrial diseases affect most commonly brain, pancreas and muscle-tissues with high energy demands (Prayson & Wang, 1998; Youssoufian & Pyeritz, 2002; Wallace, 2005; Fattal et al., 2006; Shao et al., 2008). Due to reduced oxidative phosphorylation and ATP production, common symptoms of mitochondrial disease include seizures, retinal degeneration, encephalopathy, myopathy, exercise intolerance, hearing loss and diabetes (Prayson & Wang, 1998; Wallace, 1999; Kato & Kato, 2000; Silva et al., 2000; Campos et al., 2001; Kato, 2001; Sorensen et al., 2001; Wredenberg et al., 2002; Siciliano et al., 2003; Bai et al., 2004; Wallace, 2005; Fattal et al., 2006; Grover et al., 2006; Ashley et al., 2008; DiMauro & Schon, 2008; Mancuso et al., 2008; Rocher et al., 2008; Clay Montier et al., 2009).

Of particular interest is the high prevalence of mood disturbances and psychiatric conditions in mitochondrial diseases (Prayson & Wang, 1998; Kato & Kato, 2000; Kato, 2001; Siciliano et al., 2003; Fattal et al., 2006; Grover et al., 2006; DiMauro & Schon, 2008; Mancuso et al., 2008; Shao et al., 2008). Because the enzymes needed for β-oxidation, an alternative to oxidative phosphorylation, have low activity in the brain, disturbances of electron transport can severely affect brain function (Yang et al., 1987). Depression is commonly associated with chronic progressive external ophthalmoplegia (CPEO), (Shao et al., 2008), a mitochondrial disease that presents with ptosis and progressive bilateral ocular immobility (Caballero et al., 2007). Individuals with mitochondrial illnesses also have a higher rate of relatives with mood disturbances or psychosis (Campos et al., 2001; Boles et al., 2005; DiMauro & Schon, 2008; Mancuso et al., 2008). Like bipolar disorder, many mitochondrial diseases do not appear until early adulthood (Wallace, 1999 2005), and bipolar disorder patients have higher rates of diabetes, a condition associated with mitochondrial abnormalities (Kato & Kato, 2000).

In addition to overlapping symptoms, a subset of bipolar disorder patients shows matrilineal inheritance (Gershon et al., 1982; McMahon et al., 1995; Kato et al., 1996; Kato & Kato, 2000; Kornberg et al., 2000; Kato, 2007 2008), although this finding has not been consistently observed (Kato et al., 1996; Kirk et al., 1999; Kornberg et al., 2000; Lan et al., 2007). Lack of matrilineal inheritance does not exclude mitochondrial pathology in bipolar disorder since many mitochondrial proteins are encoded in the nucleus, mtDNA mutations can be acquired during early embryogenesis (He et al., 2010), and heteroplasmy could affect different tissues in parents and offspring, (Wallace, 2005; Clay et al., 2010).

It is not known whether the pathophysiology of bipolar disorder overlaps with classical mitochondrial diseases. Mosaicism would restrict mtDNA mutations to a subset of tissues, which in some cases might include brain tissue. These factors are more difficult to assess and could in some cases have their predominant impact in brain areas involved in mood regulation. The energy demands of different neuronal subtypes and their selective exposure to oxidative stressors could determine the degree to which mtDNA

**Similarities between Bipolar Disorder and Mitochondrial Disease**

- Bona fide mitochondrial disorders have a high prevalence of mood disturbances and psychiatric conditions

- A subset of bipolar disorder patients shows matrilineal inheritance, suggesting an involvement of mitochondrial-encoded genes

- Lack of matrilineal inheritance does not exclude mitochondrial pathology in bipolar disorder

- Brain areas involved in mood regulation might be particularly vulnerable to fluctuations in ATP levels

mutations affect their function, particularly in the presence of aberrant mtDNA maintenance systems. Brain regions that modulate mood may be more vulnerable to these factors and manifest clinically as bipolar disorder.

## MTDNA VARIANTS AND BIPOLAR DISORDER

Based on findings that maternal inheritance may be involved in the transmission of bipolar disorder, the whole mtDNA genome was sequenced in nine probands from maternally transmitted pedigrees of bipolar disorder probands (McMahon et al., 2000). No statistically significant differences in the frequency of any variants between probands and healthy comparison subjects was found, but four variants showed odds ratios higher than 2 or lower than 0.5. In a similar study, the mtDNA of 25 probands from bipolar disorder pedigrees in which maternal transmission was suspected was sequenced and examined for polymorphisms. Polymorphisms identified more than once were examined in association studies of 94 bipolar disorder cases and healthy subjects, but did not yield any significant findings (Kirk et al., 1999).

Kato and colleagues found that the mtDNA single-nucleotide polymorphism 10,398A was associated with bipolar disorder (Kato et al., 2001). Interestingly, mtDNA 10,398A was one of the four variants nominally associated with bipolar disorder in a study by McMahon et al. (McMahon et al., 2000). In a comprehensive search for mtDNA variants with functional significance, this variant was found to elevate mitochondrial calcium levels (Kazuno et al., 2006). However, association of this variant with bipolar disorder was not replicated in an independent sample set (Munakata et al., 2004). A haplogroup analysis (group of similar mtDNA sequences that share a common ancestor) showed that haplogroup N9a was over-represented in bipolar disorder. The mtDNA 12,358G variant that characterizes the N9a haplogroup and increases cytosolic calcium levels was associated with bipolar disorder in the initial sample set, but it was not replicated in an independent sample set (Kazuno et al., 2009).

Munakata and colleagues sequenced the mtDNA of six patients with bipolar I disorder who had somatic symptoms suggestive of mitochondrial disease (Munakata et al., 2004). Among the variants identified in these cases, mtDNA 3644C was associated with bipolar I disorder, which was confirmed in an extended sample set. This variant is rare, but is found throughout East Asia (Kong et al., 2006). MtDNA 3644C was found to decrease mitochondrial membrane potential, and may have pathophysiological significance.

Whereas in the previously mentioned studies mutations affected all mtDNA plasmids within an organism, in many cases mutations may only affect a subset of mtDNA. These heteroplasmic mtDNA mutations include point mutations and large-scale deletions or duplications. Accumulation of mtDNA deletions is a hallmark of chronic progressive external ophthalmoplegia (CPEO), which can be accompanied by mood disorders (Suomalainen et al., 1992; Siciliano et al., 2003; Shao et al., 2008). The levels of mtDNA deletions in the brains of patients with bipolar disorder and depression were found to be normal when analyzed by Southern blot (Stine et al., 1993), but a highly sensitive PCR method used in the same brain samples found increases in the number of mtDNA deletions in brains of subjects with bipolar disorder (Kato et al., 1997).

Two groups studied the levels of mtDNA deletions in Stanley Foundation brain bank samples, which includes bipolar subjects, but did not find an accumulation of the common deletion (Kakiuchi et al., 2005; Sabunciyan et al., 2007; Fuke et al., 2008). On the other hand, Shao and colleagues found that the common deletion of mtDNA was accumulated in the postmortem brains of patients with bipolar disorder (Shao et al., 2008).

Whereas homoplasmic mtDNA variants and heteroplasmic point mutations in mtDNA are usually maternally transmitted, deletions of mtDNA can be caused secondary to mutations in nuclear genes related to mtDNA maintenance. The causative genes of mtDNA deletion syndrome include polymerase γ 1, adenine nucleotide translocator 1, Twinkle, polymerase γ 2, OPA1, and ribonucleotide reductase M2B. Among them, mutations of polymerase γ 1,

---

**mtDNA Variants are Associated with Bipolar Disorder**

- A number of mtDNA mutations have been associated with bipolar disorder

- Variants associated with bipolar disorder affect intracellular calcium signaling and mitochondrial membrane potential

- The percentage of mtDNA deletions in the brains of subjects with bipolar disorder and depression has been found to be increased

- The number of subjects in these studies was small and results have been difficult to replicate

adenine nucleotide translocator 1, Twinkle and ribonucleotide reductase M2B are associated with CPEO and its accompanying mood disorder.

## ALTERED MITOCHONDRIAL GENE AND PROTEIN EXPRESSION IN BIPOLAR DISORDER

The expression of mitochondrial genes and proteins encoded in the nucleus is reportedly altered in bipolar disorder. In the prefrontal cortex, several components of the electron transport chain were down-regulated in bipolar disorder (Iwamoto et al., 2005; Sun et al., 2006; Kato, 2007; Andreazza et al., 2010; Konradi et al., 2011a). In hippocampus, 43% of all down-regulated genes in bipolar disorder samples were mitochondria-related, including a majority of genes of the respiratory chain (Konradi et al., 2004). Analysis of postmortem brains showed the confounding effects of medication and sample pH (Iwamoto et al., 2005). However, preliminary evidence suggests that these effects were not due to medication, although more detailed studies in unmedicated bipolar disorder patients are needed for solid evidence.

The expression of nuclear-encoded mitochondria-related genes can be affected by brain pH, which was significantly lower in some brain bank samples (Iwamoto et al., 2005; Sun et al., 2006). Brain pH tends to be lower in bipolar than healthy subjects, presumably due to a shift from oxidative phosphorylation to glycolysis to maintain adequate levels of ATP production (Stork & Renshaw, 2005; Shao et al., 2008). The imbalance between glycolysis and oxidative phosphorylation can lead to to accumulation of lactic acid, the acidification of tissue, and a decrease in pH (Konradi et al., 2011a). When corrected for pH, bipolar disorder brain samples still exhibited reductions in a number of mitochondria-related genes (Iwamoto et al., 2005; Vawter et al., 2006), although the data are less strong, because the removal of samples with low pH excludes samples with the most pronounced downregulation of mitochondria-related genes and shift to glycolysis. Moreover, in a study that showed global down-regulation of mitochondria-related genes in the hippocampus, there was no significant difference in cerebellum pH between the brains of healthy and bipolar disorder subjects (Konradi et al., 2004). It is possible that low sample pH is a reflection of the pathophysiology of bipolar disorder (Sun et al., 2006), although this suggestion is still controversial (Vawter et al., 2006).

Alternative tissue types were examined to circumvent some of the issues affecting post-mortem samples, such as changes in pH. Using this approach, it was shown that lymphocytes from bipolar patients exhibit an abnormal mitochondria-related gene expression response to low-glucose stress: While control lymphocytes upregulated nuclear-encoded mitochondrial genes during low-glucose stress, lymphocytes from bipolar disorder subjects had no change in mitochondria-related gene expression (Naydenov et al., 2007). These observations cast some light on the findings of reduced mitochondria-related gene expression in the hippocampus of bipolar patients (Konradi et al., 2004) and suggest that agonal and post-mortem events might have led to increased levels of mitochondrial mRNAs in healthy brains, whereas bipolar disorder tissue failed to respond similarly. Consequently, different levels of mitochondrial gene expression in the hippocampus might not be caused by a down-regulation of mitochondrial genes in bipolar patients, but rather may reflect an inability of bipolar disorder tissue to up-regulate these genes in response to perimortem hypoxia. The hypothesis of the normal response is in line with the observation that mtDNA replication, too, is increased by agonal events (Shao et al., 2008).

**Evidence for Altered Mitochondria-related Gene Expression in Bipolar Disorder**

- Genes and proteins involved in mitochondrial respiration are altered in brains of bipolar subjects

- Indicators of energy production and reserves are diminished in bipolar subjects

- Cells from bipolar subjects respond abnormally to energy deprivation

## ALTERED ENERGY METABOLISM IN BIPOLAR DISORDER SUBJECTS

In addition to changes in mitochondrial gene expression, abnormalities in mitochondrial function have been observed in bipolar disorder (Frey et al., 2007; Kato, 2008). In the prefrontal cortex of bipolar patients, the activities of electron transport chain complexes were reduced (Andreazza et al., 2010). Magnetic resonance spectroscopy (MRS) studies demonstrated reductions in high-energy phosphates in the brains of bipolar disorder patients (Kato et al., 1998; Kato & Kato, 2000; Kato, 2001, 2005; Stork & Renshaw, 2005; Young, 2007; Quiroz et al., 2008; Schloesser et al., 2008; Shao et al., 2008). Phosphocreatine, a molecule that stores and transports high-energy phosphates from sites of ATP production to sites of ATP consumption, and creatine kinase, the enzyme involved in creatine metabolism, were also decreased in the brains of bipolar disorder patients (Deicken et al., 1995; Dager et al., 2004; MacDonald et al., 2006; Frey et al., 2007; Ongur et al., 2009).

Mitochondrial morphology is also abnormal in bipolar disorder: Electron microscopy studies of prefrontal cortex and caudate found swollen and bulky mitochondria, with an overall reduction in mitochondrial number (Cataldo et al., 2010) as compared with healthy subjects. Fibroblasts and lymphocytes of patients with bipolar disorder also showed altered distribution within the cell (Cataldo et al., 2010).

## INCREASED OXIDATIVE STRESS, CALCIUM DYSREGULATION AND APOPTOSIS IN THE TISSUE OF BIPOLAR DISORDER SUBJECTS

Bipolar disorder patients showed increased markers of oxidative stress in prefrontal cortex and in anterior cingulate cortex (Wang et al., 2009; Andreazza et al., 2010). Reactive oxygen species in prefrontal cortex correlate negatively with complex I activity, independent of medication status, indicating a link between excess reactive oxygen species activity and electron transport chain dysfunction in a brain area important for the pathophysiology of bipolar illness (Andreazza et al., 2010).

Calcium dysregulation is a well-replicated finding in bipolar disorder. Platelets and lymphocytes from bipolar disorder patients have elevated calcium levels both at baseline and after stimulation (Dubovsky et al., 1992; Kusumi et al., 1992; Kato et al., 2003). As discussed above, an mtDNA polymorphism, 10,398A, reportedly associated with bipolar disorder and neurodegenerative disorders, altered baseline calcium levels (Kazuno et al., 2006; Kato, 2008; Kazuno et al., 2009). Elevated calcium levels were seen in cultured lymphoblastoid cell lines from bipolar disorder patients, indicating that calcium dysregulation is independent of medication and affective state (Kato et al., 2003; Wasserman et al., 2004; Kato, 2008). The calcium abnormality may be specific to bipolar disorder type I, as higher baseline calcium levels were not seen in bipolar patients (Emamghoreishi et al., 1997). Interestingly, bipolar disorder-associated calcium abnormalities returned to healthy control levels after lithium treatment (Wasserman et al., 2004). Calcium abnormalities seem to be specific for mood disorders and were not seen in non-affective psychiatric diseases (Emamghoreishi et al., 1997).

Since deficits in mitochondrial function can lead to apoptotic cell death, brain volumes could be decreased in bipolar disorder. Magnetic resonance imaging (MRI) studies of bipolar disorder patients showed enlarged ventricles and reduced frontal gray matter and basal ganglia volumes (Lyoo et al., 2004; Young, 2007; Quiroz et al., 2008; Schloesser et al., 2008; Machado-Vieira et al., 2009). Recent meta-analyses showed reduced volume of anterior cingulate and insular cortices (Bora et al., 2010; Ellison-Wright & Bullmore, 2010). At the cellular level, bipolar patients exhibited reductions in prefrontal cortical thickness and in the numbers of GAD-65- and GAD-67-positive GABAergic interneurons in the hippocampus (Vawter et al., 2000; Heckers et al., 2002; Konradi et al., 2004; Konradi et al., 2011b). Counts of nonpyramidal hippocampal neurons also indicate cell loss in bipolar disorder (Benes et al., 1998; Knable et al., 2004; Konradi et al., 2011b). Interestingly, glial densities are reduced in the prefrontal cortex of brains of bipolar disorder patients as well (Vawter et al., 2000; MacDonald et al., 2006; Schloesser et al., 2008; Machado-Vieira et al., 2009). Finally, n-acetyl-aspartate (NAA) is a marker of neuronal and glial metabolism and an indicator of neuronal density (Ouyang and Giffard, 2004; Quiroz et al., 2008; Shao et al., 2008), and NAA peaks were reduced in the frontal cortex and hippocampus in bipolar disorder compared with healthy subjects (Kato, 2005; Quiroz et al., 2008; Shao et al., 2008).

> **Several Mitochondria-related Functions Are Abnormal in Bipolar Disorder**
>
> - Energy metabolism is altered in bipolar disorder
> - Bipolar disorder samples exhibit disturbed calcium homeostasis
> - Oxidative stress and apoptosis are enhanced in bipolar disorder
> - Mitochondrial morphology is altered in bipolar disorder

## MITOCHONDRIA IN ANIMAL MODELS OF BIPOLAR DISORDER

As of yet, there is no established animal model for bipolar disorder. Rather, most laboratories model mania and depression separately, and a number of these models affect mitochondrial function (Kato et al., 2007; Chen et al., 2010; Clay et al., 2010). A commonly used mania model, amphetamine exposure, impairs mitochondrial electron transport chain function (Valvassori et al., 2010). Amphetamine administration reduced activities of complexes II, III, and

IV in hippocampus, prefrontal cortex and striatum, an effect that was reversible by treatment with either of the mood stabilizers valproic acid or lithium (Valvassori et al., 2010).

Other animal models manipulate genes regulated by lithium treatment such as GSK-3β, which promotes expression of pro-apoptosis proteins. A 40% knockdown of the gene for the anti-apoptosis protein Bcl-2 in mice resulted in an increase in anxiety-related behavioral phenotypes (Einat et al., 2005). Overexpression of Bcl-2-associated athanogene 1 (BAG1), a protein that promotes cell survival through interaction with Bcl-2, resulted in decreased anxiety in mice (Schloesser et al., 2008; Chen et al., 2010), while heterozygous BAG1 knockout mice did not recover from helplessness behavior at the same rate as their wild-type controls (Maeng et al., 2008).

Kasahara et al. created a mouse with a brain-specific polymerase γ mutation that abolished its 3'-to-5' exonuclease activity (Kasahara et al., 2006; Kasahara et al., 2008). The resultant phenotype included accelerated mtDNA mutation rate and increases in the occurrence of the common mtDNA deletion (Kasahara et al., 2006; Kasahara et al., 2008). Polymerase γ mutant mice exhibited abnormal circadian rhythms that improved with lithium treatment, electroconvulsive shock, or cyclophilin D inhibition (Kasahara et al., 2006; Kasahara et al., 2008; Kubota et al., 2010). Polymerase γ mutant mice showed no alteration in mitochondrial membrane potential, but did have higher calcium uptake rates (Kubota et al., 2006; Kato et al., 2007).

> **Mitochondrial Changes in Animal Models of Bipolar Disorder**
>
> - There are no established animal models of bipolar disorder
> - Most animal models employ pharmacological probes to study mania, or mood stabilizers to study their mechanism of action
> - Polymerase γ mutant mice display bipolar disorder-like behaviors
> - More transgenic animal models are needed to study the effect of mitochondrial dysfunction on mood regulation

## MOOD STABILIZERS INCREASE MITOCHONDRIAL FUNCTION

Lithium and valproic acid are two of the more commonly used mood stabilizers in the treatment of bipolar disorder.

Improvement happens gradually, suggesting that gene and protein expression changes are components of their mechanisms of action (Wasserman et al., 2004; Quiroz et al., 2008; Schloesser et al., 2008).

Lithium and valproic acid both exhibit neuroprotective effects and prevent apoptosis (Chuang, 2005; Lai et al., 2006; Michaelis et al., 2006; Schloesser et al., 2008; Pietruczuk et al., 2009). These effects are at least partially mediated through mitochondria. Lithium and valproic acid were found to upregulate Bcl-2, an antiapoptotic protein on the mitochondrial outer membrane, after treatment in frontal cortex, anterior cingulate cortex, hippocampus, and striatum (Chen et al., 1999; Wei et al., 2001; Schloesser et al., 2008; Quiroz et al., 2010). Lithium also reportedly upregulates nuclear respiratory factor-1, nuclear respiratory factor-2, and transcription factor A, which correlates with an increase in mitochondria-related mRNA levels and mtDNA copy number (Struewing et al., 2007). Lithium and valproic acid increased the expression of electron transport chain subunits, as well as the activities of electron transport chain complexes in rat prefrontal cortex, hippocampus, and striatum (Maurer et al., 2009; Valvassori et al., 2010). In bipolar disorder patients, lithium treatment increased expression of complex I subunits in the prefrontal cortex, and valproic acid-treated lymphoblastoids showed increased expression of the complex I subunit gene NDUFV2 (Sun et al., 2006; Washizuka et al., 2009). Along with enhanced activities of individual mitochondrial enzymes, lithium and valproic acid increased overall respiratory chain activity, as evidenced by increased oxygen consumption and ATP production (Plant et al., 2002; Struewing et al., 2007; Young, 2007; Bachmann et al., 2009). Lithium and valproic acid support the mitochondrial membrane potential in culture (Shalbuyeva et al., 2007; Struewing et al., 2007; Bachmann et al., 2009; Pietruczuk et al., 2009), and they stimulate the ERK/MAPK pathway, which results in upregulation of cell survival factors such as Bcl-2 and brain-derived neurotrophic factor (BDNF), (Chen & Chuang, 1999; Michaelis et al., 2006; Young, 2007; Schloesser et al., 2008; Machado-Vieira et al., 2009; Quiroz et al., 2010). Lithium and valproic acid inhibit GSK-3 and downregulate p53, molecules that promote apoptosis (Chen & Chuang, 1999; King et al., 2001; Bezchlibnyk & Young, 2002; Yuan, 2006; Quiroz et al., 2008; Schloesser et al., 2008; Galluzzi et al., 2009; Machado-Vieira et al., 2009; Quiroz et al., 2010). Furthermore, mood stabilizers have antioxidant effects, upregulating the expression of the enzyme glutathione-S-transferase, and reducing hydrogen peroxide production at baseline and during calcium-mediated stress (Wang et al.,

2004; Shalbuyeva et al., 2007; Young, 2007; Machado-Vieira et al., 2009).

Additionally, lithium regulates intracellular calcium dynamics, preventing excess calcium release from the endoplasmic reticulum and enhancing mitochondrial calcium uptake capacity (Kato and Kato, 2000; Shalbuyeva et al., 2007). Lithium reduces peak calcium responses in B-lymphoblastoid cell lines of both healthy and bipolar disorder subjects after stimulation with thapsigargin or lysophosphatidic acid (Wasserman et al., 2004). The normally elevated calcium responses seen in B-lymphoblastoid cell lines of bipolar disorder patients were at normal control levels after lithium treatment (Wasserman et al., 2004). Lithium also protects cells from calcium-mediated damage such as membrane depolarization and swelling (Shalbuyeva et al., 2007). Lithium and valproic acid prevent cytochrome c and caspase release from mitochondria after calcium treatment, respiratory chain inhibition, amphetamine administration, or glutamate exposure (Chen & Chuang, 1999; King et al., 2001; Lai et al., 2006; Michaelis et al., 2006; Shalbuyeva et al., 2007; Bachmann et al., 2009). These effects are likely the result of Bcl-2 upregulation and Bax downregulation, two factors involved in promoting cell survival and cell death, respectively (Chen & Chuang, 1999; Bachmann et al., 2009). In humans, these anti-apoptotic effects could explain the relatively higher frontal and hippocampal volumes, and higher NAA peaks in patients taking mood stabilizers compared to non-medicated patients (Kato, 2005; Schloesser et al., 2008; Machado-Vieira et al., 2009; Quiroz et al., 2010).

As discussed previously, mood stabilizers have a variety of different actions that feed into mitochondrial health and function, thereby increasing cellular health overall. Together with the plethora of data from human and animal studies, mechanisms of mood stabilizers do support a role for mitochondrial dysfunction in bipolar disorder.

---

### Mitochondrial Effects of Mood Stabilizers

- Mood stabilizers are neuroprotective

- Mitochondrial function and energy production are enhanced following mood stabilizer treatment

- Mood stabilizers counteract cellular stress

---

## CONCLUDING REMARKS

With the advent of novel technologies such as high-throughput screening, we are beginning to understand that mitochondrial mutations are more common than was previously believed, and that they might be responsible for pathologies beyond classical mitochondrial disorders. Environmental impacts during early embryogenesis as well as polymorphisms in nuclear genes that regulate mtDNA replication can increase the rate of mutations and affect tissues derived from a single founder cell while sparing tissue derived from neighboring cells. While the impact of these early mutations might be largely uneventful, they could have deleterious effects if the founder cell gives rise to tissues with high energy demands, such as brain tissue. Although the cells with these mtDNA deletions might be subsisting almost normally, they could malfunction during times of increased energy demand and interfere with organized information processing, affecting human behavior.

Many lines of bipolar disorder research suggest mitochondrial and bioenergetic abnormalities, from an increase in mtDNA mutations, decrease in RNA and protein levels of the respiratory chain, and altered energy metabolism, and many different routes could lead to similar disease phenotypes. Mitochondrial abnormalities might not underlie all bipolar disorder cases, and they might be secondary to different disease-causing factors, but genetic, functional, and anatomical evidence points to a role for mitochondria in a significant number of bipolar disorder cases. A promising treatment route would involve drugs that stabilize mitochondrial function. These drugs are not available yet, but their development seems to be a worthy goal for drug discovery programs. Such a program might revolutionize how bipolar disorder is managed in the future.

## Abbreviations

APAF1—apoptotic protease activating factor 1
ATP—padenosine-5'-triphosphate
ATP6—mitochondrially encoded ATP synthase 6
ATP8—mitochondrially encoded ATP synthase 8
BAG1—Bcl-2-associated athanogene 1
CO1—mitochondrially encoded cytochrome c oxidase I
CO2—mitochondrially encoded cytochrome c oxidase II
CO3—mitochondrially encoded cytochrome c oxidase III
CPEO—chronic progressive external ophthalmoplegia
Cyt b—mitochondrially encoded cytochrome b
mtDNA—mitochondrial DNA (circular)
ND1—mitochondrially encoded NADH dehydrogenase 1
ND2—mitochondrially encoded NADH dehydrogenase 2
ND3—mitochondrially encoded NADH dehydrogenase 3
ND4—mitochondrially encoded NADH dehydrogenase 4

ND4L—mitochondrially encoded NADH dehydrogenase 4L

ND5—mitochondrially encoded NADH dehydrogenase 5

ND6—mitochondrially encoded NADH dehydrogenase 6

PGC-1α—peroxisome proliferator-activated receptor gamma (PPARγ), coactivator 1 alpha

RITOLS—ribonucleotide incorporation throughout the lagging strand

rRNA—ribosomal RNA

tRNA—transfer RNA

## ACKNOWLEDGMENTS

The work was supported by MH084131, MH67999, and T32MH064913. The content is solely the responsibility of the authors and does not necessarily represent the official views of the funding institutes or the National Institutes of Health.

## REFERENCES

Alam, T. I., Kanki, T., Muta, T., Ukaji,.K, Abe, Y., Nakayama, H., . . . Kang, D. 2003. Human mitochondrial DNA is packaged with TFAM. *Nucleic Acids Research*, 31: 1640–1645.

Andreazza, A. C., Shao, L., Wang, J. F., & Young, L. T. 2010. Mitochondrial complex I activity and oxidative damage to mitochondrial proteins in the prefrontal cortex of patients with bipolar disorder. *Archives of General Psychiatry*, 67: 360–368.

Ashley, N., O'Rourke, A., Smith, C., Adams, S., Gowda, V., Zeviani, M., . . . Poulton, J. 2008. Depletion of mitochondrial DNA in fibroblast cultures from patients with POLG1 mutations is a consequence of catalytic mutations. *Human Molecular Genetics*, 17: 2496–2506.

Bachmann, R. F., Wang, Y., Yuan, P., Zhou, R., Li, X., Alesci, S., Manji, H. K. 2009. Common effects of lithium and valproate on mitochondrial functions: protection against methamphetamine-induced mitochondrial damage. *International Journal of Neuropsychopharmacology*, 12: 805–822.

Bai, R. K., Perng, C. L., Hsu, C. H., & Wong, L. J. 2004. Quantitative PCR analysis of mitochondrial DNA content in patients with mitochondrial disease. *Annals of the New York Academy of Sciences*, 1011: 304–309.

Baughman, J. M., Perocchi, F., Girgis, H. S., Plovanich, M., Belcher-Timme, C. A., Sancak, Y., Bao, X. R.,. . . Mootha, V. K. 2011. Integrative genomics identifies MCU as an essential component of the mitochondrial calcium uniporter. *Nature*, 476(7360): 341–345.

Bender, A., Krishnan, K. J., Morris, C. M., Taylor, G. A., Reeve, A. K., Perry, R. H., . . . Turnbull, D. M. 2006. High levels of mitochondrial DNA deletions in substantia nigra neurons in aging and Parkinson disease. *Nature Genetics*, 38: 515–517.

Benes, F. M., Kwok, E. W., Vincent, S. L., & Todtenkopf, M. S. 1998. A reduction of nonpyramidal cells in sector CA2 of schizophrenics and manic depressives. *Biological Psychiatry*, 44: 88–97.

Bezchlibnyk, Y., & Young. L. T. 2002. The neurobiology of bipolar disorder: focus on signal transduction pathways and the regulation of gene expression. *Canadian Journal of Psychiatry*, 47: 135–148.

Bogenhagen, D. F., Rousseau, D., & Burke, S. 2008. The layered structure of human mitochondrial DNA nucleoids. *Journal of Biological Chemistry*, 283: 3665–3675.

Boles, R. G., Burnett, B. B., Gleditsch, K., Wong, S., Guedalia, A., Kaariainen, A., . . . Brumm, V. 2005. A high predisposition to depression and anxiety in mothers and other matrilineal relatives of children with presumed maternally inherited mitochondrial disorders. *American Journal of Medical Genetics. Part B*, Neuropsychiatric Genetics, 137B: 20–24.

Bora, E., Fornito, A., Yucel, M., & Pantelis, C. 2010. Voxelwise meta-analysis of gray matter abnormalities in bipolar disorder. *Biological Psychiatry*, 67 (11): 1097–1105.

Bowmaker, M., Yang, M. Y., Yasukawa, T., Reyes, A., Jacobs, H. T., Huberman, J. A., & Holt, I. J. 2003. Mammalian mitochondrial DNA replicates bidirectionally from an initiation zone. *Journal of Biological Chemistry*, 278: 50961–50969.

Brown, J. M., & Yamamoto, B. K. 2003. Effects of amphetamines on mitochondrial function: role of free radicals and oxidative stress. *Pharmacology and Therapeutics*, 99 (1): 45–53.

Caballero, P. E., Candela, M. S., Alvarez, C. I., & Tejerina, A. A. 2007. Chronic progressive external ophthalmoplegia: a report of 6 cases and a review of the literature. *Neurologist*, 13 (1): 33–36.

Campos, Y., Garcia, A., Eiris, J., Fuster, M., Rubio, J. C., Martin, M. A., . . . Arenas, J. 2001. Mitochondrial myopathy, cardiomyopathy and psychiatric illness in a Spanish family harbouring the mtDNA 3303C > T mutation. *Journal of Inherited Metabolic Disease*, 24(6): 685–687.

Cataldo, A. M., McPhie, D. L., Lange, N. T., Punzell, S., Elmiligy, S., Ye, N. Z., . . . Cohen, B. M. 2010. Abnormalities in Mitochondrial Structure in Cells from Patients with Bipolar Disorder. *American Journal of Clinical Pathology*, *177* (2): 575–585.

Chang, D. D., & Clayton, D. A. 1984. Precise identification of individual promoters for transcription of each strand of human mitochondrial DNA. *Cell*, 36 (3): 635–643.

Chen, G., Henter, I. D., & Manji, H. K. 2010. Translational research in bipolar disorder: emerging insights from genetically based models. *Molecular Psychiatry*, 15 (9): 883–895.

Chen, G., Zeng, W. Z., Yuan, P. X., Huang, L. D., Jiang, Y. M., Zhao, Z. H., & Manji, H. K. 1999. The mood-stabilizing agents lithium and valproate robustly increase the levels of the neuroprotective protein bcl-2 in the CNS. *Journal of Neurochemistry*, 72(2): 879–882.

Chen, R. W., & Chuang, D. M. 1999. Long term lithium treatment suppresses p. 53 and Bax expression but increases Bcl-2 expression. A prominent role in neuroprotection against excitotoxicity. *Journal of Biological Chemistry*, 274 (10): 6039–6042.

Chipuk, . J. E., & Green, D. R. 2008. How do BCL-2 proteins induce mitochondrial outer membrane permeabilization? *Trends in Cell Biology*, 18 (4): 157–164.

Chuang, D. M. 2005. The antiapoptotic actions of mood stabilizers: molecular mechanisms and therapeutic potentials. *Annals of the New York Academy of Sciences*, 1053: 195–204.

Clay, H. B., Sillivan, S., & Konradi, C. 2010. Mitochondrial dysfunction and pathology in bipolar disorder and schizophrenia. *International Journal of Developmental Neuroscience*, 3(29): 311–324.

Clay Montier, L. L., Deng, J. J., & Bai, Y. 2009. Number matters: control of mammalian mitochondrial DNA copy number. *Journal of Genetics and Genomics*, 36 (3): 125–131.

Corral-Debrinski, M., Horton, T., Lott, M. T., Shoffner, J. M., Beal, M. F., & Wallace, D. C. 1992. Mitochondrial DNA deletions in human brain: regional variability and increase with advanced age. *Nature Genetics*, 2 (4): 324–329.

Crews, S., Ojala, D., Posakony, J., Nishiguchi, J., & Attardi, G. 1979. Nucleotide sequence of a region of human mitochondrial DNA containing the precisely identified origin of replication. *Nature*, 277 (5693): 192–198.

Dager, S. R., Friedman, S. D., Parow, A., Demopulos, C., Stoll, A. L., Lyoo, I. K., . . . Renshaw, P. F. 2004. Brain metabolic alterations in medication-free patients with bipolar disorder. *Archives of General Psychiatry*, 61: 450–458.

Danan, C., Sternberg, D., Van Steirteghem, A., Cazeneuve, C., Duquesnoy, P., Besmond, C., . . . Amselem, S. 1999. Evaluation of parental mitochondrial inheritance in neonates born after intracytoplasmic sperm injection. *American Journal of Human Genetics*, 65(2): 463–473.

Deicken, R. F., Fein, G., & Weiner, M. W. 1995. Abnormal frontal lobe phosphorous metabolism in bipolar disorder. *American Journal of Psychiatry*, 152(6): 915–918.

De Stefani, D., Raffaello, A., Teardo, E., Szabò, I., Rizzuto, R. 2011. A forty-kilodalton protein of the inner membrane is the mitochondrial calcium uniporter. *Nature*, 476(7360): 336–340.

DiMauro, S., & Schon, E. A. 2008. Mitochondrial disorders in the nervous system. *Annual Review of Neuroscience*, 31: 91–123.

Dubovsky, S. L., Murphy, J., Thomas, M., & Rademacher, J. 1992. Abnormal intracellular calcium ion concentration in platelets and lymphocytes of bipolar patients. *American Journal of Psychiatry*, 149(1): 118–120.

Einat, H., Yuan, P., & Manji, H. K. 2005. Increased anxiety-like behaviors and mitochondrial dysfunction in mice with targeted mutation of the Bcl-2 gene: further support for the involvement of mitochondrial function in anxiety disorders. *Behavioural Brain Research*, 165(2): 172–180.

Ekstrand, M. I., Falkenberg, M., Rantanen, A., Park, C. B., Gaspari, M., Hultenby, K., . . . Larsson, N. G. 2004. Mitochondrial transcription factor A regulates mtDNA copy number in mammals. *Human Molecular Genetics*, 13: 935–944.

Ellison-Wright, I., & Bullmore, E. 2010. Anatomy of bipolar disorder and schizophrenia: a meta-analysis. *Schizophrenia Research*, 117(1): 1–12.

Emamghoreishi, M., Schlichter, L., Li, P. P., Parikh, S., Sen, J., Kamble, A., & Warsh, J. J. 1997. High intracellular calcium concentrations in transformed lymphoblasts from subjects with bipolar I disorder. *American Journal of Psychiatry*, 154: 976–982.

Endo, T., Yamamoto, H., & Esaki, M. 2003. Functional cooperation and separation of translocators in protein import into mitochondria, the double-membrane bounded organelles. *Journal of Cell Science*, 116(16): 3259–3267.

Esser, C., Ahmadinejad, N., Wiegand, C., Rotte, C., Sebastiani, F., Gelius-Dietrich, G., . . . Martin, W. 2004. A genome phylogeny for mitochondria among alpha-proteobacteria and a predominantly eubacterial ancestry of yeast nuclear genes. *Molecular Biology and Evolution*, 21: 1643–1660.

Falkenberg, M., Gaspari, M., Rantanen, A., Trifunovic, A., Larsson, N. G., & Gustafsson, C. M. 2002. Mitochondrial transcription factors B1 and B2 activate transcription of human mtDNA. *Nature Genetics*, 31: 289–294.

Fattal, O., Budur, K., Vaughan, A. J., & Franco, K. 2006. Review of the literature on major mental disorders in adult patients with mitochondrial diseases. *Psychosomatics*, 47(1): 1–7.

Fernandez-Silva, P., Enriquez, J. A., & Montoya, J. 2003. Replication and transcription of mammalian mitochondrial DNA. *Experimental Physiology*, 88: 41–56.

Fisher, R. P., Lisowsky, T., Parisi, M. A., & Clayton, D. A. 1992. DNA wrapping and bending by a mitochondrial high mobility group-like transcriptional activator protein. *Journal of Biological Chemistry*, 267: 3358–3367.

Frahm, T., Mohamed, S. A., Bruse, P., Gemund, C., Oehmichen, M., & Meissner, C. 2005. Lack of age-related increase of mitochondrial DNA amount in brain, skeletal muscle and human heart. *Mechanisms of ageing and Development*, 126: 1192–1200.

Frey, B. N., Stanley, J. A., Nery, F. G., Monkul, E. S., Nicoletti, M. A., Chen, H. H., . . . Soares, J. C. 2007. Abnormal cellular energy and phospholipid metabolism in the left dorsolateral prefrontal cortex of medication-free individuals with bipolar disorder: an in vivo 1H MRS study. *Bipolar Disorders*, 9 (Suppl 1): 119–127.

Fuke, S., Kametani, M., & Kato, T. 2008. Quantitative analysis of the 4977-bp common deletion of mitochondrial DNA in postmortem frontal cortex from patients with bipolar disorder and schizophrenia. *Neuroscience Letters*, 439(2): 173–177.

Fuke, S., Kubota-Sakashita, M., Kasahara, T., Shigeyoshi, Y., & Kato, T. 2011. Regional variation in mitochondrial DNA copy number in mouse brain. *Biochimica Biophysica Acta*, 1807: 270–274.

Fuste, J. M., Wanrooij, S., Jemt, E., Granycome, C. E., Cluett, T. J., Shi, Y., . . . Falkenberg, M. 2010. Mitochondrial RNA polymerase is needed for activation of the origin of light-strand DNA replication. *Molecular Cell*, 37(1): 67–78.

Galluzzi, L., Blomgren, K., & Kroemer, G. 2009. Mitochondrial membrane permeabilization in neuronal injury. *Natural Reviews of Neuroscience*, 10: 481–494.

Garrido, N., Griparic, L., Jokitalo, E., Wartiovaara, J., van der Bliek, A. M., & Spelbrink, J. N. 2003. Composition and dynamics of human mitochondrial nucleoids. *Molecular Biology of the Cell*, 14: 1583–1596.

Gershon, E. S., Hamovit, J., Guroff, J. J., Dibble, E., Leckman, J. F., Sceery, W., . . . Bunney, W. E., Jr. 1982. A family study of schizoaffective, bipolar I, bipolar II, unipolar, and normal control probands. *Archives of General Psychiatry*, 39(10): 1157–1167.

Gilkerson, R. W. 2009. Mitochondrial DNA nucleoids determine mitochondrial genetics and dysfunction. *International Journal of Biochemistry and Cell Biology*, 41(10): 1899–1906.

Graziewicz, M. A., Longley, M. J., & Copeland, W. C. 2006. DNA polymerase gamma in mitochondrial DNA replication and repair. *Chem Rev*, 106(2): 383–405.

Grover, S., Padhy, S. K., Das, C. P., Vasishta, R. K., Sharan, P., & Chakrabarti, S. 2006. Mania as a first presentation in mitochondrial myopathy. *Psychiatry and Clinical Neurosciences*, 60: 774–775.

He, Y., Wu, J., Dressman, D. C., Iacobuzio-Donahue, C., Markowitz, S. D., Velculescu, V. E., . . . Papadopoulos, N. 2010. Heteroplasmic mitochondrial DNA mutations in normal and tumour cells. *Nature*, 464(7288): 610–614.

Heckers, S., Stone, D., Walsh, J., Shick, J., Koul, P., & Benes, F. M. 2002. Differential hippocampal expression of glutamic acid decarboxylase 65 and 67 messenger RNA in bipolar disorder and schizophrenia. *Archives of General Psychiatry*, 59(6): 521–529.

Holt, I. J., Lorimer, H. E., & Jacobs, H. T. 2000. Coupled leading- and lagging-strand synthesis of mammalian mitochondrial DNA. *Cell*, 100: 515–524.

Hotchkiss, R. S., Strasser, A., McDunn, J. E., & Swanson, P. E. 2009. Cell death. *New England Journal of Medicine*, 361: 1570–1583.

Iborra, F. J., Kimura, H., & Cook, P. R. 2004. The functional organization of mitochondrial genomes in human cells. *BMC Biology*, 2: 9.

Isaev, N. K., Stelmashook, E. V., Dirnagl, U., Plotnikov, E. Y., Kuvshinova, E. A., & Zorov, D. B. 2008. Mitochondrial free radical production induced by glucose deprivation in cerebellar granule neurons. *Biochemistry (Moscow)*, 73(2): 149–155.

Iwamoto, K., Bundo, M., & Kato, T. 2005. Altered expression of mitochondria-related genes in postmortem brains of patients with bipolar disorder or schizophrenia, as revealed by large-scale DNA microarray analysis. *Human Molecular Genetics*, 14: 241–253.

Jou, M. J., Peng, T. I., Wu, H. Y., & Wei, Y. H. 2005. Enhanced generation of mitochondrial reactive oxygen species in cybrids containing 4977-bp mitochondrial DNA deletion. *Annals of the New York Academy of Sciences*, 1042: 221–228.

Kakiuchi, C., Ishiwata, M., Kametani, M., Nelson, C., Iwamoto, K., & Kato, T. 2005. Quantitative analysis of mitochondrial DNA deletions in the brains of patients with bipolar disorder and schizophrenia. *International Journal of Neuropsychopharmacology*, 8: 515–522.

Kasahara, T., Kubota, M., Miyauchi, T., Ishiwata, M., & Kato, T. 2008. A marked effect of electroconvulsive stimulation on behavioral aberration of mice with neuron-specific mitochondrial DNA defects. *PLoS One*, 3(3): e1877.

Kasahara, T., Kubota, M., Miyauchi, T., Noda, Y., Mouri, A., Nabeshima, T., & Kato, T. 2006. Mice with neuron-specific accumulation of mitochondrial DNA mutations show mood disorder-like phenotypes. *Molecular Psychiatry*, 11: 577–593, 523.

Kasamatsu, H., Robberson, D. L., & Vinograd, J. 1971. A novel closed-circular mitochondrial DNA with properties of a replicating intermediate. *Proceedings of National Academy of Science U S A*, 68(9): 2252–2257.

Kato, T. 2001. The other, forgotten genome: mitochondrial DNA and mental disorders. *Mol Psychiatry*, 6: 625–633.

Kato, T. 2005. Mitochondrial dysfunction in bipolar disorder: from 31P-magnetic resonance spectroscopic findings to their molecular mechanisms. *International Review of Neurobiology*, 63: 21–40.

Kato, T. 2007. Molecular genetics of bipolar disorder and depression. *Psychiatry and Clinical Neurosciences*, 61: 3–19.

Kato, T. 2008. Role of mitochondrial DNA in calcium signaling abnormality in bipolar disorder. *Cell Calcium*, 44 (1): 92–102.

Kato, T., Ishiwata, M., Mori, K., Washizuka, S., Tajima, O., Akiyama, T., & Kato, N. 2003. Mechanisms of altered Ca2 + signalling in transformed lymphoblastoid cells from patients with bipolar disorder. *International Journal of Neuropsychopharmacoogyl*, 6(4): 379–389.

Kato, T., & Kato, N. 2000. Mitochondrial dysfunction in bipolar disorder. *Bipolar Disorders*, 2: 180–190.

Kato, T., Kubota, M., & Kasahara, T. 2007. Animal models of bipolar disorder. *Neuroscience and Biobehavioral Reviews*, 31: 832–842.

Kato, T., Kunugi, H., Nanko, S., & Kato, N. 2001. Mitochondrial DNA polymorphisms in bipolar disorder. *Journal of Affective Disorders*, 62: 151–164.

Kato, T., Murashita, J., Kamiya, A., Shioiri, T., Kato, N., & Inubushi, T. 1998. Decreased brain intracellular pH measured by 31P-MRS in bipolar disorder: a confirmation in drug-free patients and correlation with white matter hyperintensity. *Eur Arch Psychiatry Clinical Neuroscience*, 248(6): 301–306.

Kato, T., Stine, O. C., McMahon, F. J., & Crowe, R. R. 1997. Increased levels of a mitochondrial DNA deletion in the brain of patients with bipolar disorder. *Biological Psychiatry*, 42(10): 871–875.

Kato, T., Winokur, G., Coryell, W., Keller, M. B., Endicott, J., & Rice, J. 1996. Parent-of-origin effect in transmission of bipolar disorder. *American Journal of Medical Genetics*, 67: 546–550.

Kaufman, B. A., Durisic, N., Mativetsky, J. M., Costantino, S., Hancock, M. A., Grutter, P., Shoubridge, E. A. 2007. The mitochondrial transcription factor TFAM coordinates the assembly of multiple DNA molecules into nucleoid-like structures. *Molecular Biologyof the Cell*, 18(9): 3225–3236.

Kazuno. A. A., Munakata, K., Mori, K., Nanko, S., Kunugi, H/., Nakamura, K., . . . Kato, T. 2009. Mitochondrial DNA haplogroup analysis in patients with bipolar disorder. *Am J Med Genet B Neuropsychiatric Genetics*, 150B(2): 243–247.

Kazuno, A. A., Munakata, K., Nagai, T., Shimozono, S., Tanaka, M., Yoneda, M., . . . Kato, T. 2006. Identification of mitochondrial DNA polymorphisms that alter mitochondrial matrix pH and intracellular calcium dynamics. *PLoS Genetics*, 2(8): e128.

Kelly, D. P., & Scarpulla, R. C. 2004. Transcriptional regulatory circuits controlling mitochondrial biogenesis and function. *Genes and Development*, 18(4): 357–368.

King, T. D., Bijur, G. N., & Jope, R. S. 2001. Caspase-3 activation induced by inhibition of mitochondrial complex I is facilitated by glycogen synthase kinase-3beta and attenuated by lithium. *Brain Research*, 919(1): 106–114.

Kirk, R., Furlong, R. A., Amos, W., Cooper, G., Rubinsztein, J. S., Walsh, C., . . . Rubinsztein, D. C. 1999. Mitochondrial genetic analyses suggest selection against maternal lineages in bipolar affective disorder. *American Journal of Human Genetics*, 65(2): 508–518.

Knable, M. B., Barci, B. M., Webster, M. J., Meador-Woodruff, J., & Torrey, E. F. 2004. Molecular abnormalities of the hippocampus in severe psychiatric illness: postmortem findings from the Stanley Neuropathology Consortium. *Molecular Psychiatry*, 9(6): 609–620, 544.

Kong, Q. P., Bandelt, H. J., Sun, C., Yao, Y. G., Salas, A., Achilli, A., . . . Zhang, Y. P. 2006. Updating the East Asian mtDNA phylogeny: a prerequisite for the identification of pathogenic mutations. *Human Molecular Genetics*, 15(13): 2076–2086.

Konradi, C., Eaton, M., MacDonald, M. L., Walsh, J., Benes, F. M., & Heckers, S. 2004. Molecular evidence for mitochondrial dysfunction in bipolar disorder. *Archives of General Psychiatry*, 61(6): 300–308.

Konradi, C., Sillivan, S. E., & Clay, H. B. 2011a. Mitochondria, oligodendrocytes and inflammation in bipolar disorder: evidence from transcriptome studies points to intriguing parallels with multiple sclerosis. *Neurobiology of Disease*, (in press).

Konradi, C., Zimmerman, E. I., Yang, C. K., Lohmann, K. M., Gresch, P., Pantazopoulos, H., . . . Heckers, S. 2011b. Reduced number of hippocampal interneurons in bipolar disorder. *Archives of General Psychiatry*, epub.

Korhonen, J. A., Pham, X. H., Pellegrini, M., & Falkenberg, M. 2004. Reconstitution of a minimal mtDNA replisome in vitro. *EMBO Journal*, 23(12): 2423–2429.

Kornberg, J. R., Brown, J. L., Sadovnick, A. D., Remick, R. A., Keck, P. E., Jr., McElroy, S. L., . . . Kelsoe, J. R. 2000. Evaluating the parent-of-origin effect in bipolar affective disorder. Is a more penetrant subtype transmitted paternally? *Journal of Affective Disorders*, 59(3): 183–192.

Kraytsberg, Y., Kudryavtseva, E., McKee, A. C., Geula, C., Kowall, N. W., & Khrapko, K. 2006. Mitochondrial DNA deletions are abundant and cause functional impairment in aged human substantia nigra neurons. *Nature Genetics*, 38(5): 518–520.

Krishnan, K. J., Reeve, A. K., Samuels, D. C., Chinnery, P. F., Blackwood, J. K., Taylor, R. W., . . . Turnbull, D. M. 2008. What causes mitochondrial DNA deletions in human cells? *Nature Genetics*, 40: 275–279.

Kubota, M., Kasahara, T., Iwamoto, K., Komori, A., Ishiwata, M., Miyauchi, T., & Kato, T. 2010. Therapeutic implications of downregulation of cyclophilin D in bipolar disorder. *International Journal of Neuropsychopharmacology*, 13: 1355–1368.

Kubota, M., Kasahara, T., Nakamura, T., Ishiwata, M., Miyauchi, T., & Kato, T. 2006. Abnormal Ca2 + dynamics in transgenic mice with neuron-specific mitochondrial DNA defects. *Journal of Neuroscience*, 26(47): 12314–12324.

Kukat, C., Wurm, C. A., Spåhr, H., Falkenberg, M., Larsson, N. G., Jakobs, S. 2011. Super-resolution microscopy reveals that mammalian mitochondrial nucleoids have a uniform size and frequently contain a single copy of mtDNA. *Proceedings of the National Academy of Sciences of the United States of America*, 108(33): 13534–13539.

Kusumi, I., Koyama, T., & Yamashita, I. 1992. Thrombin-induced platelet calcium mobilization is enhanced in bipolar disorders. *Biological Psychiatry*, 32: 731–734.

Kutik, S., Stroud, D. A., Wiedemann, N., & Pfanner, N. 2009. Evolution of mitochondrial protein biogenesis. *Biochimica et Biophysica Acta*, 1790(6): 409–415.

Lai, J. S., Zhao, C., Warsh, J. J., Li, P. P. 2006. Cytoprotection by lithium and valproate varies between cell types and cellular stresses. *European Journal of Pharmacology*, 539(1-2): 18–26.

Lan, T. H., Beaty, T. H., DePaulo, J. R., & McInnis, M. G. 2007. Parent-of-origin effect in the segregation analysis of bipolar affective disorder families. *Psychiatric Genetics*, 17: 93–101.

Lebon, S., Chol, M., Benit, P., Mugnier, C., Chretien, D., Giurgea, I., . . . Munnich, A. 2003. Recurrent de novo mitochondrial DNA mutations in respiratory chain deficiency. *Journal of Medical Genetics*, 40(12): 896–899.

Lee, H. C., & Wei, Y. H. 2005. Mitochondrial biogenesis and mitochondrial DNA maintenance of mammalian cells under oxidative stress. *International Journal of Biochemistry and Cell Biology*, 37(4): 822–834.

Legros, F., Malka, F., Frachon, P., Lombes, A., & Rojo, M. 2004. Organization and dynamics of human mitochondrial DNA. *Journal of Cell Science*, 117(Pt 13): 2653–2662.

Liu, C. Y., Lee, C. F., Hong, C. H., & Wei, Y. H. 2004. Mitochondrial DNA mutation and depletion increase the susceptibility of human cells to apoptosis. *Annals of the New York Academy of Sciences*, 1011: 133–145.

Liu, C. Y., Lee, C. F., & Wei, Y. H. 2007. Quantitative effect of 4977 bp deletion of mitochondrial DNA on the susceptibility of human cells to UV-induced apoptosis. *Mitochondrion*, 7(1-2): 89–95.

Lyoo, I. K., Kim, M. J., Stoll, A. L., Demopulos, C. M., Parow, A. M., Dager, S. R., . . . Renshaw, P. F. 2004. Frontal lobe gray matter density decreases in bipolar I disorder. *Biological Psychiatry*, 55(6): 648–651.

MacDonald, M. L., Naydenov, A., Chu, M., Matzilevich, D., & Konradi, C. 2006. Decrease in creatine kinase messenger RNA expression in the hippocampus and dorsolateral prefrontal cortex in bipolar disorder. *Bipolar Disorders*, 8: 255–264.

Machado-Vieira, R., Manji, H. K., & Zarate, C. A. 2009. The role of the tripartite glutamatergic synapse in the pathophysiology and therapeutics of mood disorders. *Neuroscientist*, 15(5): 525–539.

Maeng, S., Hunsberger, J. G., Pearson, B., Yuan, P., Wang, Y., Wei, Y., . . . Manji, H. K. 2008. BAG1 plays a critical role in regulating recovery from both manic-like and depression-like behavioral impairments. *Proc Natl Acad Sci U S A*, 105(25): 8766–8771.

Mancuso, M., Ricci, G., Choub, A., Filosto, M., DiMauro, S., Davidzon, G., . . . Siciliano, G. 2008. Autosomal dominant psychiatric disorders and mitochondrial DNA multiple deletions: report of a family. *Journal of Affective Disorders*, 106(1-2): 173–177.

Marchington, D. R., Macaulay, V., Hartshorne, G. M., Barlow, D., & Poulton, J. 1998. Evidence from human oocytes for a genetic bottleneck in an mtDNA disease. *American Journal of Human Genetics*, 63: 769–775.

Maurer, I. C., Schippel, P., & Volz, H. P. 2009. Lithium-induced enhancement of mitochondrial oxidative phosphorylation in human brain tissue. *Bipolar Disorders*, 11(5): 515–522.

McCulloch, V., & Shadel, G. S. 2003. Human mitochondrial transcription factor B1 interacts with the C-terminal activation region of h-mtTFA and stimulates transcription independently of its RNA methyltransferase activity. *Molecular and Cellular Biology*, 23(16): 5816–5824.

McFarland, R., Kirby, D. M., Fowler, K. J., Ohtake, A., Ryan, M. T., Amor, D. J., . . . Thorburn, D. R. 2004. De novo mutations in the mitochondrial ND3 gene as a cause of infantile mitochondrial encephalopathy and complex I deficiency. *Annals of Neurology*, 55(1): 58–64.

McInerny, S. C., Brown, A. L., & Smith, D. W. 2009. Region-specific changes in mitochondrial D-loop in aged rat CNS. *Mechanisma of Ageing and Development*, 130: 343–349.

McMahon, F. J., Chen, Y. S., Patel, S., Kokoszka, J., Brown, M. D., Torroni, A., . . . Wallace, D. C. 2000. Mitochondrial DNA sequence diversity in bipolar affective disorder. *American Journal of Psychiatry*, 157: 1058–1064.

McMahon, F. J., Stine, O. C., Meyers, D. A., Simpson, S. G., & DePaulo, J.R. 1995. Patterns of maternal transmission in bipolar affective disorder. *American Journal of Human Genetics*, 56(6): 1277–1286.

Michaelis, M., Suhan, T., Michaelis, U. R., Beek, K., Rothweiler, F., Tausch, L., . . . Cinatl, J., Jr. 2006. Valproic acid induces extracellular signal-regulated kinase 1/2 activation and inhibits apoptosis in endothelial cells. *Cell Death and Differentiation*, 13(3): 446–453.

Munakata, K., Tanaka, M., Mori, K., Washizuka, S., Yoneda, M., Tajima, O., . . . Kato, T. 2004. Mitochondrial DNA 3644T—> C mutation associated with bipolar disorder. *Genomics*, 84(6): 1041–1050.

Naydenov, A. V., MacDonald, M. L., Ongur, D., & Konradi, C. 2007. Differences in lymphocyte electron transport gene expression levels between subjects with bipolar disorder and normal controls in response to glucose deprivation stress. *Archives of General Psychiatry*, 64(5): 555–564.

Naydenov, A. V., Vassoler, F., Luksik, A. S., Kaczmarska, J., & Konradi, C. 2010. Mitochondrial abnormalities in the putamen in Parkinson's disease dyskinesia. *Acta Neuropathologica*, 120(5): 623–631.

Ongur, D., Prescot, A. P., Jensen, J. E., Cohen, B. M., & Renshaw, P. F. 2009. Creatine abnormalities in schizophrenia and bipolar disorder. *Psychiatry Research*, 172: 44–48.

Orrenius, S., Zhivotovsky B., & Nicotera, P. 2003. Regulation of cell death: the calcium-apoptosis link. *Nature Reviews Molecular Cell Biology*, 4(7): 552–565.

Ouyang, Y. B., & Giffard, R. G. 2004. Cellular neuroprotective mechanisms in cerebral ischemia: Bcl-2 family proteins and protection of mitochondrial function. *Cell Calcium*, 36: 303–311.

Pagliarini, D. J., Calvo, S. E., Chang, B., Sheth, S. A., Vafai, S. B., Ong, S. E., . . . Mootha, V. K. 2008. A mitochondrial protein compendium elucidates complex I disease biology. *Cell*, 134(1): 112–123.

Parisi, M. A., & Clayton, D. A. 1991. Similarity of human mitochondrial transcription factor 1 to high mobility group proteins. *Science*, 252(5008): 965–969.

Pietruczuk, K., Jozwik, A., Ruckemann-Dziurdzinska, K., Bryl, E., & Witkowski, J. M. 2009. Cytoprotective effect of lithium against spontaneous and induced apoptosis of lymphoid cell line MOLT-4. *Folia Histochem Cytobiol*, 47(4): 639–646.

Plant, N., Barber, P., Horner, E., Cockburn, C. L., Gibson, G., Bugelski, P., & Lord, P. 2002. Differential gene expression in rats following subacute exposure to the anticonvulsant sodium valproate. *Toxicology and Applied Pharmacology*, 183: 127–134.

Pohjoismaki, J. L., Holmes, J. B., Wood, S. R., Yang, M. Y., Yasukawa, T., Reyes, A., . . . Holt, I. J. 2010. Mammalian mitochondrial DNA replication intermediates are essentially duplex but contain extensive tracts of RNA/DNA hybrid. *Journal of Molecular Biology*, 397(5): 1144–1155.

Prayson, R. A., & Wang, N. 1998. Mitochondrial myopathy, encephalopathy, lactic acidosis, and strokelike episodes (MELAS) syndrome: an autopsy report. *Archives of Pathology & Laboratory Medicine*, 122(11): 978–981.

Pulkes, T., Liolitsa, D., Nelson, I. P., & Hanna, M. G. 2003. Classical mitochondrial phenotypes without mtDNA mutations: the possible role of nuclear genes. *Neurology*, 61(8): 1144–1147.

Pysh, J. J., & Khan, T. 1972. Variations in mitochondrial structure and content of neurons and neuroglia in rat brain: an electron microscopic study. *Brain Research*, 36(1): 1–18.

Quiroz, J. A., Gray, N. A., Kato, T., & Manji, H. K. 2008. Mitochondrially mediated plasticity in the pathophysiology and treatment of bipolar disorder. *Neuropsychopharmacology*, 33(11): 2551–2565.

Quiroz, J. A., Machado-Vieira, R., Zarate, C. A., Jr., & Manji, H. K. 2010. Novel insights into lithium's mechanism of action: neurotrophic and neuroprotective effects. *Neuropsychobiology*, 62(1): 50–60.

Rizzuto, R., & Pozzan, T. 2006. Microdomains of intracellular Ca2 +: molecular determinants and functional consequences. *Physiological Reviews*, 86(1): 369–408.

Rocher, C., Taanman, J. W., Pierron, D., Faustin, B., Benard, G., Rossignol, R., . . . Letellier, T. 2008. Influence of mitochondrial DNA level on cellular energy metabolism: implications for mitochondrial diseases. *Journal of Bioenergetics and Biomembranes*, 40(2): 59–67.

Russell, J. W., Golovoy, D., Vincent, A. M., Mahendru, P., Olzmann, J. A., Mentzer, A., Feldman, E. L. 2002. High glucose-induced oxidative stress and mitochondrial dysfunction in neurons. *FASEB Journal*, 16(13): 1738–1748.

Sabunciyan, S., Kirches, E., Krause, G., Bogerts, B., Mawrin, C., Llenos, I. C., & Weis, S. 2007. Quantification of total mitochondrial DNA and mitochondrial common deletion in the frontal cortex of patients with schizophrenia and bipolar disorder. *Journal of Neural Transmission*, 114(5): 665–674.

Schloesser, R. J., Huang, J., Klein, P. S., & Manji, H. K. 2008. Cellular plasticity cascades in the pathophysiology and treatment of bipolar disorder. *Neuropsychopharmacology*, 33(1): 110–133.

Shadel, G. S., & Clayton, D. A. 1997. Mitochondrial DNA maintenance in vertebrates. *Annual Review of Biochemistry*, 66: 409–435.

Shalbuyeva, N., Brustovetsky, T., & Brustovetsky, N. 2007. Lithium desensitizes brain mitochondria to calcium, antagonizes permeability transition, and diminishes cytochrome C release. *Journal of Biological Chemistry*, 282(25): 18057–18068.

Shao, L., Martin, M. V., Watson, S. J., Schatzberg, A., Akil, H., Myers, R. M., . . . Vawter, M. P. 2008. Mitochondrial involvement in psychiatric disorders. *Annals of Medicine*, 40(4): 281–295.

Siciliano, G., Tessa, A., Petrini, S., Mancuso, M., Bruno, C., Grieco, G. S., Malandrini, A., . . . Murri, L. 2003. Autosomal dominant external ophthalmoplegia and bipolar affective disorder associated with a mutation in the ANT1 gene. *Neuromuscular Disorders*, 13(2): 162–165.

Silva, J. P., Kohler, M., Graff, C., Oldfors, A., Magnuson, M. A., Berggren, P. O., Larsson, N. G. 2000. Impaired insulin secretion and beta-cell loss in tissue-specific knockout mice with mitochondrial diabetes. *Nature Genetics*, 26(3): 336–340.

Smoly, J. M., Kuylenstierna, B., & Ernster, L. 1970. Topological and functional organization of the mitochondrion. *Proceedings of the National Academy of Science U S A*, 66(1): 125–131.

Soong, N. W., Hinton, D. R., Cortopassi, G., & Arnheim, N. 1992. Mosaicism for a specific somatic mitochondrial DNA mutation in adult human brain. *Nature Genetics*, 2(4): 324–329.

Sorensen, L., Ekstrand, M., Silva, J. P., Lindqvist, E., Xu, B., Rustin, P., . . . Larsson, N.G. 2001. Late-onset corticohippocampal neurodepletion attributable to catastrophic failure of oxidative phosphorylation in MILON mice. *J Neurosci*, 21: 8082–8090.

Starkov, A. A. 2008. The role of mitochondria in reactive oxygen species metabolism and signaling. *Annals of the New York Academy of Sciences*, 1147: 37–52.

Stelmashook, E. V., Isaev, N. K., Plotnikov, E. Y., Uzbekov, R. E., Alieva, I. B., Arbeille, B., Zorov, D. B. 2009. Effect of transitory glucose deprivation on mitochondrial structure and functions in cultured cerebellar granule neurons. *Neuroscience Letters*, 461(2): 140–144.

Stine, O. C., Luu, S. U., Zito, M., & Casanova, M. 1993. The possible association between affective disorder and partially deleted mitochondrial DNA. *Biol Psychiatry*, 33(2): 141–142.

Stork, C., & Renshaw, P. F. 2005. Mitochondrial dysfunction in bipolar disorder: evidence from magnetic resonance spectroscopy research. *Molecular Psychiatry*, 10: 900–919.

Struewing, I. T., Barnett, C. D., Tang, T., & Mao, C. D. 2007. Lithium increases PGC-1alpha expression and mitochondrial biogenesis in primary bovine aortic endothelial cells. *FEBS Journal*, 274(11): 2749–2765.

Sun, X., Wang, J. F., Tseng, M., & Young, L. T. 2006. Downregulation in components of the mitochondrial electron transport chain in the postmortem frontal cortex of subjects with bipolar disorder. *Journal of Psychiatry and Neuroscience*, 31(3): 189–196.

Suomalainen, A., Majander, A., Haltia, M., Somer, H., Lonnqvist, J., Savontaus, M. L., Peltonen, L. 1992. Multiple deletions of mitochondrial DNA in several tissues of a patient with severe retarded depression and familial progressive external ophthalmoplegia. *Journal of Clinical Investigation*, 90(1): 61–66.

Szydlowska, K., & Tymianski, M. 2010. Calcium, ischemia and excitotoxicity. *Cell Calcium*, 47(2): 122–129.

Tapper, D. P., & Clayton, D. A. 1981. Mechanism of replication of human mitochondrial DNA. Localization of the 5' ends of nascent daughter strands. *Journal of Biological Chemistry*, 256(10): 5109–5115.

Thomas, J. O., & Travers, A. A. 2001. HMG1 and 2, and related "architectural" DNA-binding proteins. *Trendsin Biochemical Sciences*, 26: 167–174.

Tiranti, V., Savoia, A., Forti, F., D'Apolito, M. F., Centra, M., Rocchi, M., & Zeviani, M. 1997. Identification of the gene encoding the human mitochondrial RNA polymerase (h-mtRPOL) by cyberscreening of the Expressed Sequence Tags database. *Human Molecular Genetics*, 6: 615–625.

Valvassori, S. S., Rezin, G. T., Ferreira, C. L., Moretti, M., Goncalves, C. L., Cardoso, M. R., . . . Quevedo, J. 2010. Effects of mood stabilizers on mitochondrial respiratory chain activity in brain of rats treated with d-amphetamine. *Journal of Psychiatric Research*, 44(14):903–909.

Vawter, M. P., Freed, W. J., & Kleinman, J. E. 2000. Neuropathology of bipolar disorder. *Biological Psychiatry*, 48(6): 486–504.

Vawter, M. P., Tomita, H., Meng, F., Bolstad, B., Li, J., Evans, S., . . . Bunney, W. E. 2006. Mitochondrial-related gene expression changes are sensitive to agonal-pH state: implications for brain disorders. *Molecular Psychiatry*, 11(7): 615, 663–679.

Wallace, D. C. 1999. Mitochondrial diseases in man and mouse. *Science* 283(5407): 1482–1488.

Wallace, D. C. 2005. A mitochondrial paradigm of metabolic and degenerative diseases, aging, and cancer: a dawn for evolutionary medicine. *Annual Review of Genetics*, 39: 359–407.

Wallace, D. C., & Fan, W. 2010. Energetics, epigenetics, mitochondrial genetics. *Mitochondrion*, 10(1): 12–31.

Wang, J., & Lu, Y. Y. 2009. Mitochondrial DNA 4977-bp deletion correlated with reactive oxygen species production and manganese superoxidedismutase expression in gastric tumor cells. *Chinese Medical Journal (Engl)*, 122(4): 431–436.

Wang, J. F., Shao, L., Sun, X., & Young, L. T. 2004. Glutathione S-transferase is a novel target for mood stabilizing drugs in primary cultured neurons. *Journal of Neurochemistry*, 88: 1477–1484.

Wang, J. F., Shao, L., Sun, X., & Young, L. T. 2009. Increased oxidative stress in the anterior cingulate cortex of subjects with bipolar disorder and schizophrenia. *Bipolar Disorders*, 11: 523–529.

Washizuka, S., Iwamoto, K., Kakiuchi, C., Bundo, M., & Kato, T. 2009. Expression of mitochondrial complex I subunit gene NDUFV2 in the lymphoblastoid cells derived from patients with bipolar disorder and schizophrenia. *Neuroscience Research*, 63(3): 199–204.

Wasserman, M. J., Corson, T. W., Sibony, D., Cooke, R. G., Parikh, S. V., Pennefather, P. S., . . . Warsh, J. J. 2004. Chronic lithium treatment attenuates intracellular calcium mobilization. *Neuropsychopharmacology*, 29(4): 759–769.

Wei, H., Qin, Z. H., Senatorov, V. V., Wei, W., Wang, Y., Qian, Y., & Chuang, D. M. 2001. Lithium suppresses excitotoxicity-induced striatal lesions in a rat model of Huntington's disease. *Neuroscience*, 106(3): 603–612.

Wredenberg, A., Wibom, R., Wilhelmsson, H., Graff, C., Wiener, H. H., Burden, S.J., . . . Larsson, N. G. 2002. Increased mitochondrial mass in mitochondrial myopathy mice. *Proceedings of the National Academy of Sciences U S A*, 99: 15066–15071.

Yang, M. Y., Bowmaker, M., Reyes, A., Vergani, L., Angeli, P., Gringeri, E., . . . Holt, I. J. 2002. Biased incorporation of ribonucleotides on the mitochondrial L-strand accounts for apparent strand-asymmetric DNA replication. *Cell*, 111: 495–505.

Yang, S. Y., He, X. Y., & Schulz, H. 1987. Fatty acid oxidation in rat brain is limited by the low activity of 3-ketoacyl-coenzyme A thiolase. *Journal of Biological Chemistry*, 262: 13027–13032.

Yasukawa, T., Reyes, A., Cluett, T. J., Yang, M. Y., Bowmaker, M., Jacobs, H. T., & Holt, I. J. 2006. Replication of vertebrate mitochondrial DNA entails transient ribonucleotide incorporation throughout the lagging strand. *EMBO Journal*, 25: 5358–5371.

Yasukawa, T., Yang, M. Y., Jacobs, H. T., & Holt, I. J. 2005. A bidirectional origin of replication maps to the major noncoding region of human mitochondrial DNA. *Mol Cell*, 18: 651–662.

Ylikallio, E., Tyynismaa, H., Tsutsui, H., Ide, T., & Suomalainen, A. 2010. High mitochondrial DNA copy number has detrimental effects in mice. *Human Molecular Genetics*, 19: 2695–2705.

Young, L. T. 2007. Is bipolar disorder a mitochondrial disease? *Journal of Psychiatry and Neuroscience*, 32: 160–161.

Youssoufian, H., & Pyeritz, R. E. 2002. Mechanisms and consequences of somatic mosaicism in humans. *Nature Reviews Genetics*, 3(10): 748–758.

Yuan, J. 2006. Divergence from a dedicated cellular suicide mechanism: exploring the evolution of cell death. *Molecular Cell*, 23: 1–12.

Zhang, H., Barcelo, J. M., Lee, B., Kohlhagen, G., Zimonjic, D. B., Popescu, N. C., & Pommier, Y. 2001. Human mitochondrial topoisomerase I. *Proceedings of National Academy of Sciences U S A*, 98: 10608–10613.

# PART III

## INTEGRATION AND FUTURE DIRECTIONS

# 12.

# INTEGRATING IMAGING AND GENETIC RESEARCH
## TOWARD PERSONALIZED MEDICINE

## Roy H. Perlis and Hilary P. Blumberg

## INTRODUCTION

Earlier chapters reviewed in detail the remarkable progress toward identifying consistent associations with bipolar disorder (BD) among neuroimaging and genetic studies. The neuroimaging studies discussed in Section I of this volume demonstrate a convergence of findings across research groups in showing structural and functional abnormalities in a corticolimbic system including the ventral prefrontal and anterior cingulate cortices and amygdala, their limbic, striatothalamic, and cerebellar connections sites, and in the connections between these brain regions in this system. The genetic studies reviewed in part II implicate the involvement of a broad and growing number of genes, some of which may moderate development, plasticity and functioning of the corticolimbic system. The integration of imaging and genetic research holds promise for further elucidating the molecular mechanisms that contribute to the brain changes of bipolar disorder. As these associations are confirmed and extended, they should enable more focused investigations of the pathophysiology underlying this illness at systems, cellular, or molecular levels. In parallel, these findings may begin to directly bear on clinical practice, fulfilling the promise of personalized medicine invoked frequently over the past decade.

This chapter begins by reviewing the relatively small number of studies that have combined imaging and genetics in bipolar disorder. In addition to considering their implications for understanding the pathophysiology of this illness, it addresses how such studies may inform future investigations by establishing more biologically homogeneous patient populations. The second section of the chapter takes an even broader perspective and considers the point at which such integrated studies may be directly applied to guide clinical practice and personalized treatment.

## INTEGRATED GENETIC-IMAGING STUDIES OF BIPOLAR DISORDER

### IMAGING AND STUDY OF CANDIDATE GENES

Initial imaging-genetic studies focused on the influence of candidate genes 1) related to mechanisms identified in preclinical studies to mediate brain changes that were homologous with the brain changes observed in mood disorders, 2) associated with mood symptoms, 3) correlated with effects of medications to treat mood disorders, or 4) found to be associated with bipolar disorder specifically. Relationships have been demonstrated between variations in these genes and the structure, function or connectivity of the corticolimbic system implicated in bipolar disorder.

In a structural imaging study example, Chepenik et al. (2009) investigated the relationship between the brain-derived neurotrophic growth factor (BDNF) gene *Val66Met* polymorphism and hippocampus morphology in bipolar disorder. BDNF has been demonstrated repeatedly in preclinical models to have corticolimbic neurotrophic effects, especially within the hippocampus; these effects appear to mediate antidepressant effects of pharmacotherapies used to treat mood disorders (Duman, 2002). The *val66met* BDNF polymorphism is a functional variation associated with diminished intracellular trafficking and activity-dependent release of BDNF protein (Chen et al., 2004). Consistent with the preclinical findings, Chepenik et al. (2009) found that both healthy individuals and those with bipolar disorder who carried the *BDNF met* allele had smaller hippocampus volumes. Those with bipolar disorder who carried the *BDNF met* allele had the lowest hippocampus volumes. Volume decreases were detected in anterior regions of left hippocampus (Figure 12.1) that are associated with verbal memory functions and hypothalamic-pituitary-adrenal axis stress responses. These findings suggest a genetic mechanism that may modify the expression of bipolar disorder and may help to explain one or more heterogeneous features of the condition. Cognitive dysfunction and stress-related impairments may be found in individuals with bipolar disorder, but may not be present in all individuals (Bearden & Freimer, 2006). We speculate that individuals with bipolar disorder who carry the *BDNF met* allele are especially vulnerable to cognitive dysfunction and stress effects. These effects may continue to progress during the adult years as *met* allele carriers with bipolar disorder showed larger decreases in temporal lobe volumes over a four-year interval than BDNF non-carriers (McIntosh et al., 2007). It is possible that *met* carriers may benefit most from treatments designed to compensate for BDNF deficiencies, such as antidepressant and mood-stabilizing pharmacotherapies, as well as exercise that has been shown in preclinical models to upregulate BDNF and increase its neurotrophic effects in hippocampus (Manji & Lenox, 2000; Duman & Monteggia, 2006). Lithium salts have been demonstrated to increase hippocampus volume in individuals with bipolar disorder (Bearden et al., 2008). However, the imaging-genetic finding is not specific to bipolar disorder, as decreased hippocampus volume in association with the *BDNF met* allele was also reported in major depressive disorder (Frodl et al., 2007) and schizophrenia (Szeszko et al., 2005). This suggests that rather than target a specific DSM-IV diagnosis with a treatment with a specific mechanism, it may be helpful to target the brain and behavioral expression associated with a specific genetic variation across disorders.

In a functional imaging study example, Shah et al. (2009) investigated the relationship between variations in a functional polymorphism for a serotonin transporter promoter protein (5-HTTLPR, locus *SLC6A4*) and regional brain response to emotional face stimuli. The short "s" allele,

associated with lower serotonin transporter mRNA transcription, and previously associated with decreased functional connectivity between the ventral anterior cingulate cortex and amygdala in healthy individuals (Pezawas et al., 2005), was associated with lower ventral anterior cingulate response to faces depicting both fearful and happy expressions. Similar to the BDNF study noted previously, the effects of the genetic variation were observed in both the healthy and bipolar groups, and there were no significant gene-by-diagnosis effects; however, the bipolar disorder "s" subgroup had the lowest ventral anterior cingulate cortex response (Figure 12.2). This finding suggests a genetic effect at another node within the corticolimbic circuitry that might be especially related to abnormalities in processing of emotional faces, a recognized characteristic of the disorder (Getz et al., 2003). The *SLC6A4* variation has been studied more extensively in major depressive disorder, with findings of associations with corticolimbic structure and function that also show interactions with stress (Williams et al., 2009). As discussed in chapter 6 in this volume, the ventral anterior cingulate has been identified previously as a region that may predict response to treatment for mood disorders, although this has been most studied for major depressive disorder (Mayberg et al., 2005). There have been reports that the "s" allele is associated with greater vulnerability to switching to a manic episode with an antidepressant (Ferreira Ade et al., 2009) and is associated with more favorable to response to lithium augmentation for depression (Stamm et al., 2008). Epistatic interactions between the BDNF and 5-HTTLPR genes in response to lithium prophylaxis for bipolar disorder have been suggested (Rybakowski et al., 2007). However, limitations in these studies are reviewed subsequently in this chapter.

In a third neuroimaging-genetics study example, that examined white matter connectivity using white matter density T1-weighted MRI and diffusion tensor imaging (DTI) methods to study healthy individuals, McIntosh et al. (McIntosh et al., 2008) observed decreased frontal-striatothalamic subcortical white matter density and structural connectivity in association with homozygosity for the "T" risk allele for the neuregulin (*NRG1*) single nucleotide polymorphism (SNP) rs6994992 (SNP8NRG243177) locus (Figure 12.3). This gene has been associated with altered type IV promoter activity in vitro, as well as binding of myelin transcription factor-1 and increased levels of type-IV NRG1 mRNA in post-mortem tissue (Law et al., 2006; Tan et al., 2007). A case-control association study demonstrated an association of the *NRG1* haplotype with susceptibility to bipolar disorder, especially in individuals with psychotic features; this association was first identified

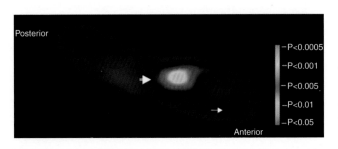

*Figure 12.1* Brain-Derived Neurotrophic Growth Factor *Val66Met* Variation and Hippocampus Morphology. The image demonstrates a three-dimensional morphometric map of the anterior hippocampus regions in which volume was smaller in met carriers for the *Val66Met* brain-derived neurotrophic growth factor gene, than in individuals homozygous for the val allele. (Source: Used with permission from the journal *Neuropsychopharmacology*; Chepenik et al. 2009.)

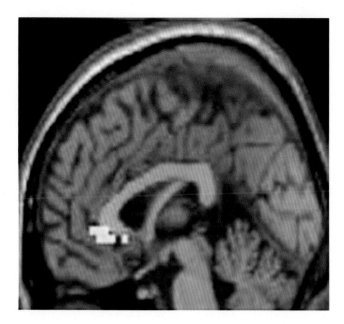

*Figure 12.2* Serotonin Transporter Promoter Protein Gene and Ventral Anterior Cingulate Function in Bipolar Disorder. The sagittal image demonstrates the ventral anterior cingulate region where individuals with bipolar disorder carrying the short "s" allele for the gene had lower response to faces depicting fearful expressions than individuals homozygous for the long "l" allele. (Source: Used with permission from the journal *Neuropsychopharmacology*; Shah et al., 2009.)

in schizophrenia (Green et al., 2005). As discussed in chapter 7 in this volume, abnormalities in white matter connections are increasingly implicated in bipolar disorder by reports of reductions in glia, and especially oligodendrocytes, as well as down-regulation of oligodendrocyte- and

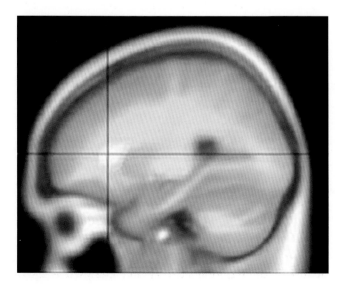

*Figure 12.3* Neuregulin 1 Gene and Frontotemporal White Matter Density. The sagittal image demonstrates the region where there was a decrease in white matter density in individuals homozygous for the T allele, compared to individuals carrying the C allele, for the neuregulin gene, rs6994992 locus. (Source: Used with permission from the journal *Molecular Psychiatry*; McIntosh et al., 2008.)

myelination-related genes (Ongur et al., 1998; Rajkowska 2002; Tkachev et al., 2003; Uranova et al., 2004; Vostrikov et al., 2007; Kim & Webster, 2008). Preclinical studies demonstrated NRG1 effects on oligodendrocyte-related structure and function, and myelin thickness (Park et al., 2001; Mei & Xiong, 2008). Social behaviors, that model symptoms of bipolar disorder, have been reported in *NRG1*-conditional-knockout mice (O'Tuathaigh et al., 2007). Interestingly, although very preliminary, small studies suggest that glial pathology in bipolar disorder may be attenuated by lithium, valproate or antipsychotic pharmacotherapy (Hamidi et al., 2004; Toro et al., 2006). This finding raises questions about subsets of individuals with bipolar disorder who may be especially vulnerable to glial pathology and who may benefit from mood-stabilizing medications. As with the other genes discussed previously in this chapter, effects of *NRG1* may not be specific to bipolar disorder. *NRG1* in particular has been associated with susceptibility to schizophrenia, and a different SNP of this gene has been associated with corticolimbic white matter connectivity in schizophrenia (Wang et al., 2009).

**Integrated Imaging and Candidate Gene Research:**

- Small studies suggest associations between specific genetic variations and specific phenotypic features of bipolar disorder

- A *BDNF* variation may influence hippocampus *structure* and associated mnemonic and stress-related functions

- A serotonin transporter promoter variation may influence ventral anterior cingulate *function* and response to emotional stimuli

- An *NRG1* variation may influence frontal-subcortical white matter *connectivity*

## IMAGING AND GENOME-WIDE ASSOCIATION STUDIES

As discussed in chapters 8 and 9, more recent availability of genome-wide association studies (GWAS) offers opportunities to identify novel genes associated with bipolar disorder. Despite limitations imposed by the need to account for multiple comparisons, such studies have begun to reliably identify variants that show statistically significant association to bipolar disorder. Among the first associations to be identified, as noted previously, was with a variant in a gene coding for a subunit of the L-type voltage-gated calcium channel, *CACNA1C*. Variation in the *CACNA1C* gene has now been demonstrated in independent genome-wide association studies to be significantly associated with bipolar disorder (Ferreira et al., 2008; Sklar et al., 2008). The rs1006737 SNP has been associated with alterations in prefrontal *CACNA1C* expression (Bigos et al., 2010), although the function of that variant *in vitro* has not been directly established.

The subsequent investigation of *CACNA1C* in imaging studies illustrates a key advantage of the combined imaging-genetic approach. That is, this approach provides a key avenue by which genetic association results may be explored and refined, complementing traditional *in vitro* approaches such as those used in gene expression studies. In fact, several studies of healthy individuals have demonstrated effects of *CACNA1C* on the structure and function of the corticolimbic neural system implicated in bipolar disorder. These findings include associations between allelic variation at rs1006737 and gray matter (GM) morphology, including total GM volume (Kempton et al., 2009) and GM volume specifically in amygdala in individuals with bipolar disorder (Perrier et al., 2011). Functional neuroimaging studies demonstrate associations between *CACNA1C* variation and functioning of the prefrontal cortex, amygdala, and hippocampus (Bigos et al., 2010; Erk et al., 2010; Wessa et al., 2010; Jogia et al., 2011). A recent study (Wang et al., 2011) demonstrated an association between a *CACNA1C* variation (rs1006737) and both frontotemporal GM morphology and ventral prefrontal-amygdala functional connectivity implicated in bipolar disorder. Together, these demonstrations of effects of the *CACNA1C* variation on many of the core neural system findings of bipolar disorder suggest that this variation may have an important role in contributing to the neural circuitry of the condition for at least a subset of individuals with bipolar disorder. Chapter 9 summarizes several additional genes suggested to be associated with bipolar disorder in GWAS studies, which are being actively investigated in current imaging-genetic studies.

---

**Integrated Imaging and GWAS Research:**

- GWAS studies have identified a few common genetic variants associated with bipolar disorder

- *CACNA1C* is an example of a gene that has repeatedly shown association to bipolar disorder, as well as with structure, function and connectivity of the corticolimbic neural system

---

## IMAGING AND OTHER GENETIC APPROACHES IN BIPOLAR DISORDER

Many more studies of relationships between imaging measures and specific genes in bipolar disorder are emerging. These relationships include recent studies of the Val158Met catechol-O-methyltransferase, D-amino acid oxidase activator and disrupted-in-schizophrenia-1 (*DISC1*) genes and corticolimbic structure, function and connectivity (Chakirova et al., 2011; Lelli-Chiesa et al., 2011; Prata et al., 2011). Each of these is associated with different aspects of the corticolimbic neural system. It is possible that there are multiple paths to the development of disruptions in the corticolimbic circuitry underlying bipolar disorder. Disruption within a particular node could contribute to overall system dysfunction. However, it is likely that multiple genes contribute to the bipolar phenotype for most individuals, and that this combination of genes differs across individuals leading to heterogeneous presentations.

Caution in drawing conclusions is needed at this early time in this field, as will be elaborated subsequently in this chapter. For example, many of the studies include small sample sizes, and the studies differ substantially in methods. However, overall, the studies suggest that genetic variations related to the development, structure and functioning of the corticolimbic neural system may have substantial effects on this system, impacting the expression of bipolar disorder. These effects appear to cut across diagnostic boundaries and map more closely onto aspects of particular brain regions and their functions. As has been highlighted throughout this volume, bipolar disorder is a highly heterogeneous disorder. Imaging-genetic studies may be first steps in understanding these heterogeneous features, such as how specific genes may lead to specific brain changes and specific features of bipolar illness. Therefore, these studies may comprise an important first step towards personalized medical approaches in which treatment for an individual may be targeted to his/her specific biological vulnerabilities. At minimum, even if the combination of imaging and genetics does not directly enable personalization, it may elucidate the biology sufficiently to allow for development of the next generation of more targeted interventions.

## CHALLENGES AND FUTURE DIRECTIONS FOR THE FIELD

With parallel advances in imaging and genetics that are applied to studying bipolar disorder, it is appealing to consider when these techniques can be deployed for clinical use. That is, can the combination be directly applied to personalize treatment, at minimum by clarifying diagnosis, and ideally by identifying optimal treatment. Because we live in a highly exciting time in the field and the field is moving toward a future of personalized medicine, there has been a recent explosion in the amount of data rapidly emerging that requires careful interpretation in order to advance our goals of personalized medicine, rather than cloud the landscape with confusion. Before such clinical translation can become reality, numerous challenges remain. Past experience with biomarkers in mood disorders suggests that clinical application may be misleading if these obstacles are not addressed systematically and explicitly, early in the course of investigation (Purcell et al., 2009). The sections that follow establish a framework for analyzing and interpreting neuroimaging, genetic, and integrated studies of bipolar disorder within a clinical context.

> **Combination of Neuroimaging and Genetics May Advance Treatment of Bipolar Disorder in Two Ways:**
>
> - By elucidating new treatment targets
>
> - By allowing more precise matching of treatments to patient subgroups, defined by biomarkers

## DEFINING SIGNIFICANCE

The customary framework for evaluating both genetic and neuroimaging studies invokes statistical significance, a measure of probability—typically of the observed data under the null hypothesis. Identifying *statistical* significance is useful for hypothesis-testing and guiding subsequent investigations, but it does not lend itself to determining *clinical* significance. Even considering effect sizes—that is, standardized differences between groups—does not in and of itself indicate whether a given association will have clinical utility. If two groups are very different on average, but exhibit substantial overlap on a particular biomarker (as has been the case for many imaging studies, for example), even a large effect may not ensure useful discrimination between those groups. To adequately assess utility, two additional kinds of information are required.

First, the performance of many tests can be described in terms of their discrimination using a two-by-two table—that is, false positives, false negatives, true positives, and true negatives—and consequently sensitivity and specificity. An extension of these metrics considers the performance of a given test in a given population; that is, the test's positive predictive value and negative predictive value. Importantly, all of these approaches require dichotomizing

measures that may be continuous—for example, blood oxygen level dependent (BOLD) signal in a functional magnetic resonance (fMRI) study—by defining a particular threshold. In order to incorporate a range of thresholds, it is possible to consider the performance of a diagnostic test in terms of sensitivity and specificity across a range of thresholds, yielding a receiver operating characteristic (ROC) curve (for examples, see Figure 12.5). An advantage of area under the ROC curve as a metric is that it combines (and integrates over) a range of sensitivity and specificity, yielding a single value; a disadvantage is that its interpretation is less obvious clinically. (For further discussion of traditional metrics of diagnostic performance, and their limitations, see Perlis, 2011).

These measures are at least interpretable in a clinical context. As an example, a diagnostic test for bipolar disorder using fMRI might have a sensitivity of 0.3 and specificity of 0.9. Such a test would not seem especially useful for identifying bipolar individuals, given its low sensitivity, which will lead it to miss many cases of bipolar disorder. On the other hand, among those testing positive, the relatively high specificity indicates it might still be a useful confirmation of diagnosis. Studies of bipolar disorder that focus on these issues have been increasingly emerging in the past few years. For example, in a study using fMRI analyses of both temporal lobe and default mode networks to discriminate individuals with bipolar disorder, schizophrenia and healthy controls (Calhoun et al., 2007), the investigators found that the combination provided average sensitivity and specificity from 90%–95%. This type of study suggests that combining different measures may increase the value over single measures alone, even though study designs and analytic approaches tend to date have tended to focus on the latter.

A measure of effect which has become popular in the effectiveness literature is number needed to treat (NNT); that is, how many patients would need to receive a given treatment to prevent (or achieve) a specific outcome for one additional patient. (For one application of this approach, see Bridge et al., 2007). This metric can be applied to testing as well: the number needed to test refers to the number of patients who need to be tested to identify a relevant outcome for one patient, which might be remission or a given adverse effect.

These examples hint at the second sort of information required to evaluate a novel diagnostic: the context. A very common misconception is that achieving a particular threshold, such as a sensitivity and specificity of 0.9, or an NNT of 3, is required to establish a useful test. In reality, there are numerous examples of clinically viable tests with far poorer discrimination. The key question is: How is the test likely to be applied? Will it be used for all patients newly-diagnosed with bipolar disorder? How about treatment-resistant patients? Or individuals with highly recurrent illnesses? And, if an accurate prediction can be made, can it be acted on, for example by selecting an alternative treatment? For example, if the goal of the test is simply to perform more efficient research by improving sample homogeneity, even a modestly discriminative tool could be useful.

Given the paucity of useful diagnostic tests in psychiatry, the temptation is great to accept any biomarker as helpful. However, if a test actually leads to more patients being exposed to a potentially toxic or expensive medication, or provides a false sense of security that leads to inadequate treatment or compromises patient safety, this approach might not be the case. On the other hand, in other circumstances in which two competing strategies have similar utility and the decision is a toss-up (Kassirer & Pauker, 1981), tests with modest performance might be valuable (Steyerberg et al., 2010).

Two related methodologies can be helpful in evaluating the clinical utility of a test once it has been validated (shown to measure what it purports to measure), and after its performance in an independent population can be estimated. One is decision analysis, which requires knowledge of the probability of specific test results and outcomes as well as their relative utility; that is, how beneficial is one outcome compared to another. These parameters can often be estimated from large clinical data sets, but a limitation of this approach is its reliance on sometimes arbitrary numbers, necessitating sensitivity analysis to examine how important each assumption might be. For an example of decision analysis for antipsychotic prescribing, see Perlis et al. (2005).

A related approach is cost-effectiveness analysis, which builds on decision analysis by incorporating costs and assigning monetary values to different outcomes (affairs). Such models can yield measures such as cost per quality-adjusted life year (i.e., how many additional years of life are "purchased" by spending an additional amount). Provided these costs are determined systematically and empirically, tools such as this can be invaluable to policymakers trying to evaluate novel technologies for clinical application. While rarely applied in this way, they can also be helpful to researchers trying to develop novel biomarkers by providing a data-based answer to questions such as: How good a test is required for clinical usefulness? For antidepressant pharmacogenomics, one such application is illustrated in (Perlis et al., 2009).

Because of the numerous assumptions required in these models, characterizing the performance of a biomarker in clinical populations may ultimately require prospective investigation. The optimal design for such studies—for example, the role of randomization and the use of historical controls—remains an area of active discussion (Perlis, 2011).

**Key Considerations Towards Using Imaging or Genetics to Personalize Care of Bipolar Disorder:**

- Statistical significance does not necessarily imply clinical significance

- A standard approach to describing diagnostic tests can also be applied to interpret imaging and genetic associations in clinical terms

- Means of describing the performance of a biomarker include area under the receiver operating characteristic curve as well as number needed to test

- The threshold at which imaging or genetic markers alone or in combination become clinically useful depends critically on context

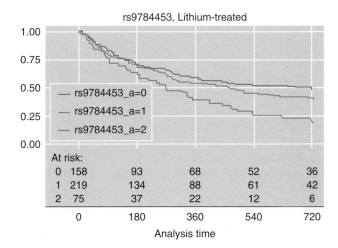

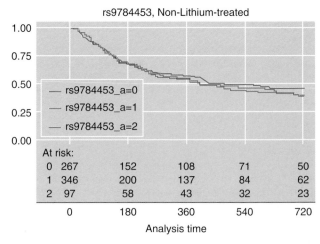

*Figure 12.4* Example of genetic association with treatment response, in this case time to mood episode recurrence in bipolar patients on lithium (top) and not on lithium (bottom). (Source: Used with permission from the journal *American Journal of Psychiatry*; Perlis et al. 2010.)

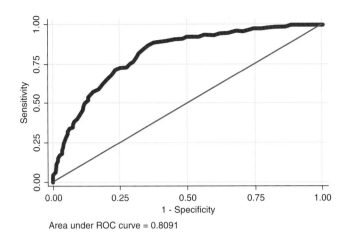

Area under ROC curve = 0.8091

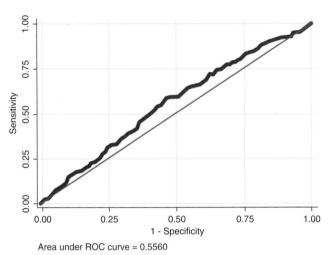

Area under ROC curve = 0.5560

*Figure 12.5* Examples of receiver operating characteristic curves for two models, based on clinical data. (Source: Used with permission from the journal *Molecular Psychiatry*; Perlis, 2011.)

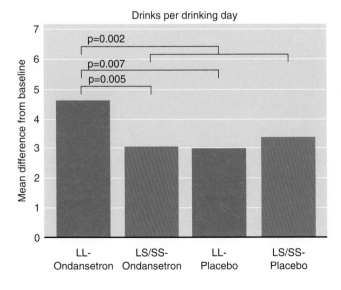

*Figure 12.6* Example of a biomarker-stratified design, used to examine ondansetron for alcohol use disorder. (Source: Used with permission from the journal *American Journal of Psychiatry*; Johnson et al. 2011.)

## DIAGNOSTIC, PROGNOSTIC, AND PREDICTIVE TESTS

In general, there are three broad categories in which biomarkers might be used to guide practice. The first is diagnosis—does a given patient have bipolar disorder, or something else? A caveat here is that distinguishing bipolar disorder from health may be more straightforward than distinguishing it from other psychiatric conditions, for example, schizophrenia. While most studies focused on discovery (whether of genes or brain structure or function) compare cases to healthy subjects, in practice discrimination from another diagnosis is more likely to be required. That is, for a patient presenting with depressive or psychotic symptoms, which may be nonspecific, is it possible to make a prediction regarding the actual disorder? Chapters 6 (Tables 6.1, 6.2, and 6.3) and 7 (Table 7.1–7.4) discuss recent studies in which direct comparisons have been performed between groups with bipolar disorder and major depressive disorder or schizophrenia respectively. These studies have suggested neural circuitry differences between conditions, such as the presence of right uncinate abnormalities in bipolar, but not major depressive, disorder or more prominent lateral prefrontal abnormalities in schizophrenia as compared to bipolar disorder. On the other hand, while these studies identify group differences, they do not typically discriminate strongly between individual cases with the diagnoses; one exception that found excellent discrimination between bipolar, schizophrenic, and healthy subjects using fMRI data has been reported (Calhoun et al., 2007).

As these studies continue to emerge, two special cases for diagnosis bear consideration. One is identification of phenocopies, presentations which may mimic bipolar disorder but in which the etiology (or at least pathology) is known. A simple example in imaging might be identification of a frontal lobe tumor in a patient presenting with manic symptoms. In genetics, individuals with velocardiofacial syndrome (DiGeorge syndrome, a deletion at 22q11) may present with symptoms of psychosis and mood disorder. In both cases, there would be distinct aspects of the management of the illness needed that would differ from those for mania arising from idiopathic bipolar disorder, even if elements of treatment are similar; consequently, recognizing the phenocopy early in the course of illness could be extremely important. Another consideration is identification of individuals at high risk for illness while they are presymptomatic, critical for developing interventions for illness prevention. It should be noted that, for bipolar disorder, family history itself is a strong predictor of risk (Smoller & Finn, 2003), but far from a perfect one. If the application of a biomarker could generate more reliable prediction, it would be more feasible and ethically viable to study interventions that carry greater risk than purely behavioral strategies. Here again, even modest prediction could greatly accelerate development of personalized interventions.

Beyond diagnosis, another potential application is prediction of treatment response. A major challenge cited by patients and clinicians is the trial and error required to identify an effective and well-tolerated treatment, despite (or perhaps because of) a growing number of pharmacotherapies with demonstrated efficacy compared to placebo. Ideally such a test would allow selection of specific treatments—that is, rather than simply estimating probability of response to a given medication, it would be useful to know whether probability of success is greater with a different treatment (Simon & Perlis, in press). Unfortunately, to date, the genetic investigation of treatment response in bipolar disorder has little to say regarding specificity. This limitation arises primarily from a paucity of large-scale randomized, controlled trials using active comparators rather than placebo (Hirschfeld et al., 2002).

There have been a small number of candidate-based association studies of lithium response, implicating neurotransmitter genes such as *DRD1* (Rybakowski et al., 2009) and *SLC6A4* (Rybakowski et al., 2005), second messenger systems involving CREB (Mamdani et al., 2008) and glycogen synthase kinase (GSK) 3 (Benedetti et al., 2005), among many others. A recent review highlights substantial methodological limitations (Smith et al., 2010), including sample heterogeneity, small sample size, variable definitions of responsiveness, and absence of replication. To date, one recent genome-wide association study has examined lithium responsiveness (Perlis et al., 2009). That study examined two cohorts of lithium-treated patients with bipolar I or II disorders, and identified suggestive evidence of association for a region including the gene coding for glutamate/AMPA receptor (*GRIA2*). This association was not observed in a cohort of non-lithium-treated subjects, perhaps suggesting some degree of specificity. Association results also did not support previously reported candidate gene studies.

The 5-HTTLPR polymorphism, in the serotonin transporter SCL6A4, previously implicated in phenotypes ranging from rapid-cycling bipolar disorder (Cusin et al., 2001) to personality trait features such as neuroticism (Jacob et al., 2004), has also been investigated as a predictor of antidepressant-associated mania. Despite individual small positive studies, a meta-analysis (Biernacka et al., 2011) did not support the latter association. Finally, one small candidate-gene based study examined olanzapine/fluoxetine and lamotrigine in the treatment of depression in bipolar disorder.

That study examined common variants primarily in neurotransmitter-related genes, and suggested associations for dopamine receptor 3 (*DRD3*) and histamine H1 receptor genes with olanzapine/fluoxetine combination response, and a different set (though with HRH1 in common) with lamotrigine (Perlis et al., 2010). To date, however, these findings have not been replicated.

Still, even in the absence of specific predictors, prognostic tests may also inform practice. A nonspecific predictor of greater risk could play a central role in targeting interventions and allocating resources. For example, individuals at greatest risk for manic recurrence might be triaged to receive more aggressive antimanic treatment (perhaps higher dosages, or combination treatments), even if the optimal antimanic treatment cannot be determined a priori. Those at high risk for depressive symptom chronicity, or for cognitive symptoms, might be triaged to receive behavioral interventions early in their illness course. Patients and families may benefit directly from even limited information about the likely course of illness, perhaps giving them a better sense of control.

---

**Considerations Toward Using Genetics and Imaging for Personalize Care of Bipolar Disorder:**

- One way in which imaging and genetics may be applied for diagnosis is in the identification of phenocopies—specific disease entities which may mimic a psychiatric disorder

- Biomarkers combined with known risk factors for bipolar disorder (e.g., family history) may be more useful than either alone

- Biomarkers also offer promise in predicting treatment response in bipolar disorder, if preliminary studies can be replicated

- No genes have yet been identified that reliably predict treatment response

---

## OVERFITTING AND THE IMPORTANCE OF INDEPENDENT DATA SETS

A tremendous diversity of approaches exist to building predictive models, from regression to complex machine learning approaches such as support vector machines as discussed in chapter 6. Common among these approaches is finding some optimal combination of predictor variables to model a specific data set. These algorithms are developed, or trained, using a given data set, so they will essentially always have the best fit for that data set. An important distinguishing feature among machine learning techniques is the extent to which they are likely to "overfit" a data set, incorporating variables which are actually noise but improve prediction in the discovery data (Ioannidis, 2008). Unfortunately, if model performance is reported for the same data set to which the model was fitted, the performance is highly likely to be optimistic, or to overestimate model performance.

A rule of thumb in developing predictive models holds one-third of a data set in reserve and builds the model from the remaining two-thirds. As reviewers and journal editors increasingly recognize the problem of type I error and insist upon replication of discoveries in genetics and neuroimaging, researchers face a dilemma: conduct the best-powered analysis using all of their data, or work with a smaller discovery sample to ensure access to a replication data set. While practical in large data sets (for example, population-based studies of disease), this latter approach may be infeasible in the smaller data sets more common in psychiatric biomarker studies. At minimum, the use of cross-validation—for example, iteratively holding out 10% of the sample to estimate model performance, then repeating with each subsequent 10%—can help reduce overfitting.

A common example in both psychiatric genetics and neuroimaging is to report the test parameters of a given variant or region after a series of univariate tests—those with smallest p-values are then used to distinguish (for example) cases and controls. As a rough measure of relevance, this approach is not unreasonable, provided that these results are not misinterpreted as indicating how a model is likely to perform in subsequent data sets. The problem is that such claims are tautological: A marker is selected because it allows detection of some difference between groups, then shown to detect separation between groups. If the goal is to make a claim about how a given predictor really performs, an independent data set is required (Steyerberg et al., 2010).

In interpreting model results, another important indicator is generalizability—that is, how well do the results generalize to other populations? Clinical trial populations may differ markedly from general clinical populations (Wisniewski et al., 2009); even individual clinical populations may be very different in terms of features that would influence treatment outcomes, such as socioeconomic status or extent of medical comorbidity. This challenge may be particularly great in genetic studies, which have often been limited to very homogeneous populations by design. The extent to which findings in large Caucasian cohorts in mood or psychotic disorders may be applicable in other ethnic groups remains to be determined.

## COMPARING MODELS

At times, researchers or clinicians will want to directly compare two alternate models, such as different biomarker-based tests. A first step is defining model performance in terms of some common measure that is independent of sample size and composition. Alternatively, performance in a reference or gold-standard data set can be reported—the need for such data sets, ideally encompassing a broad range of biomarkers, is acute. One common figure is area under ROC curve (AUC), a measure of discrimination; two AUCs can be compared to determine if they are statistically significantly different. Comparing ROC curves may not be sensitive to more modest improvements; however, single variables with strong evidence of univariate association may minimally impact AUC (Cook, 2007).

A practical way of comparing two biomarkers might be to contrast sensitivity for a given specificity, or vice versa. While comparing AUCs indicates performance over a range of thresholds, ultimately a single threshold will be selected for implementation, so it is reasonable to examine performance at that threshold. Notably, a test with a lesser AUC may still have superior performance at a given threshold, depending on the shapes of the ROC curves.

It should also be noted that discrimination is only one aspect of model performance, albeit a crucial one. It is also important to consider model calibration: that is, how well does predicted risk match observed risk? While in some cases a dichotomous determination is required—"does this patient have bipolar disorder?"—in others a probability is more useful. For example, one might ask how likely a patient is to experience a second manic episode within six months; while a definite yes or no probably overstates the case, a figure like 60% from a well-calibrated model can guide clinical decision-making. Models with similar discrimination overall may have very different calibration, which could influence their mode of application. While an optimal test would perform well on both measures, it many cases there is some tradeoff between them (Diamond, 1992).

## A BETTER MEANS OF INTEGRATING BIOMARKERS: THE NET RECLASSIFICATION INDEX

Biomarker investigators in psychiatry often see themselves as working from scratch—trying to develop prediction models that are simply superior to chance. In other areas of medicine, where numerous clinical and biological markers have been identified and clinically applied, the perspective is somewhat different. Here, techniques have been developed to characterize the improvement in a model achieved by adding a new set of predictors, referred to as the net reclassification index (NRI). (For a review, see Pencina et al., 2008). In other words, rather than beginning with chance, investigators can begin with the best available model and examine whether adding additional biomarkers improves performance. Essentially, the NRI measures how much the addition of a marker is able to move subjects to more accurate classifications (that is, higher-risk subjects move up, lower-risk subjects move down). An extension of this approach eliminates the need to specify categories a priori (Pencina et al., 2008). To illustrate the application of the NRI, adding a genetic score for cardiovascular risk based on cholesterol studies failed to improve AUC over a standard clinical measure, but did yield significant reclassification improvement (Kathiresan et al., 2008).

---

**Considerations for Biomarker Model Building:**

- A key challenge in extending research findings to practice is the risk of overfitting—building models that fit the initial data set well but do not perform well in subsequent cohorts

- Techniques for measuring the improvement in test performance with addition of new markers, including the net reclassification index, may be particularly useful in integrating imaging and genetic results

- Biomarkers also offer promise in predicting treatment response in bipolar disorder, if preliminary studies can be replicated

---

## INTEGRATING NEUROIMAGING, GENETIC, AND CLINICAL DATA

The extant data from genetic association studies in bipolar disorder suggest that no single locus is likely to account for a large proportion of variance in disease risk. Aggregating over multiple markers is one strategy to improve prediction; a 2009 report demonstrated that even variants of rather modest association could still increase variance accounted for (Purcell et al., 2009); indeed, model fit improved with inclusion of many thousands of variants of modest statistical significance. With the rapid fall in cost for genome-wide genotyping, it is no longer necessary to focus only on the two or three "best" variants; the incremental cost for models incorporating thousands of variants is modest.

More generally, assuming that predictors are not completely correlated, there is no reason one cannot combine

modalities to achieve better performance in diagnostic tests. This approach may be particularly relevant for neuroimaging and genetics, which probably capture somewhat different markers of or diatheses for illness. While the studies reviewed earlier suggest associations between genes and brain structure or function, such correlation does not preclude the combination of these measures to derive more predictive markers. Moreover, there is no reason clinical data cannot be integrated with these kinds of data to further improve prediction. The application of NRI and related concepts could help guide this sort of integration, by determining which combinations improve performance and which do not, when reliance on (for example) model fit alone is not well-suited.

A key next step will be to begin to report sufficient results in imaging and genetic studies to allow their performance to be established. In this way, future studies can try to improve upon previous work by adding additional clinical, genetic, or phenotypic data.

## BIOMARKERS IN CLINICAL TRIALS

Biomarkers may be especially useful in designing more efficient clinical trials, and both imaging and genetics offer promise for this application. At present, the route from target discovery to clinical availability is long, tortuous, and costly. If trials could be made more efficient, this process might be accelerated and new treatments brought to the clinic more rapidly. One such approach relies on identifying markers that could serve as surrogate endpoints (Hampel et al., 2010). Here, of course, genetic variation (as a trait marker which does not change over time) would not be useful, but neuroimaging or other markers may well be, as has been the case in Alzheimer's disease (Dickerson & Sperling, 2005), for example.

Alternatively, markers could be used to improve drug-placebo separation in clinical trials. Two categories of designs to do so are biomarker-enriched and biomarker-stratified. In the first design, subjects are characterized at study entry for a predefined set of markers. Only subjects with a given profile (presumably, those more likely to respond to drug, or less likely to respond to placebo) would be randomized. This yields a study that is enriched for (in fact, limited to) that population. A limitation of this approach is that it assumes that the putative biomarker is correct, which can rarely be established with confidence. In addition, a successful study still does not establish the value of the biomarker—it is possible that those subjects who were excluded would have responded just as well, necessitating a follow-up study.

By comparison, a biomarker-stratified trial enrolls all eligible subjects, but stratifies randomization by a particular marker to ensure equal representation in treatment and comparison arms. One recent example in psychiatry examined ondansetron response in alcohol dependence, stratifying groups by variation in the *SLC6A4* gene ( Johnson et al., in press). This study found a significant benefit versus placebo in one group, but not the other. An advantage of this approach is that it allows determination of overall treatment effects as well as treatment-by-biomarker interactions. A major disadvantage, however, is the need for large sample sizes in order to have adequate statistical power to detect true differences. That is, if the goal is first to identify significant differences in the marker-positive group, that group must be powered accordingly.

Essentially, enriched and stratified trials may be considered as conducting the necessary trials in serial (enriched) versus parallel (stratified), trading off resources (cost) for time. In other words, a negative result from an enriched trial might lead to a decision not to proceed, saving at least the cost of a second (marker-negative) trial, but a positive result will likely entail a second trial, with additional expenditure of time.

One final point relevant to both designs is often overlooked. Most trials use some form of a screen-baseline design, often with a one-week interval preceding randomization. In order for either study type to be feasible, it must be possible to collect the necessary data to stratify or determine eligibility in the interval between screen and baseline. While most biomarkers allow for rapid turnaround, in practice this speed may be challenging to operationalize—for example, getting DNA extracted and genotyped, or scheduling a neuroimaging appointment, sufficiently quickly to inform treatment selection or randomization.

---

**Additional Considerations for Imaging and Genetic Biomarker Development:**

- Combinations of imaging and genetic data with other biomarkers or clinical data may further improve performance of a test

- Integrating imaging and genetics may also facilitate more efficient clinical investigation, yielding more homogeneous patient populations for study

- Applying putative biomarkers to clinical trial designs might both refine biomarkers as well as facilitate novel drug identification/development

---

## HIGH-PRIORITY AREAS FOR DIAGNOSTIC DEVELOPMENT IN BIPOLAR DISORDER

Any number of approaches could be used to prioritize areas in which a biomarker-based test in bipolar disorder might be most useful. Experience in developing guidelines for the treatment of bipolar disorder (Hirschfeld et al., 2002) suggests a number of areas where practice could be impacted with an appropriate diagnostic, predictive, or prognostic test. As an interim step, integrating imaging and genetics might at least establish initial models, facilitating development of subsequent tests with greater precision.

High priority areas for these types of approaches include:

1. *Distinguishing bipolar disorder from major depressive disorder*: Identifying bipolar disorder among individuals presenting in a major depressive episode remains a clinical challenge, particularly in the absence of collateral or historic data or early in an individual's illness course. A test that distinguishes these two could be very useful in planning treatment and understanding likely course, and may be especially important as incorrect treatment may have major adverse effects on prognosis.

2. *Diagnosing bipolar disorder in youth*: Some research groups consider chronic irritable symptoms sufficient for the diagnosis when there can be substantial overlap with the symptoms of other disorders such as attention deficit hyperactivity disorder, whereas other groups consider the presence of a distinct episode, euphoria and grandiosity necessary conditions (Geller et al., 1998; Leibenluft et al., 2003). Longitudinal follow-up suggests that the latter is associated with a full bipolar disorder course in adulthood (Findling et al., 2010). Several neuroimaging studies have emerged to directly compare youths with different subsets of symptoms (Brotman et al., 2010). Differences have been identified but such studies are highly challenging and these findings have not yet been replicated. It has been argued that these children should be considered and treated differently. There, however, remains much debate over whether this is premature. On the other hand the stakes are high as incorrect treatment can have serious consequences.

3. *Antipsychotic-associated weight gain and metabolic symptoms*: The atypical antipsychotics have shown significant efficacy in acute and longer-term treatment of bipolar disorder (Hirschfeld et al., in press), but at present those drugs with the most supportive data are also among those with the greatest metabolic risk. A test that could stratify weight gain risk might allow for more

confident prescribing, with more metabolically toxic treatments reserved for those at low risk for weight gain.

4. *Estimating suicide risk*: While bipolar individuals may be ~20 times more likely to die by suicide than the general population (Osby et al., 2001), clinical tools for assessing this risk are extremely limited, particularly for the longer-term. For example, one key predictor of suicide attempts is past attempts, but of course this assumes that the patient survives the initial attempt. As the majority of suicide attempts, though by no means all, appear to come early in the course of illness (Osby et al., 2001), a tool for rapidly stratifying suicide risk could be invaluable.

Of course, numerous other clinical scenarios in bipolar disorder would benefit from identification and validation of biomarkers, whether genetic, neuroimaging, or another emerging technology. As such biomarkers emerge, it will be critical that researchers and clinicians understand how markers are validated, how their performance can be quantified, and how their utility can be established.

## CONCLUSIONS

There have been substantial advances in understanding bipolar disorder from the fields of neuroimaging and genetics research. Joining these two research fields holds considerable promise for revealing genetic mechanisms that contribute to the brain system abnormalities that underlie the disorder and for the development of treatments that can be better targeted for individuals based on their underlying biology. The imaging data may help to characterize the function *in vivo* of genetic effects, while the genetic data may help to elucidate mechanisms contributing to the observed imaging findings. By defining more homogeneous groups, the combination of imaging and genetics may facilitate further characterization of biology necessary to drive discovery of treatments or diagnostic tools. From a clinical/translational perspective, such an integrated approach also offers potential benefit. Even if a single modality is insufficient to define a patient subgroup, combining multiple modalities—which may include imaging, genetics, other biomarkers, and even clinical data—may overcome this limitation.

Research combining diverse technologies, like neuroimaging and genetics, is in its youth and there are major challenges ahead. An exciting aspect of this combination, however, is the increasing ability to explore numerous hypotheses simultaneously, and thereby drive discovery; unfortunately, this approach also contributes to a substantial risk of *false* discovery. One traditional method to manage this problem requires replication of initial findings in larger samples, which may pose challenges in feasibility and lead to prematurely abandoning promising findings. As multiple genetic factors likely contribute to the bipolar disorder phenotype, and these likely differ across individuals with the disorder, the field will need to find solutions to address this high level of complexity. The framework discussed in this chapter reviews some of the concepts important in interpreting and integrating biomarkers where clinical application is contemplated. Ultimately, such integrated measures may allow for true personalized medicine in psychiatry, as a tool for matching patients with the interventions most likely to be effective for them.

## REFERENCES

Affairs, U. D. o. V. Introduction to Cost-Effectiveness Analysis (CEA).

Bearden, C. E. and N. B. Freimer 2006. Endophenotypes for psychiatric disorders: ready for primetime? *Trends in Genetics*, 22(6): 306–313.

Bearden, C. E., P. M. Thompson, . . . et al. 2008. Three-dimensional mapping of hippocampal anatomy in unmedicated and lithium-treated patients with bipolar disorder. *Neuropsychopharmacology*, 33(6): 1229–1238.

Benedetti, F., A. Serretti, Pontiggia, A., Bernasconi, A., Lorenzi, C., Colombo, C., & Smeraldi, E. 2005. Long-term response to lithium salts in bipolar illness is influenced by the glycogen synthase kinase 3-beta -50 T/C SNP. *Neuroscience Letters*, 376(1): 51–55.

Biernacka, J. M., McElroy, S. L., Crow, S., Sharp, A., Benitez, J., Veldic, M., . . . Frye, M. A. (2011). Pharmacogenomics of antidepressant induced mania: A review and meta-analysis of the serotonin transporter gene (5HTTLPR) association. *Journal of Affective Disorders*.

Bigos, K. L., Mattay, V. S., Callicott, J. H., Straub, R. E., Vakkalanka, R., Kolachana, B., . . . Weinberger, D. R. (2010). Genetic variation in CACNA1C affects brain circuitries related to mental illness. *Archives of General Psychiatry*, 67(9): 939–945.

Bridge, J. A., Iyengar, S., Salary, C. B., Barbe, R. P., Birmaher, B., Pincus, H. A., . . . Brent, D. A. (2007). Clinical response and risk for reported suicidal ideation and suicide attempts in pediatric antidepressant treatment: a meta-analysis of randomized controlled trials. *JAMA*, 297(15): 1683–1696.

Brotman, M. A., Rich, B. A., Guyer, A. E., Lunsford, J. R., Horsey, S. E., Reising, M. M., . . . , Leibenluft, E. 2010. Amygdala activation during emotion processing of neutral faces in children with severe mood dysregulation versus ADHD or bipolar disorder. *The American journal of Psychiatry*, 167(1): 61–69.

Calhoun, V. D., Maciejewski, P. K., Pearlson G.D., & Kiehl K. A. 2007. Temporal lobe and "default" hemodynamic brain modes discriminate between schizophrenia and bipolar disorder. *Human Brain Mapping*.

Chakirova, G., Whalley, H. C., Thomson, P. A., Hennah, W., Moorhead, T. W., Welch, K. A. . . . McIntosh, A. M. 2011. The effects of DISC1 risk variants on brain activation in controls, patients with bipolar disorder and patients with schizophrenia. *Psychiatry Research*, 192(1): 20–28.

Chen, Z. Y., Patel, P. D., Sant, G., Meng, C. X., Teng, K. K., Hempstead, B. L., & Lee, F. S. 2004. Variant brain-derived neurotrophic factor (BDNF) (Met66) alters the intracellular trafficking and activity-dependent secretion of wild-type BDNF in neurosecretory cells and cortical neurons. *The Journal of neuroscience: The Official Journal of the Society for Neuroscience*, 24(18): 4401–4411.

Chepenik, L. G., Fredericks, C., Papademetris, X., Spencer, L., Lacadie, C., Wang F. . . . Blumberg, H. P. 2009. Effects of the brain-derived neurotrophic growth factor val66met variation on hippocampus morphology in bipolar disorder. *Neuropsychopharmacology*. Mar;34(4):944–51.

Cook, N. R. 2007. Use and misuse of the receiver operating characteristic curve in risk prediction. *Circulation*, 115(7): 928–935.

Cusin, C., Serretti, A., Lattuada, E., Lilli, R., Lorenzi, C., Mandelli, L., . . . Smeraldi, E. 2001. Influence of 5-HTTLPR and TPH variants on illness time course in mood disorders. *Journal of Psychiatric Research*, 35(4): 217–223.

Diamond, G. A. 1992. What price perfection? Calibration and discrimination of clinical prediction models. *Journal of Clinical Epidemiology*, 45(1): 85–89.

Dickerson, B. C. and Sperling, R. A. 2005. Neuroimaging biomarkers for clinical trials of disease-modifying therapies in Alzheimer's disease. *NeuroRx: The Journal of the American Society for Experimental NeuroTherapeutics*, 2(2): 348–360.

Duman, R. S. 2002. Synaptic plasticity and mood disorders. *Molecular Psychiatry*, 7 (Suppl 1): S29–34.

Duman, R. S. and Monteggia, L. M. 2006. A neurotrophic model for stress-related mood disorders. *Biological Psychiatry*, 59(12): 1116–1127.

Erk, S., Meyer-Lindenberg, A., Schnell, K., Opitz von Boberfeld, C., Esslinger, C., Kirsch, P., . . . Walter H. 2010. Brain function in carriers of a genome-wide supported bipolar disorder variant. *Archives of General Psychiatry*, 67(8): 803–811.

Ferreira Ade, A., Neves, F. S., da Rocha, F. F., Silva, G. S., Romano-Silva, M. A., Miranda, D. M., . . . Correa, H. 2009. The role of 5-HTTLPR polymorphism in antidepressant-associated mania in bipolar disorder. *Journal of Affective Disorders*, 112(1–3): 267–272.

Ferreira, M. A., O'Donovan, M. C., Meng, Y. A., Jones, I. R., Ruderfer, D. M., Jones, L., . . . et al. 2008. Collaborative genome-wide association analysis supports a role for ANK3 and CACNA1C in bipolar disorder. *Nature Geneicst*, 40(9): 1056–1058.

Findling, R. L., Youngstrom, E. A., Fristad, M. A., Birmaher, B., Kowatch, R. A., Arnold, L. E., . . . Horwitz, S. M. 2010. Characteristics of children with elevated symptoms of mania: the Longitudinal Assessment of Manic Symptoms (LAMS) study. *The Journal of Clinical Psychiatry*, 71(12): 1664–1672.

Frodl, T., Schüle, C., Schmitt, G., Born, C., Baghai, T., Zill, P., Bottlender, R., . . . Meisenzahl, E.M. 2007. Association of the brain-derived neurotrophic factor Val66Met polymorphism with reduced hippocampal volumes in major depression. *Archives of General Psychiatry*, 64(4): 410–416.

Geller, B., Williams, M., Zimerman, B., Frazier, J., Beringer, L. and Warner, K. L. 1998. Prepubertal and early adolescent bipolarity differentiate from ADHD by manic symptoms, grandiose delusions, ultra-rapid or ultradian cycling. *Journal of Affective Disorders*, 51(2): 81–91.

Getz, G. E., Shear, P. K. and Strakowski, S. M. 2003. Facial affect recognition deficits in bipolar disorder. *Journal of the International Neuropsychological Society*, 9(4): 623–632.

Green, E. K., Raybould, R., Macgregor, S., Gordon-Smith, K., Heron, J., Hyde, S., . . . Craddock, N. 2005. Operation of the schizophrenia susceptibility gene, neuregulin 1, across traditional diagnostic boundaries to increase risk for bipolar disorder. *Archives of General Psychiatry*, 62(6): 642–648.

Hamidi, M., Drevets, W. C. and Price, J. L. 2004. Glial reduction in amygdala in major depressive disorder is due to oligodendrocytes. *Biological Psychiatry*, 55(6): 563–569.

Hampel, H., Frank, R., Broich, K., Teipel, S. J., Katz, R. G., Hardy, J., . . . Blennow, K. 2010. Biomarkers for Alzheimer's disease: academic, industry and regulatory perspectives. *Nature Reviews Drug Discovery*, 9(7): 560–574.

Hirschfeld, R. A., C. L. Bowden, . . . et al. 2002. Practice guideline for the treatment of patients with bipolar disorder (revision). *American Journal of Psychiatry*, 159(4 Supp.).

Hirschfeld, R. A., M. J. Gitlin, . . . et al. In press. Practice Guideline for the Treatment of Patients with Bipolar Disorder. Arlington, VA: American Psychiatric Association.

Ioannidis, J. P. 2008. Why most discovered true associations are inflated. *Epidemiology*, 19(5): 640–648.

Jacob, C. P., Strobel, A., Hohenberger, K., Ringel, T., Gutknecht, L., Reif, A., . . . Lesch, K. P. 2004. Association between allelic variation of serotonin transporter function and neuroticism in anxious cluster C personality disorders. *The American Journal of Psychiatry*, 161(3): 569–572.

Jogia, J., Ruberto, G., Lelli-Chiesa, G., Vassos, E., Maierú, M., Tatarelli, R., . . . Frangou, S. 2011. The impact of the CACNA1C gene polymorphism on frontolimbic function in bipolar disorder. *Molecular Psychiatry*.

Johnson, B. A., Ait-Daoud, N., Seneviratne, C., Roache, J. D., Javors, M. A., Wang, X. Q., . . . Li, M. D. In press. Pharmacogenetic Approach at the Serotonin Transporter Gene as a Method to Reduce the Severity of Drinking Alcohol. *American Journal of Psychiatry*.

Kassirer, J. P. and Pauker, S. G. 1981. The toss-up. *New England Journal of Medicine*, 305(24): 1467–1469.

Kathiresan, S., Melander, O., Anevski, D., Guiducci, C., Burtt, N. P., Roos, C., . . . Orho-Melander, M. 2008. Polymorphisms associated with cholesterol and risk of cardiovascular events. *New England Journal of Medicine*, 358(12): 1240–1249.

Kempton, M. J., Ruberto, G., Vassos, E., Tatarelli, R., Girardi, P., Collier, D., & Frangou, S. 2009. Effects of the CACNA1C risk allele for bipolar disorder on cerebral gray matter volume in healthy individuals. *American Journal of Psychiatry*, 166(12): 1413–1414.

Kim, S. and Webster, M. J. 2008. Correlation analysis between genome-wide expression profiles and cytoarchitectural abnormalities in the prefrontal cortex of psychiatric disorders. *Molecular Psychiatry*.

Law, A. J., Lipska, B. K., Weickert, C. S., Hyde, T. M., Straub, R. E., Hashimoto, R., . . . Weinberger, D. R. 2006. Neuregulin 1 transcripts are differentially expressed in schizophrenia and regulated by 5' SNPs associated with the disease. *Proceedings of National Academy of Science U S A*, 103(17): 6747–6752.

Leibenluft, E., Charney, D. S., Towbin, K. E., Bhangoo, R. K. and Pine, D. S. 2003. Defining clinical phenotypes of juvenile mania. *The American Journal of Psychiatry*, 160(3): 430–437.

Lelli-Chiesa, Kempton, M. J., Jogia, J., Tatarelli, R., Girardi, P., Powell, J., . . . Frangou, S. 2011. The impact of the Val158Met catechol-O-methyltransferase genotype on neural correlates of sad facial affect processing in patients with bipolar disorder and their relatives. *Psychological Medicine*, 41(4): 779–788.

Mamdani, F., Alda, M., Grof, P., Young, L. T., Rouleau, G., & Turecki, G. 2008. Lithium response and genetic variation in the CREB family of genes. *American Journal of Medical Genetics. Part B, Neuropsychiatric Genetics: The Official Publication of the International Society of Psychiatric Genetics*, 147B(4): 500–504.

Manji, H. K. and Lenox, R. H. 2000. Signaling: cellular insights into the pathophysiology of bipolar disorder. *Biological Psychiatry*, 48(6): 518–530.

Mayberg, H. S., Lozano, A. M., Voon, V., McNeely, H. E., Seminowicz, D., Hamani, C., . . . Kennedy, S. H. 2005. Deep brain stimulation for treatment-resistant depression. *Neuron*, 45(5): 651–660.

McIntosh, A. M., Moorhead, T. W., McKirdy, J., Sussmann, J. E., Hall, J., Johnstone, E. C., & Lawrie, S. M. 2007. Temporal grey matter reductions in bipolar disorder are associated with the BDNF Val66Met polymorphism. *Molecular Psychiatry*, 12(10): 902–903.

McIntosh, A. M., Moorhead, T. W., Job, D., Lymer, G. K., Muñoz Maniega, S., McKirdy, J., . . . Hall, J. 2008. The effects of a neuregulin 1 variant on white matter density and integrity. *Molecular Psychiatry*, 13(11): 1054–1059.

Mei, L. and Xiong, W. C. 2008. Neuregulin 1 in neural development, synaptic plasticity and schizophrenia. *Nature Reviews Neuroscience*, 9(6): 437–452.

O'Tuathaigh, C. M., Babovic, D., O'Sullivan, G. J., Clifford, J. J., Tighe, O., Croke, D. T., . . . Waddington, J. L. 2007. Phenotypic characterization of spatial cognition and social behavior in mice with 'knockout' of the schizophrenia risk gene neuregulin 1. *Neuroscience*, 147(1): 18–27.

Ongur, D., Drevets, W. C. and Price, J. L. 1998. Glial reduction in the subgenual prefrontal cortex in mood disorders. *Proceedings of National Academy of Science U S A*, 95(22): 13290–13295.

Osby, U., Correia, N., Ekbom, A. and Sparén, P. 2001. Excess mortality in bipolar and unipolar disorder in Sweden. *Archives of General Psychiatry*, 58(9): 844–850.

Park, S. K., Solomon, D. and Vartanian, T. 2001. Growth factor control of CNS myelination. *Developmental Neuroscience*, 23(4–5): 327–337.

Pencina, M. J., D'Agostino, R. B. Sr., D'Agostino, R. B. Jr., Vasan R. S. 2008. Evaluating the added predictive ability of a new marker: from area under the ROC curve to reclassification and beyond. *Stat Medical*, 27(2): 157–172; discussion 207–112.

Perlis, R. H. 2011. Translating biomarkers to clinical practice. *Molecular psychiatry*.

Perlis, R. H., Patrick, A., Smoller, J. W. and Wang, P. S. 2009. When is pharmacogenetic testing for antidepressant response ready for the clinic? A cost-effectiveness analysis based on data from the STAR*D study. *Neuropsychopharmacology*, 34(10): 2227–2236.

Perlis, R. H., Ganz, D. A., Avorn, J., Schneeweiss, S., Glynn, R. J., Smoller, J. W. and Wang, P. S. 2005. Pharmacogenetic testing in the clinical management of schizophrenia: a decision-analytic model. *Journal of Clinical Psychopharmacology*, 25(5): 427–434.

Perlis, R. H., Adams, D. H., Fijal, B., Sutton, V. K., Farmen, M., Breier, A. and Houston, J. P. 2010. Genetic association study of treatment response with olanzapine/fluoxetine combination or lamotrigine in bipolar I depression. *The Journal of Clinical Psychiatry*, 71(5): 599–605.

Perlis, R. H., Smoller, J. W., Ferreira, M. A., McQuillin, A., Bass, N., Lawrence, J., . . . Purcell, S. 2009. A genomewide association study of response to lithium for prevention of recurrence in bipolar disorder. *American Journal of Psychiatry*, 166(6): 718–725.

Perrier, E., Pompei, F., Ruberto, G., Vassos, E., Collier, D. and Frangou, S. 2011. Initial evidence for the role of CACNA1C on subcortical brain morphology in patients with bipolar disorder. *European Psychiatry*, 26(3): 135–137.

Pezawas, L., Meyer-Lindenberg, A., Drabant, E. M., Verchinski, B. A., Munoz, K. E., Kolachana, B. S., . . . Weinberger, D. R. 2005. 5-HTTLPR polymorphism impacts human cingulate-amygdala interactions: A genetic susceptibility mechanism for depression. *Nature Neuroscience*, 8: 828–834.

Prata, D. P., Papagni, S. A., Mechelli, A., Fu, C. H., Kambeitz, J., Picchioni, M., . . . McGuire, P. K. 2011. Effect of D-amino acid oxidase activator (DAOA; G72) on brain function during verbal fluency. *Human Brain Mapping*, 33(1): 143–153.

Purcell, S. M., Wray, N. R., Stone, J. L., Visscher, P. M., O'Donovan, M. C., Sullivan, P. F. and Sklar, P. 2009. Common polygenic variation contributes to risk of schizophrenia and bipolar disorder. *Nature*, 460(7256): 748–752.

Rajkowska, G. 2002. Cell pathology in mood disorders. *Semin Clin Neuropsychiatry*, 7(4): 281–292.

Rybakowski, J. K., Suwalska, A., Czerski, P.M., Dmitrzak-Weglarz, M., Leszczynska-Rodziewicz, A. and Hauser, J. 2005. Prophylactic effect of lithium in bipolar affective illness may be related to serotonin transporter genotype. *Pharmacological Reports*, 57(1): 124–127.

Rybakowski, J. K., Suwalska, A., Skibinska, M., Dmitrzak-Weglarz, M., Leszczynska-Rodziewicz, A. and Hauser, J. 2007. Response to lithium prophylaxis: interaction between serotonin transporter and BDNF genes. *American Journal of Medical Genetics. Part B, Neuropsychiatric Genetics: The Official Publication of the International Society of Psychiatric Genetics*, 144B(6): 820–823.

Rybakowski, J. K., Dmitrzak-Weglarz, M., Suwalska, A., Leszczynska-Rodziewicz, A. and Hauser, J. 2009. Dopamine D1 receptor gene polymorphism is associated with prophylactic lithium response in bipolar disorder. *Pharmacopsychiatry*, 42(1): 20–22.

Shah, M. P., Wang, F., Kalmar, J. H., Chepenik, L. G., Tie, K., Pittman, B., Jones, M. M., . . . Blumberg, H. P. 2009. Role of variation in the serotonin transporter protein gene (SLC6A4) in trait disturbances in the ventral anterior cingulate in bipolar disorder. *Neuropsychopharmacology*, 34(5): 1301–1310.

Simon, G. and Perlis, R. In press. Personalized treatment of major depressive disorder. *American Journal of Psychiatry*.

Sklar, P., Smoller, J. W., Fan, J., Ferreira, M. A., Perlis, R. H., Chambert, K., . . . Purcell, S. M. 2008. Whole-genome association study of bipolar disorder. *Molecular Psychiatry*, 13(6): 558–569.

Smith, D. J., Evans, R. and Craddock, N. 2010. Predicting response to lithium in bipolar disorder: a critical review of pharmacogenetic studies. *Journal of Mental Health*, 19(2): 142–156.

Smoller, J. W. and Finn, C. T. 2003. Family, twin, and adoption studies of bipolar disorder. *American Journal of Medical Genetics*, 123C(1): 48–58.

Stamm, T. J., Adli, M., Kirchheiner, J., Smolka, M. N., Kaiser, R., Tremblay, P. B. and Bauer, M. 2008. Serotonin transporter gene and response to lithium augmentation in depression. *Psychiatric Genetics*, 18(2): 92–97.

Steyerberg, E. W., Vickers, A. J., Cook, N. R., Gerds, T., Gonen, M., Obuchowski, N., . . . Kattan, M. W. 2010. Assessing the performance of prediction models: a framework for traditional and novel measures. *Epidemiology*, 21(1): 128–138.

Szeszko, P. R., R. Lipsky, . . . et al. 2005. Brain-derived neurotrophic factor val66met polymorphism and volume of the hippocampal formation. *Molecular Psychiatry*, 10(7): 631–636.

Tan, W., Y. Wang, . . . et al. 2007. Molecular cloning of a brain-specific, developmentally regulated neuregulin 1 (NRG1) isoform and identification of a functional promoter variant associated with schizophrenia. *Journal of Biological Chemistry*, 282(33): 24343–24351.

Tkachev, D., M. L. Mimmack, . . . et al. 2003. Oligodendrocyte dysfunction in schizophrenia and bipolar disorder. *Lancet*, 362(9386): 798–805.

Toro, C. T., J. E. Hallak, . . . et al. 2006. Glial fibrillary acidic protein and glutamine synthetase in subregions of prefrontal cortex in schizophrenia and mood disorder. *Neurosci Lett*, 404(3): 276–281.

Uranova, N. A., V. M. Vostrikov, . . . et al. 2004. Oligodendroglial density in the prefrontal cortex in schizophrenia and mood disorders: a study from the Stanley Neuropathology Consortium. *Schizophrenia Research*, 67(2–3): 269–275.

Vostrikov, V. M., N. A. Uranova, . . . et al. 2007. Deficit of perineuronal oligodendrocytes in the prefrontal cortex in schizophrenia and mood disorders. *Schizophrenia Research*, 94(1–3): 273–280.

Wang, F., T. Jiang, . . . et al. 2009. Neuregulin 1 genetic variation and anterior cingulum integrity in patients with schizophrenia and healthy controls. *Journal of Psychiatry and Neuroscience*, 34(3): 181–186.

Wang, F., McIntosh, A. M., He, Y., Gelernter, J., Blumberg, H. P. (2011). The effects of risk-associated genetic variation in **CACNA1C** on the structure and function of a frontotemporal system. *Bipolar Disorders*, 13(7–8): 696–700.

Wessa, M., J. Linke, . . . et al. 2010. The CACNA1C risk variant for bipolar disorder influences limbic activity. *Molecular Psychiatry*, 15(12): 1126–1127.

Williams, L. M., J. M. Gatt, . . . et al. 2009. "Negativity bias" in risk for depression and anxiety: brain-body fear circuitry correlates, 5-HTT-LPR and early life stress. *Neuroimage*, 47(3): 804–814.

Wisniewski, S. R., A. J. Rush, . . . et al. 2009. Can phase III trial results of antidepressant medications be generalized to clinical practice? A STAR*D report. *American Journal of Psychiatry*, 166(5): 599–607.

# 13.

# INTEGRATION AND CONSOLIDATION
## A NEUROPHYSIOLOGICAL MODEL OF BIPOLAR DISORDER

## Stephen M. Strakowski

Bipolar disorder has accompanied humanity throughout recorded history. For example, over 3,000 years ago King Saul exhibited mania and depression, as recorded in the Bible (Ben-Noun, 2003). Saul was not alone; throughout history bipolar disorder has affected kings, queens, politicians, celebrities, and millions of people worldwide (e.g., Jamison, 1993). Despite its constant presence, bipolar disorder was not really described until Emil Kraepelin separated manic-depressive insanity from dementia praecox, based primarily on the former exhibiting recovery between exacerbations rather than the chronic deterioration of the latter (Kraepelin, 1921). The term "bipolar disorder" was coined in 1957 by Karl Leonhard, in order to distinguish patients with recurrent affective episodes that included mania from those people who only experienced depression (Goodwin & Jamison, 2007). Since then, the diagnosis of bipolar disorder has been refined to include bipolar I and II subtypes, as well as potentially related conditions such as cyclothymia.

Bipolar disorder is common. Bipolar I disorder occurs in 1%–2% of the population, a similar percent suffer from bipolar II disorder, and even a larger fraction experience so-called subthreshold symptoms that do not meet full DSM-IV criteria for the illness (Narrow et al., 2002; Judd & Akiskal, 2003; Hirschfeld et al., 2003). Bipolar disorder is the sixth leading cause of disability worldwide, and it is also a lethal illness since up to 15% of affected individuals commit suicide; bipolar disorder is also associated with a shorter life span than would be expected otherwise (Murray & Lopez, 1996; Goodwin & Jamison, 2007). Nonetheless, despite being historical, common, potentially debilitating, and lethal, only during the last two to three decades has investigation into the neurophysiological basis of bipolar disorder really flourished. Indeed, the previous chapters in this book describe the significant progress made toward this end, particularly in the current decade. Even with this progress, integrated neurophysiological models of bipolar disorder are relatively rarely discussed. The goal of this chapter, then, is to synthesize neuroimaging and genetic data in order to present such a model that can then serve to inform future investigations that further clarify the etiological basis of bipolar illness.

## RELEVANT CLINICAL FEATURES OF BIPOLAR DISORDER

Any neurophysiological model of bipolar disorder must include consideration of the key clinical features that characterize the illness. Bipolar disorder type I is defined by the occurrence of mania. Bipolar II disorder is characterized by the occurrence of hypomania plus at least one episode of depression. Mania is a syndrome that includes extreme mood states (euphoria, irritability, or expansive/labile mood) accompanied by cognitive impairments (e.g., grandiose thinking, distractibility, racing thoughts, flight of ideas), neurovegetative symptoms and signs (e.g., decreased need for sleep), and impulsive or agitated behavior. Hypomania is simply a less disabling form of the same symptoms. Most individuals who experience mania also experience recurrent depressive episodes that are also associated with mood, cognitive, neurovegetative, and other behavioral symptoms. Moreover, psychosis (delusions, hallucinations, thought disorder) is common in mania and may occur during bipolar depression. However, the term bipolar disorder is somewhat misleading as it suggests that patients exist on distinct manic or depressive poles, when actually it is common for both illness phases to co-occur in mixed states. Consequently, although defined by mania and hypomania, bipolar disorder is characterized as a dynamic condition with oscillations among extreme mood states accompanied by cognitive impairments, neurovegetative symptoms and signs, and psychosis (at times), as well as other impulsive and characteristic behaviors. Any neurophysiological model of bipolar disorder, then, must be able to potentially explain this dynamic, diverse set of symptoms.

In addition to being dynamic, the course of bipolar disorder is progressive, at least during the first several years of illness (Angst & Sellaro, 2000). For example, in his classic text *Manic-Depressive Insanity,* Kraepelin (1921) observed that "the shortening of the intervals, at first rapid then slower, with the number of the repetitions <of attacks> is clearly seen" (Figure 13.1). More recently, Roy-Byrne and colleagues (1985) used life-chart methods to identify cycle lengths in 95 bipolar patients recruited at the NIMH. Their findings were similar to those of Kraepelin (Figure 13.1). As Angst and Sellaro (2000) stated in their review of the last century's research: "So far, then, it would seem to have been established that the course of bipolar disorder is recurrent and progressive." Specifically, the interval between affective recurrences tends to rapidly shorten between the first few (i.e., three to five) episodes, followed by a relative flattening of changes in cycle length subsequently (Goodwin & Jamison, 2007). Together, these findings suggest that the early course of bipolar disorder is characterized by cycle progression during which the underlying neurophysiology of this long-term, recurrent and dynamic illness is established. Neurophysiological models of bipolar disorder, then, must account for this progression.

Although bipolar disorder is a life-long condition that persists to senescence, the onset of illness is typically in late adolescence or young adulthood. Data from the Systematic Treatment Enhancement Program for Bipolar Disorder (STEP-BD) found a mean age at onset of 17 years, and two-thirds of cases had an onset prior to age 18 (Perlis et al., 2004). The World Mental Health Survey Initiative found that more than half of bipolar I disorder subjects had a first manic episode prior to age 25. The most common age at onset appears to be between 15–19 years (Goodwin & Jamison, 2007); however, patients may have mood dysregulation and other behavioral symptoms for years prior to the first affective episode (McNamara et al., 2010; Skjelstad, Malt, & Holte, 2010). Consequently, the onset of bipolar disorder appears to be progressive and developmental, consistent with the early course progression of the illness noted previously. Neurophysiological models of bipolar, then, must consider the apparent developmental nature of the onset of bipolar disorder (McNamara et al., 2010).

Bipolar disorder runs in families; this longstanding observation was formally acknowledged at least as far back as Kraepelin (1921) and was strongly substantiated by studies from more than 30 years ago, including adoption studies that helped to separate the effects of genes and environment (as reviewed in chapter 9 in this volume). The heritability of bipolar disorder is very high, up to 80%–85% (Bienvenu, Davydow, & Kendler 2010). Taken together, these data indicate that bipolar disorder is genetic. These potential genetic effects must be considered in developing a neurophysiological model of bipolar disorder.

In the remainder of this chapter, then, we will develop a neurophysiological model of bipolar disorder, specifically type I (i.e., with full manic episodes). We will focus on bipolar I disorder since the relevant data are much richer for this "classic" illness than the more recently defined bipolar II disorder subtype and related conditions. Consequently, for the rest of this chapter, the term bipolar disorder will refer only to the type I condition.

---

**Clinical Features to be Considered for Neurophysiological Models of Bipolar Disorder**

- The occurrence of mania

- Dynamic dysregulation of mood, cognition and neurovegetative functions

- Progressive shortening of euthymic periods early in the illness course

- Onset in adolescence

- Strong heritability

---

## EMOTIONAL NETWORKS

As noted, bipolar disorder is defined by the occurrence of at least one manic episode, although it is characterized by

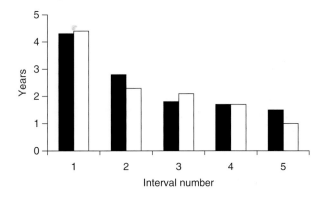

*Figure 13.1* Chart illustrating decreasing length of intervals between successive affective episodes. (Source: Dark bar = Kraepelin 1921; light bar = Roy-Byrne et al., 1985).

dynamic changes in mood, cognition, and neurovegetative symptoms. Despite the relatively broad clinical presentation, bipolar disorder has been assumed to be a primary disorder of mood and affect regulation, rather than of cognitive or neurovegetative control. This assumption is based upon decades of clinical experience and, to date, there is no convincing evidence to suggest otherwise. That said, the possibility that bipolar disorder instead results primarily from abnormalities in cognition, sleep, or other neurovegetative functions has not been completely disproven, although recent imaging studies tend to be more supportive of the mood dysregulation assumption, as will be discussed later in this chapter. Consequently, as a starting point, we will follow clinical convention and hypothesize that bipolar disorder results from a primary abnormality in the regulation of mood and affect.

To begin building a model based on this hypothesis, it would be useful if the neurophysiology of the modulation of emotion was completely understood; it is not. However, recent work suggests the presence of two parallel networks in which emotional and reward stimuli processed by amygdala and ventral striatum are modulated by ventral prefrontal cortex (Chen et al., 1995; Lane et al., 1998; Phan et al., 2002; Yamasaki, LaBar & McCarthy, 2002). These can be described as the ventromedial and ventrolateral prefrontal emotional networks and are illustrated in Figure 13.2.

The first of these networks, the ventromedial, involves connections between amygdala and medial ventral prefrontal cortex Brodmann Area 11 (BA11), along with rostral insula and subgenual anterior cingulate (BA 25). As is common to prefrontal architecture, regions of the ventral prefrontal cortex are connected to specific and unique corresponding regions in ventral striatum, thalamus and pallidum that then connect back to the originating prefrontal area to form an iterative feedback (and perhaps sometimes feed-forward) loop. These ventral prefrontal-striato-pallido-thalamic loops modulate emotional and behavioral responses. In particular, this ventromedial prefrontal network appears to process internally referenced emotional states (Yamasaki, LaBar & McCarthy, 2002), so it is activated in studies using induced emotion paradigms.

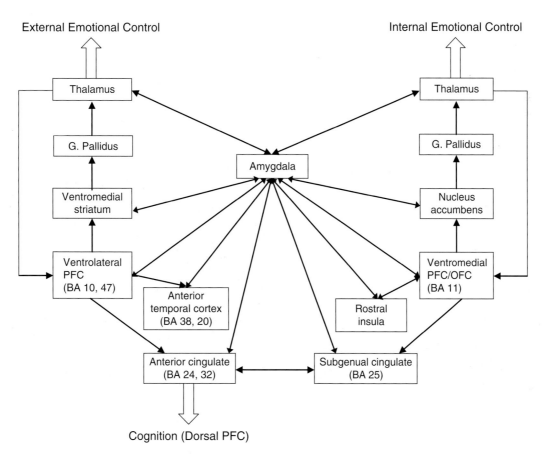

Figure 13.2 Schematic of the proposed ventrolateral and ventromedial prefrontal networks underlying human emotional control. PFC=prefrontal cortex; OFC=orbitofrontal cortex, BA=Brodmann area; G.=globus.

The second emotional pathway is formed from connections among amygdala and inferotemporal regions with lateral ventral prefrontal cortex (BA10/47) and rostral anterior cingulate (BA24/32). Again, these prefrontal regions map to specific striatal, thalamic, and pallidal areas forming an iterative loop. In contrast to the medial pathway, this ventrolateral prefrontal network seems to be responsible for managing external emotional cues, so is commonly activated within behavioral paradigms that involve external emotional stimuli; for example, affective faces.

Thinking evolutionarily, one could propose that these networks serve to nuance the more primitive fight or flight instinct and reward seeking behaviors modulated by amygdala and ventral striatum, respectively, in other animals in order to produce the more complex and subtle emotional-social behaviors that characterize human interactions (Kim et al., 2011). It is this emotional nuance that is one product of the excessively enlarged prefrontal cortex that distinguishes humans from other animal species. However, during the course of bipolar disorder, the prefrontal nuance or modulation of amygdala and iterative control of ventral striatum appears to be disrupted, thereby leading to extreme mood states and emotional and behavioral instability. Dysfunction within these prefrontal networks, then, can be hypothesized to underlie the emotional dysregulation that characterizes bipolar disorder.

From studies in depression, Mayberg et al. (1999) postulated that emotional networks originating in ventral prefrontal areas are reciprocally connected to dorsal prefrontal systems that provide non-emotional cognitive functions. In other words, when ventral (emotional) prefrontal systems are activated, they deactivate dorsal (cognitive) brain, and the converse also occurs. A recent study by Yamasaki and colleagues (2002), using a continuous performance task with emotional and neutral distracters (CPT-END), as well as other studies (e.g., Fichtenholtz et al., 2004), supported this reciprocal dorsal-ventral prefrontal organization and

also supported suggestions that this reciprocal connection is modulated within anterior cingulate. This ventral-dorsal organization of the prefrontal cortex provides a model for the cognitive symptoms observed in bipolar disorder; namely, with dysregulated ventral (emotional) networks, dorsal prefrontal networks are reciprocally disrupted, leading to the cognitive symptoms observed during mania and depression—namely, impaired attentional, memory, and executive processes. The next step in developing this model, then, is to examine whether neuroimaging studies support this hypothesized dysregulation.

## SUMMARY OF STRUCTURAL NEUROIMAGING

### MORPHOMETRICS

Structural neuroimaging abnormalities in bipolar disorder have been reviewed extensively in this book (see chapter 2 in its entirety and the appropriate sections in chapter 5), so we will focus on a few key points from those reviews in order to address the proposed model. One key finding from structural neuroimaging of bipolar disorder is the presence of abnormalities in amygdala volume and development. The amygdala is a key structure, integrated with ventral prefrontal areas as noted, for managing human emotional responses (Kim et al., 2011). In young patients with bipolar disorder, studies have consistently demonstrated decreased volumes compared with healthy subjects (Pfeifer et al., 2008). Moreover, Bitters et al., (2011) recently demonstrated that, during the first year after a manic episode, bipolar adolescents demonstrate failure of healthy amygdala growth (i.e., enlargement) and appear to, conversely, experience loss of amygdala volume. In contrast, studies of amygdala are mixed when comparing bipolar and healthy adults, although amygdala enlargement in the former may be the more common finding (see chapter 2). Moreover, amygdala enlargement with healthy-sized hippocampus may be a relatively specific finding to adult bipolar disorder that differentiates it from schizophrenia (Altshuler et al., 1998). This observation suggests that after an amygdala developmental anomaly of adolescence, that is, failure to grow along a healthy trajectory, there is a subsequent overgrowth of the structure. This subsequent enlargement may be due to lithium or other medication exposure, although that is not certain (Hallahan et al., 2011). Since studies have not observed amygdala abnormalities prior to illness onset in at-risk subjects (Singh et al., 2008; Ladouceur et al., 2008), and report decreased volumes in first-episode patients (Rosso et al., 2007), amygdala enlargement may be a consequence of

> **The Neurophysiology of Emotion**
>
> · Is not completely understood
>
> · Appears to be modulated within two prefrontal-striatopallidothalmic networks: a ventral-lateral network that manages external emotional stimuli, and a ventral-medial network that manages internal emotional cues
>
> · Involves modulation of amygdala function by these two prefrontal networks

bipolar illness rather than a cause. Future longitudinal studies in at-risk subjects are needed to clarify the time sequence of structural amygdala changes in the course of bipolar disorder. Regardless, structural neuroimaging data support abnormal amygdala growth and structure as a component of the neurophysiology of bipolar disorder.

The striatum includes the caudate, putamen, and nucleus accumbens. The nucleus accumbens receives substantial dopaminergic input from the ventral tegmentum and is widely recognized as modulating reward and novelty seeking behaviors that are clearly relevant to the symptoms of bipolar disorder. Closely linked to these structures is the globus pallidus, which, with the striatum, forms the basal ganglia. As noted previously, the ventral (emotional) prefrontal cortex specifically projects to the ventral, rather than dorsal, striatum, so that the regions of these structures that might contribute to the pathophysiology of bipolar disorder are those of the ventral striatum, which is comprised of the nucleus accumbens, ventral putamen, and ventromedial caudate. The ventral striatum receives extensive input not only from the ventral prefrontal cortex, but also from the amygdala (Marchand & Yurgelun-Todd, 2010). Consequently, the ventral striatum plays an integrative role in the prefrontal networks that process emotional functions (Marchand & Yurgelun-Todd, 2010).

Abnormalities in the structure of the striatum have been observed in a number of neuroimaging studies of bipolar disorder. Specifically, a meta-analysis by Hallahan et al. (2011) found enlargement of the putamen and a meta-analysis by Arnone et al., (2009) observed globus pallidus enlargement in bipolar compared with healthy subjects. As reviewed by Marchand and Yurgelun-Todd (2010), confounding interpretation of these results is that antipsychotic medications may cause striatal volume increases. However, striatal enlargement was observed by Strakowski et al. (2002) in first-episode patients, and DelBello et al. (2004), Wilke et al. (2004), Dickstein et al. (2005), and Lopez-Larson et al. (2009) in adolescents with minimal prior antipsychotic exposure, suggesting that this finding is not necessarily iatrogenic. Moreover, Noga, Vladar and Torrey (2001) found caudate enlargement in both bipolar subjects and their unaffected co-twins compared with healthy twin pairs, suggesting that structural abnormalities in the striatum predate illness onset and may serve as an endophenotypic marker of bipolar disorder. Bora et al. (2010) found that basal ganglia gray matter volumes may increase with longer illness duration, and Sanches et al. (2005) observed that age may affect striatal volumes. Together, these data suggest that striatal structural abnormalities occur early in the course of bipolar illness, perhaps prior to onset of mania,

but may also progress with exposure to medications and illness course. Given the critical juncture of the striatum in emotional processing networks among various contributing brain regions, these structural abnormalities may reflect functional impairments in mood regulation and illness progression in bipolar disorder.

As noted, the prefrontal cortex in humans is dramatically enlarged relative to other animal species and this enlargement is a new event in the course of human evolution, occurring approximately 50,000 years ago. Consequently, it is not surprising that the prefrontal cortex seems to be particularly relevant for modulating human complex emotional and social behaviors, as well as advanced executive and cognitive functions. Similarly, then, it would not be surprising that the prefrontal cortex is likely involved in the expression of a uniquely human illness like bipolar disorder. Supporting this suggestion, several structural imaging studies identified abnormalities in bipolar compared with healthy subjects.

Meta-analyses suggested that decreased gray matter volumes in the peri- and sub-genual anterior cingulate, as well as ventral prefrontal regions that overlap into the insula, are present in bipolar disorder compared with healthy individuals (Ellison-Wright et al., 2010; Bora et al., 2010). Lateral ventricular enlargement appears to be a common finding in bipolar disorder as well, which seems to be secondary to decreases in the corresponding white matter volumes of prefrontal cortical areas (Strakowski et al., 2002; Hallahan et al., 2010; Arnone et al., 2009). However, studies in first-episode patients do not observe these changes (Strakowski et al., 1993; Vita et al., 2009), suggesting that prefrontal volume decreases may occur during the course of illness progression and with age, rather than being present at the outset (Blumberg et al., 2006; Bora et al., 2010). In a small study of children who initially presented with atypical psychosis and went on to develop bipolar disorder, regionally specific decreases in anterior cingulate volume were observed over time. Together, these findings suggest that progressive losses of prefrontal gray and white matter may contribute to illness progression and onset. These structural abnormalities within emotion-control networks are illustrated in Figure 13.3 and extend our model of bipolar neurophysiology.

### DIFFUSION TENSOR IMAGING (DTI)

Diffusion tensor imaging (DTI) provides a means to examine white matter tracts using MRI. Specifically, because water movement is constrained along white matter tracts, changes in white matter structure impact water flow

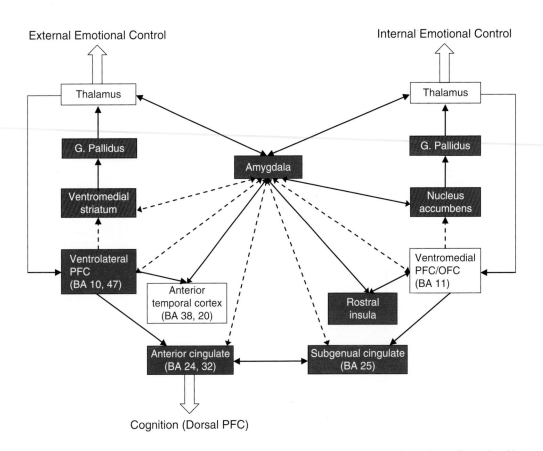

External Emotional Control

Internal Emotional Control

Cognition (Dorsal PFC)

*Figure 13.3* Abnormalities identified within emotional networks in bipolar disorder using structural neuroimaging methods. Rust-colored boxes = regional abnormalities that appear to post-date the onset of illness (i.e., first manic episode); blue boxes = regional abnormalities that may predate illness onset. All of these regions exhibit progressive changes with age and illness course; amygdala appears to exhibit developmental abnormalities in adolescence/young adulthood as well. Dashed arrows represent potential connectivity abnormalities identified in bipolar disorder using diffusion tensor imaging (DTI).

in the brain. Two standard measures are commonly reported describing this water movement. Fractional anisotropy (FA) indicates how freely water flows in three dimensions—that is, the higher the FA value the less isotropic the flow and the more structured the region. Trace apparent diffusion coefficient, or TADC, is a measure of the amount of diffusion water demonstrates in a brain region: higher values indicate water diffuses more freely. DTI, then, has been used to compare white matter structure in bipolar and healthy subjects.

As noted in chapters 2 (Table 2.2) and 5, DTI findings in bipolar disorder have been somewhat variable. However, a recent meta-analysis found decreased FA in two primary brain regions in bipolar disorder—the anterior/subgenual cingulate and the parahippocampal gyrus, although this report was limited to whole brain studies (Vederine et al., 2011). These findings suggest loss of healthy white matter structure in these critical brain regions that are involved with emotional regulation; in particular, parahippocampal

gyrus contains important white matter fibers that connect amygdala to cortical and other subcortical brain regions. A number of studies observed both FA and TADC abnormalities in ventral prefrontal and periventricular regions in bipolar disorder, suggesting disruption of connections among prefrontal cortex, striatum and amygdala, that is, the major components of emotion regulatory networks (Figure 13.2) (Adler et al., 2004a; Beyer et al., 2005; Adler et al., 2006; Kantanfaris et al., 2009). Abnormalities have also been observed in the anterior commissure and corpus callosum in bipolar disorder, suggesting loss of integration between prefrontal regions across the right and left hemispheres (Wang et al., 2008; Adler et al., 2004a; Yurgelun-Todd et al., 2007; Bruno, Cercignani, & Ron, 2008). DTI can also be used to specifically delineate white matter tracts connecting two or more brain regions, a technique called "tractography." Using this approach, Lin et al. (2011) observed abnormal connections specifically among prefrontal, medial temporal (i.e., amygdala) and subcortical brain structures consistent with disruption of the normal connectivity of the emotional networks illustrated in Figure 13.2.

Moreover, studies in subjects at risk for bipolar disorder, by virtue of having bipolar parents, suggest that these white matter abnormalities predate illness onset. Specifically, DTI-observed white matter abnormalities in many of the same regions noted in bipolar subjects are already present in at risk individuals (reviewed in detail in chapter 5) as well as unaffected relatives (Sprooten et al., 2011). These findings suggest that connections among regions of the emotional networks in Figure 13.2 may exist early in development in individuals with a genetic vulnerability for bipolar disorder. These abnormal network connections may contribute to emotional dysregulation, perhaps in response to environmental or development events, that eventually progresses into the first manic episode and a subsequent bipolar course of affective illness. These considerations have been added to the model we are developing (Figure 13.3).

---

**Key Structural Imaging Findings in Bipolar Disorder Include:**

- Developmental abnormalities in amygdala growth and volumes

- Striatal and basal ganglia enlargement that appears to predate illness onset

- Progressive decreases in ventral prefrontal and anterior cingulate gray and white matter with illness course and onset

- Disrupted white matter connections among prefrontal cortex, amygdala and other subcortical structures that may predate illness onset

---

## SUMMARY OF FUNCTIONAL NEUROIMAGING

Functional neuroimaging may involve a number of modalities, including positron emission tomography (PET), single-photon emission computed tomography (SPECT), electroencephalography (EEG), and now most commonly blood oxygen-level dependent (BOLD) functional magnetic resonance imaging (fMRI). These techniques were reviewed elsewhere in this textbook (chapter 1), so will not be discussed further here. Additionally, since detailed reviews of functional neuroimaging findings are presented in chapter 3 in its entirety, and sections in chapter 5, 6, and 7, we will focus on regional abnormalities identified by those reviews as they extend across phases of illness and

different cognitive tasks, in order to refine our model illustrated in Figure 13.2.

Although functional neuroimaging findings are often difficult to replicate across studies in psychiatry, the most consistent functional neuroimaging finding in bipolar disorder is excessive activation during mania of emotional brain regions, namely amygdala and surrounding medial temporal cortex, as compared to healthy subjects and other patient groups. This observation is particularly true during tasks involving facial affect recognition (e.g., Althshuler et al., 2005; Blumberg et al., 2005; Almeida et al., 2010; Whalley et al., 2009). Additionally, amygdala hyperactivity has been reported in both manic adolescents and adults (Pavuluri et al., 2007, 2008, 2009), so does not appear to be developmentally specific. Amygdala over-activation has also been observed in unaffected relatives of bipolar patients, suggesting that it may represent an illness endophenotype (Whalley et al., 2011). Importantly, not all studies find over-activation in amygdala in response to all tasks in bipolar disorder, as under-activation relative to healthy subjects is also reported, typically in tasks that do not overtly require emotional processing. For example, we (Strakowski et al., 2011) used a relatively complex continuous performance task that included emotional and neutral distracters (CPT-END; Yamasaki et al., 2002) and observed relatively blunted amygdala response to distracters in bipolar manic compared with healthy subjects. In this task, emotional images were predominantly affectively negative and were buried within the primary attentional component, namely, identifying nonemotional targets. We suggested from this finding that if amygdala was over-activated throughout the task (including the non-emotional attentional component, e.g., Strakowski et al., 2004), then the relative increase during distracters might be limited, compared with healthy subjects, as the physiological response could already be approaching a maximum. This restriction in amygdala flexibility might then contribute to loss of emotional control or the ability to correct emotional extremes.

Amygdala over-activation is not restricted to the manic phase of bipolar disorder, as it may also occur during euthymia in bipolar subjects (Strakowski et al., 2004). During bipolar depression amygdala abnormalities are frequently observed, but they are inconsistent in direction (i.e., over- or under-activated). For example, Almeida et al. (2010) suggested that amygdala may be over-reactive to mild, particularly negative, affective expressions in depressed bipolar subjects, but then under-reactive to other types of stimuli. Increased amygdala activation was also observed by Lawrence et al. (2004) in depressed bipolar patients during an emotional faces task. Conversely, Altshuler et al. (2008)

did not observe amygdala over-activation during a facial affect matching task in depressed bipolar subjects, and suggested, coupled with findings in mania, that amygdala over-activation may be state dependent. Even with these inconsistencies across studies, most investigators report that amygdala function is disrupted during the course of bipolar disorder.

Indeed, one challenge in interpreting fMRI studies is that activation is never truly an absolute measure, but rather, represents a difference between an active task and a baseline, presumably non-active, task. Variability in tasks introduces complexity comparing results across studies, so that it can be difficult to determine if group differences reflect differences in response to the experimental or baseline task. With these considerations in mind, perhaps a more parsimonious view of fMRI findings to date is that, independent of the direction of abnormalities, across bipolar mood states amygdala exhibits abnormal reactivity, or perhaps response flexibility, to both emotional and non-emotional cognitive stimuli (Strakowski et al., 2011). In other words, the amygdala response to both direct and indirect stimuli is dysregulated compared with healthy subjects. Moreover, abnormalities in amygdala function, particularly in response to tasks that require emotional processing, may distinguish bipolar disorder from related conditions, namely schizophrenia and unipolar depression (please see relevant sections in chapters 6, and 7).

Another relatively consistent functional neuroimaging finding in bipolar disorder, particularly during mood episodes, is decreased ventral prefrontal activation. Specifically, decreased activation in both lateral and medial (orbitofrontal) ventral prefrontal brain regions has been observed in bipolar disorder across a wide variety of emotional and non-emotional tasks (see, e.g., Foland et al., 2008; Yurgelun-Todd et al., 2000; Strakowski et al., 2011). Ventral prefrontal under-activation has also been observed with positron emission tomography (PET; Blumberg et al., 1999), in which, in contrast to fMRI, an absolute measure of blood flow can be made. Similar findings, particularly during emotional tasks, were observed in adolescents as well as adults (Pavuluri et al., 2008), so this finding extends across ages groups and therefore may not be developmental *per se;* however, some studies in bipolar youth observed increased prefrontal activation to various cognitive tasks, different from what is observed in adults (e.g., Rich et al., 2006; Dickstein et al., 2005. These latter observations suggest that it is likely that prefrontal activation abnormalities in bipolar disorder involve developmental components, given the changes in prefrontal structure during adolescence, that are reflected in these apparently discordant findings. Unlike amygdala

hyperactivation, ventral prefrontal hypoactivation does not appear to occur differentially in bipolar versus unipolar depression (Strakowski, 2002) or versus schizophrenia (reviewed in chapter 7), suggesting a lack of specificity of this finding. Regardless, when coupled with amygdala hyperactivation, hypoactivation of ventral prefrontal cortex may reflect a relatively specific disinhibition of amygdala in bipolar disorder that indicates failure of healthy ventral prefrontal network modulation of the limbic brain (Foland et al., 2008); this failure may provide the functional neuroanatomic basis for bipolar disorder symptoms.

In contrast, during euthymia, increased ventrolateral prefrontal cortical activation has been reported (Strakowski et al., 2004; Adler et al., 2004b). Specifically, during performance of a simple non-emotional continuous performance task (CPT) in medication-free, early course, euthymic bipolar patients Strakowski et al. (2004) observed increased activation in ventrolateral prefrontal cortex (BA 10) in addition to increased amygdala activation. In this study, patients were asymptomatic for at least one month prior to and one month after the fMRI scan. They were also off all medications for at least one month prior to the scan (and most for considerably longer), and they performed the CPT essentially the same as the healthy subjects. The increased ventrolateral prefrontal cortical activation in the bipolar subjects may reflect a compensatory response to amygdala over-activation (which was not expected in this non-emotional attention task); over-activation in posterior attentional brain regions was also observed that similarly might reflect compensatory mechanisms to maintain cognitive function in response to amygdala over-activation in order to maintain euthymia. Similar findings were reported by Adler et al. (2004b) during a working memory task. These results suggest that when euthymic, bipolar subjects may exhibit recovery of prefrontal activation, even to the point of over-activation, to compensate for ongoing amygdala over-activation. However, if during euthymia bipolar patients exhibit compensatory responses in prefrontal and other brain regions to manage amygdala over-activation, there may be insufficient reserves to respond to stress or cognitive challenges, thereby leading to failure of these compensatory mechanisms and the development of mood episodes. Additional studies of recovering patients are needed to substantiate this suggestion.

Supporting this suggestion, several studies reported abnormalities in functional connectivity between ventral prefrontal regions and amygdala in bipolar disorder. Functional connectivity can be measured in several ways (e.g., Adler et al., 2004b, 2006; Beyer et al., 2005; Lin et al., 2011; Almeida et al., 2009), but in general it provides an assessment of how brain activation correlates among different regions over time. Higher temporal correlations between two or more brain areas suggest that they are more strongly linked—that is, functionally connected. Specifically, during mania, functional connectivity is decreased between amygdala and lateral ventral prefrontal cortex, consistent with a loss of prefrontal modulation of limbic brain, thereby leading to the emotional dysregulation and the affective extremes of mania (Foland et al., 2008; Chepenik et al., 2010).

During bipolar depression, functional connectivity abnormalities between ventral prefrontal cortex and amygdala also appear to occur, but are more complex. For example, investigators at the University of Pittsburgh examined effective connectivity during bipolar and unipolar depression while subjects viewed affective faces (N.B. effective connectivity is a more advanced analytic approach modeling the direction of functional connectivity beyond simple correlations; Almeida et al., 2009). They found a relatively specific inverse functional relationship between right amygdala and medial ventral prefrontal (orbitofrontal) cortex during happy emotion processing in bipolar depression that was not present in either unipolar depressed or healthy subjects; that is, the bipolar depressed group specifically exhibited decreasing amygdala activity with increasing orbitomedial prefrontal cortex activity that did not occur in the other two groups. In contrast, both unipolar and bipolar depressed subjects exhibited decreased effective connectivity between these structures on the left that differed from healthy subjects. This finding does not reconcile clearly with the loss of prefrontal modulation of amygdala commonly observed in mania, although may reflect affective state-specific abnormalities in effective connectivity between these brain regions. Regardless, this finding suggests that the manner in which ventral prefrontal cortex and amygdala interact during depression might distinguish bipolar and unipolar depressed groups.

It is not clear if functional connectivity abnormalities persist into euthymia. Moreover, abnormalities in functional connectivity may or may not reflect actual changes in the structural connections in the brain. However, the previously reviewed DTI findings of white matter tract abnormalities within prefrontal networks of bipolar subjects are consistent with fMRI observations of functional connectivity abnormalities in bipolar disorder. Consequently, the functional disruption of prefrontal modulation of amygdala and other limbic structures may have a neuroanatomic basis. Studies in at-risk individuals (i.e., those with bipolar parents who are not yet ill) suggest that white matter connections may be disrupted even before illness onset

(Frazier et al., 2007; Versace et al., 2010), and then progress over time (e.g., Strakowski et al., 2002; Versace et al., 2008), perhaps contributing to the progression in the frequency of affective episodes (Figure 13.1).

Several other brain regions are commonly observed to differentially activate between healthy and bipolar subjects during functional imaging studies, including the insula, anterior cingulate, and striatum. The insula is thought to be particularly involved in processing disgust and other negative emotions (Fusar-Poli et al., 2009). Lennox et al., (2004) observed increased insula activation during mania in response to sad faces. Insula over-activation persists into euthymia (Wessa et al., 2007) and occurs in bipolar adolescents (Chang et al., 2004). The insula is heavily innervated by both the ventral medial prefrontal cortex and the anterior cingulate, and abnormalities in functional connectivity between medial prefrontal cortex and insula have been observed (Chai et al., 2011).

The anterior cingulate provides an integrative role in information processing, so consequently appears to localize, at least in part, the reciprocal relationship between cognitive and emotional processing, that is, ventral and dorsal brain (Yamasaki et al., 2002; Strakowski et al., 2011). In imaging studies, the anterior cingulate has consistently demonstrated abnormalities in both adults and adolescents with bipolar disorder versus healthy subjects (e.g., Strakowski et al., 2011; Strakowski et al., 2008; Altshuler et al., 2005; Pavuluri et al., 2007). During mania and euthymia, the anterior cingulate excessively activates in bipolar subjects to a variety of stimuli, but particularly emotional stimuli, compared with healthy subjects, whereas the converse occurs in bipolar depression (Wessa et al., 2007; Marchand et al., 2007; Strakowski et al., 2008; Altshuler et al., 2005). Recent studies more specifically suggest that during euthymia, the emotional aspects of the anterior cingulate may be over-activated (Kronhaus et al., 2006), whereas the more cognitive aspects are under-activated (Gruber et al., 2004), indicating a possible dissociation within the anterior cingulate of different types of abnormal responses in bipolar subjects. Moreover, during mania the anterior cingulate exhibits abnormal functional connectivity with amygdala, further supporting the suggestion that regions of the prefrontal cortex are failing to effectively modulate limbic brain during the course of bipolar illness (Wang et al., 2009).

As discussed earlier in this chapter, and illustrated in Figure 13.2, prefrontal brain regions involved in emotional modulation function within the context of relatively independent prefrontal-striatal-pallidal-thalamic iterative circuits. Consistent with this organization and the observed prefrontal abnormalities in bipolar disorder, several functional imaging studies have identified striatal and thalamic abnormalities in bipolar subjects as well. As reviewed by Marchand and Yurgelun-Todd (2010), excessive striatal (particularly caudate) and thalamic activation have been commonly reported in bipolar disorder, especially during mania and euthymia, (Strakowski et al., 2005; Kaladjian et al., 2009a,b). This observation is in contrast to studies of unipolar depression, in which striatum and thalamus tend to be hypoactive (Marchand & Yurgelun-Todd, 2010). Consistent with this observation, Strakowski (2002; Strakowski et al., 2002) suggested that striatal over-activation, coupled with striatal structural abnormalities, might distinguish unipolar and bipolar depression. The striatum and thalamus are critical integrative structures within prefrontal iterative circuits and provide cross-talk among otherwise relatively independent prefrontal regions. Consequently, these findings in bipolar disorder suggest dysregulation of these integrative activities, contributing to dysregulation of prefrontal modulation of emotional processes.

Taken together, then, functional imaging studies in bipolar disorder suggest a loss of prefrontal modulation of limbic brain systems that include amygdala and insula. Hyper-activation in some regions (e.g., amygdala) coupled with hypoactivation in specific ventral prefrontal areas may be relatively specific for bipolar disorder. This disruption in the healthy balance between prefrontal and limbic brain function may occur, at least in part, from abnormalities in white matter connections among these regions. These white matter abnormalities may occur prior to illness onset, then progress over time, leading to changes in functional connectivity and activation abnormalities in bipolar disorder that are reflected by progression in the illness as illustrated in Figure 13.1. These considerations add functional components to our evolving model (Figure 13.4).

---

**Key Functional Imaging Findings in Bipolar Disorder Include:**

- Consistently abnormal amygdala function, frequently over-activation, across mood states and cognitive tasks, compared with healthy subjects

- Decreased ventral prefrontal activation across mood states and tasks that may reflect loss of prefrontal modulation of limbic brain areas

- Abnormalities in functional connectivity among emotional brain regions possibly secondary to or reflecting white matter abnormalities identified with DTI

---

## SUMMARY OF BRAIN NEUROCHEMICAL FINDINGS FROM MRS

Magnetic resonance spectroscopy (MRS) provides a technique for studying the molecular substrate of the brain *in vivo* in human subjects. Various MRS methods are described in chapter 1 and therefore will not be repeated here. However, features of MRS relevant to this discussion are that it can be performed on the same systems used to generate fMRI and structural MRI data, and it can also be used to study different atomic nuclei, permitting measurements of a large variety of molecules. Chapter 4 provides a comprehensive review of MRS studies in bipolar disorder, which are clearly summarized in Tables 4.1, 4.2, and 4.3. Consequently, in this section we will focus on several key findings to further expand our model of bipolar disorder.

The MRS technique most commonly applied to study bipolar disorder is referred to as [1]H-MRS or proton MRS, because it is based on the magnetic properties of hydrogen atoms. Proton MRS is widely used in biomedical research because hydrogen is the most common atom in the body, particularly as a component of water, so that the [1]H-MRS signal is relatively large. The manner in which hydrogen is bound to other atoms alters its MRS signal, which allows different molecules to be separately identified. Although many molecules can be measured (as long as they include hydrogen), the most commonly reported neurochemicals of interest in studies of bipolar disorder are: n-acetyl-aspartate (NAA), choline, creatine, *myo*-inositol, and so-called Glx. Glx is a peak within the proton-MRS spectrum that includes glutamate, GABA, glutamine and smaller amounts of other molecules; newer high-field scanners and techniques can separately distinguish the glutamate component of this peak specifically, but older reports typically do not, so that they report the combined Glx concentration. Regardless, each of these molecules has been found to exhibit differences in concentrations between bipolar and healthy subjects (chapter 4, Table 4.1).

As noted, MRS is not restricted to studying hydrogen, as other atoms can be examined, although in general, these are less common than hydrogen and so are harder to measure. Nonetheless, one relatively common MRS technique is to study molecules containing phosphorus ($^{31}$P). $^{31}$P-MRS permits measurement of a number of molecules involved in cellular energetics: α-, β-, and γ-adenosine triphosphate (ATP), creatine phosphate (PCr), and high-energy membrane metabolism, that is, phosphomonoesters (PME) and phosphodiesters (PDE). Studies using 31P-MRS often find abnormalities, relative to healthy subjects,

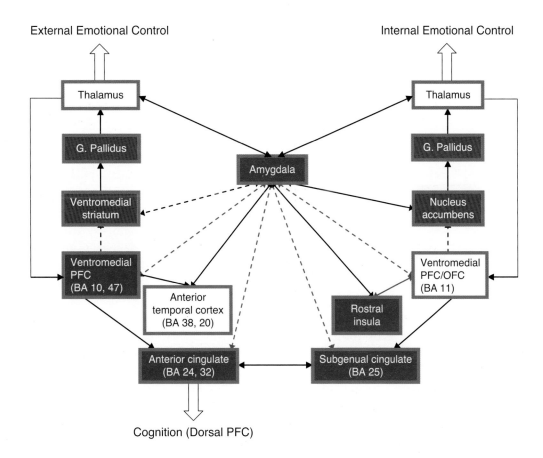

External Emotional Control

Internal Emotional Control

Cognition (Dorsal PFC)

*Figure 13.4* Abnormalities identified within emotional networks in bipolar disorder using functional neuroimaging methods, superimposed over those from structural neuroimaging (Figure 13.3). Brain regions exhibiting relatively consistent functional differences between bipolar and healthy subjects are indicated by the bright green border around the structure. Functional connectivity abnormalities are indicated by blue arrows. N.B. all of these regions have been found to exhibit functional abnormalities in studies of bipolar disorder. Other characteristics of the figure from structural imaging are described with Figure 13.3 as follows: rust-colored boxes = regional abnormalities that appear to post-date the onset of illness (i.e., first manic episode); blue boxes = regional abnormalities that may predate illness onset; dashed arrows = potential connectivity abnormalities identified in bipolar disorder using diffusion tensor imaging (DTI).

in bipolar disorder, consistent with disruptions in cellular energy processes (see chapter 4, Table 4.2).

Indeed, as reviewed in chapter 4, results from both [1]H- and [31]P-MRS studies suggest that disrupted neuronal bioenergetics may underlie the functional and structural abnormalities within emotional networks and, consequently, the expression of bipolar disorder (Dager et al., 2004, Kato & Kato, 2000, Lyoo et al., 2003, Modica-Napolitano & Renshaw, 2004, Stork & Renshaw, 2005). For example, Dager et al., (2004) used [1]H-MRS to compare medication-free, predominantly depressed bipolar and healthy subjects. They found elevated gray matter lactate and Glx levels in the bipolar patients, particularly in anterior cingulate and insula. Lactate is typically not visible with [1]H-MRS; its presence suggested a shift in energy redox state from oxidative phosphorylation toward less efficient glycolysis. Since glycolysis tends to predominate in highly

activated states, this finding in bipolar patients might reflect hypermetabolism in brain areas that modulate mood or disruptions in healthy metabolic processes (Stork & Renshaw, 2005). The frequently observed elevated glutamate or Glx levels also support this conclusion.

Elevated glutamate concentrations identified using [1]H-MRS in bipolar disorder during affective episodes have been frequently reported (chapter 4, Table 4.1), and these elevations appear to improved with treatment (chapter 4, Table 4.3) and may not be present during euthymia (Change et al., 2003, Winsberg et al., 2000). Glutamate is the most abundant amino acid in the brain and is the primary excitatory neurotransmitter; it is ubiquitous within the prefrontal-striatal-pallidal-thalamic networks reviewed in this chapter. Therefore, affective episodes may be associated with elevated levels of glutamate, and consequently, resulting glutamatergic excitotoxicity can be hypothesized to potentially underlie progressive functional and structural changes in the brain as well as in markers of neuronal health (e.g., neuronal density) in bipolar disorder.

[1]H-MRS levels of NAA provide one measure of neuronal health. NAA is the second most common amino acid in the central nervous system, and it is relatively restricted to neurons and glia. In bipolar disorder compared with healthy subjects, differences in NAA are variable, but perhaps most commonly, NAA is decreased, particularly in medial temporal (hippocampal), striatal, and dorsolateral prefrontal cortical regions (Table 4.1). Moreover, recent work increasingly suggests that NAA plays an integral role in the energetics of neuronal mitochondria (Stork & Renshaw, 2005, Madhavarao et al., 2003). Therefore, metabolic inefficiencies or hypermetabolism in bipolar disorder might contribute to decreased NAA levels, particularly as patients accumulate affective episodes. Consistent with this suggestion, studies have found that NAA concentrations are inversely proportional to illness duration (Chang et al., 2003; Winsberg et al., 2000). NAA levels appear to increase in bipolar disorder with successful treatment, suggesting that metabolic processes recover (Moore et al., 2000; DelBello et al., 2006; Brennan et al., 2010). Additionally, prefrontal NAA decrements do not appear in at-risk subjects, until the development of significant mood episodes (Galleli et al., 2005; Cecil et al., 2003), although decreased NAA levels have been observed in at-risk subjects who are beginning to express behavioral symptoms in the cerebellar vermis. Consequently, there may be regional variation within the brain for metabolic abnormalities arising during development of bipolar illness.

Abnormalities in neuronal metabolism coupled with over-active glutamatergic neurotransmission would be expected to disrupt other high energy processes, such as neuronal phospholipid (membrane) metabolism (Stork & Renshaw, 2005). Indeed, several studies reported elevations of [1]H-MRS choline (Cho) levels in bipolar disorder, particularly in the striatum (chapter 4, Table 4.1). The MRS Cho peak is comprised predominantly of membrane-based choline compounds such as phosphocholine and glycerophosphocholine. Additionally, myo-inositol (mI) levels are also elevated in bipolar disorder (chapter 4, Table 4.1); myo-inositol is an important precursor to the membrane phospholipid phophatidylinositol. These choline and myo-inositol elevations suggest accelerated membrane turnover and breakdown consistent with a hypermetabolic state in bipolar disorder (Stork & Renshaw, 2005). Moreover, myo-inositol is a substrate for the phosphoinositide second-messenger system, so that abnormalities in the myo-inositol peak observed with MRS may also reflect abnormalities in

cellular communication. Cecil et al. (2003) found elevated myo-inositol levels in children without bipolar disorder, but with bipolar parents, compared to children of healthy parents. This finding suggested that elevated myo-inositol may precede other metabolic abnormalities early in the development of bipolar illness.

This finding in at-risk kids may be particularly relevant because one of the primary targets of lithium treatment is the inositol pathway. Specifically, lithium inhibits inositol monophosphatase, leading to increases in inositol-1-monophosphate and decreased inositol. Moore et al. (1999) observed a decrease in the prefrontal myo-inositol [1]H-MRS resonance five to seven days after initiating lithium treatment that persisted through at least 3 weeks. Symptom improvement did not temporally correlate with changes in myo-inositol levels. This observation might indicate that myo-inositol changes are unrelated to treatment response; alternatively, these changes may be an early marker of a cascade of events leading to normalized cellular metabolism and clinical improvement. Consistent with the latter suggestion, Davanzo et al. (2001) reported decreases in myo-inositol levels in bipolar adolescents treated with lithium, but only in treatment responders. Early changes in myo-inositol levels in at-risk children may therefore reflect the early developmental processes leading to bipolar disorder and may be altered by treatment with lithium. However, since, in a given at-risk subject, the actual risk of developing bipolar disorder cannot yet be predicted, a better understanding of the evolution of the illness is needed before premorbid intervention with lithium could be recommended.

Also supporting the suggestion that neuronal bioenergetics are disrupted in bipolar disorder are [31]P-MRS findings (chapter 4, Table 4.2). For example, phosphocreatine (PCr) is a high-energy phosphate that is formed from ATP and creatine. When ATP is consumed, PCr transfers its phosphate to adenosine diphosphate (ADP) in order to replenish ATP stores, essentially buffering the concentration of ATP. PCr concentrations decrease in response to increased energy demand. [31]P-MRS studies found lower prefrontal PCr levels in bipolar patients during affective episodes than in healthy subjects (Kato, Inubushi, & Kato, 1998; Kato et al., 1994; Murashita et al., 2000). These observations are consistent with the presence of hypermetabolic processes in bipolar patients during mood episodes.

Several studies reported that the PME signal in euthymic bipolar patients is lower than in healthy subjects (chapter 4, Table 4.2). The [31]P-MRS PME resonance consists of phospholipid membrane components, namely phosphocholine, phosphoethanolamine, phosphoserine, and sugar phosphates including inositol-1-monophosphate. Therefore, low PME levels in bipolar disorder suggest excessive membrane turnover, consistent with the previously noted choline findings. Additionally, the presence of this PME abnormality during euthymia suggests it may be a trait, rather than state, marker. As noted, lithium affects PME levels by inhibiting inositol monophosphatase (IMP), leading to increased levels of inositol-1-monophosphate and corresponding increases in PME levels, in addition to changes in *myo*-inositol previously discussed (Renshaw et al., 1986; Yildiz et al., 2001a). From these and other findings, Yildiz et al. (2001b) proposed that some bipolar patients may have genetically low levels of IMP, so that when lithium is administered, the increase in inositol-1-monophosphate reaches a threshold that up-regulates IMP production, which normalizes high-energy membrane metabolism and improves symptoms of the illness. Sudden withdrawal of lithium may then destabilize this situation, leading to relapse of symptoms, consistent with clinical studies of lithium discontinuation (Suppes et al., 1991).

In their extensive review, Stork and Renshaw (2005) concluded that the current MRS findings support a hypothesis of mitochondrial dysfunction in bipolar disorder characterized by impaired oxidative phosphorylation (or regional hypermetabolism) with a resultant shift toward glycolytic energy production (increased lactate and glutamate), a decrease in total energy production or substrate availability (decreased PCr and NAA), altered phospholipid metabolism (elevated Cho and decreased PME), and increased glutamatergic neurotransmission. The suggestion of regional hypermetabolism is consistent with functional imaging observations of over-activated brain areas, particularly amygdala. The presence of excessive glutamate may also lead to neuronal injury or death, contributing to structural changes in gray and white matter, for example, abnormalities in DTI measures of white matter tracts or decrements in prefrontal cortical volumes. These changes may therefore be related to the progression of the early course of bipolar disorder (Figure 13.1), and add to our evolving model of the neurophysiology of bipolar illness (Figure 13.5).

## SUMMARY OF BIPOLAR GENETICS

It has been recognized for centuries that mania (bipolar disorder) runs in families. In clinical practice, most patients presenting with bipolar disorder will be able to identify other family members who have experienced similar symptoms. In some families, the condition is so prevalent that for many years investigators expected to find a specific causative gene, much like was done with Huntington's disease (Egeland et al., 1987). However, this early optimism was not sustainable by genetics studies, so that it is no longer considered likely that bipolar disorder is caused by a single gene (Patel et al., 2010, Nurnberger, 2008). Nonetheless, it remains clear that genetic effects play the major role in the onset and expression of bipolar disorder (Bienvenu et al., 2011).

The specific genes causing bipolar disorder have not yet been identified, but a number of candidate genes are being investigated. Evidence to date suggests that these candidate genes confer susceptibility or risk, but no single gene seems to have a large effect, so that recent genetic models hypothesize that it is the combination of several smaller genetic effects, interacting with environmental features, that create a neurobiological substrate that creates vulnerability for the onset of bipolar disorder. Using the technique of convergent functional genomics, Patel et al. (2010) proposed a pyramid of 56 genes with varying likelihood of contributing to the risk for bipolar disorder. These genes have many different functions, but common themes include the control of neurodevelopment (BDNF, ANK3, DISC1, NCAN, MBP), calcium-channel modulation (CACNA1C), and circadian rhythm regulation (ARNTL, RORB, DBP). As reviewed in chapter 9, other genes that may confer risk of bipolar disorder involve glutamate (DAOA) and monoamine regulation (DAT, 5HTT, MAOA, COMT, TPH1&2). Moreover, as discussed previously in this chapter, MRS studies suggest disruption in mitochondrial cellular energetics, and there is substantial evidence that the function of mitochondrial genes and nuclear genes that modulate mitochondrial function are also abnormal in bipolar disorder (Konradi et al., 2004).

---

**Key Neurochemical Imaging Findings in Bipolar Disorder Include:**

- Elevated glutamate levels during mood episodes

- Decreases in MRS measured NAA & PCr, and increases in choline, lactate & *myo*-inositol consistent with hypermetabolism or disrupted neuronal energetics

- Some neurochemical abnormalities may predate illness onset

- Successful treatment appears to correct neurometabolite abnormalities

- MRS abnormalities may be explained by a mitochondrial bioenergetic dysfunction model

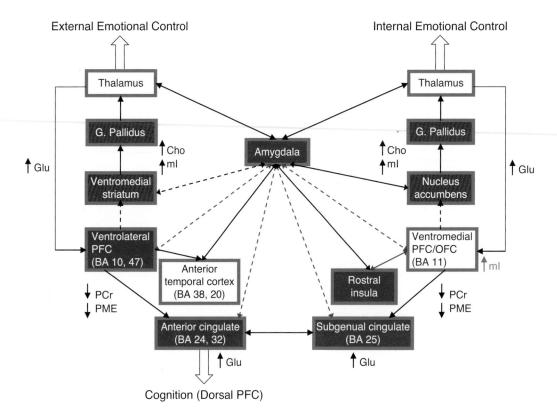

External Emotional Control

Internal Emotional Control

Cognition (Dorsal PFC)

*Figure 13.5* Abnormalities identified within emotional networks in bipolar disorder using magnetic resonance spectroscopy, superimposed over those from structural and functional neuroimaging (Figures 13.3 and 13.4). Increased glutamate (Glu) is observed in mania and depression throughout these networks. Increased *myo*-inositol (ml) and choline (Cho) are commonly observed across mood states in basal ganglia; increased ml (in red) is observed in orbitofrontal cortex prior to illness onset, in at-risk offspring of bipolar parents. Finally, decreased prefrontal phosphocreatine (PCr) and phospholipid (PME) level are also decreased, the latter in euthymia only. Other characteristics of the figure from structural and functional imaging are described with Figures 13.3 and 13.4 and are as follows: green border = brain regions exhibiting relatively consistent functional differences between bipolar and healthy subjects; rust-colored boxes = regional structural abnormalities that appear to post-date the onset of illness (i.e., first manic episode); blue boxes = regional structural abnormalities that may predate illness onset; dashed arrows = potential connectivity abnormalities identified in bipolar disorder using diffusion tensor imaging (DTI).

Together, then, these findings suggest that multiple genetic lesions might variably disrupt the emotional networks of Figure 13.2 leading to the development of bipolar disorder, perhaps in combination with specific environmental events. These environmental contributions remain unclear, but may include significant life stress or substance abuse (McNamara et al., 2010; Ostiguy et al., 2011). These genetic effects may contribute to specific components of the illness as well, that when occurring in combination culminates in a bipolar course of illness. For example, several investigators hypothesized that abnormal circadian clock genes may underlie the development of mood and neurovegetative cycling, as well as switches between mood episodes (reviewed in Patel et al., 2010). As a second example, mania has been hypothesized to arise from excessive dopamine input into the striatum and prefrontal cortex, perhaps due to hypoactive serotonergic and norepinephrine systems (Fountoulakis, Kelsoe, & Akiskal, 2011; Cousins et al., 2009; Berk et al., 2007), leading to failed

monoaminergic modulation of the emotional networks of Figure 13.2. These failures in monoamine control can be hypothesized to arise from the previously noted genes responsible for various aspects of monoamine regulation

**Key Genetic Findings in Bipolar Disorder Include:**

- Bipolar disorder is likely to arise from multi-genetic influences, rather than a single gene

- Possible risk genes impact neurodevelopment, monoamine and glutamate modulation, circadian rhythm control, and calcium-channel modulation

- Genetic effects are expected to impact emotional brain networks

- Moving the genetics of bipolar forward will require integration within functional neuroanatomic and molecular models

and metabolism (Benedetti et al., 2011; Coque et al., 2011; Pinsonneault et al., 2011). Moving forward, then, by integrating possible genetic effects within the brain networks that appear to underlie the expression of bipolar disorder, it may be possible to better identify the cascade of molecular events leading to failure of emotional, cognitive and neurovegetative modulation that characterizes this illness. These genetic considerations are integrated into Figure 13.6.

## INTEGRATION

From the considerations of this chapter (and this book), the model illustrated in Figure 13.6 was developed. This integrated neurophysiological model of bipolar disorder arises from genetic variations in the control of monoaminergic or glutamatergic regulation, mitochondrial function, brain development, or circadian rhythm regulation that disrupt the neurochemistry, structure, and function of prefrontal-amygdala brain networks that are responsible for maintaining emotional homoeostasis. It is likely the genetic etiology of bipolar disorder is heterogeneous, such that these genetic variations interact in various combinations, rather than all lesions occurring in all patients, to lead to failure of emotional networks. As noted, specific environmental events may also be necessary to impact gene expression or initiate symptoms, although what these are remain essentially unknown. Consequently, this genetic heterogeneity coupled with the likelihood that environmental effects contribute to illness onset may explain why heritability, though very high at 85%, is not 100%. Regardless, abnormal development, bioenergetics, and modulation of these emotional networks lead to emotional dysregulation, as well as other symptoms of bipolar disorder. With this brief overview, then, how might this model explain the various key clinical features we identified at the beginning of this chapter?

As noted, mania is the defining syndrome of bipolar disorder. Among psychiatric syndromes, it is relatively specific in predicting a subsequent course of illness (i.e., mood cycling) and a specific treatment response (especially lithium). In our proposed model, and as implied previously, we hypothesize that mania results from the loss of ventral prefrontal modulation of amygdala and other limbic brain areas due to developmental errors in brain structure (e.g., striatal overgrowth, disrupted prefrontal/amygdala connectivity), coupled with excessive (or incorrectly modulated) dopaminergic neurotransmission to striatum and prefrontal cortex. These abnormalities in neurotransmission might arise directly from genetic lesions or indirectly

through ineffective metabolic processes or structural abnormalities that control dopamine input and feedback into emotional networks (Cousins et al., 2009). Together these abnormalities lead to the symptoms of mania, namely extreme and labile moods from dysregulated limbic brain, coupled with characteristics known to result from dopaminergic excess, such as disinihibited reward seeking, agitation, and psychosis. Moreover, our model suggests that vulnerability for mania is likely to be multifactorial, resulting from abnormalities in genes related to brain structural formation and from genes modulating monoaminergic and glutamatergic function. Moreover, the amygdala provides significant input into monoamine control (Kim et al., 2011), so that loss of prefrontal modulation of amygdala may contribute to disruptions in dopaminergic neurotransmission. Since lithium is relatively specific for the treatment of mania and works, at least in part, through effects on inositol metabolism and bioenergy cascades, it is likely that genetic abnormalities in cellular energetics contribute to symptoms, perhaps by providing an inefficient substrate that is unable, in the face of prefrontal loss of control, to recover and re-establish equilibrium. Excessive glutamate neurotransmission, then, arises either directly (through genetic errors) or indirectly through failed energetics, thereby maintaining symptoms. Obviously, many of these considerations are speculative. Nonetheless, this model provides testable hypotheses to better define the substrate of mania.

Similar considerations underlie how this model might predict other key symptoms of bipolar disorder, namely dynamic mood cycling, cognitive impairment and disrupted neurovegetative processes. As suggested previously, abnormalities in circadian clock genes can be hypothesized to deregulate biological rhythms in bipolar disorder (Patel et al., 2010). With these biological clock systems genetically impaired or limited, the biological system may be unable to re-establish equilibrium in response to life events, substance abuse or other triggers, particularly in the setting of the previously discussed structural, functional, and metabolic abnormalities of emotional mood networks. Over time, an increasingly dysregulated and sensitized mood system may result in even minor triggers precipitating mood episodes; if so, then precipitating stressful events linked to mood episodes might be more difficult to identify later in the course of illness (McNamara et al., 2010; Paykel 2003; Dienes et al., 2006; Post 2007; Pavlova et al., 2011).

With reciprocal connections between ventral prefrontal emotional networks and dorsal cognitive networks, abnormalities in one would be expected to produce abnormalities in the other. Consequently, our model suggests that

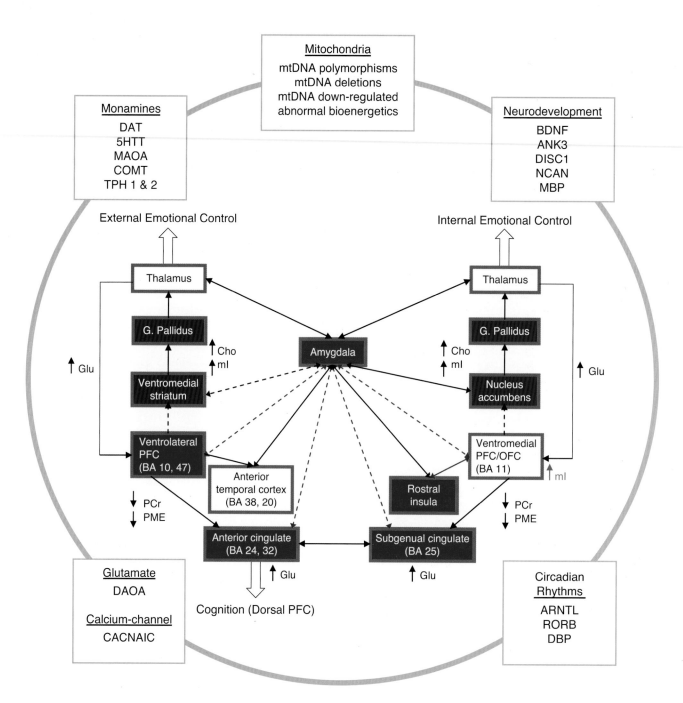

*Figure 13.6* Integration of genetics findings with abnormalities identified with neuroimaging and MRS in bipolar disorder (see Figures 13.2, 13.3, 13.4, and 13.5). Genes are linked by the orange circle and are listed by overall areas of effects; since genes have effects in multiple areas, no attempt has been made to link them to specific brain regions within the diagram. Other characteristics of the figure from neuroimaging, as described in the previous figures, include: Glu = glutamate; mI = *myo*-inositol (mI); Cho = choline; increased mI (in red) is observed in orbitofrontal cortex prior to illness onset in at-risk offspring of bipolar parents; PCr = phosphocreatine; PME = phospholipid; green border = brain regions exhibiting relatively consistent functional differences between bipolar and healthy subjects; rust-colored boxes = regional structural abnormalities that appear to post-date the onset of illness (i.e., first manic episode); blue boxes = regional structural abnormalities that may predate illness onset; dashed arrows = potential connectivity abnormalities identified in bipolar disorder using diffusion tensor imaging (DTI). Gene abbreviations: DAT = dopamine transporter; 5HTT = serotonin transporter; MAOA = monoamine oxidase A; COMT = catechol-O-methyltransferase; TPH = tryptophan hydroxylase; DAOA = D-amino acid oxidase activator; CACNA1C = calcium channel, voltage-dependent, L type, alpha 1C subunit; ARNTL = aryl hydrocarbon receptor nuclear translocator-like; RORB = RAR-related orphan receptor B; DBP = D site of albumin promoter (albumin D-box) binding protein; MBP = myelin basic protein; NCAN = neurocan; DISC1 = disrupted in schizophrenia 1; ANK3 = ankyrin 3; BDNF = brain-derived neurotrophic factor; mtDNA = mitochondrial DNA.

the cognitive symptoms of bipolar disorder are secondary to disruption from unstable and often overactive mood networks, consistent with previous suggestions by Mayberg et al. (1999). Finally, because the autonomic nervous system is closely linked to amygdala and other regions within prefrontal emotional networks (Kim et al., 2011), as well as hypothalamic regions that modulate biorhythms, abnormalities in these areas would be expected to be expressed in dynamic neurovegetative symptoms, consistent with those seen in the course of bipolar disorder (e.g., disrupted sleep, increased energy). Indeed, work in animal models and human subjects suggests that prefrontal cortex gates amygdala input into hypothalamic nuclei, so that loss of prefrontal modulation of amygdala may directly contribute to neurovegetative symptoms and signs (McNamara et al., 2010; Ohira et al., 2006; Urry et al., 2006; Quirk et al., 2003).

The proposed multi-genetic substrate underlying vulnerability to bipolar disorder, and the bioenergetic abnormalities arising from this substrate within these networks that produce over- and under-activation of key structures, are hypothesized to contribute to disruption of healthy developmental processes. This disruption is predicted to lead to inadequate structural, and consequently functional, integration among the key brain regions necessary to modulate emotional processes. Direct lesions in developmental genetics (e.g., faulty expression of BDNF), in addition to potential indirect effects of dysfunctional neural systems guiding connections may both contribute to developmental vulnerabilities. Consequently, as individuals pass through critical neurodevelopmental stages, namely the significant reorganization of prefrontal cortical regions that occurs in adolescence and young adulthood, the deficits of this disrupted system are exposed, leading to the expression of mania and the development of mood cycling in young people, consistent with the clinical observation of this period being the typical age at onset.

With increasing episodes, hypermetabolic processes and excessive glutamatergic neurotransmission can be hypothesized to injure these networks. Neurons with abnormal mitochondrial metabolism that have inadequate ability to manage reactive oxygen species that arise in the course of metabolism and maintain healthy cellular metabolic dynamics, may be particularly susceptible to injury or death during periods of hypermetabolism or excessive glutamate neurotransmission (e.g., mood episodes). Damaging or killing neurons, leading to loss of white matter neuropil and regional connectivity, may lead to deterioration of balance within emotional brain networks, causing progressively dysregulated emotional control. This loss of

structural and functional integrity over time may consequently underlie the early course progression of bipolar illness (Figure 13.1).

## MOVING FORWARD

The model illustrated in Figure 13.6 and the previous discussions are not meant to imply that we have established a complete understanding of the neurophysiology of bipolar disorder, as many of the considerations remain speculative. However, this model identifies a number of areas requiring future investigation and suggests several testable hypotheses. For example, as noted, mania is a relatively unique and specific syndrome that defines bipolar illness. However, its specific neurophysiology remains incompletely defined. Our model suggests that loss of prefrontal control of limbic brain, couple with excessive dopaminergic neurotransmission might lead to this symptom complex. With this in mind several testable hypotheses arise:

1. Ventral prefrontal functional connectivity with amygdala improves as patients recover from mania to euthymia.

2. Excessive dopaminergic neurotransmission during mania is associated with increased amygdala and decreased prefrontal activation.

3. Specific gene variations associated with dopamine neurotransmission (e.g., DAT, or the modulation of such, e.g. 5HTT) occur in at-risk subjects and are associated with abnormalities in prefrontal-amygdala connectivity prior to illness onset.

4. The combination of amygdala over-activation and prefrontal under-activation occurs in bipolar manic but not schizophrenic patients.

5. Lithium treatment decreases *myo*-inositol acutely, leading to increased prefrontal activation and decreased amygdala hyperactivity in patients with mania.

These are simply five examples, as obviously, many other questions arise from this model. However, these examples illustrate several points that will be critical to address in order to advance understanding of the neurophysiology of bipolar disorder. First, longitudinal neuroimaging studies are necessary in order to better understand how specific functional, neurochemical (i.e., MRS) and perhaps even structural changes within *individual subjects* are associated with clinical course. Bipolar disorder is dynamic and the processes underlying its dynamic nature are poorly defined, yet likely critical to really understand how this illness develops. Second, studies are needed that integrate imaging modalities, such as ligand measures coupled with activation patterns, in order to better interpret imaging findings. Third, genetic screens and neuroimaging must be combined in order to understand the molecular substrate that underlies the neuroimaging picture. Moreover, studies in at-risk and early-course patients are needed to clarify the initial progression of neurophysiological changes associated with the onset and evolution of illness. Additionally, it is not clear yet what specific neurodevelopmental events occur in adolescence that initiate mania in vulnerable subjects. These types of findings separate themselves naturally from the epiphenomena of mood episodes and help clarify the enduring components of this dynamic condition. Fourth, many of the findings observed with both imaging and genetics appear to be relatively nonspecific, as similar findings are often observed in other psychiatric conditions. More studies comparing subjects with different psychiatric conditions, beyond simple comparisons with only healthy subjects, are needed to illuminate those specific abnormalities that lead to bipolar illness instead of, for example, unipolar depression or schizophrenia. Finally, clinical interventions not only help patients, but also provide neurochemical or behavioral probes that presumably impact the neurophysiology of bipolar subjects; studies integrating treatment effects with imaging may not only better define how treatments work, but also reveal the substrate underlying these effects.

In this chapter specifically, and this book more generally, we have tried to summarize and integrate two of the most active scientific approaches to understanding bipolar disorder, namely genetics and neuroimaging. We believe that integrating these approaches is most likely to lead to discovery of the causes of this condition. We hope that this text inspires both the current and the next generation of scientists to tackle the neurophysiological basis of this fascinating, dynamic, and sometimes disabling and tragic condition in order to lead in the future to improved treatments for bipolar patients, and ultimately prevention of bipolar illness.

## REFERENCES

Adler, C. M., Adams, J., DelBello, M. P., Holland, S. K., Schmithorst, V., Levine, A., . . . Strakowski, S. M. 2006. Evidence of white matter pathology in bipolar disorder adolescents experiencing their first episode of mania: a diffusion tensor imaging study. *American Journal of Psychiatry*, 163: 322–324.

Adler, C. M., Holland, S. K., Schmithorst, V., Tuchfarber, M. J., & Strakowski, S.M. 2004. Changes in neuronal activation in patients with bipolar disorder during performance of a working memory task. *Bipolar Disorders*, 6(6): 540–549.

Adler, C. M., Holland, S. K., Schmithorst, V., Wilke, M., Weiss, K. L., Pan, H., & Strakowski, S. M. 2004. Abnormal frontal white matter tracts in bipolar disorder: a diffusion tensor imaging study. *Bipolar Disorders*, 6(3): 197–203.

Almeida, J. R., Mechelli, A., Hassel, S., Versace, A., Kupfer, D. J., & Phillips, M. L. 2009. Abnormally increased effective connectivity between parahippocampal gyrus and ventromedial prefrontal regions during emotion labeling in bipolar disorder. *Psychiatry Reearchs*, 174: 195–201.

Almeida, J. R., Versace, A., Hassel, S., Kupfer, D. J., & Phillips, M. L. 2010. Elevated amygdala activity to sad facial expressions: a state marker of bipolar but not unipolar depression. *Biological Psychiatry*, 67: 414–421.

Altshuler, L., Bookheimer, S., Proenza, M. A., Townsend, J., Sabb, F., Firestine, A., . . . Cohen, M. S. 2005. Increased amygdala activation during mania: a functional magnetic resonance imaging study. *American Journal of Psychiatry*, 162: 1211–1213.

Altshuler, L., Bookheimer, S., Townsend, J., Proenza, M. A., Sabb, F., Mintz, J., & Cohen, M. S. 2008. Regional brain changes in bipolar I depression: a functional magnetic resonance imaging study. *Bipolar Disorders*, 10: 708–717.

Altshuler, L. L., Bartzokis, G., Grieder, T., Curran, J., & Mintz. J. 1998. Amygdala enlargement in bipolar disorder and hippocampal reduction in schizophrenia: an MRI study demonstrating neuroanatomic specificity. *Archives of General Psychiatry*, 55: 663–664.

Angst, J., & Sellaro, R. 2000. Historical perspectives and natural history of bipolar disorder. *Biological Psychiatry*, 48: 445–457.

Arnone, D., Cavanagh, J., Gerber, D., Lawrie, S. M., Ebmeier, K. P., & McIntosh, A. M. 2009. Magnetic resonance imaging studies in bipolar disorder and schizophrenia: meta-analysis. *British Journal of Psychiatry*, 195(3): 194–201.

Benedetti, F., Radaelli, D., Poletti, S., Locatelli, C., Dallaspezia, S., Lorenzi, C., Pirovano, A., Colombo, C., Smeraldi, E. 2011. Association of the C(-1019)G 5-HT1A promoter polymorphism with exposure to stressors preceding hospitalization for bipolar depression. *Journal of Affective Disorders*, 132(1-2): 297–300.

Ben-Noun, L. 2003. What was the mental disease that afflicted King Saul? *Clinical Case Studies*, 2(4): 270–282.

Berk, M., Dodd, S., Kauer-Sant'anna, M., Malhi, G. S., Bourin, M., Kapczinski, F., Norman, T. 2007. Dopamine dysregulation syndrome: implications for a dopamine hypothesis of bipolar disorder. *Acta Psychiatrica Scandinavica*, 434: 41–49.

Beyer, J. L., Taylor, W. D., MacFall, J. R., Kuchibhatla, M., Payne, M. E., Provenzale, J. M., . . . Krishnan, K. R. 2005. Cortical white matter microstructural abnormalities in bipolar disorder. *Neuropsychopharmacology*, 30(12): 2225–2229.

Bienvenu, O. J., Davydow, D. S., & Kendler, K. S. 2011. Psychiatric "diseases" versus behavioral disorders and degree of genetic influence. *Psychological Medicine*, 41(1): 33–40.

Bitter, S. M., Mills, N. P., Adler, C. M., Strakowski, S. M., & DelBello, M. P. 2011. In press. Progression of Amygdala Volumetric Abnormalities in Adolescents After Their First Manic Episode. *J Am Acad Child Adolescent Psychiatry*.

Blumberg, H. P., Fredericks, C., Wang, F., Kalmar, J. H., Spencer, L., Papademetris, X., . . . Krystal, J. H. 2005. Preliminary evidence for persistent abnormalities in amygdala volumes in adolescents and young adults with bipolar disorder. *Bipolar Disorders*, 7(6): 570–576.

Blumberg, H. P., Krystal, J. H., Bansal, R., Martin, A., Dziura, J., Durkin, K., . . . Peterson, B. S. 2006. Age, rapid-cycling, and pharmacotherapy effects on ventral prefrontal cortex in bipolar disorder: a cross-sectional study. *Biological Psychiatry*, 59(7): 611–618.

Blumberg, H. P., Stern, E., Ricketts, S., Martinez, D., de Asis, J., White, T., . . . Silbersweig, D. A. 1999. Rostral and orbital prefrontal cortex dysfunction in the manic state of bipolar disorder. *American Journal of Psychiatry*, 156(12): 1986–1988.

Bora, E., Fornito, A., Yucel, M., & Pantelis, C. 2010. Voxelwise meta-analysis of gray matter abnormalities in bipolar disorder. *Biological Psychiatry*, 67(11): 1097–1105.

Brennan, B. P., Hudson, J. I., Jensen, J. E., McCarthy, J., Roberts, J. L., Prescot, A. P., ... Ongur, D. 2010. Rapid enhancement of glutamatergic neurotransmission in bipolar depression following treatment with riluzole. *Neuropsychopharmacology*, 35: 834–846.

Bruno, S., Cercignani, M., & Ron, M. A. 2008. White matter abnormalities in bipolar disorder: a voxel-based diffusion tensor imaging study. *Bipolar Disorders*, 10(4): 460–468.

Cecil, K. M., DelBello, M. P., Sellars, M. C., & Strakowski, S. M. 2003. Proton magnetic resonance spectroscopy of the frontal lobe and cerebellar vermis in children with a mood disorder and a familial risk for bipolar disorders. *Journal of Child and Adolescent Psychopharmacology*, 13: 545–555.

Chai, X. J., Whitfield-Gabrieli, S., Shinn, A. K., Gabrieli, J. D., Nieto Castañón, A., McCarthy, J. M., ... Ongür, D. 2011. Abnormal Medial Prefrontal Cortex Resting-State Connectivity in Bipolar Disorder and Schizophrenia. *Neuropsychopharmacology*. 2011 [Epub ahead of print]

Chang, K., Adleman, N., Dienes, K., Barnea-Goraly, N., Reiss, A., & Ketter, T. 2003. Decreased N-acetylaspartate in children with familial bipolar disorder. *Biological Psychiatry*, 53: 1059–1065.

Chang, K., Adleman, N. E., Dienes, K., Simeonova, D. I., Menon, V., & Reiss, A. 2004. Anomalous prefrontal-subcortical activation in familial pediatric bipolar disorder: a functional magnetic resonance imaging investigation. *Arch Gen Psychiatry*, 61(8): 781–792.

Chen, Y. C., Thaler, D., Nixon, P. D., Stern, C. E., & Passingham, R. E. 1995. The functions of the medial premotor cortex. II. The timing and selection of learned movements. *Experimental Brain Research*, 102: 461–473.

Chepenik, L. G., Raffo, M., Hampson, M., Lacadie, C., Wang, F., Jones, M. M., ... Blumberg, H. P. 2010. Functional connectivity between ventral prefrontal cortex and amygdala at low frequency in the resting state in bipolar disorder. *Psychiatry Research*, 182(3): 207–210.

Coque, L., Mukherjee, S., Cao, J. L., Spencer, S., Marvin, M., Falcon, E., Sidor, M. M., Birnbaum, S. G., Graham, A., Neve, R. L., Gordon, E., Ozburn, A. R., Goldberg, M. S., Han, M. H., Cooper, D. C., McClung, C. A. 2011. Specific role of VTA dopamine neuronal firing rates and morphology in the reversal of anxiety-related, but not depression-related behavior in the ClockΔ19 mouse model of mania. *Neuropsychopharmacology*, 36(7): 1478–1488.

Cousins, D. A., Butts, K., & Young, A. H. 2009. The role of dopamine in bipolar disorder. *Bipolar Disorders*, 11: 787–806.

Dager, S. R., Friedman, S. D., Parow, A., Hirashima, F., Demopulos, C., Stoll, A. L., ... Renshaw, P. F. 2004. Brain metabolic alterations in medication-free patients with bipolar disorder. *Arch General Psychiatry*, 61: 450–458.

Davanzo, P., Thomas, M. A., Yue, K., Oshiro, T., Belin, T., Strober, M., & McCracken, J. 2001. Decreased anterior cingulate myo-inositol/creatine spectroscopy resonance with lithium treatment in children with bipolar disorder. *Neuropsychopharmacology*, 24: 359–369.

DelBello, M. P., Cecil, K. M., Adler, C. M., Daniels, J. P., & Strakowski, S. M. 2006. Neurochemical effects of olanzapine in first-hospitalization manic adolescents: A proton magnetic resonance spectroscopy study. *Neuropsychopharmacology*, 31: 1264–1273.

DelBello, M. P., Zimmerman, M. E., Mills, N. P., Getz, G. E., & Strakowski, S. M. 2004. Magnetic resonance imaging analysis of amygdala and other subcortical brain regions in adolescents with bipolar disorder. *Bipolar Disorders*, 6: 43–52.

Dickstein, D. P., Milham, M. P., Nugent, A. C., Drevets, W. C., Charney, D. S., Pine, D. S., & Leibenluft, E. 2005. Frontotemporal alterations in pediatric bipolar disorder: results of a voxel-based morphometry study. *Arch Gen Psychiatry*, 62(7): 734–741.

Dienes, K. A., Hammen, C., Henry, R. M., Cohen, A. N., & Daley, S. E. 2006. The stress sensitization hypothesis: understanding the course of bipolar disorder. *Journal of Affective Disorders*, 95: 43–49.

Egeland, J. A., Gerhard, D. S., Pauls, D. L., Sussex, J. N., Kidd, K. K., Allen, C. R., ... Housman, D. E. 1987. Bipolar affective disorders linked to DNA markers on chromosome 11. *Nature*, 325(6107): 783–787.

Ellison-Wright, I., & Bullmore. E. 2010. Anatomy of bipolar disorder and schizophrenia: a meta-analysis. *Schizophrenia Research*, 117(1): 1–12.

Fichtenholtz, H. M., Dean, H. L., Dillon, D. G., Yamasaki, H., McCarthy, G., & LaBar, K. S. 2004. Emotion-attention network interactions during a visual oddball task. *Brain Res Cognitive Brain Research*, 20: 67–80.

Foland, L. C., Altshuler, L. L., Bookheimer, S. Y., Eisenberger, N., Townsend, J., & Thompson, P. M. 2008. Evidence for deficient modulation of amygdala response by prefrontal cortex in bipolar mania. *Psychiatry Research*, 162(1): 27–37.

Fountoulakis, K. N., Kelsoe, J. R., & Akiskal, H. 2011. Receptor targets for antidepressant therapy in bipolar disorder: An overview. *Journal of Affective Disorders*, 2011 [Epub ahead of print].

Frazier, J. A., Breeze, J. L., Papadimitriou, G., Kennedy, D. N., Hodge, S. M., Moore, C. M., ... Makris, N. 2007. White matter abnormalities in children with and at risk for bipolar disorder. *Bipolar Disorders*, 9(8): 799–809.

Fusar-Poli, P., Placentino, A., Carletti, F., Allen, P., Landi, P., Abbamonte, M., ... Politi, P. L. 2009. Laterality effect on emotional faces processing: ALE meta-analysis of evidence. *Neurosci Letters*, 452: 262–267.

Gallelli, K. A., Wagner, C. M., Karchemskiy, A., Howe, M., Spielman, D., Reiss, A., & Chang, K. D. 2005. N-acetylaspartate levels in bipolar offspring with and at high-risk for bipolar disorder. *Bipolar Disorders*, 7: 589–597.

Goodwin, F. K., & Jamison, K. R. 2007. *Manic-Depressive Illness: Bipolar Disorders and Recurrent Depression*, 2nd ed. New York: Oxford University Press.

Gruber, S. A., Rogowska, J., & Yurgelun-Todd, D. A. 2004. Decreased activation of the anterior cingulate in bipolar patients: an fMRI study. *Journal of Affective Disorders*, 82(2): 191–201.

Hallahan, B., Newell, J., Soares, J. C., Brambilla, P., Strakowski, S. M., Fleck, D. E., ... McDonald, C. 2011. Structural magnetic resonance imaging in bipolar disorder: an international collaborative mega-analysis of individual adult patient data. *Biological Psychiatry*, 69(4): 326–335.

Hirschfeld, R. M., Holzer, C., Calabrese, J. R., Weissman, M., Reed, M., Davies, M., ... Hazard, E. 2003. Validity of the mood disorder questionnaire: a general population study. *American Journal of Psychiatry*, 160: 178–180.

Jamison, K. 1993. *Touched with Fire*. New York: Free Press.

Judd, L. L., & Akiskal HS. 2003. The prevalence and disability of bipolar spectrum disorders in the US population: re-analysis of the ECA database taking into account subthreshold cases. *Journal of Affective Disorders*, 73: 123–131.

Kafantaris, V., Kingsley, P., Ardekani, B., Saito, E., Lencz, T., Lim, K., & Szeszko, P. 2009. Lower orbital frontal white matter integrity in adolescents with bipolar I disorder. *Journal of American Academy of Child Adolescent Psychiatry*, 48(1): 79–86.

Kaladjian, A., Jeanningros, R., Azorin, J. M., Nazarian, B., Roth, M., Anton, J. L., & Mazzola-Pomietto, P. 2009. Remission from mania is associated with a decrease in amygdala activation during motor response inhibition. *Bipolar Disorders*, 11(5): 530–538.

Kaladjian, A., Jeanningros, R., Azorin, J. M., Nazarian, B., Roth, M., & Mazzola-Pomietto, P. 2009. Reduced brain activation in euthymic bipolar patients during response inhibition: an event-related fMRI study. *Psychiatry Research*, 173(1): 45–51.

Kato, T., Inubushi, T., & Kato, N. 1998. Magnetic resonance spectroscopy in affective disorders. *J Neuropsychiatry*, 10: 133–147.

Kato, T., & Kato, N. 2000. Mitochondrial dysfunction in bipolar disorder. *Bipolar Disorders*, 2: 180–190.

Kato, T., Takahashi, S., Shioiri, T., Murashita, J., Hamakawa, H., & Inubushi, T. 1994. Reduction of brain phosphocreatine in bipolar II disorder detected by phosphorus-31 magnetic resonance spectroscopy. *Journal of Affective Disorders*, 31: 125–133.

Kim, M. J., Loucks, R. A., Palmer, A. L., Brown, A. C., Solomon, K. M., Marchatne, A. N., & Whalen, P. J. 2011. The structural and functional connectivity of the amygdala: from normal emotion to pathological anxiety. *Behavioural Brain Research* 223(2): 403–410.

Konradi, C., Eaton, M., MacDonald, M. L., Walsh, J., Benes, F. M., & Heckers, S. 2004. Molecular evidence for mitochondrial dysfunction in bipolar disorder. *Archives of General Psychiatry*, 61: 300–308.

Kraepelin, E. 1921. *Manic-Depressive Insanity and Paranoia.* Trans. R. M. Barclay, ed. G. M. Robertson. Edinburgh: E. and S. Livingstone. Reproduced in the series "The Classic of Psychiatry and Behavioral Sciences Library," E. T. Carlson, ed. Birmingham, AL: Gryphon Editions, Inc.

Kronhaus, D. M., Lawrence, N. S., Williams, A. M., Frangou, S., Brammer, M. J., Williams, S. C., . . . Phillips, M. L. 2006. Stroop performance in bipolar disorder: further evidence for abnormalities in the ventral prefrontal cortex. *Bipolar Disorders*, 8(1): 28–39.

Ladouceur, C. D., Almeida, J. R., Birmaher, B., Axelson, D. A., Nau, S., Kalas, C., . . . Phillips, M. L. 2008. Subcortical gray matter volume abnormalities in healthy bipolar offspring: potential neuroanatomical risk marker for bipolar disorder? *Journal of the American Academy of Child and Adolescent Psychiatry*, 47(5): 532–539.

Lane, R. D., Reiman, E. M., Axelrod, B., Yun, L. S., Holmes, A., & Schwartz, G. E. 1998. Neural correlates of levels of emotional awareness. Evidence of an interaction between emotion and attention in the anterior cingulate cortex. *Journal of Cognitive Neuroscience*, 10(4): 525–535.

Lawrence, N. S., Williams, A. M., Surguladze, S., Giampietro, V., Brammer, M. J., Andrew, C., . . . Phillips, M. L. 2004. Subcortical and ventral prefrontal cortical neural responses to facial expressions distinguish patients with bipolar disorder and major depression. *Biological Psychiatry*, 55(6): 578–587.

Lennox, B. R., Jacob, R., Calder, A. J., Lupson, V., & Bullmore, E. T. 2004. Behavioural and neurocognitive responses to sad facial affect are attenuated in patients with mania. *Psychological Medicine*, 34(5): 795–802.

Lin, F., Weng, S., Xie, B., Wu, G., & Lei, H. 2011. Abnormal frontal cortex white matter connections in bipolar disorder: a DTI tractography study. *Journal of Affective Disorders*, 131(1–3): 299–306.

Lopez-Larson, M., Michael, E. S., Terry, J. E., Breeze, J. L., Hodge, S. M., Tang, L., . . . Frazier, J. A. 2009. Subcortical differences among youths with attention-deficit/hyperactivity disorder compared to those with bipolar disorder with and without attention-deficit/hyperactivity disorder. *Journal of Child and Adolescent Psychopharmacology*, 19(1): 31–39.

Lyoo, I. K., Demopulos, C. M., Hirashima, F., Ahn, K. H., & Renshaw, P. F. 2003. Oral choline decreases brain purine levels in lithium-treated subjects with rapid-cycling bipolar disorder: a double-blind trial using proton and lithium magnetic resonance spectroscopy. *Bipolar Disorders*,; 5: 300–306.

Madhavarao, C. N., Chinopoulos, C., Chandrasekaran, K., & Namboodiri, M. A. 2003. Characterization of the N-acetylaspartate biosynthetic enzyme from rat rain. *Journal of Neurochemistry*, 86: 824–835.

Marchand, W. R., Lee, J. N., Thatcher, G. W., Jensen, C., Stewart, D., Dilda, V., . . . Creem-Regehr, S. H. 2007. A functional MRI study of a paced motor activation task to evaluate frontal-subcortical circuit function in bipolar depression. *Psychiatry Res*, 155(3): 221–230.

Marchand, W. R., & Yurgelun-Todd, D. 2010. Striatal structure and function in mood disorders: a comprehensive review. *Bipolar Disorders*, 12(8): 764–785.

Mayberg, H. S., Liotti, M., Brannan, S. K., McGinnis, S., Mahurin, R. K., Jerabek, P. A., . . . Fox, P. T. 1999. Reciprocal limbic-cortical function and negative mood: converging PET findings in depression and normal sadness. *American Journal of Psychiatry*, 156(5): 675–682.

McNamara, R. K., Nandagopal, J. J., Strakowski, S. M., & DelBello, M. P. 2010. Preventative strategies for early-onset bipolar disorder: towards a clinical staging model. *CNS Drugs*, 24(12): 983–996.

Modica-Napolitano, J. S., & Renshaw, P. F. 2004. Ethanolamine and phosphoethanolamine inhibit mitochondrial function in vitro: implications for mitochondrial dysfunction hypothesis in depression and bipolar disorder. *Biological Psychiatry*, 55(3): 273–277.

Moore, G. J., Bebchuk, J. M., Hasanat, K., Chen, G., Seraji-Bozorgzad, N., Wilds, I. B., . . . Manji, H. K. 2000. Lithium increases N-acetylaspartate in the human brain: in vivo evidence in support of bcl-2's neurotrophic effects? *Bioogicall Psychiatry*, 48(1): 1–8.

Moore, G. J., Bebchuk, J. M., Parrish, J. K., Faulk, M. W., Arfken, C. L., Strahl-Bevacqua, J., & Manji, H. K. 1999. Temporal dissociation between lithium-induced changes in frontal lobe myo-inositol and clinical response in manic-depressive illness. *American Journal of Psychiatry*, 156: 1902–1908.

Murashita, J., Kato, T., Shioiri, T., Inubushi, T., & Kato, N. 2000. Altered brain energy metabolism in lithium-resistant bipolar disorder detected by photic stimulated 31P-MR spectroscopy. *Psychological Medicine*, 30: 107–115.

Murray, C. J., & Lopez, A. D. 1996. The Global Burden of Disease: A Comprehensive Assessment of Mortality and Disability from Diseases, Injuries and Risk Factors in 1990 and Projected to 2020. Cambridge, MA: Harvard School of Public Health (Global Burden of Disease and Injury Series, vol. I).

Narrow, W. E., Rae, D. S., Robins, L. N., & Regier, D. A. 2002. Revised prevalence estimates of mental disorders in the United States: Using a clinical significance criterion to reconcile 2 surveys' estimates. *Archives of General Psychiatry*, 59: 115–123.

Noga, J. T., Vladar, K., & Torrey, E. F. 2001. A volumetric magnetic resonance imaging study of monozygotic twins discordant for bipolar disorder. *Psychiatry Research*, 106(1): 25–34.

Nurnberger, Jr., J. I. 2008. A simulated genetic structure for bipolar illness. *American Journal of Medical Genetics: B. Neuropsychiatric Genetics*, 147B(6): 952–956.

Ohira, H., Nomura, M., Ichikawa, N., Isowa, T., Iidaka, T., Sato, A., . . . Yamada, J. 2006. Association of neural and physiological responses during voluntary emotion suppression. *Neuroimage*, 29(3): 721–733.

Ostiguy, C. S., Ellenbogen, M. A., Walker, C. D., Walker, E. F., & Hodgins, S. 2011. Sensitivity to stress among the offspring of parents with bipolar disorder: a study of daytime cortisol levels. *Psychological Medicine*, 28: 1–11.

Patel, S. D., Le-Niculescu, H., Koller, D. L., Green, S. D., Lahiri, D. K., McMahon, F. J., . . . Niculescu, A. B. III. 2010. Coming to grips with complex disorders: genetic risk prediction in bipolar disorder using panels of genes identified through convergent functional genomics. *American Journal of Medical Genetics: B. Neuropsychiatric Genetics*, 153B(4): 850–877.

Pavlova, B., Uher, R., Dennington, L., Wright, K., & Donaldson, C. 2011. Reactivity of affect and self-esteem during remission in bipolar affective disorder: An experimental investigation. *Journal of Affective Disorders*, 134(1-3):102–11.

Pavuluri, M. N., O'Connor, M. M., Harral, E., & Sweeney, J. A. 2007. Affective neural circuitry during facial emotion processing in pediatric bipolar disorder. *Biological Psychiatry*, 62(2): 158–167.

Pavuluri, M. N., O'Connor, M. M., Harral, E. M., & Sweeney, J. A. 2008. An fMRI study of the interface between affective and cognitive neural circuitry in pediatric bipolar disorder. *Psychiatry Res*, 162(3): 244–255.

Pavuluri, M. N., Passarotti, A. M., Harral, E. M., & Sweeney, J. A. 2009. An fMRI study of the neural correlates of incidental versus directed emotion processing in pediatric bipolar disorder. *J Am Acad Child Adolesc Psychiatry*, 48(3): 308–319.

Paykel, E. S. 2003. Life events and affective disorders. *Acta Psychiatria Scandanavica Supplement*, 418: 61–66.

Perlis, R. H., Miyahara, S., Marangell, L. B., Wisniewski, S. R., Ostacher, M., DelBello, M. P., . . . STEP-BD Investigators. 2004. Long-term implications of early onset in bipolar disorder: data from the first 1000 participants in the systematic treatment enhancement program for bipolar disorder (STEP-BD). *Biological Psychiatry*, 55(9): 875–881.

Pfeifer, J. C., Welge, J., Strakowski, S. M., Adler, C. M., & DelBello, M. P. 2008. Meta-analysis of amygdala volumes in children and adolescents with bipolar disorder. *Journal of American Academy of Child and Adolescent Psychiatry*, 47(11): 1289–1298.

Phan, K. L., Wager, T., Taylor, S. F., & Liberzon, I. 2002. Functional neuroanatomy of emotion: a meta-analysis of emotion activation studies in PET and fMRI. *Neuroimage*, 16: 331–348.

Pinsonneault, J. K., Han, D. D., Burdick, K. E., Kataki, M., Bertolino, A., Malhotra, A. K., . . . Sadee, W. 2011. Dopamine Transporter Gene Variant Affecting Expression in Human Brain is Associated with Bipolar Disorder. *Neuropsychopharmacology*, 36: 1644–1655.

Post, R. M. 2007. Kindling and sensitization as models for affective episode recurrence, cyclicity, and tolerance phenomena. *Neuroscience and Biobehavioral Reviews*, 31(6): 858–873.

Quirk, G. J., Likhtik, E., Pelletier, J. G., & Paré, D. 2003. Stimulation of medial prefrontal cortex decreases the responsiveness of central amygdala output neurons. *Journal of Neuroscience*, 23(25): 8800–8807.

Renshaw, P. F., Summers, J. J., Renshaw, C. E., Hines, K. G., & Leigh, J. S., Jr. 1986. Changes in the $^{31}$P-NMR spectra of cats receiving lithium chloride systemically. *Biological Psychiatry*, 21: 694–698.

Rich, B. A., Vinton, D. T., Roberson-Nay, R., Hommer, R. E., Berghorst, L. H., McClure, E. B., . . . Leibenluft, E. 2006. Limbic hyperactivation during processing of neutral facial expressions in children with bipolar disorder. *Proceeds of the National Academy of Science U S A*, 103(23): 8900–8905.

Rosso, I. M., W. D. Killgore, C. M. Cintron, S. A. Gruber, M. Tohen, and D. A. Yurgelun-Todd. 2007. Reduced amygdala volumes in first-episode bipolar disorder and correlation with cerebral white matter. *Biological Psychiatry*, 61(6): 743–749.

Roy-Byrne, P. P., Post, R. M., Uhde, T. W., Porcu, R. M., & Davis, D. 1985. The longitudinal course of recurrent affective illness: life chart data from research patients at the NIMH. *Acta Psychiatrica Scandinavia*, 71 (Suppl 317): 1–34.

Sanches, M., Roberts, R. L., Sassi, R. B., Axelson, D., Nicoletti, M., Brambilla, P., . . . Soares, J. C. 2005. Developmental abnormalities in striatum in young bipolar patients: a preliminary study. *Bipolar Disorders*, 7(2): 153–158.

Singh, M. K., DelBello, M. P., Stanford, K., & Strakowski, S. M. 2008. Neuroanatomical characterization of child offspring of parents with bipolar disorder. *Journal of American Academy of Child and Adolescent Psychiatry*, 47(5): 526–531.

Skjelstad, D. V., & Malt, U. F, 2010. Holte A.Symptoms and signs of the initial prodrome of bipolar disorder: a systematic review. *Journal of Affective Disorders*, 126(1–2): 1–13.

Sprooten, E., Sussmann, J. E., Clugston, A., Peel, A., McKirdy, J., Moorhead, T.W.J., . . . McIntosh, A. M. 2011. White matter integrity in individuals at high genetic risk of bipolar disorder. *Biologicl Psychiatry*, 70: 350–356.

Stork, C., & Renshaw, P. F. 2005. Mitochondrial dysfunction in bipolar disorder: evidence from magnetic resonance spectroscopy research. *Molecular Psychiatry*, 10(10): 900–919.

Strakowski, S. M. 2002. Differential brain mechanisms in bipolar and unipolar disorders: Considerations from brain imaging. In: JC Soares, ed. *Brain Imaging in Affective Disorders*. NY: Marcel Dekker.

Strakowski, S. M., Adler, C. M., Cerullo, M. A., Eliassen, J. C., Lamy, M., Fleck, D. E., . . . DelBello, M. P. 2008. MRI brain activation in first-episode bipolar mania during a response inhibition task. *Early Intervention in Psychiatry*, 2: 225–233.

Strakowski, S. M., Adler, C. M., Holland, S. K., Mills, N., & DelBello, M. P. 2004. A preliminary FMRI study of sustained attention in euthymic, unmedicated bipolar disorder. *Neuropsychopharmacology*, 29(9): 1734–1740.

Strakowski, S. M., Adler, C. M., Holland, S. K., Mills, N., DelBello, M. P., & Eliassen, J. C. 2005. Abnormal fMRI brain activation in euthymic bipolar disorder during a counting Stroop task. *American Journal of Psychiatry*, 162: 1697–1705.

Strakowski, S. M., DelBello, M. P., Zimmerman, M. E., Getz, G. E., Mills, N. P., Ret. J., . . . Adler, C. M. 2002. Ventricular and periventricular structural volumes in first- versus multiple-episode bipolar disorder. *American Journal of Psychiatry*, 159: 1841–1847.

Strakowski, S. M., Eliassen, J. C., Lamy, M., Cerullo, M. A., Allendorfer, J. B., Madore, M., . . . Adler, C. M. 2011. Functional magnetic resonance imaging brain activation in bipolar mania: evidence for disruption of the ventrolateral prefrontal-amygdala emotional pathway. *Biological Psychiatry*, 69(4): 381–388.

Strakowski, S. M., Wilson, D. R., Tohen, M., Woods, B. T., Douglass, A. W., & Stoll, A. L. 1993. Structural brain abnormalities in first-episode mania. *Biological Psychiatry*, 33: 602–609.

Suppes, T., Baldessarini, R. J., Faedda, G. L., & Tohen, M. 1991. Risk of recurrence following discontinuation of lithium treatment in bipolar disorder. *Archives of General Psychiatry*, 48: 1082–1088.

Urry, H. L., van Reekum, C. M., Johnstone, T., Kalin, N. H., Thurow, M. E., & Schaefer, H. S., . . . Davidson, R. J. 2006. Amygdala and ventromedial prefrontal cortex are inversely coupled during regulation of negative affect and predict the diurnal pattern of cortisol secretion among older adults. *Journal of Neuroscience*, 26: 4415–4425.

Vederine, F. E., Wessa, M., Leboyer, M., & Houenou, J. 2011. A meta-analysis of whole-brain diffusion tensor imaging studies in bipolar disorder. *Prog Neuropsychopharmacol Biol Psychiatry*, 35(8): 1820–1826.

Versace, A., Almeida, J.R.C., Hassel, S., Walsh, N. D., Novelli, M., Klein, C. R., . . . Phillips, M. L. 2008. Elevated left and reduced right orbitomedial prefrontal fractional anisotropy in adults with bipolar disorder revealed by tract-based spatial statistics. *Archives of General Psychiatry*, 65(9): 1041–1052.

Versace, A., Ladouceur, C. D., Romero, S., Birmaher, B., Axelson, D. A., Kupfer, D. J., Phillips, M. L. 2010. Altered development of white matter in youth at high familial risk for bipolar disorder: a diffusion tensor imaging study. *Jornal of American Academy of Child and Adolescent Psychiatry*, 49(12): 1249–1259.

Vita, A., De Peri, L, & Sacchetti, E. 2009. Gray matter, white matter, brain, and intracranial volumes in first-episode bipolar disorder: a meta-analysis of magnetic resonance imaging studies. *Bipolar Disorders*, 11(8): 807–814.

Wang, F., Jackowski, M., Kalmar, J. H., Chepenik, L. G., Tie, K., Qiu, M., . . . Blumberg, H. P. 2008. Abnormal anterior cingulum integrity in bipolar disorder determined through diffusion tensor imaging. *British Journal of Psychiatry*, 193(2): 126–129.

Wang, F., Kalmar, J. H., He, Y., Jackowski, M., Chepenik, L. G., Edmiston, E. E., . . . Blumberg, H. P. 2009. Functional and structural connectivity between the perigenual anterior cingulate and amygdala in bipolar disorder. *Biological Psychiatry*, 66(5): 516–521.

Wessa, M., Houenou, J., Paillère-Martinot, M. L., Berthoz. S., Artiges, E., Leboyer, M., & Martinot, J. L. 2007. Fronto-striatal overactivation in euthymic bipolar patients during an emotional go/nogo task. *American Journal of Psychiatry*, 164: 638–646.

Whalley, H. C., McKirdy, J., Romaniuk, L., Sussmann, J., Johnstone, E. C., Wan, H., . . . Hall, J. 2009. Functional imaging of emotional memory in bipolar disorder and schizophrenia. *Bipolar Disorders*, 11: 840–856.

Whalley, H. C., Sussmann, J. E., Chakirova, G., Mukerjee, P., Peel, A., McKirdy, J., . . . McIntosh, A. M. 2011. The neural basis of familial risk and temperamental variation in individuals at high risk of bipolar disorder. *Biological Psychiatry*, 70: 343–349.

Wilke, M., Kowatch, R. A., DelBello, M. P., Mills, N. P., & Holland, S. K: 2004. Voxel-based morphometry in adolescents with bipolar disorder: first results. *Psychiatry Residence*, 131: 57–69.

Winsberg, M. E., Sachs, N., Tate, D. L., Adalsteinsson, E., Spielman, D., & Ketter, T. A. 2000. Decreased dorsolateral prefrontal N-acetyl aspartate in bipolar disorder. *Biol Psychiatry*, 47(6): 475–481.

Yamasaki, H., LaBar, K. S., & McCarthy, G. 2002. Dissociable prefrontal brain systems for attention and emotion. *Proceedings of the National Academy of Science USA*, 2002; 99: 11447–11451.

Yildiz, A., Demopolus, C. M., Moore, C. M., Renshaw, P. F., & Sachs, G. S. 2001. Effect of chronic lithium on phosphoinositide metabolism in human brain: a proton-decoupled (31)P-magnetic resonance spectroscopy study. *Biological Psychiatry*, 50: 3–7.

Yildiz, A., Sachs, G. S., Dorer, D. J., & Renshaw, P. F. 2001. 31P Nuclear magnetic resonance spectroscopy findings in bipolar illness: a meta-analysis. *Psychiatry Research*, 106: 181–191.

Yurgelun-Todd, D. A., Gruber, S. A., Kanayama, G., Killgore, W. D., Baird, A. A., & Young, A. D. 2000. fMRI during affect discrimination in bipolar affective disorder. *Bipolar Disorders*, 2(3 Pt 2): 237–248.

Yurgelun-Todd, D. A., Silveri, M. M., Gruber, S. A., Rohan, M. L., & Pimentel, P. J. 2007. White matter abnormalities observed in bipolar disorder: a diffusion tensor imaging study. *Bipolar Disorders*, 9(5): 504–512.

# INDEX

Page numbers followed by *f* or *t* indicate figures or tables, respectively.